OXFORD MEDICAL PUBLICATIONS

Practical Radiation Protection in Healthcare

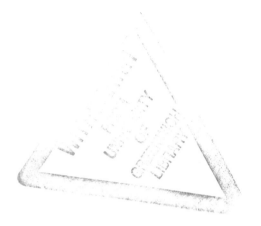

Practical Radiation Protection in Healthcare

Edited by

Dr Colin J Martin

Head of Health Physics
Department of Clinical Physics & Bio-Engineering,
North Glasgow University Hospitals
NHS Trust

and

Dr David G Sutton

Head of Radiation Physics,
Department of Medical Physics,
Ninewells Hospitals & Medical School, Dundee.

OXFORD
UNIVERSITY PRESS

This book has been printed digitally and produced in a standard specification in order to ensure its continuing availability

OXFORD
UNIVERSITY PRESS

Great Clarendon Street, Oxford OX2 6DP

Oxford University Press is a department of the University of Oxford.
It furthers the University's objective of excellence in research, scholarship,
and education by publishing worldwide in

Oxford New York

Auckland Cape Town Dar es Salaam Hong Kong Karachi
Kuala Lumpur Madrid Melbourne Mexico City Nairobi
New Delhi Shanghai Taipei Toronto
With offices in
Argentina Austria Brazil Chile Czech Republic France Greece
Guatemala Hungary Italy Japan South Korea Poland Portugal
Singapore Switzerland Thailand Turkey Ukraine Vietnam

Oxford is a registered trade mark of Oxford University Press
in the UK and in certain other countries

Published in the United States
by Oxford University Press Inc., New York

Reprinted 2006

ISBN 0-19-263082-2

Printed and bound by CPI Antony Rowe, Eastbourne

Preface

The application of radiation to medical problems plays a major role in diagnosis and treatment of disease. However, there is an attendant risk from the exposure to radiation. The practices of radiation protection have been developed in order to minimise radiation exposure and so keep the risks to a minimum. Requirements have been established in legislation to ensure that all individuals are afforded adequate protection and that standards are applied uniformly. This textbook is designed to provide a practical guide for medical physicists and others whose work involves any aspect of ionising and non-ionising radiation protection in the healthcare environment. It gives guidance on methods that may be used in tackling the wide range of practical tasks that may need to be performed while working in these areas.

The book is divided into four sections. The first covers background physics, radiobiology and instrumentation, emphasises points of relevance to radiation protection practice and provides information that might be required for interpretation of results. The second part deals with the general principles of ionising radiation protection and legislative controls applicable to all fields of radiation use. Although detailed requirements are determined by national legislation, these are based on recommendations by international committees and the book describes general implementation of processes to meet these requirements. Examples of guidance linked to UK legislation are included, in order to provide illustrations of the approach to be adopted. The third part of the book encompasses the specific applications of ionising radiation within healthcare and it is this section which contains most of the practical methodology required for day-to-day work in the healthcare environment. Many radiation protection practitioners also provide advice concerning the risks and hazards from non-ionising radiation and protection against these is detailed in the last section of the book. Although the procedural controls used may be similar to those for ionising radiations, the physics, effects and measurement techniques require a different area of knowledge. The book attempts to provide sufficient background information to enable the radiation protection practitioner to deal with the range of practical problems likely to be encountered.

The text has been arranged in order to facilitate its use as a practical reference manual. Background information, which the reader may wish to refer to, has been included in boxes. Worked examples and assessments have also been placed in boxes so that they do not disrupt the flow of text. Some tables of data are given to allow the reader to carry out calculations for situations encountered frequently without reference to further texts.

Since radiation protection practice is founded on the current recommendations of the International Commission for Radiological Protection, the methods described in the book are based on the principles set out in current recommendations and guidance. The editors acknowledge that ideas about the validity of current radiation risk models are a subject of discussion and conjecture, but did not consider it appropriate to include anything about this in a text designed to be a practical guide to current radiation protection methodology.

C J Martin & D G Sutton
July 2002

Acknowledgements

The editors wish to thank the following for helpful information, advice, discussion, and comment during the preparation of the book:

Ben Archer
Andy Brennan
Ron Corrigall
Jim Gemmill
Chris Goddard
John Kennedy
John LeHeron
Caoimhe McIntyre
Brian McParland
Helen Morgan
Kwan Ng
Janice O'Neill
John Robertson
Julie Smyth
Paul Shrimpton
Barry Wall
Helen Warren-Forward

Contents

Contributors

P. J. Allisy-Roberts
Bureau International des Poids et Mesures
Pavilion de Breteuil
F-92312 Sevres
Cedex, France

S. Batchelor
Medical Physics Department
Guy's and St Thomas' NHS Trust
St Thomas Street
London SE1 9RT, UK

A. R. Denman
Medical Physics Department
Northampton General Hospital Trust
Cliftonville
Northampton NN1 5BD, UK

K. E. Goldstone
East Anglian Regional Radiation Protection Service
Box 191
Addenbrooke's NHS Trust
Hills Road
Cambridge CB2 2QQ, UK

S. Green
Department of Medical Physics and Clinical Engineering
Queen Elizabeth Medical Centre
Metchlay Lane
Edgbaston
Birmingham
West Midlands B15 2TH, UK

J. W. Hand
Radiological Sciences Unit
Hammersmith Hospital
Du Cane Road
London W12 OHS, UK

G. C. Hart
Medical Physics Department
Bradford Royal Infirmary
Duckworth Lane
Bradford
West Yorkshire BD12 9AA, UK

R. M. Harrison
Regional Medical Physics Department
Newcastle General Hospital
Westgate Road
Newcastle-upon-Tyne NE4 6BE, UK

A. P. Hufton
North Western Medical Physics Department
Christie Hospital NHS Trust
Withington
Manchester M20 4BX, UK

T. M. Kehoe
Oncology Physics
Clinical Oncology Directorate
Western General Hospital
Crewe Road
Edinburgh EH4 2XU, UK

G. D. Lambert
Regional Medical Physics Department
Newcastle General Hospital
Westgate Road
Newcastle-upon-Tyne NE4 6BE, UK

C. J. Martin
Health Physics Service
Department of Clinical Physics and Bio-Engineering
Divisional Headquarters (West)
Lower Ground Floor
Western Infirmary
Dumbarton Road
Glasgow G11 6NT, UK

H. Moseley
Photobiology Unit
Dundee Teaching Hospitals NHS Trust
Ninewells Hospital
Dundee DD1 9SY, UK

P. J. Mountford
Medical Physics Directorate
North Staffordshire Hospital
Princes Road
Hartshill
Stoke-on-Trent
Staffordshire ST4 7LN, UK

J. M. Parry
Medical Physics Department
Ninewells Hospital and Medical School
Dundee DD1 9SY, UK

E. M. Pitcher
Medical Physics and Bioengineering Department
Bristol General Hospital
Guinea Street
Bristol BS1 6SY, UK

S. D. Pye
Medical Physics Department
Western General Hospital
Crewe Road
Edinburgh EH4 2XU, UK

H. Smith
Formerly of the National Radiological Protection Board and Secretary to the International Commission on Radiological Protection

J. W. Stather
National Radiological Protection Board
Chilton
Didcot
Oxon OX11 ORQ, UK

D. G. Sutton
Medical Physics Department
Ninewells Hospital and Medical School
Dundee DD1 9SY, UK

D. K. Taylor
Medical Physics Department
Gloucester Royal Hospital
Great Western Road
Gloucester GL1 3NN, UK

D. H. Temperton
Regional Radiation Physics and Protection Service
PO Box 803
Edgbaston
Birmingham
West Midlands B15 2TB, UK

J. R. Williams
Medical Physics Department
Western General Hospital
Crewe Road
Edinburgh EH4 2XU, UK

R. G. Zamenhof
Radiological Physics Section
Beth Israel Deaconess Medical Center
Harvard Institutes of Medicine
Suite 147
77 Avenue Louis Pasteur
Boston
MA 02115, USA.

B. Zeqiri
Centre for Mechanical and Acoustical Metrology
National Physical Laboratory
Queens Road
Teddington
Middlesex TW11 OLW, UK

Abbreviations

AAPM	American Association of Physicists in Medicine
ABCC	Atomic Bomb Casualty Commission
ACGIH	American Conference of Governmental Industrial Hygienists
ACXRP	Advisory Committee on X-ray and Radium Protection (US)
AEC	Automatic Exposure Control
AEGIS	Advanced Extremity Gamma Instrumentation System
AEL	Accessible exposure limit
AERE	Atomic Energy Research Establishment
ALARA	As low as reasonably achievable
ALARP	As low as reasonably practicable
ALI	Annual limit on intake
AKR	Air kerma rate constant
AMAD	Average mean aerodynamic diameter
AP	Antero-posterior
ARPANSA	Australian Radiation Protection and Nuclear Safety Act
ARSAC	Administration of Radioactive Substances Advisory Committee (UK)
AURPO	Association of University Radiation Protection Officers (UK)
BCC	Basal cell carcinoma
BEIR	Biological effects of ionising radiation
BIR	British Institute of Radiology
BMUS	British Medical Ultrasound Society
BNR	Beam non-uniformity ratio
BPM	Best practicable means
BSF	Backscatter factor
BSS	Basic Safety Standards
BXRPC	British X-ray and Radium Protection Committee
CBI	Confederation of British Industries
CCD	Charge-coupled device
CCTV	Closed-circuit television
CE	Conformité Européene
CEC	Commission of the European Community
CFR	Codes of Federal Regulation (US)
CIDI	Central Index of Dose Information (UK)
CIE	Commission Internationale de l'Éclairage
CNSC	Canadian Nuclear Safety Commission
CoR	College of Radiographers
COSHH	Control of Substances Hazardous to Health
cps	Counts per second
CR	Computed radiography
CSP	Chartered Society of Physiotherapists
CT	Computed tomography
CTDI	Computed tomography dose index
$CTDI_w$	Weighted computed tomography dose index
CTG	Cardiotocograph
DAP	Dose–area product

DC	Direct current
DETR	Department of the Environment, Transport, and the Regions
DDREF	Dose and dose-rate effectiveness factor
DG	Directorate General (EU)
DIS	Direct ion storage
DLP	Dose–length product (for CT dosimetry)
DMSA	2,3-Dimercaptosuccinic acid
DNA	Deoxyribonucleic acid
DOE	Department of Energy (US)
DOELAP	Department of Energy Laboratory Accreditation Program (US)
DR	Digital radiography
DRL	Diagnostic reference level
DTPA	Diethylenetriaminepentaacetic acid
DXA	Dual X-ray absorptiometry (bone mineral densitometry)
EC	Electron capture
EC	European Commission
ECMUS	European Committee for Ultrasound in Medicine
ECRP	Endoscopic retrograde cholangiopancreatatogram
EDTA	Ethylenediaminetetraacetic acid
EEC	European Economic Community
ELF	Extremely low frequency
EM	Electromagnetic
EMI	Electromagnetic interference
ENT	Ear, nose, and throat
EPA	Environment Protection Agency (US)
EPD	Electronic personal dosimeter
ERA	Effective radiating area
ESD	Entrance surface dose
ESWL	Extracorporeal shockwave lithotripsy
EU	European Union
FAO	Food and Agricultural Organization
FDA	Food and Drug Administration (US)
FDG	^{18}F-fluorodeoxyglucose
FFD	Focus to film distance
FID	Focus to intensifier distance
FSD	Focus to skin distance
FWD	Focus to wall distance
GEMS	Gamma extremity monitoring system
GI	Gastrointestinal
GM	Geiger–Müller
GSD	Genetically significant dose
HCN	Health Council of the Netherlands
HDR	High dose rate
HIG	Human polyclonal immunoglobulin
HMPAO	Hexamethylpropyleneamine oxime
HMSO	Her Majesty's Stationery Office
HpGe	Hyperpure germanium
HSC	Health and Safety Commission (UK)
HSE	Health and Safety Executive (UK)
HVL	Half-value layer
IAEA	International Atomic Energy Agency
IAK	Incident air kerma
IATA	International Air Transport Association
ICAO	International Civil Aviation Organization
ICNIRP	International Commission on Non-Ionising Radiation Protection

ICRP	International Commission on Radiological Protection
ICRU	International Commission on Radiation Units and Measurements
IDR	Instantaneous dose rate
IEC	International Electrotechnical Commission
IEEE	Institute of Electrical and Electronic Engineers
IF	Fraction of incident radiation imparted to patient
ILO	International Labour Organization
IMO	International Maritime Organization
ImPACT	Imaging Performance Assessment of CT scanners (MDA, UK)
INIRC	International Non-Ionising Radiation Committee
IPEM	Institute of Physics and Engineering in Medicine (UK)
IQ	Intelligence quotient
IR	Infrared (bands IR-A, IR-B, and IR-C)
IR(ME)R	Ionising Radiation (Medical Exposure) Regulations (UK)
IRAC	Ionising Radiations Advisory Committee (UK)
IRPA	International Radiation Protection Association
ISO	International Organization for Standardization
IT	Isomeric transition
IVU	Intravenous urogram
KTP	$K_{1-x} Na_xTiOPO_4$ laser material
kV	Kilovoltage
Lat	Lateral
LDR	Low dose rate
LED	Light-emitting diode
LET	Linear energy transfer
LMP	Last menstrual period (date of)
LPA	Laser protection adviser
LPS	Laser protection supervisor
LSA	Low specific activity
LSJ	Lumbar sacral joint
LSO	Laser safety officer
LSS	Life Span Study (A-bomb survivors)
MAA	Human albumin macroaggregates
MAG3	Benzoylmercaptoacetyltriglycerine
MARS	Medical Administration of Radioactive Substances (UK)
mAs	milliamp seconds (exposure current × time)
MDA	Medical Devices Agency
MDP	Methylene diphosphonate
MED	Medical Exposures Directive (EU)
MED	Minimal erythema dose
MGD	Mean glandular dose (mammography)
MIBG	^{123}I labelled meta-iodobenzyl guanidine
MIBI	2-Methoxy-isobutyl-isonitrile
MIRD	Medical Internal Radiation Dose Committee of American Society of Nuclear Medicine
MPD	Maximum permissible dose
MPD	Minimal phototoxic dose
MPE	Medical physics expert
MPE	Maximum permissible exposure
MR	Magnetic resonance
MRI	Magnetic resonance imaging
MSAD	Multiple scan average dose (CT)
MSSD	Multi-slice surface dose (CT)
MUGA	Multiple gated acquisition
MW	Microwave

NAIR	National Arrangements for Incidents involving Radioactivity
NCRP	National Council on Radiation Protection and Measurements (US)
Nd:YAG	Neodymium: Yttrium Aluminium Garnet
NE	Nuclear Enterprises
NEA	Nuclear Energy Agency
NHS	National Health Service (UK)
NIR	Non-ionising radiation
NIREP	Nuclear Industry Road Emergency Response Plan (UK)
NMS	National measurement system
NOHD	Nominal ocular hazard distance
NOHSC	National Health and Medical Research Council (Australia)
NPL	National Physical Laboratory (UK)
NRC	Nuclear Regulatory Commission (US)
NRPB	National Radiological Protection Board (UK)
NRRW	National Registry of Radiation Workers (UK)
NVLAP	National Voluntary Laboratory Accreditation Program (US)
OD	Optical density
ODS	Output display standard
OECD	Organization for Economic Development
OHSA	Occupational Safety and Health Agency (US)
OPT	Orthopantomographic
OSL	Optically stimulated luminescence
PA	Postero-anterior
PADC	Polyallyl diglycol carbonate
PAEC	Potential α-energy concentration (concentration of radon decay products)
PAHO	Pan-American Health Organization
PAS	Personal air samplers
PDD	Percentage depth dose
PDR	Pulsed dose rate
PDT	Photodynamic therapy
PET	Positron emission tomography
PMMA	Polymethylmethacrylate (perspex)
PMT	Photomultiplier tube
POSL	Pulsed optically stimulated luminescence
PRK	Photorefractive keratectomy
PTB	Physikalisch-Technische Bundesanstalt
PTCA	Percutaneous transluminal coronary angiography
PTFE	Polytetrafluoroethylene
PUVA	Psoralen ultraviolet-A
PVDF	Polyvinylidene fluoride
PZT	Lead zirconate titanate
QART	Quality assurance in radiotherapy
QCT	Quantitative computed tomography (bone mineral densitometry)
RA	Radiographic absorptiometry (bone mineral densitometry)
RAKR	Reference air kerma rate (at 1 m used instead of activity in radiotherapy)
RAL	Remote afterloading
RANDO	Anthropomorphic phantom
RBE	Relative biological effectiveness
RCR	Royal College of Radiologists (UK)
REPPIR	Radiation (Emergency Preparedness and Public Information) Regulations (UK)
RERF	Radiation Effects Research Foundation
RF	Radiofrequency

RIMNET	Radioactive Incident Monitoring Network
RMS	Root mean square
RNA	Ribonucleic acid
RPA	Radiation protection adviser
RPL	Radiophotoluminescence
RPS	Radiation protection supervisor
RRPPS	Regional Radiation Physics and Protection Service (UK)
SAR	Specific absorption rate
SAS	Static air sampler
SCC	Squamous cell carcinoma
Si(Li)	Lithium drifted silicon
SID	Source to isocentre distance
SPECT	Single-photon emission computed tomography
SSL	Sealed-source laboratory
SSNTD	Solid-state nuclear track detector
SXA	Single X-ray absorptiometry (bone mineral densitometry)
TADR	Time-averaged dose rate
TAR	Tissue–air ratio
TIPS	Transjugular intrahepatic portosystemic shunt
TL	Thermoluminescence
TLD	Thermoluminescence dosimeter
UNSC	United States National Research Council
UNSCEAR	United Nations Scientific Committee on the Effects of Radiation
UV	Ultraviolet (bands UV-A, UV-B, and UV-C)
WHO	World Health Organization

List of Boxes

Part I

Ionising radiations: hazards, detection, and measurement

The first part of *Practical Radiation Protection* provides a background to the subject and a knowledge of the basic science and technology required by a radiation protection physicist. Chapter 1 traces the history of radiation in healthcare from the early applications to medical problems to the development of standards and legislation to control the hazard. Chapter 2 contains an outline of the fundamental physics governing the interaction of radiations with matter. Chapter 3 sets out current knowledge of the biological effects of radiation from the cellular interactions to effects on the whole body and Chapter 4 deals with the fundamentals of ionising radiation measurement.

Symbols

absorbed dose in air	D_{air} (Gy)
absorbed dose in material m	D_m (Gy)
absorbed dose (mean) (ICRP)	$D_{T,R}$ (Gy)
air kerma	K_{air} (Gy)
ambient dose equivalent	$H^*(d)$ (Sv)
angle of incidence	α (degree or radian)
angle of scatter	θ (degree or radian)
angular frequency	ω (s^{-1})
area of spherical element	da (m^2)
atomic number	Z
atomic number effective	Z_{eff}
branching ratio	BR (Bq emissions^{-1})
calibration factor (contamination monitor)	S (emissions s^{-1} cm^{-2} cps^{-1})
count rate	n (cps)
dead time	τ (s)
decay constant	λ (s^{-1})
density	ρ (kg m^{-3})
depth	d (mm)
directional dose equivalent	$H'(d,\alpha)$ (Sv)
dose equivalent (ICRU)	H (Sv)
effective dose	E (Sv)
electric charge	q (C)
energy of β-particle	E_β (eV)
energy of photon	E (eV)
energy fluence	ψ (J m^{-2})
equivalent dose (ICRP)	$H_{T,R}$ (Sv)
equivalent power density	S_{eq} (W m^{-2})
Fano factor	F
fluence	φ (m^{-2})
frequency	f (Hz)
geometric factor	P
half-life (radioactive decay)	$T_{1/2}$ (years, days, h, s)
instrument response (contamination monitor)	R (cps (Bq $cm^{-2})^{-1}$)
kerma	K (Gy)
linear attenuation coefficient	μ (m^{-1})
Compton scattering coefficient	σ_c (m^{-1})
elastic scattering coefficient	σ_{coh} (m^{-1})
pair production coefficient	κ (m^{-1})
photoelectric effect coefficient	τ (m^{-1})
linear energy transfer	L (keV μm^{-1})
mass	m (kg), M (kg)
mass attenuation coefficient	μ/ρ (kg^{-1} m^2)
mass energy absorption coefficient	μ_{en}/ρ (kg^{-1} m^2)
mass energy transfer coefficient	μ_{tr}/ρ ($kg^{-1}m^2$)
mass of electron	m_e
neutron	n
number of atoms	N
personal dose equivalent	$H_p(d)$
Planck constant	h (J s)
propagation constant	γ (m^{-1})
quality factor	Q
radiation type	R
radiation weighting factor	w_R
radionuclide activity	A (Bq)
tissue type	T
tissue weighting factor	w_T
speed of light	c (m s^{-1})
velocity	v (m s^{-1})
wavelength	λ (m)

Chapter 1
The development of radiation protection

C. J. Martin

1.1 Historical perspective

1.1.1 Early applications of ionising radiation in medicine

The potential for the application of ionising radiations in medicine was realized almost as soon as Wilhelm Roentgen discovered X-rays in 1895. Roentgen determined the basic properties of X-rays, such as their ability to penetrate light materials and the dependence of absorption on density, within a few weeks of his discovery. He also found that X-rays affected photographic plates, and six weeks after his initial discovery he used X-rays to form an image of his wife's hand, the first radiograph. The use of X-rays for medical diagnosis developed rapidly and many radiological techniques were applied within the first year of Roentgen's discovery. Fluorescent screens were used to enhance radiographic images, and in 1897 W. B. Cannon at Harvard reported a study of 'Movements of the stomach by means of Roentgen X-rays', the first fluoroscopic examination. Radiology departments were established to aid diagnosis in most major hospitals in the last few years of the nineteenth century. During this period, clinicians tried to use X-rays for treatment of a variety of conditions including lupus, ringworm, tuberculosis, epithelioma, port-wine stain, and cancer. The first proven cure of a cancer patient by X-ray treatment was as early as 1899 by Tage Sjorgen in Sweden.

Roentgen's discovery stimulated the interest of other scientists working in related fields and in 1896 Henri Becquerel discovered radioactivity when he found that uranium salts gave off penetrating radiation which blackened photographic film. Understanding of the nature of the radiations emitted developed gradually over succeeding years. Many scientists contributed to this, of whom Marie Curie made some of the most significant discoveries, establishing that radiation was emitted by compounds containing the elements uranium, thorium, and radium, and in 1898 separating radium which became widely used for therapy.

1.1.2 Early radiation protection

As the use of X-rays became widespread, evidence that radiation might be harmful began to accumulate. Skin burns and dermatitis were reported among scientists and medical practitioners working with X-rays and the Roentgen Society set up a Committee of Inquiry to look into 'the alleged injurious effects of Roentgen rays' in March 1898. Radiation protection facilities for most early workers were rudimentary or non-existent and a number of reports of hazards from overexposure to radiation appeared during the period 1897–1907. It became apparent that there was a need for measures to protect operators and patients from unnecessary exposure. During the early years of the twentieth century many protective devices, such as shielding around X-ray tubes, aprons and gloves containing lead, mobile lead screens, and lead protection in walls, began to be used by some workers, and in 1915 the Roentgen Society produced recommendations for the use of X-ray operators. These measures marked the beginning of formal radiation protection. Box 1.1 lists some of the events in the evolution of radiation protection.

1.1.3 The development of radiation safety standards

X-rays were used extensively during the First World War and many cases of leukaemia and aplastic anaemia were reported among operators and radiologists. These effects emphasized the need for radiation protection and criteria for limiting exposure to ionising radiations were proposed by various groups and individuals. The British X-ray and Radium Protection Committee (BXRPC) published formal recommendations on radiation protection measures in 1921. For diagnostic radiology these included shielding of X-ray tubes with 2 mm of lead, use of rubber gloves providing protection equivalent to 0.5 mm of lead, and provision of a shielded enclosure for the operator. For radium therapy the use of forceps when handling radioactive sources and the use of lead-lined boxes for transporting sources were recommended. It was also in 1921 that the BXRPC suggested the first tolerance dose of X-rays equivalent to one-tenth of the erythema dose per month. This was the first attempt to introduce a formal dose restriction.

In 1925 the International Commission on Radiological Units and Measurements (ICRU) was set up at the First International Congress of Radiology in London. The aim of the ICRU is the development of a framework of scientific concepts relevant to the assessment of radiation for its safe and effective use. It recommends radiation quantities and units, measuring procedures, and numerical values for physical data. In 1928 the International Commission on X-ray and Radium Protection was established to consider radiation protection problems and issue recommendations on safety measures and practices. This was later to become the International Committee on Radiological Protection (ICRP). Once the roentgen had been established as the unit of exposure, radiation doses could be quantified and limits set for exposure. Techniques were required to measure doses received by radiation workers so that limits could be

Box 1.1 Events in the first 100 years of ionising radiation protection

1896	Grubbe's published paper describing X-ray dermatitis of the hands
1897	Roentgen Society founded
1911	Adoption of international radium standard and Curie as unit of activity
1915	Roentgen Society (London) recommends X-ray protection measures
1920	American Roentgen Ray Society founded
1921	BXRPC presents first radiation protection rules
1925	First International Congress of Radiology (London) establishes ICRU
1925	Tolerance dose of 0.01 skin erythema per month proposed (about 50 mSv per month)
1926	Dutch Board of Health adopts first regulatory exposure limit (1 skin erythema dose per 90 000 working hours)
1928	International Committee on X-ray and Radium Protection established, later to become the ICRP
1928	ICRU adopts roentgen as unit of exposure
1929	ACXRP formed, which becomes the NCRP in 1946
1931	ACXRP proposes body dose limit of 0.2 R per day (about 2 mSv per day)
1933	Irene Curie discovers that artificial radionuclides can be produced when elements are bombarded with particle radiations
1934	ICXRP proposes 'safe threshold' exposure of 0.2 R per day
1934	ACXRP recommends separate dose limit for hands of 5 R per day (about 50 mSv)
1937	National Physical Laboratory (NPL) set up first radiation monitoring service
1941	ACXRP recommends maximum body burden of radium of 0.1 μCi
1942	Start of Manhattan project with first reactor at University of Chicago
1942	Concept of maximum permissible dose for inhaled radioactivity introduced, together with rem (roentgen equivalent man)
1945	Atomic bombs dropped on Hiroshima and Nagasaki on 6th and 9th August
1947	US National Academy of Sciences establishes ABCC to initiate long-term studies of Japanese A-bomb survivors
1948	First UK Radioactive Substances Act implemented
1949	NCRP lowers maximum permissible dose (MPD) for workers to 0.3 R per week
1950	ICRP recommends 0.3 R per week MPD for low linear energy transfer (LET) radiation and highlights potential risks from leukaemia, malignancy, genetic effects, superficial injury, and cataract
1953	ICRU introduces concept of absorbed dose
1953	ICRP introduces maximum permissible concentration for 90 radionuclides
1954	Atomic Energy Act allows private commercial companies to use radioactive materials under licence in the USA
1955	ICRP rejects concept of 'safe threshold' and recommends MPD set to reduce exposure to 'lowest possible level'
1955	UNSCEAR established
1955	NCRP recommends occupational MPD of 5 R (50 mSv) per year
1957	IAEA set up by General Assembly of United Nations with remit relating to use of radioactive materials

applied successfully. The National Physical Laboratory (NPL) in Britain set up a radiation dose-monitoring service for their employees in 1937 using dental X-ray film, and this was extended to hospitals in 1942. In 1948 the BXRPC recommended use of photographic film or condensers for assessment of doses for radiation workers, together with regular medical examinations including blood counts.

The first attempt to establish restrictions on intake of a radionuclide was made after radium poisoning was recognized among luminous dial painters who frequently died from leucopenia or bone tumours during the 1930s. A maximum body burden of 0.1 μg of radium was proposed in 1941.

During the early 1950s committees were set up by the ICRP to consider permissible doses from external and internal radiation, protection against X-rays and high-energy radiation, and handling and disposal of radioactive materials. In 1954 the NCRP made the statement: 'exposure to radiation should be kept at the lowest practicable level in all cases'. This concept was subsequently adopted by the ICRP who stated that all radiation doses should be kept 'as low as reasonably practicable', the ALARP principle. For general radiation safety, a Code of Practice for the Protection of Persons Exposed to Ionising Radiations was issued to National

Box 1.1 *(continued)*

1957	Windscale accident in UK in which cloud of radioactive iodine released
1958	First UNSCEAR report on exposure sources and biological hazards
1958	ICRP recommends MPD of 50 mSv per year
1958	Oxford survey of childhood malignancies suggests link with fetal exposure
1959	ICRP states that doses should be 'as low as practicable' and recommends limitation of genetically significant dose to population
1960	Adrian Committee publishes results of survey of doses from medical exposures
1962	First remote afterloading brachytherapy machine built in Sweden
1968	FDA regulates X-ray equipment in US
1970	NRPB formed from amalgamation of Radiological Protection Service (formed 1953) and division of UK AEA
1972	Initial report by BEIR Committee
1973	ICRP adopts concept of 'as low as reasonably achievable' (Report 22)
1975	ABCC replaced by RERF to continue studies of Japanese A-bomb survivors
1977	ICRP adopts 'effective dose equivalent' terminology and introduces principles which become 'justification, optimisation, and dose limitation' (Report 26)
1978	UK MARS regulations require certification of those prescribing radiopharmaceuticals through ARSAC
1979	Three Mile Island accident on 28th March
1980	Euratom Directive 80/836 sets out radiation safety requirements for workers and public, including limit of 500 mSv per year for extremities
1980	Society for Radiological Protection and Hospital Physicists Association set up schemes for certification of radiation protection practitioners
1984	Euratom Directive 84/466 sets out requirements for medical exposures
1985	First Ionising Radiations Regulations implemented in the UK
1986	Dosimetry System 1986 (DS86) developed by RERF for A-bomb survivors
1986	Chernobyl accident on 26th April
1986	NRPB publishes results of survey of patient doses in English hospitals
1989	NRPB proposes reference doses for common radiological examinations
1989	RCR issues guidelines on making best use of a Department of Radiology
1990	BEIR V report provides new estimates of risks from ionising radiation
1991	IAEA report on health effects from the Chernobyl accident
1991	ICRP proposes major revision of practices, reduction in occupational dose limit to 20 mSv, and adopts effective dose terminology (Report 60)
1994	FDA issues guidance relating to risk of skin erythema from fluoroscopy
1996	IAEA publishes international BSS for ionising radiation
1997	IPEM, CoR, and NRPB issue recommended standards for performance testing of X-ray equipment in the UK
1997	Euratom Directive 97/43 issues revised guidance on medical exposures

Abbreviations are given at the start of Part I of the book.

Health Service (NHS) hospitals in the UK in 1957. Ionising radiation safety continued through voluntary implementation of codes of practice until the 1980s.

1.1.4 The application of radionuclides to imaging

Shortly after the USA entered the Second World War, President Roosevelt approved the programme to construct an atomic bomb (Manhattan Project). The first reactor was built at the University of Chicago and this provided experience in the production of radionuclides. After the war, radionuclides were made available to qualified physicians outside the Manhattan Project. ^{131}I was employed in the treatment of thyroid cancer and to image the thyroid gland using a point-by-point counting technique. Subsequently, large sodium iodide crystals became available and were used by Hal Anger to construct the first scintillation gamma camera in 1957. A method for enabling hospitals to obtain a supply of ^{99m}Tc, a radionuclide with a short half-life ideal for imaging applications, became available in 1961 with the manufacture of a generator containing ^{99}Mo. These two developments led to the beginning of radionuclide imaging and the founding of nuclear medicine.

Formal regulation by national governments of the use of radionuclides began in about 1950. The first Radioactive Substances Act dealing with holding, use, and disposal of radioactive material came into force in the UK in 1948. The Atomic Energy Act regulating the use of reactor-produced radionuclides in the United States was enacted in 1954.

1.2 Standards and legislation for protection against ionising radiations

1.2.1 Review of evidence on biological effects of radiation

Evidence has been accumulated slowly to document the harmful effects of ionising radiations. Threshold doses were determined for skin erythema and other so-called 'deterministic' effects (§3.3). However, the question of most importance in occupational use of ionising radiation concerns the risk from exposure to very low levels of radiation dose received over long periods of time. The dropping of a ^{235}U bomb on Hiroshima and a ^{239}Pu bomb on Nagasaki exposed an immense number of individuals to substantial whole-body doses of radiation. The United Nations Scientific Committee on the Effects of Radiation (UNSCEAR) was set up in 1955 to study evidence on the effects of radiation exposure. The United States National Research Council (USNRC) commissioned a study of survivors of the atomic bombs and other groups who had been either accidentally exposed to large doses of radiation or routinely exposed over many years and the results were published in 1972 in the Biological Effects of Ionising Radiation (BEIR) report. Reports by the BEIR, III (1980), IV (1988), and V (1990), together with ones from UNSCEAR collated evidence on effects of long-term exposure to low levels of ionising radiation. The knowledge gained from the study of radiation effects is used by ICRP to recommend standards that will prevent deterministic effects and limit the risk of radiation-induced cancer and genetic effects. The current recommendations of the ICRP issued in 1991 are based largely on the BEIR V report, which included data on the health of the Japanese survivors for a period of over 40 years after the atomic bombs were dropped. The standards for individuals working with radiation are designed to provide an occupational risk that is lower than that found in areas of work normally considered as 'safe' industries.

1.2.2 Implementation of radiation protection standards

Organizations such as the ICRU and ICRP are independent bodies composed of specialists from a wide range of related disciplines, whose aims are to put forward recommendations based on international consensus. They have no affiliation to national governments and have no legal authority to enforce the recommendations they make. National governments have responsibility for implementation of radiation protection programmes, taking account of social, political, and economic considerations. National radiological protection bodies such as the National Radiological Protection Board (NRPB) in the UK and the National Council on Radiation Protection and Measurements (NCRP) in the USA provide guidance on implementation of recommendations made by the ICRP and may advise on and contribute to the development of national legislation.

Legislation in the European Economic Community is drawn up to fulfil requirements laid down in Euratom Directives (§5.2). These set out safety standards to minimize divergence between the national legislation of member states, although each is allowed to decide how the regulations should be incorporated into their national legal framework. Regulations are supplemented by approved codes of practice which give guidance on general requirements set out in the legislation. Failure to comply with an approved code of practice is held to be proof of a contravention of a requirement of the code unless a defendant can show that compliance was achieved in another equally appropriate way. Guidance notes accompany legislation and set out opinions on good practice in particular applications. Government bodies may issue guidance notes as opinions on good practice in specific activities; professional bodies may also be a source of guidance for their particular field. Guidance notes do not in themselves have legal force, but because of their origin and the experience of the individuals involved in their production, they are in practice persuasive documents in lower courts and are useful in establishing reasonable standards prevailing in a particular industry.

1.2.3 Medical radiation exposure

Concerns about the potential harmful consequences of medical exposures were raised in 1957 by UNSCEAR, who stated that 'the medical use of radiation is clearly of the utmost value in prevention, diagnosis, investigation and treatment of human disease, but the possible effects of irradiation of individuals requires examination'. The main concern at this time was the potential risk of genetic defects in future generations from irradiation of the gonads. Some evaluations of radiation levels from medical exposures were made during the 1950s. The Adrian Committee reported results of a UK survey in 1960, which found that 21 million medical examinations were performed each year, with an associated mean genetically significant dose (GSD) to the population of 0.123 mGy. A survey carried out by the NRPB in the early 1980s showed that the number of medical examinations had risen to 30 million per year and the GSD was 0.120 mGy.

Meanwhile, a study in Oxford by Alice Stewart reported in 1958 suggested that the level of childhood malignancies was higher among individuals whose mothers were X-rayed during pregnancy. This finding, coupled with results of further studies, led to restrictions on fetal exposures. The Adrian Committee expressed concern about the variation in doses at different hospitals in their 1960 report and recommended strategies for dose reduction, many of which are still applicable today. The variations were highlighted by an NRPB survey report in 1986 and, based on these results, reference doses were recommended in 1989 which could be utilized by hospitals in evaluating local practice. This principle has subsequently been taken up in a Euratom Directive in the form of diagnostic reference levels which are now embodied in legislative requirements of European countries. These topics are discussed in more detail in Chapter 11.

1.3 Public perception of ionising radiation

Deaths of radiation workers aroused concern in the early part of the century. The destructive potential of atomic weapons with the grim aftermath of the bombs dropped on Japan left an indelible image in the minds of the developed world. Following on from its destructive beginnings, the peaceful use of nuclear power has been dogged by bad press linked to the arms race and concern about potential hazards around nuclear establishments. Nuclear accidents at Windscale (1957), Three Mile Island (1979), and Chernobyl (1986) have reinforced public awareness of the dangers from radiation. The tendency to a lack of openness has contributed to public distrust and uncertainty. Public outcry over atomic weapons tests and the potential hazards during the 1950s was dismissed in early reports of BEIR and UNSCEAR, which regarded the risks as small. During the 1970s reports of a high incidence of leukaemia among veterans proved that risks had been underestimated. Errors in radiotherapy treatments delivered to patients in the 1980s and 1990s have raised public concern about hospital applications.

With this background, it is hardly surprising that radiation conjures up alarm and distrust in the public mind. Public concern is raised because radiation is unfamiliar and its effects are poorly understood. In addition, radiation has a number of other 'fright factors' which further help to trigger public anxiety. The risks are imposed rather than being a matter of individual choice and are seen as involuntary, inescapable, and unequally distributed. They also cause hidden damage, which may lead to cancer, an illness arousing particular dread, many years after exposure. Moreover, there is a particular danger to small children or pregnant women and a risk of damage to future generations.

All these factors arouse public concern about radiation exposure. The public impression of the danger is often disproportionate to the measurable harm. There tends to be a large discrepancy between the perception of the size of the risk and values estimated from the available data. For example, people are usually surprised to learn that the atomic bombs dropped on Japan caused less than 500 deaths from cancer among about 50 000 exposed survivors. This is less than 5% of all deaths from cancer even in that highly exposed population, and only 1% of all deaths.

In order to retain the confidence of the general public, openness is required about the risks from radiation and a proper emphasis on justification and optimisation of medical procedures involving radiation is necessary.

1.4 Non-ionising radiations

Electromagnetic radiation photons can be divided into two categories: those that have sufficient energy to produce ionisation (X-rays and γ-rays) and those with energies less than 12 eV which are referred to as non-ionising radiations (NIRs). The spectrum of electromagnetic radiation, together with some applications of the different parts in medicine and elsewhere, is shown in Box 1.2. Non-ionising electromagnetic radiations can be divided into optical radiations and electromagnetic fields, and the energy/wavelength/frequency ranges to which these correspond are shown in Box 1.2. Other forms of NIR are high-frequency mechanical waves or ultrasound waves, which can be propagated through the body and the energy absorbed by tissue.

NIRs usually interact with tissue through the generation of heat. The hazards depend on the ability to penetrate the human body and the absorption characteristics of different tissues (Box 1.3). There is much uncertainty about the severity of the effects of both acute and chronic exposure to various types of NIRs. Questions raised in relation to each type of NIR are different because of the variation in properties with wavelength. Public concern about NIR has been greatest about the longer wavelength radiations defined as electromagnetic fields (Box 1.2), which include microwaves and radiofrequency radiations. However, the greatest risk to public health probably arises from natural ultraviolet radiation (Box 1.3).

1.4.1 Optical radiations

The optical radiations are centred around visible light; photons having higher energies are termed ultraviolet radiation and those with lower energies infrared radiation. Intensities of optical radiations decline according to an inverse square law with distance from a point source and the radiations are capable of being focused and interact with matter in a similar way to visible light.

Ultraviolet phototherapy has been used for many years to treat a variety of conditions. Treatment of psoriasis has been carried out since the 1920s, but only during the latter part of the twentieth century were attempts made to optimise treatment and establish accurate dosimetry. The first laser was produced in 1960 by Mainman. The potential value of lasers in medicine with the high-intensity beam, which could be coupled into an optical fibre and delivered to the treatment site, was realized immediately and by 1964 lasers were being employed as a microsurgical tool.

Damage from optical radiations is largely confined to the eye and skin. Despite having insufficient energy to ionise atoms, single photons of ultraviolet radiation can damage tissue through disruption of bonds within DNA molecules and give a long-term risk of cancer. This must be borne in mind when determining allowable exposures. Visible light and infrared only produce damage through high-intensity multi-photon interactions. For radiation protection, a distinction is made between lasers and non-coherent sources. The biological effects induced are essentially the same for both, but lasers are capable of producing higher irradiances and can heat localized volumes of tissue to a high enough temperature to produce rapid physical change.

1.4.2 Electromagnetic fields

The term electromagnetic fields describes a wide range of lower energy electromagnetic waves (Box 1.2). The wavelengths range from 1 mm up to thousands of kilometres. The term ‘fields’ is used because of the need to consider effects of the electric and magnetic components separately, because of their different interactions. Radiofrequency (RF) electromagnetic fields are used in medicine to heat tissue to aid healing, with shortwave diathermy (27 MHz) being applied widely by physiotherapists and in a few centres oncologists using microwave heating (e.g. 912 MHz) to treat tumours by hyperthermia. High static electromagnetic fields with RF pulses are used in magnetic resonance imaging (MRI) and hazards of these must also be considered. Radiofrequency radiations are used extensively in communications and the potential for electromagnetic interference with electro-medical equipment has to be borne in mind.

Energy densities of long-wavelength electromagnetic fields vary in a non-uniform manner at distances from sources at which operators might typically be working because of interference effects between emissions from different parts of a source. RF radiations present the greatest perceived risk of any non-ionising radiation, although studies so far performed do not provide statistical evidence of long-term effects at levels encountered in occupational exposure.

1.4.3 Ultrasound

Ultrasound became an established technique for medical imaging in the middle of the twentieth century. The risks from diagnostic ultrasound are generally agreed to be much lower than for X-rays and there have been no adverse effects observed following the routine diagnostic exposure of children *in utero* over a period of 50 years. Higher intensity ultrasound has been used for applications in physiotherapy, lithotripsy, and surgery. Because of its safe record, the establishment of recommended limits on intensity levels has been slow, but these are now being introduced.

1.4.4 Standards and guidance for non-ionising radiations

The earliest recommendations for exposure limitation for NIRs were made in the 1950s and 1960s for microwave and RF radiations produced by military radar and communication equipment. Recommendations relating to protection of the eye from lasers were made in the 1970s. The growing importance of all forms of NIRs led

Box 1.2 The electromagnetic spectrum

Radiations in different parts of the electromagnetic spectrum can be defined in terms of energy (E), wavelength (λ), or frequency (f). Conventionally, ionising radiations are described in terms of photon energy in electron volts (eV) [1 eV = 1.6×10^{-19} joules], optical radiations are described by the wavelength, and electromagnetic fields are characterized in terms of the radiation frequency. The relationships between these quantities are given by:

$E = hf$ where h is the Planck constant = 6.626×10^{-34} J s

and $c = f\lambda$ where c is the velocity of light = 3×10^{8} m s^{-1}.

The parts into which the spectrum is divided and some applications in medicine (italics) and in other areas are given in the table. The values of energy, wavelength, and frequency given for optical radiations and electromagnetic fields mark the boundaries between radiation subgroups, but those included for ionising radiations are linked to applications.

Radiation		Energy	Wavelength	Frequency	Applications
Ionising radiations					
	X-rays	**15 MeV**	80 fm	4 ZHz	*Linac radiotherapy*
	and				*Brachytherapy*
	γ-rays	**150 keV**	8 pm	40 EHz	*Nuclear medicine*
					Diagnostic radiology
		15 keV	80 pm	4 EHz	
Optical radiations		12.4 eV	**100 nm**	3 PHz	
	UVC				*Corneal surgery lasers*
Ultraviolet (UV)		4.43 eV	**280 nm**	1.07 PHz	*Sterilization*
	UVB				
		3.94 eV	**315 nm**	952 THz	*UVB phototherapy*
	UVA				*PUVA*/sunbeds
Visible	Visible	3.10 eV	**400 nm**	750 THz	*Neonate phototherapy*
					Ophthalmic lasers
Infrared (IR)		1.59 eV	**780 nm**	385 THz	*Surgical and therapy lasers*
	IRA				*Physiotherapy heat lamps*
Near IR		886 meV	**1.4 μm**	214 THz	*Nd:YAG surgical laser*
	IRB				
		413 meV	**3 μm**	100 THz	*Thermographic imaging*
Far IR	IRC				*CO_2 surgical laser*
Electromagnetic		1.24 meV	1 mm	**300 GHz**	
fields ↑	EHF				MW telecommunications
↑		124 μeV	10 mm	**30 GHz**	*Microwave radiometry*
Microwaves	SHF				Radar/satellite links
		12.4 μeV	100 mm	**3 GHz**	Mobile phones/MW ovens
↓	UHF				*Microwave hyperthermia*
		1.24 μeV	1 m	**300 MHz**	TV transmitters
	VHF				Emergency service radios
Radiofrequency (RF)		124 neV	10 m	**30 MHz**	*Therapeutic diathermy*
Shortwave	HF				*MRI RF pulses*
		12.4 neV	100 m	**3 MHz**	
Mediumwave	MF				*Surgical diathermy*
		1.24 neV	1 km	**300 kHz**	AM radio
Longwave	LF				Shop/airport security
		124 peV	10 km	**30 kHz**	Visual display units
	VLF				Television sets
		12.4 peV	100 km	**3 kHz**	
	Voice-F				Induction heaters
		1.24 peV	1000 km	**300 Hz**	
↓	ELF				Electricity supply
		124 feV	10 000 km	**30 Hz**	Power lines
	Static			**0 Hz**	*MRI magnetic field*

HF, high frequency; MF, medium frequency; LF, low frequency; E, extremely; S, super; U, ultra; V, very; MW, microwave; FM, frequency modulated; AM, amplitude modulated; MRI, magnetic resonance imaging.

Box 1.3 Biological effects of different electromagnetic radiations

Radiation		Energy, wavelength, frequency	Biological effects
Ionising radiations	X-rays and γ-rays	>12 eV	Skin erythema, cataract, sterility Death from acute high doses *Cancer in radiosensitive organs, Genetic effects*
Optical radiations		100 nm	
	UVC		Skin—Erythema, increased pigmentation
		280 nm	Eye—Photokeratitis (inflammation of cornea)
			Skin—Erythema, increased pigmentation
Ultraviolet	UVB		*Skin cancer*
		315 nm	Eye—Photochemical cataract
			Photosensitive skin reactions
	UVA		Skin—Erythema, increased pigmentation
		400 nm	*Skin photo-ageing, Skin cancer*
Visible	Visible		Eye—Photochemical and thermal retinal injury
		780 nm	Eye—Thermal retinal injury
	IRA		Eye—Thermal retinal injury, thermal cataract
		1.4 μm	Skin burn
Infrared	IRB		Eye—Corneal burn, cataract
		3 μm	Skin burn
	IRC		Eye—Corneal burn, cataract
		1 mm	Heating of body surface
Electromagnetic fields		300 GHz	
	Microwaves		Heating of body surface
		1 GHz	Heating with 'penetration depth' of 10 mm
			Raised body temperature
		<100 kHz	Cumulation of charge on body surface
			Disturbance of nerve and muscle responses
	Static	0 Hz	Magnetic field—vertigo/nausea
			Electric field—charge on body surface

Long-term effects are given in italics.

to the setting up of the International Non-Ionising Radiation Committee (INIRC) at an International Radiation Protection Association (IRPA) congress in 1977 to develop guidance for NIR protection programmes. The committee produced guidelines on limitation to exposure from ultrasound, lasers, and optical radiations in 1982 and for low-frequency electromagnetic fields in 1984 and 1987. The INIRC became independent from the IRPA in 1992 and was renamed the International Commission on Non-Ionising Radiation Protection (ICNIRP). The ICNIRP works with the World Health Organization (WHO) to assess health effects of NIRs and to develop international guidelines on limits to exposure and protection measures, which are science based and independent. The American Conference of Governmental Industrial Hygienists (ACGIH) set threshold limit values relating to exposure across the whole electromagnetic spectrum in 1992, which are revised annually and have been influential in the development of recommendations by the ICNIRP. The NRPB make recommendations and the Medical Devices Agency issues guidance on NIRs relating to the UK. The American National Standards Institution publish guidance on recommended practices in the USA.

The practical implementation of health-based exposure standards requires inputs from bodies responsible for the development of standards for measurement, product design, NIR emission, and safety, such as the International Electrotechnical Commission (IEC), the International Organization for Standardization (ISO), and the Commission Internationale de l'Éclairage [Illumination] (CIE). The ICNIRP guidelines are concerned with the basic principles of protection and it is the responsibility of national governments to implement appropriate radiation protection programmes. The United States Radiation Control Health and Safety Act 1968 administers emission standards for ionising and non-ionising radiations for many types of equipment through the Food and Drug Administration (FDA). There is currently little legislation relating directly to NIRs in Europe. This gap is expected to be addressed by adoption of requirements of the CEC Directive on Physical Agents, which covers occupational protection from non-ionising radiations. A draft proposal was published in 1994 but its final form is still under debate. Lack of specific legislation does not release the user from responsibility or immunity from prosecution. Good practice must be adopted, usually in accordance with accepted standards, recommendations, and guidelines.

1.5 Further reading

Harding, L. K. (1997). Radiation protection—lessons from the past. *Br. J. Radiol.*, **70**, S10–S16.

Mould, R. F. (1993). *A century of X-rays and radioactivity in medicine.* IOP, Bristol.

Oliver, R. (1973). Seventy-five years of radiation protection. *Br. J. Radiol.*, **46**, 854–60.

Thomas, A. M. K. (ed.) (1995). *The invisible light.* Blackwell Science, Oxford.

Chapter 2
Interaction of ionising radiations with matter

C. J. Martin

2.1 Introduction

The whole of radiation protection is involved with the interaction of ionising radiations with matter. It is important for the radiation protection physicist to have a thorough knowledge of the physics of these processes in order to understand why particular techniques and materials are used for different applications and to enable him/her to develop solutions for new problems as they present themselves. This chapter gives an overview of the physics relating to ionising radiation. Radioactive decay is discussed briefly for completeness and the remainder of the chapter deals with interactions of radiation with matter. Areas of medical physics where properties resulting from different interactions are important are highlighted. More in-depth treatments can be found in texts on radiological physics [1,2] and radiation dosimetry [3].

2.2 Radioactive decay

The mode of decay of a radioactive atom or radionuclide depends on whether the ratio of neutrons to protons in the parent nucleus is too high or too low and on the mass–energy relationship between parent and daughter nuclides. The various modes of decay and particles that can be emitted are described in Box 2.1. Individual atoms of a particular radionuclide may decay by emission of particles with different energies (Box 2.2) or even through more than one mode of decay. Data on emissions from different radionuclides are summarized in various handbooks [4–7]. The changes in activity with time for all radioactive decay processes are governed by the same simple law. A physical half-life in which the activity will have dropped to one-half of the original value can be defined for every radionuclide. The half-life ($T_{½}$) is a statistical property and the law is only valid because of the large numbers of atoms involved.

From the definition of half-life:

$$A_n = A_0/2^n \tag{2.1}$$

where A_0 is the original activity and A_n the activity after n half-lives.

The activity A_t at time t after the original activity A_o was measured can be expressed as an exponential:

$$A_t = A_0\,\mathrm{e}^{-\lambda t}. \tag{2.2}$$

The decay constant

$$\lambda = \ln 2/T_{\frac{1}{2}} = 0.693/T_{\frac{1}{2}} \tag{2.3}$$

or

$$\lambda = -(1/N)(\mathrm{d}N/\mathrm{d}t) \tag{2.4}$$

where $\mathrm{d}N$ is the change in the number of atoms (N) of a radionuclide during a short time interval $\mathrm{d}t$. Useful rules of thumb are that the activity of any radionuclide is reduced to less than 1% in 7 half-lives and less than 0.1% in 10 half-lives.

Activity is measured in terms of the becquerel (Bq), which is the amount of material in which one disintegration of a radioactive atom occurs every second. The old unit is the curie (Ci), equal to 3.7×10^{10} Bq. The specific activity is the number of becquerels per unit mass $[(0.693 \times 6.02 \times 10^{26})/(T_{\frac{1}{2}} \times \text{atomic mass})\ \text{Bq kg}^{-1}]$ for a pure sample of the radionuclide.

2.3 Electron interactions

When a particle or a photon passes through a material it may interact with the electrons or the nucleus of an atom. The electrons surrounding the nucleus are arranged in orbitals or shells with discrete 'binding' energies. Successive shells are labelled alphabetically and can contain the following maximum numbers of electrons: K 2, L 8, M 18, N 32, and O 50. The binding energy of an

Box 2.1 Radionuclide emission

Modes of decay

α-particle

α-particles consist of two protons (p) and two neutrons (n) and are emitted from heavy nuclei when the n/p ratios are too low. α-particles are monoenergetic because the energy released is shared entirely between the product nucleus and the α-particle.

β-particle

A β-particle is a high-energy electron emitted when a neutron is transformed into a proton within the nucleus. The energy released in the transition is shared between the β-particle and an anti-neutrino, so the β-particles from a particular decay may have an energy anywhere from zero up to the maximum (Figure B2.1). The average β-particle energy is about one-third of the maximum.

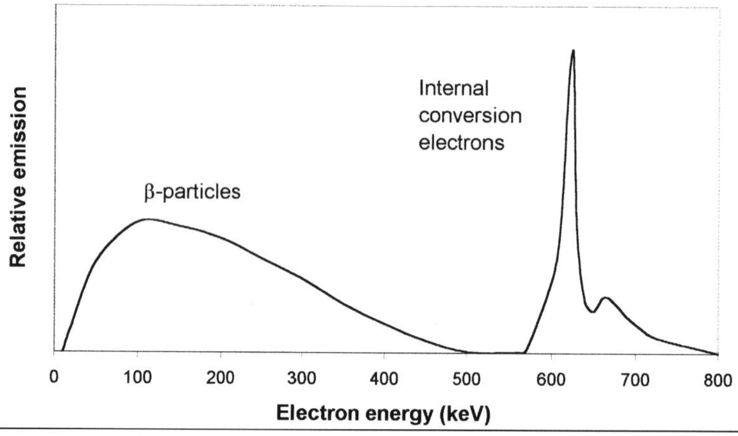

Figure B2.1 Electron energy spectrum for ^{137}Cs showing the broad range of energies from β-particle emission with narrow peaks at 624 and 656 keV from internal conversion electrons.

electron in a particular shell depends on the charge on the nucleus and so is greater for elements with higher atomic numbers (Figure 2.1). These energies are characteristic of each element and are important in determining particle and photon interactions with different materials.

Energetic electrons may undergo a large number of interactions in matter [1–5]. They collide with atomic electrons producing excitation and ionisation and they lose a small amount of energy each time. A small percentage of the interactions results in the production of X-ray photons.

2.3.1 Bremsstrahlung X-rays

A bremsstrahlung X-ray may be produced as an energetic electron undergoes a violent change in direction, when it comes close to an atomic nucleus. This is the most important mechanism involved in the production of X-rays in an X-ray tube, although the proportion of the energy from an electron beam that is converted into X-rays is less than 1%. The yield of bremsstrahlung X-rays is proportional to atomic number, so metals such as tungsten are used for X-ray tube anodes.

Bremsstrahlung X-ray photons have a range of energies from zero up to the energy of the interacting electron. When an electron strikes a thin sheet of metal, the probability of bremsstrahlung production at every energy up to the maximum is the same. However, when electrons hit the surface of a thick object, X-ray emissions may occur at some depth below the surface, and this alters the energy distribution. The electrons lose energy through minor interactions as they penetrate deeper, so the maximum photon energy decreases with depth. In addition, the X-rays are attenuated before they emerge from the material, with the low-energy photons being attenuated more. Further attenuation occurs in the body of the X-ray tube itself. The net result is a continuous spectrum of X-ray energies between about 15 keV and the maximum electron energy, with a peak near the middle (see Figure 2.8). The form of the spectrum and its implications for radiology are considered in §12.3. Bremsstrahlung X-rays are also produced when high-energy β-particles interact with heavier materials. The average energy (E_{av}) of bremsstrahlung produced by

Box 2.1 (*continued*)

Positron

A positron (β^+) is a β-particle with a positive charge. It results from the transformation of a proton into a neutron and is accompanied by emission of a neutrino. The positron will dissipate its energy locally and then amalgamate with an electron to produce two γ-rays travelling in opposing directions (annihilation radiation) with energies equal to the mass equivalent of the positron and the electron (511 keV).

Orbital electron capture

A neutron-deficient atom may decay by capturing an orbital electron, which combines with an intranuclear proton to form a neutron. A characteristic X-ray will be emitted as an electron falls from an outer orbit into the energy level formerly occupied by the captured electron (§2.3.2).

Emission of excitation energy

Following a radioactive decay process, the nucleus may be left in an excited state. The nucleus can lose this excitation energy by emission of either γ-rays or internal conversion electrons.

γ-ray emission

γ-rays emitted during radioactive decay are monoenergetic and are characteristic of the decay occurring. The lifetimes of nuclear excited states are typically of the order of 10^{-10} s, so γ-rays are usually emitted effectively at the same time as the nuclear transformations. However, in some cases quantum mechanical selection rules prevent photon emission for an extended period. The excited state of ^{99}Tc following the decay of ^{99}Mo has a half-life of 6.02 h before it makes the isomeric transition to the ground state. A nuclear excited state with a long half-life is termed metastable and is designated by the symbol m, e.g. ^{99m}Tc.

Internal conversion

Internal conversion is a process in which a tightly bound electron absorbs nuclear excitation energy and is ejected from the atom. Internal conversion electrons are monoenergetic (Figure B2.1). Characteristic X-rays are emitted during the process as outer orbital electrons fill the vacancies left by the internal conversion electrons (§2.3.2). Internal conversion occurs more frequently in heavy nuclei and γ-ray emission predominates in lighter ones.

Box 2.2 Energy level diagrams

Nuclear transitions can be portrayed as energy level diagrams. Comprehensive diagrams for all radionuclides are collected in ICRP 38 [7]. Figure B2.2 shows a much simplified example for ^{131}I. Ninety per cent of the atoms emit β-particles with an energy of 0.61 MeV, and 10% with an energy of 0.33 MeV. Both leave the daughter nuclide in an excited state and the additional energy is lost by emission of γ-rays (Box 2.1).

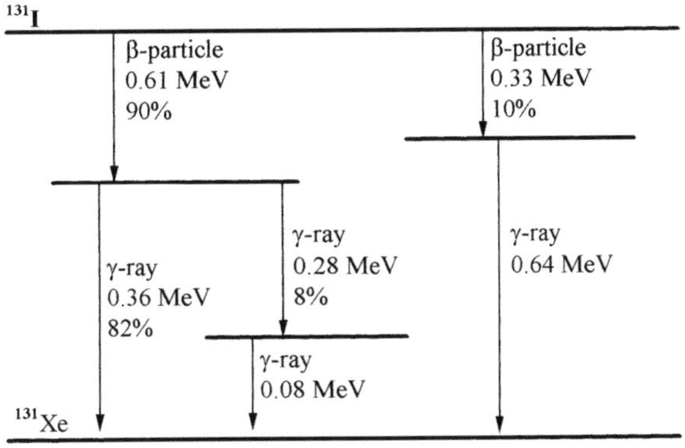

Figure B2.2 Energy level diagram showing decay scheme for ^{131}I. This is a simplification of the scheme in which each of the energy levels is split into subsidiary levels separated by a few tens of keV [7].

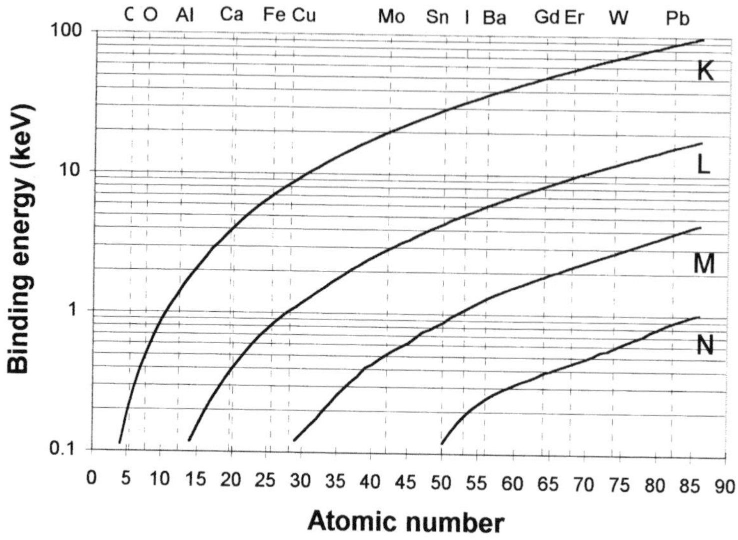

Figure 2.1 Binding energies for electrons in the K, L, M, and N atomic shells as a function of atomic number. The energies equate to photoelectric absorption edges (§2.4.2) and the difference between energies of individual shells relate to energies of characteristic X-rays (§2.3.2). Positions of elements which are important for medical applications are marked.

β-particles with a maximum energy E_β keV, when interacting with a material of atomic number Z, will be approximately

$$E_{av} = 1.4 \times 10^{-7} Z E_\beta^2 \text{ keV}. \tag{2.5}$$

2.3.2 Characteristic X-rays

When an electron from an inner K or L shell of an atom has been ejected or excited, this leaves a vacancy which may be filled by an electron falling from a shell with a lower binding energy (L, M, or outer shells). The excess energy is emitted in the form of an X-ray photon. The energies of each shell vary with the atomic number (Figure 2.1) and the energies of the X-rays emitted are characteristic of that element. For low atomic number elements in soft tissue, the energies are small and the X-rays are absorbed rapidly.

2.3.3 Auger electrons

An atom in which an L electron makes a transition to fill a vacancy in the K shell does not always emit a characteristic X-ray, particularly in low atomic number elements. The energy may be transferred to another L electron which is then ejected from the atom (KLL emission). The ejected electron is called an Auger electron and the process leaves an additional vacancy in the L shell. As the atomic number increases, LMM and MNN transitions can also occur.

2.4 Interactions of X-rays and γ-rays with matter

The interaction of photons with atoms in matter is random, but it is possible to specify the probability of an interaction occurring. Each atom can be regarded as having a cross-section or an apparent area which if traversed will lead to an interaction. One consequence of this is that a thickness of a material can be specified in which there will be a certain fractional change in radiation intensity. This can be expressed in terms of a linear attenuation coefficient (μ) or a mass attenuation coefficient (μ/ρ) as

$$I_x = I_o \, e^{-\mu x} = I_o \, e^{-(\mu/\rho)\rho x} \tag{2.6}$$

where I_0 is the incident intensity and I_x is the intensity after traversing thickness x of the material (density ρ) [1–5].

X-rays and γ-rays covering a range of energies may interact with matter through several mechanisms. Five processes will be considered; Rayleigh or coherent scattering, the photoelectric effect, Compton scattering, pair production, and photonuclear interactions, which have linear attenuation coefficients represented by σ_{coh}, τ, σ_c, κ, and τ_{nucl}, respectively.

2.4.1 Rayleigh scattering

An incident photon collides with an electron which is bound tightly enough to the nucleus for the whole atom

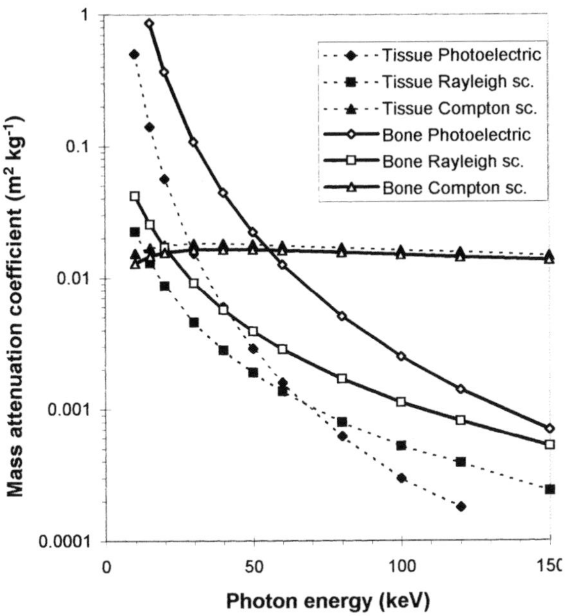

Figure 2.2 Attenuation coefficients for photoelectric absorption, and Compton and Rayleigh scattering for interactions with soft tissue and cortical bone as a function of photon energy [8].

to absorb the recoil. The photon is scattered in a different direction but the transfer of energy to the atom is negligible. The interaction occurs more frequently when the atomic number (Z) of the scattering material is high ($\sigma_{coh}/\rho \propto Z^2$) and is only important in tissue for photons with energies (E) < 10 keV ($\sigma_{coh}/\rho \propto 1/E^2$) (Figure 2.2).

2.4.2 Photoelectric effect

This effect dominates at low photon energies. All the energy from an incident photon is absorbed and transferred to an electron which is ejected from an inner shell of the atom. A characteristic X-ray is emitted as an electron from a higher orbital fills the vacancy (§2.3.2). There are discontinuities in the variation of the photoelectric absorption coefficient with photon energy at the binding energies of the ejected electrons. When the photon energy is slightly greater than that required to remove an electron from a particular shell, there is a sharp increase in the photoelectric absorption coefficient (Figure 2.3), which is referred to as an absorption edge. The probability of interaction decreases rapidly as photon energy increases above an absorption edge ($\tau/\rho \propto E^{-3}$). Energies of absorption edges associated with K shells of elements with atomic numbers greater than 30 lie in the diagnostic X-ray range (10–100 keV) (Figure 2.1). They are important in the selection of materials for intensifying screens, contrast agents, and filters.

Mass attenuation coefficients for some materials used for shielding diagnostic X-ray rooms are shown in Figure 2.4. Since the K-edge of lead lies in the upper part of the diagnostic energy range and the attenuation falls to one quarter at energies below the K-edge, care is required in considering relative attenuation properties of different shielding materials.

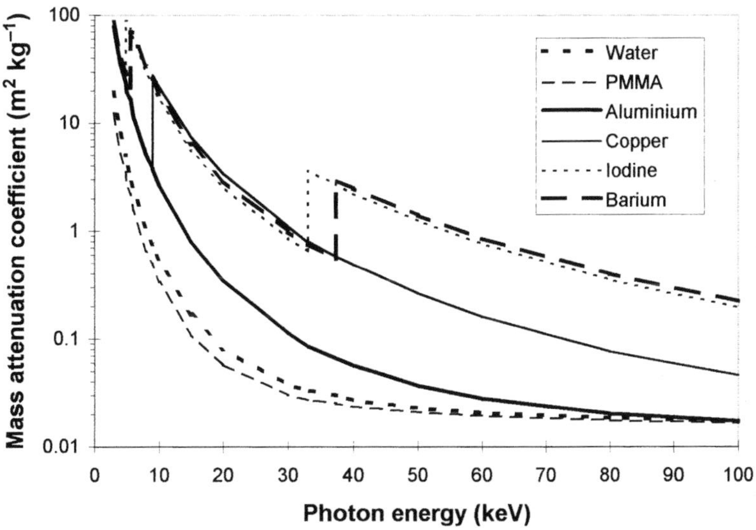

Figure 2.3 Plots of mass attenuation coefficients (μ/ρ) (m^2 kg^{-1}) against photon energy for materials used in X-ray test phantoms (water, PMMA, or perspex), beam filters (aluminium, copper), and contrast agents (iodine, barium) [5].

Contrast in diagnostic radiology

K-edges of elements present in tissue are below the diagnostic X-ray energy range (Figure 2.1) and so the probability of photoelectric interaction decreases rapidly with photon energy (Figure 2.2). Photoelectric absorption is the most important mode of interaction for elements in soft tissue up to 30 keV. The probability of photoelectric interaction in this energy range increases with atomic number ($\tau/\rho \propto Z^3$). It is the mechanism responsible for the large difference in attenuation between calcium (which makes up 14% of bone) and the lighter elements in soft tissue (Figure 2.2) and thus primarily responsible for the contrast in an X-ray image. Preparations containing elements with their K-edges in the diagnostic energy range (iodine 33 keV, barium 37 keV) are used to enhance X-ray contrast for the study of vessels in the body (Figure 2.3). The best contrast in an X-ray image is obtained where the photoelectric effect predominates, but because the energy absorption is high, the radiation dose to the tissue is also greater.

2.4.3 The Compton effect

The Compton effect involves an interaction in which a portion of the energy from a photon is transferred to a loosely bound or free electron (i.e. the electron binding energy (Figure 2.1) is much less than the energy of the photon). Energy and momentum are conserved and the angles at which the electron and scattered photon travel are determined by the amount of energy transferred. Compton scattering is the predominant mode of interaction in soft tissue between 30 keV and 10 MeV. The Compton mass attenuation coefficient (σ_c/ρ) is approximately constant in the energy range of diagnostic X-rays (Figure 2.2). Thus attenuation by Compton scattering is closely related to the tissue density, but is independent of atomic number Z. This relationship is utilized in computed tomography in which images relating to tissue density are reconstructed from X-ray transmission measurements. A higher energy X-ray beam (120–140 kVp) is used, which is heavily filtered to remove the majority of the lower energy photons that would interact via the photoelectric effect.

The Compton mass attenuation coefficient starts to decline at photon energies above 100 keV ($\sigma_c/\rho \propto E^{-1}$). This decline can be seen in Figure 2.4 for the mass attenuation coefficients for concrete and iron between 200 and 2000 keV, for which attenuation is predominantly due to Compton scattering.

It is instructive to consider the variation in Compton interactions with scattering angle, as this is relevant to radiation protection. The collision differential cross-section of the Klein–Nishina equation for the Compton effect can be used to predict the angular distribution of scattered photons for different incident photon energies resulting from interaction with a free electron (Figure 2.5a). This shows that:

- the probabilities of forward or backward scatter are greater than that through 90°
- the number of photons scattered in the forward and backward directions is almost symmetrical for low-

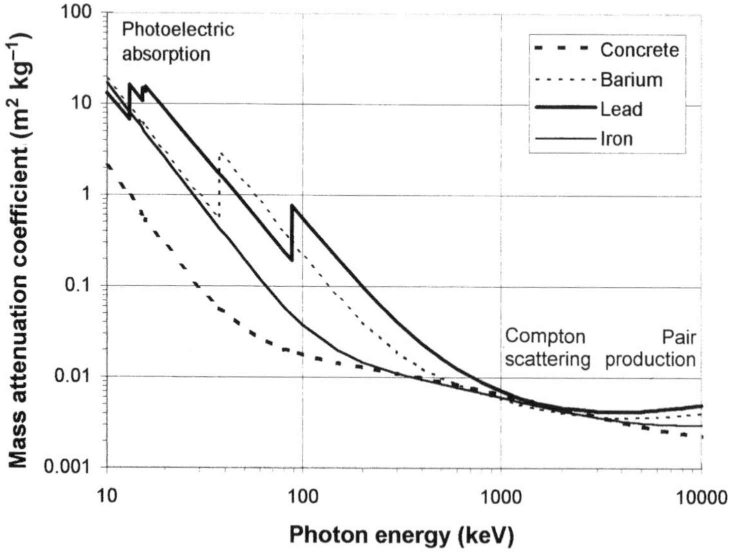

Figure 2.4 Plots of mass attenuation coefficients (μ/ρ) ($m^2\ kg^{-1}$) against photon energy for various shielding materials used in diagnostic radiology and radiotherapy. Positions where photoelectric absorption, Compton scattering, and pair production predominate are marked [5].

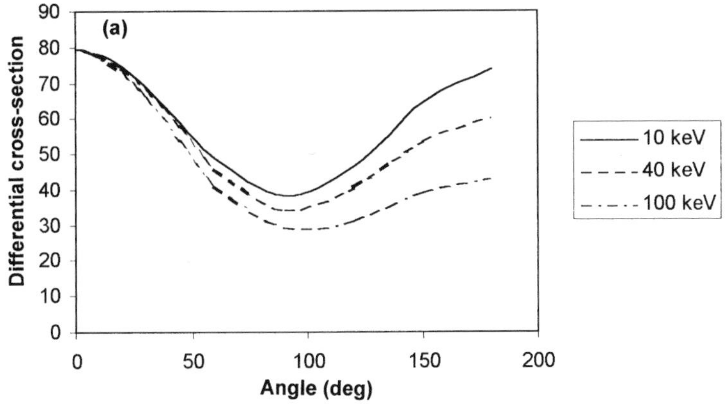

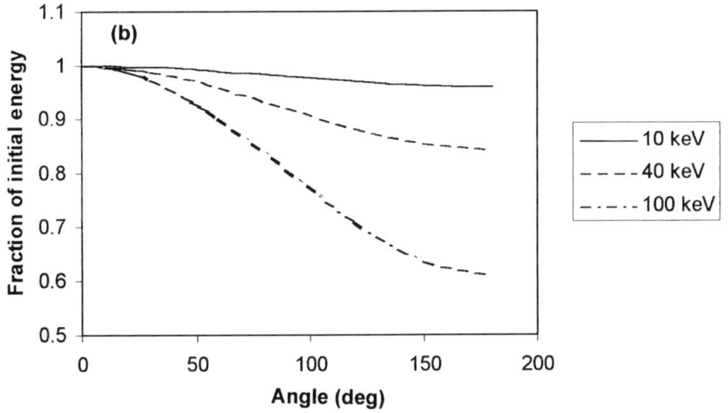

Figure 2.5 Variation of Compton scatter from a single unbound electron with angle of scatter (0° = no deflection) for monoenergetic photons: (a) differential collision cross-section in units of 10^{-31} m^2 steradian^{-1} per electron; (b) proportion of the interaction energy retained by the photon following scattering.

energy X-rays (10–40 keV), but as photon energy increases, more are scattered in the forward direction.

The change in wavelength ($\Delta\lambda$) for a photon scattered through angle θ is given by:

$$\Delta\lambda = (h/m_e c)(1 - \cos\theta). \quad (2.7)$$

The energy loss increases with scattering angle and with photon energy as shown in Figure 2.5b. Some consequences of this relationship are:

- photons scattered in the forward direction only lose a small proportion of their energy;
- photons that are scattered back towards the surface have a lower energy than those scattered in the forward direction;
- the proportion of the energy lost by the incident photon increases with photon energy, e.g. for a photon scattered at 60°, the proportion of the energy taken up by the electron varies from 5% at 60 keV, to 9% at 100 keV, and 50% at 1 MeV.

The relationships considered are for interactions with a free electron. However, where the body is irradiated, the distribution of photons is determined by attenuation of the scattered photons in the body tissues and the implications of this for radiation protection are considered in §2.5.2.

2.4.4 Pair production

Pair production is the conversion of a photon to an electron–positron pair. This effect dominates at high photon energies (> 5–50 MeV). An energy greater than 1.02 MeV is required, which is the energy equivalence of the masses of a positron and an electron. Additional energy is distributed evenly between the two particles. The positron amalgamates with an electron to produce annihilation radiation (Box 2.1). Thus 1.02 MeV of energy is radiated again and only the kinetic energy of the electron and positron is absorbed. The probability of pair production (κ/ρ) increases with photon energy [$\kappa/\rho \propto (E - 1.02\ \text{MeV})$], unlike the other three types of process.

The interaction is more likely to occur in the vicinity of a heavy nucleus and the mass attenuation coefficient is proportional to Z. As a result, differences in mass attenuation coefficients between heavier and lighter shielding materials are more pronounced above 3000 keV, where pair production predominates for heavier materials (Figure 2.4).

2.4.5 Photonuclear interactions

Photons interacting with a nucleus may induce the emission of a neutron or proton, if the photon energy is sufficient. For most stable nuclei heavier than carbon the threshold energy lies between 6 and 16 MeV. The threshold is 6.3 MeV for ^{235}U, 7.4 MeV for ^{108}Pb, and 10.8 MeV for ^{63}Cu, but tends to be higher for lower atomic number materials. The cross-section for neutron production rises to a maximum at 12–24 MeV, falling off at higher energies, but the interaction never makes up more than a few per cent of the total attenuation. Significant numbers of neutrons are produced through this mechanism by linear accelerators operating above 10 MV.

2.4.6 Attenuation and absorption coefficients

The interaction processes occur independently and the resultant transmitted intensity can be expressed in terms of the linear attenuation coefficient μ as:

$$I_x = I_o\, e^{-\mu x} = I_o\, e^{-\sigma_{coh} x}\, e^{-\tau x}\, e^{-\sigma_c x}\, e^{-\kappa x} \qquad (2.8)$$

or in terms of the mass attenuation coefficient (μ/ρ) where ρ is the density [9]:

$$I_x = I_o\, e^{-(\mu/\rho)\rho x} = I_o\, e^{-(\sigma_{coh}/\rho + \tau/\rho + \sigma_c/\rho + \kappa/\rho)\rho x}. \qquad (2.9)$$

The mass attenuation coefficient includes energy carried away by the scattered Compton photon and lost as annihilation radiation from pair production. It is useful to define a mass transfer coefficient μ_{tr}/ρ, excluding these components, that relates to the photon energy transferred to charged particles as kinetic energy which is linked to kerma (§2.7.3) [3]. Not all the energy transferred to charged particles is absorbed, as a small fraction g is converted again to photon energy (bremsstrahlung, §2.3.1), so the coefficient for mass energy absorption μ_{en}/ρ is given by

$$\mu_{en}/\rho = (\mu_{tr}/\rho)(1-g). \qquad (2.10)$$

2.5 Practical implications of photon interactions

The interactions of photons of different energy with matter affect diagnostic radiology imaging techniques, influence the choice of materials for use with X-rays, and have implications for radiation protection. This section deals with some of these issues.

2.5.1 Influence of photoelectric interaction on materials for filters and phantoms

Interaction mechanisms and the resulting attenuation and absorption coefficients influence the choice of materials for applications such as filters and phantoms. Materials which have K-edges at the bottom of the diagnostic X-ray energy range will absorb low-energy photons more strongly through the photoelectric effect. Aluminium (K-edge 1.6 keV) has traditionally been used to filter X-ray beams, but copper (K-edge 9.0 keV) attenuates photons in the energy range above 9 keV more strongly (Figure 2.3) and is used to reduce skin dose. Some rare earth materials with L absorption edges in this range and K-edges at the upper end of the diagnostic X-ray energy range (e.g. Er: L-edge, 8.7 keV; K-edge, 57.5 keV) have been used for filters to produce a beam with a narrower photon energy spread. Copper is used to harden X-ray beams for equipment tests, such as measurement of image intensifier dose rates (§12.6.4). The high attenuation due to the photoelectric effect enables a smaller amount of material to be used and gives a much smaller scattered component than tissue. However, there will be differences in the spectrum of X-rays transmitted by copper and tissue (Figure 2.3), and where this is important, because of differences in detector energy sensitivities (e.g. testing of AEC system, §12.6.4), more tissue equivalent materials should be used.

The energies of absorption edges, which equate to removal of an electron from an atom, are slightly greater than the energies of the characteristic X-rays, which are equal to the difference in energy between the energy level and higher energy states (§2.3.2). As a result, materials are relatively transparent to their own characteristic X-rays. This property is used in mammographic equipment, where a molybdenum anode is used with a filter of the same material to enable the characteristic X-ray peaks to be utilized.

2.5.2 Scattered radiation in diagnostic radiology

As well as degrading the diagnostic quality of the radiograph, Compton scatter is the source of the majority of the radiation dose to staff in diagnostic radiology. Knowledge of the distribution of scattered radiation around a patient is important for the protection of staff and for determining shielding requirements. Variations in the scattering cross-section and energy for monoenergetic photons scattered from single unbound electrons are shown in Figure 2.5. However, the X-ray spectrum is not monoenergetic and, in addition, all photons scattered following an interaction in a patient will undergo further

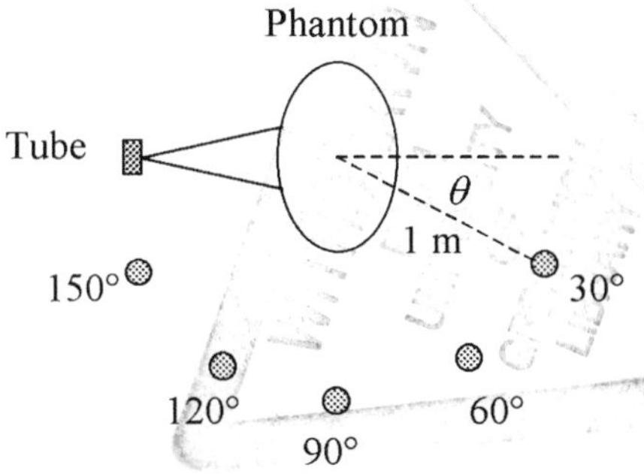

Figure 2.6 Arrangement used to simulate and measure scatter of an X-ray beam from a body.

interactions, both photoelectric and Compton, within the patient. As a result, it is not possible to use simple analytical techniques to describe the distribution of scattered radiation around a patient. The problem must be approached either by using direct measurements or by seeking numerical solutions using Monte Carlo methods.

Numerical and experimental determinations of the distribution of scattered radiation have been determined using the geometry shown in Figure 2.6 and both yield similar results [10–12]. Figure 2.7 shows a generalized form of the distribution of scatter around the phantom. Since the amount of scatter produced depends on the volume irradiated, it is proportional to the area of the X-ray beam at the surface of the phantom. Therefore, scatter dose is shown normalized with respect to the easily measured quantity dose–area product (§12.2.1). For all values of kVp, the lowest scatter dose (i.e. fluence) occurs at small angles and the greatest as the scattering angle approaches 180°. It is possible to fit a polynomial to describe analytically the scatter distribution function and thus define the scatter fluence at any angle. This approach has been used to determine the scatter levels against which shielding is required for X-ray rooms (see Chapter 13).

The spectrum of the scattered radiation will vary with direction because of the characteristics of the Compton interaction process (§2.4.3) and also because of the differing levels of attenuation within the phantom in different directions. Plots of the distribution of photon energies in the incident beam and scattered radiation in two directions are shown in Figure 2.8. The radiation that is scattered at 30° has a greater proportion of higher energy photons than that scattered at 120° and consequently a higher average energy, although the scatter fluence at 120° will be much greater.

The same pattern is observed for all accelerating potentials. The variation of the photon energy distribution (or quality) of the scattered radiation is shown in Figure 2.9. The quality is commonly expressed in terms of the thickness of aluminium to reduce the air kerma by half, or the half-value layer (HVL). The HVL of the scattered radiation is described by a curve which is opposite in sense to that observed for scatter fluence. These results show that for scattering of X-rays from a body:

- the greater the scattering angle, the greater the scattered air kerma

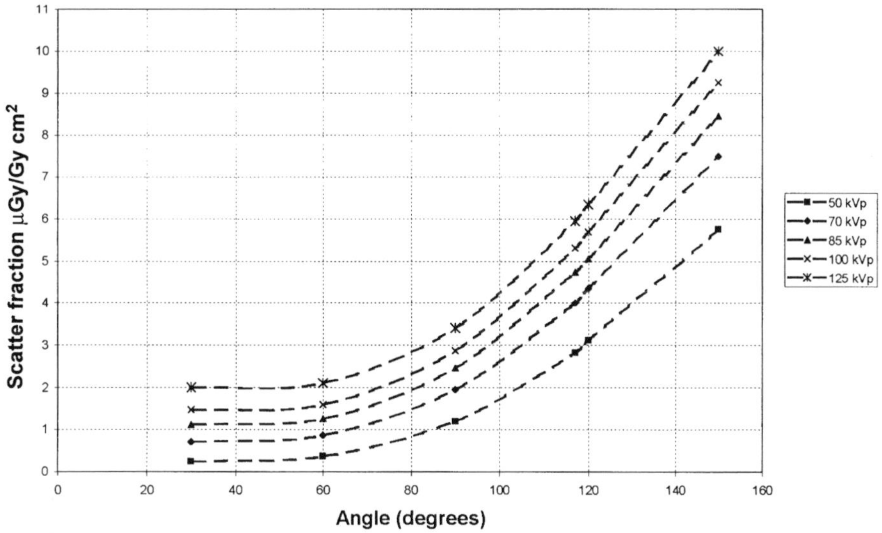

Figure 2.7 Variation in scattered air kerma per unit dose–area product with angle of scatter for X-ray beams of different energies.

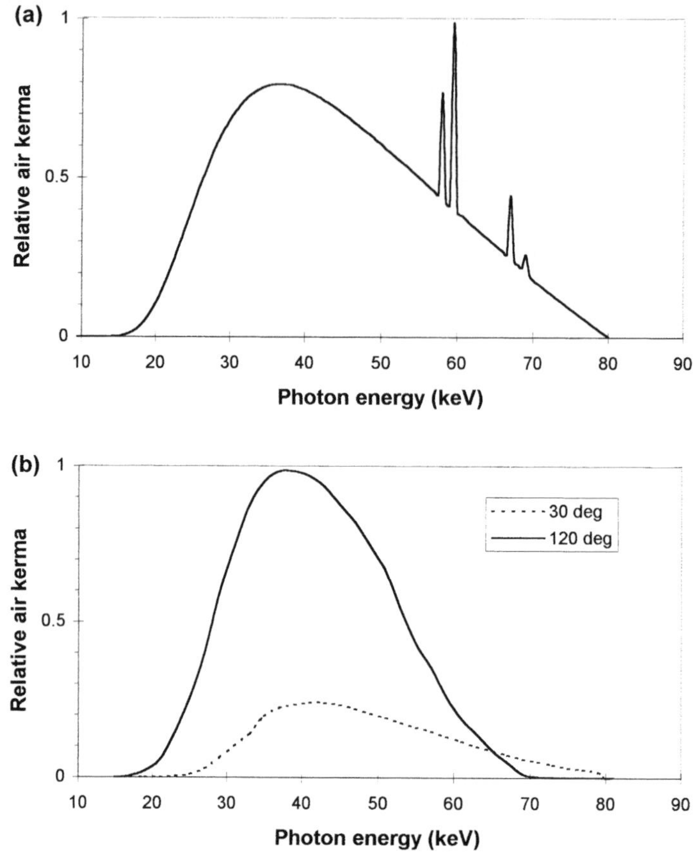

Figure 2.8 Spectra of (a) an 80 kVp X-ray beam produced from a tungsten target filtered by 3 mm of aluminium and (b) the radiation scattered at angles of 30 and 120 from a phantom simulating a human trunk. Units are arbitrary.

- the greater the scattering angle, the lower the HVL of the scattered radiation
- the spectrum of X-rays scattered back from the patient is softer than the incident X-ray beam (lower HVL) as the proportion of high-energy photons is lower
- the spectrum of X-rays passing through a patient after scattering through angles less than 60° is harder then the incident X-ray beam.

2.6 Neutrons

2.6.1 Neutron production

There are no radionuclides that emit neutrons, other than a few nuclear fission fragments with very short half-lives and certain heavy radionuclides, which decay by spontaneous fission, such as ^{252}C. Neutrons are produced by nuclear reactions and the largest sources of neutrons are nuclear reactors and particle accelerators. The interaction of α-particles with certain nuclides such as ^{9}Be can be used to make small neutron sources. The α-particle enters the Be nucleus to form a compound nucleus which disintegrates, emitting a neutron. Thus a neutron source can be made by mixing ^{9}Be with an α-particle source such as ^{241}Am. The neutrons produced by this type of source have a range of high energies.

$$^{9}_{4}\mathrm{Be} + {}^{4}_{2}\mathrm{He} \rightarrow {}^{13}_{6}\mathrm{C} \rightarrow {}^{12}_{6}\mathrm{C} + \mathrm{n} \qquad [^{9}\mathrm{Be}\,(\alpha, \mathrm{n})\,^{12}\mathrm{C}]$$

compound nucleus

2.6.2 Neutron interactions

Neutrons are divided into two classes, fast neutrons which have energies over 0.1 MeV and thermal neutrons which have the same average kinetic energy as gas molecules in the environment. All neutrons produced by nuclear reactions are fast. They lose energy by collision with atomic nuclei and when they have been slowed down to thermal energies, they are captured by nuclei. The most important collision interaction is elastic scattering in

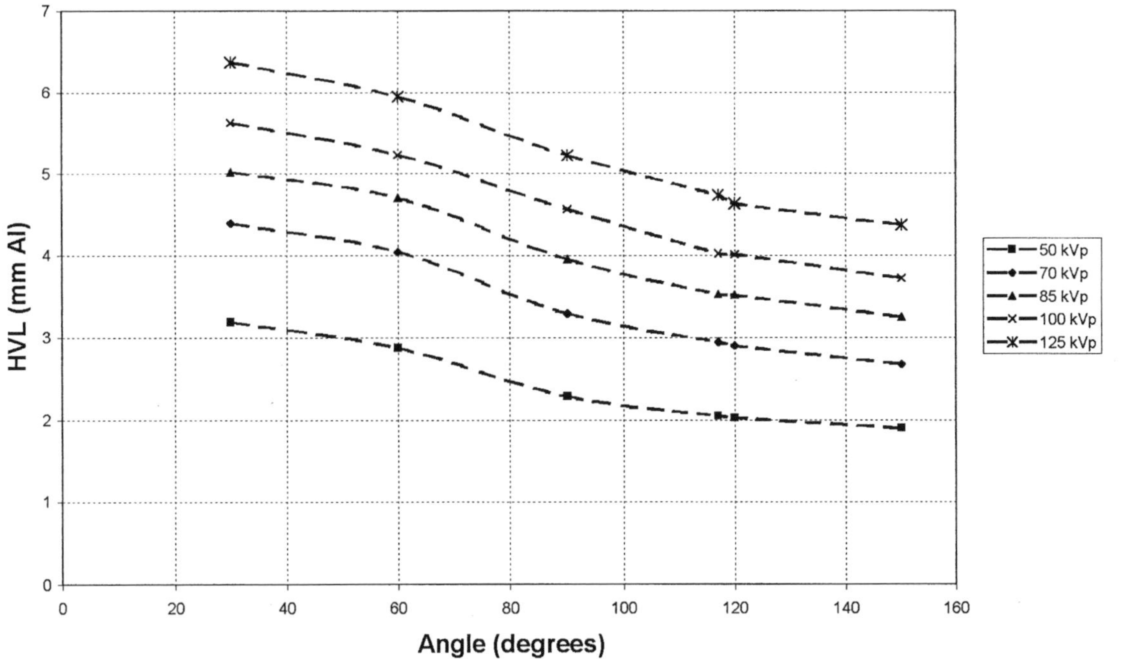

Figure 2.9 Variation in the half-value layer (HVL) for scattered radiation with the angle of scatter for X-ray beams with different energies.

which the kinetic energy of the neutron is shared with the collision nucleus. When a neutron undergoes an elastic interaction, the energy change is given by

$$\Delta E = E_0 - E_f = E_0[1 - (M-m)^2/(M+m)^2]\cos^2\theta = E_0\, 4Mm/(M+m)^2\cos^2\theta \qquad (2.11)$$

where E_0 is the initial energy of the incident neutron, E_f is the final energy of the neutron, θ is the angle of recoil, and M and m are the masses of the scattering nucleus and the incident neutron, respectively.

As can be seen, a larger fraction of the neutron's energy is transferred in interactions with smaller nuclei, and the hydrogen nucleus, which has a similar mass to a neutron, is the most efficient nuclei for slowing down neutrons. Neutrons are damaging to biological tissue, which has a large component of hydrogen atoms, and hydrogen-rich materials such as water and paraffin are used as neutron moderators. Fast neutrons may also interact via inelastic scattering in which the atomic nucleus is left in an excited state. The excitation energy will be radiated rapidly in the form of a γ-ray or if the neutron energy is greater than 10 MeV, a second high-energy neutron may be produced.

Neutrons that have been slowed down to thermal energies of the order of 0.025 eV are captured by a nucleus. The neutron absorption cross-section is inversely proportional to the square root of the neutron energy above 0.025 eV. Neutron-shielding materials contain atoms such as ^{10}B which have a large neutron absorption cross-section. Neutron capture may be followed by γ-ray emission or may transform the nucleus to a radionuclide (activation), usually of short half-life, which decays by emission of particle radiation. It is important to ensure that materials used in areas exposed to neutron fluxes do not contain atoms which may be transformed to radionuclides with significant half-lives (e.g. $^{59}Co(n)^{60}Co$, 5.3 years half-life).

2.7 The radiation field and radiation dose

The damage to biological tissue produced by the interaction of ionising radiations described in §2.4 is quantified in terms of the deposition of energy. Dosimetric quantities are determined by the interaction of a radiation field with a material and can be expressed in terms of the product of a radiation field quantity and an interaction coefficient [9].

2.7.1 The radiation field

The passage of particles through a radiation field is described in terms of the fluence φ, which is defined as $\varphi = dN/da$, where dN particles are incident on a sphere of cross-sectional area d*a* [5, 9]. A sphere is used to avoid the need to take account of the beam direction or to specify the orientation of the area. Other important quantities for specifying a radiation field are the fluence rate (m^{-2} s^{-1}), which is the number of particles that cross unit area in unit time, the energy fluence ψ (J m^{-2}), which is the energy that passes through unit area, and the energy fluence rate, which is the rate of energy flow per unit area, the energy flux density or the intensity (J m^{-2} s^{-1} or W m^{-2}).

2.7.2 Absorbed dose

Absorbed dose quantifies the transfer of energy from ionising radiation to matter and is equal to the mean energy per unit mass imparted to a small volume of a material. It is measured in units of gray (Gy), equal to the absorption of 1 joule (J) in 1 kilogram of matter (1 Gy = 1 J kg^{-1}). The absorbed dose (D_m) in a material (m) is equal to the product of the energy fluence and the mass energy absorption coefficient:

$$D_{\rm m} = \psi(\mu_{\rm en}/\rho). \qquad (2.12)$$

Absorbed dose in a small volume has been adopted by the ICRU and used in defining operational quantities for dose measurement (Box 4.1 and §8.1.1). However, for assessment of harm from radiation exposure, the dose averaged over a tissue or an organ is more appropriate and this definition is used by ICRP for dose evaluation (§3.2.2).

2.7.3 Kerma

Kerma (acronym for kinetic energy released in matter) is a measure of all the kinetic energy of charged ionising particles liberated by uncharged ionising particles per unit mass of material. It is also measured in units of gray and is equal to the product of the energy fluence ψ (§2.7.1) and the coefficient of mass energy transfer (μ_{tr}/ρ) (§2.4.6):

$$K = \psi(\mu_{\rm tr}/\rho). \qquad (2.13)$$

Kerma quantifies the first stage of energy absorption, i.e. the transfer of energy from photons or neutrons to charged particles. The second stage in which energy is imparted to matter by the charged particles is described by absorbed dose. This does not include energy lost as bremsstrahlung from electron interactions and so not deposited in the material.

The relationship between absorbed dose in air and air kerma is given by

$$D_{\rm air} = K_{\rm air}(\mu_{\rm en}/\rho)_{\rm air}/(\mu_{\rm tr}/\rho)_{\rm air} = K_{\rm air}(1-g). \qquad (2.14)$$

The difference between $(\mu_{en}/\rho)_{air}$ and $(\mu_{tr}/\rho)_{air}$ results from energy lost in bremsstrahlung production (§2.3.1 and §2.4.6). For air and water, the difference between absorbed dose and kerma (g) is less than 0.4% for photon energies under 1 MeV but increases with energy, rising to 4% at 10 MeV.

2.7.4 Radiation measurement

Since the amounts of energy deposited in matter by ionising radiations are small, measurements related to absorbed dose for X- and γ-radiations are based on the number of ion-pairs created. The charge generated by photon interactions in a defined mass of air includes both ions produced directly by the incident photons and those produced by the secondary electrons. Some electrons produced by photon interactions within the measurement volume will escape and not be detected, while some electrons from photon interactions outside the measurement volume will be collected. Practical measurement systems are designed so that these two components are approximately equal, so that there is no net loss of charge. Under these conditions electronic equilibrium is said to exist. The mean energy to produce an ion-pair in air is constant except at very low energies and so energy deposition can be determined from the number of ion-pairs formed. Kerma is the quantity determined by radiation measuring instruments.

The energy absorbed per unit mass of materials subjected to the same energy fluence will be proportional to the mass energy absorption coefficients (μ_{en}/ρ) of those materials. Thus the absorbed dose (D_m) in a material other than air can be calculated from the equation

$$D_{\rm m} = D_{\rm air}(\mu_{\rm en}/\rho)_{\rm m}/(\mu_{\rm en}/\rho)_{\rm air} = K_{\rm air}(\mu_{\rm en}/\rho)_{\rm m}/(\mu_{\rm tr}/\rho)_{\rm air}. \qquad (2.15)$$

The ratio $(\mu_{en}/\rho)_m/(\mu_{en}/\rho)_{air}$ only varies slowly with photon energy for materials with atomic numbers close to that of air (Figure 2.10a), so the photon energy does not have to be known accurately to determine dose in tissue. However, this is no longer true for materials with higher atomic number such as bone (Figure 2.10b) or with large numbers of hydrogen atoms such as fat (Figure 2.10a). The ratio for water is 1.08±0.03 between 100 keV and 10 MeV, and that for lithium fluoride, which is used for dose measurement in the diagnostic X-ray energy range (Box 4.7), is about 1.1. Average mass energy absorption coefficient ratios for a range of X-ray spectra, which may be used for making adjustments to LiF dose measurements made at different X-ray tube potentials, are given in Table 2.1.

2.7.5 Exposure

Exposure in air is the term given to the amount of charge of one sign produced when all the electrons liberated by photons in unit mass of air have been stopped completely (C kg^{-1}) [9]. This includes the ions produced directly by the incident photons and those produced by all the secondary electrons, but not ionisation resulting from bremsstrahlung. It is the quantity formerly used for measurement of ionising radiation.

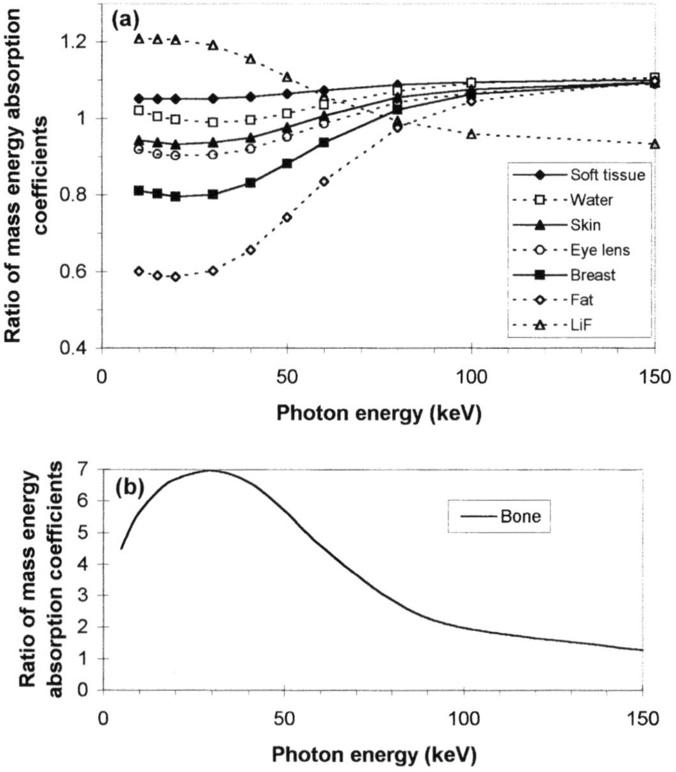

Figure 2.10 Ratios of the mass energy absorption coefficients for tissues relative to that of air $[(\mu_{en}/\rho)_m{:}(\mu_{en}/\rho)_{air}]$ as a function of photon energy: (a) various tissues, water, fat, and lithium fluoride; (b) bone [5, 9].

2.7.6 *Absorbed doses from charged particles*

Charged particles are strongly attenuated in matter, so will primarily affect the surface layer of tissues. α-particles with energies less than 7.5 MeV cannot penetrate the outer layer of the skin and do not give rise to an external hazard, although they present a severe hazard if taken into the body. However, β-particle radiation may give significant doses to the skin. A radionuclide deposited on a surface with a concentration of 100 Bq cm^{-2} (1 MBq m^{-2}) emitting β-particles with energies over 0.6 MeV will give a dose rate of 250 μGy h^{-1} through the protective layer of the skin.

Table 2.1 Average ratios of mass energy absorption coefficients for LiF and various tissues (m) with respect to air $[(\mu_{en}/\rho)_m/(\mu_{en}/\rho)_{air}]$ for X-ray spectra of different energies. Each result was derived by summing relative contributions (Figure 2.10) across the air kerma spectra for a constant potential X-ray unit filtered by 3 mm of aluminium. Factors can be used to adjust X-ray patient dosimetry TLD calibration factors to allow for different tube potentials (see Box 4.7)

Tube potential (kVp)	Lithium fluoride	ICRU soft tissue	Fat
60	1.178	1.054	0.638
70	1.168	1.055	0.655
80	1.157	1.057	0.673
90	1.147	1.058	0.691
100	1.137	1.060	0.709
110	1.127	1.062	0.727

2.8 References

1 Johns, H. E. and Cummingham, J. R. (1983). *The physics of radiology* (4th edn). Charles C. Thomas, Springfield, USA.
2 Dendy, P. P. and Heaton, B. (1999). *Physics for diagnostic radiology*. Medical Science Series. Institute of Physics, Bristol.
3 Greening, J. R. (1985). *Fundamentals of radiation dosimetry*. Adam Hilger, Bristol.
4 Longworth, G. (ed.) (1998). *The radiochemical manual*. AEA Technology, Harwell.
5 Shleien, B., Slaback Jr, L. A., and Birky, B. K. (eds) (1998). *Handbook of health physics and radiological health* (3rd edn). Williams and Williams, Baltimore.

6 Delcroix, D., Guevre, J. P., Leblanc, P., and Hickman, C. (1998). Radionuclide and radiation protection data handbook. *Radiat. Prot. Dosim.*, **76**, (1–2).

7 International Committee on Radiological Protection (1983). Radionuclide transformations: energies and intensities of emissions. ICRP Publication 38. *Ann. ICRP*, **11–13**.

8 International Commission on Radiological Units and Measurements (1989). *Tissue substitutes in radiation dosimetry and measurement*. ICRU Report 44. ICRU, Bethesda, MD.

9 International Commission on Radiological Units and Measurements (1998). *Fundamental quantities and units for ionising radiation*. ICRU Report 60. ICRU, Bethesda, MD.

10 Williams, J. R. (1996). Scatter dose estimation based on dose–area product and the specification of radiation barriers. *Br. J. Radiol.*, **69**, 1032–7.

11 Marshall, N. W., Faulkner, K., and Warren, H. (1996). Measured scattered X-ray energy spectra for simulated irradiation geometries in diagnostic radiology. *Med. Phys.*, **23**, 1271–6.

12 Sutton, D. G. and Williams, J. R. (2000). *Radiation shielding for diagnostic X-rays*. BIR/IPEM report. BIR, London.

Chapter 3
Biological effects of ionising radiation

J. W. Stather and H. Smith

3.1 Introduction

Ionising radiations have the potential to disrupt the structure of organic molecules in cells. This chapter looks at this damage at the cellular level, reviews evidence on the effects that may result in humans, and outlines how the risks are quantified. *In vitro* studies using proliferating cells have provided information on the primary physicochemical effects and on the relative biological effectiveness of different types of radiation. *In vivo* studies and follow-up of individuals after radiation exposure have shown the effects of radiation on the organism.

Acute exposure of the whole or parts of the body to doses of radiation equivalent to a few thousands of times that from naturally-occurring background radiation may result in the functional impairment of tissues and organs. This response is referred to by the International Commission on Radiological Protection (ICRP) as a 'deterministic effect'. The probability of the effect occurring and the severity of damage is related to dose, duration of exposure, and the amount of tissue irradiated. It is known from extensive experience in radiotherapy that there are tissue-specific threshold doses below which damage does not occur. Radiation effects seen above these thresholds include bone marrow aplasia, degeneration of the lining of the gastrointestinal tract, inflammation of the lining of the lungs, atrophy of the gonads, and skin burns. The replacement of functional tissue with non-functional connective tissue occurs as a late effect. If tissue damage is extensive, death of the organism may occur.

With an increasing understanding of dose–response relationships for radiation exposure, interest in radiation protection has focused increasingly on the effects of low doses, that is, up to a few tens of times the natural background radiation. The manifestation of this type of damage is not the loss of functional tissue but damage to the genetic make-up of cells leading to the induction of cancer in the organism or hereditary disease in subsequent generations. In radiological protection terminology, these diseases are referred to collectively as 'stochastic effects'. It is assumed that the probability of these effects, but not their severity, depends on the radiation dose, without a dose threshold.

The chapter reviews the biological effects of radiation on the adult organism and the developing conceptus. The risks associated with radiation exposure are also reviewed in relation to radiological protection criteria for acceptable exposure of workers and members of the general public. More detailed information on biological effects and risks may be obtained from the 1990 Recommendations of the ICRP [1] and publications of the United Nations Scientific Committee on the Effects of Atomic Radiation (UNSCEAR) [2–4].

3.2 Cellular effects

3.2.1 Primary physical and chemical events following exposure

When radiation passes through matter, it deposits energy in the material concerned. Radiations can be classified as *directly* or *indirectly ionising*. Charged particles (α-particles and β-particles emitted from radionuclides) are directly ionising and deposit energy through electrical interactions with electrons in the material. Other types of radiation (X-rays generated artificially or γ-rays from nuclear transitions) are indirectly ionising. When passing through matter, they lose energy in various ways but each results in giving up some of their energy to atoms with which they collide and electrons are ejected from these target atoms leaving behind positive ions. These high-velocity electrons move randomly through matter and may ionise atoms in their path. More electrons are then ejected, the incident electrons continuing on their trajectories with decreased energy and velocity until they eventually come to rest. Neutrons also lose energy in

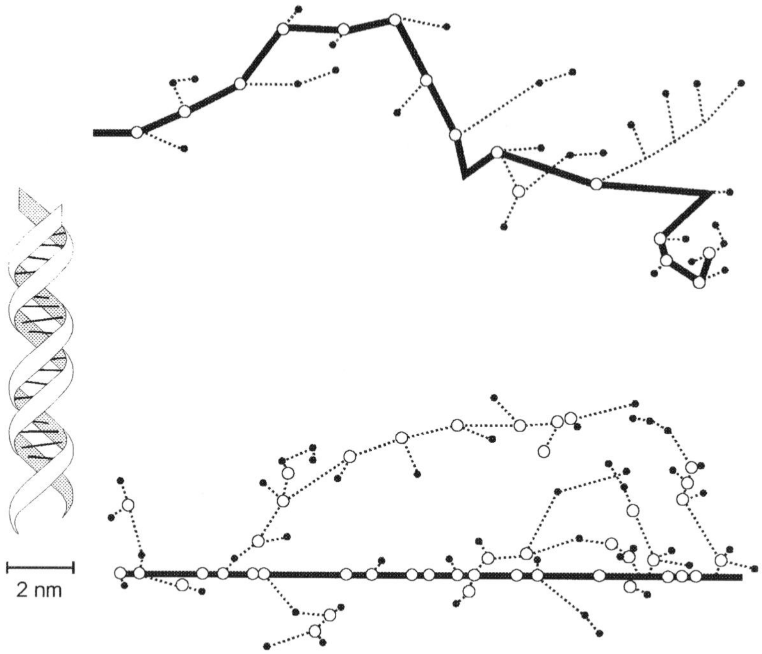

Figure 3.1 Simulated low-energy electron track (*upper trace*, initial energy 500 eV) and simulated short portion of an α-particle track (*lower trace*, 4 MeV). Open circles are ionisations, filled circles are excitations. A section of DNA is shown to give a perspective on dimensions [6]. Reproduced from the *International Journal of Radiation Biology* with permission from Taylor & Francis Ltd (http://www.tandf.co.uk/journals).

various ways, an important means being through collisions with hydrogen nuclei, which are single protons: the protons are set in motion and, being charged, they again deposit energy through electrical interactions. So in all cases, the radiation ultimately produces electrical interactions in the material. Another process, *excitation*, may occur if the energy transferred transiently moves orbiting electrons to a higher energy level in the atom. In biological terms, excitation is considered of less significance than ionisation. These physical processes are completed within 10^{-12} s.

The unique feature of ionising radiation is the highly localized release of energy along a *particle track* in sufficient amounts to alter atomic and molecular structure. The particle track is the ensemble of ionisations and excitations along the trajectory of electrons and protons. The random nature of the particle track can be simulated by computer analysis using Monte Carlo techniques. A two-dimensional clustering of ionisations is shown diagrammatically in Figure 3.1. It is stressed that this is a gross approximation of the more complex three-dimensional events that involve random clustering of ionisations on a sub-atomic scale. Nevertheless, the figure suffices to illustrate the concept that low-energy electrons are *sparsely ionising* because the individual ionisations are well separated. Alpha-particles, in contrast, are *densely ionising* because the ionisations are closely packed together along the track and have the potential to cause more damage to tissues.

The energy lost by a charged particle per unit path length is referred to as the unrestricted *linear energy transfer* (LET or *L*), expressed as kiloelectron volts per micrometre (keV μm^{-1}). In general terms, photons (X- and γ-rays) and electrons have LET values in the range of about 0.2 to 10 keV μm^{-1}. Protons, α-particles, and neutrons have higher LET values, between about 10 and 100 keV μm^{-1}; and heavy charged particles (e.g. nuclei of elements such as carbon, neon, and silicon) have values of up to a few thousands of kilo electron volts per micrometre.

LET does not define the amount of energy lost to matter in the *volume* of interest. This can be expressed as *mean lineal energy* which, in concept, is more meaningful in physical terms than LET [5]. Nor does it address the size of the individual energy-loss events that occur along the particle track, that is the microdistribution of dose at the sub-atomic level. This approach, using other radiation quantities based upon the statistical distribution of events at a molecular level may well be adopted in the future for assessing the biological consequences of radiation exposure.

3.2.2 Dose quantities

The fundamental dosimetric quantity presently used in radiological protection is the *absorbed dose*, D (§2.7.2 and Box 3.1). The ICRP define this as the mean energy absorbed per unit mass of tissue or organ, in contrast to the International Commission on Radiological Units and Measurements (ICRU) who define it as the mean energy absorbed at the point of interest in matter. The SI unit for average absorbed dose in a tissue, D_T, is the gray (Gy), which is equal to 1 joule per kilogram.

It has been calculated that a particle track of low-LET radiation (e.g. 1 MeV γ-rays) passing through an $8 \mu m$ diameter spherical nucleus in a cell delivers an absorbed dose of about 1 mGy [6]. In contrast, a high-LET radiation (e.g. 1 MeV neutrons) would deliver an estimated absorbed dose of a few hundred mGy in the same volume. The probability of stochastic effects occurring depends, then, not only on the absorbed dose but also on the type and energy of the radiation. This is taken into account by weighting the absorbed dose by a factor related to the quality of the radiation. Called the *quality factor* (Q) by ICRU, it is related to L by the so-called Q–L relationship to reflect higher values for intermediate energy neutrons. The dose equivalent (H) at a point in tissue is given by

$$H = QD. \tag{3.1}$$

In comparing the biological damage caused by radiations of different 'quality', the term *relative biological effectiveness* (RBE) is frequently used. This is defined as the ratio of an absorbed dose of a reference low-LET radiation to a dose of the test radiation that gives an *identical biological endpoint* [7]. RBE values are influenced by variations in LET, dose, and dose rate. RBE values increase from unity in relation to LET values up to about 100 keV μm^{-1}, decreasing thereafter because of the 'overkill effect' when more energy is deposited than is necessary to cause damage. Thus some radiation is effectively 'wasted'. The absolute value of the RBE is not unique but depends on the level of biological damage and, therefore, on the absorbed dose. For tumour induction, for example, the RBEs for fission neutrons at the most biologically effective energy, versus 1 MeV γ-rays, are generally taken to be between about 15 and 60 and for a particles in the range from about 5 to 40. For cytogenetic effects, the RBE value for neutrons falls between about 35 and 55 [8]. For deterministic effects, however, lower RBE values between about 5 and 10 are generally found.

The ICRP have selected weighting factors to be representative of values of relative biological effectiveness of that radiation for the induction of stochastic effects at low doses. Called *radiation-weighting factors*, w_R, they are numerically similar to values of Q but are conceptually different. Radiation weighting factors recommended by ICRP are given in Table 3.1. The weighted absorbed dose is called the *equivalent dose*, $H_{T,R}$, and the name of the special unit is the sievert, Sv.

$$H_{T,R} = w_R \mathrm{R} D_{T,R} \tag{3.2}$$

where $D_{T,R}$ is the average absorbed dose from radiation R in tissue T. Defined in this way, the equivalent dose provides an index of the risk of harm to a particular tissue

Table 3.1 Radiation weighting factors

Type and energy range[a]	Radiation weight factor, w_R[b]
Photons, all energies	1
Electrons and muons, all energies[c]	1
Neutrons, energy < 10 keV	5
10 keV to 100 keV	10
> 100 keV to 2 MeV	20
> 2 MeV to 20 MeV	10
> 20 MeV	5
Photons, other than recoil protons, energy > 2 MeV	5
α particles, fission fragments, heavy nuclei	20

[a] [1].
[b] All values relate to the radiation incident on the body or, for internal sources, emitted from the source.
[c] Excluding Auger electrons emitted from nuclei bound to DNA.

Box 3.1 *Hierarchy of dose quantities based on mean dose values*

Absorbed dose
Energy imparted by radiation to unit mass of tissue

Equivalent dose
Absorbed dose weighted for harmfulness of different radiations

Effective dose
Equivalent dose weighted for susceptibility to harm of different tissues

or organ from exposure to various radiations, regardless of their type or energy. So 1 Sv of α-radiation to the lung would give the same risk of induced fatal cancer as 1 Sv of β- or γ-radiation. The total equivalent dose, H_T, is the sum of $H_{T,R}$ over all radiation types:

$$H_T = \sum_R H_{T,R}. \quad (3.3)$$

The risk to the various parts of the human body varies from organ to organ: for example, the risk of fatal malignancy per unit equivalent dose is lower for the thyroid than for the lung. Moreover, there are other important types of harm such as non-fatal cancers or the risk of serious hereditary disease caused by irradiation of the testes or ovaries. These effects are different in kind and in magnitude and we must take them into account when assessing the overall detriment to health of an exposed individual. This is taken into account by taking the equivalent dose in each of the major organs and tissues and multiplying it by a *tissue weighting factor*, w_T, related to the risk associated with that tissue or organ. The sum of these weighted doses is a quantity called the *effective dose*, *E*; it allows the risk to the whole body from either whole of partial body exposure to be expressed as a single number:

$$E = \sum_T w_T H_T. \quad (3.4)$$

Generally, the effective dose gives a broad indication of the detriment to health from any exposure to ionising radiation regardless of the energy of the radiation or the number of organs exposed. It applies equally to external and internal exposure and to uniform and non-uniform irradiation.

Another quantity that is frequently calculated in relation to exposure to internally incorporated radionuclides is the *committed dose*. This is the dose calculated over the remaining lifespan of the individual and is taken to represent the total risk resulting from an intake of a radionuclide. In the case of a worker this is normally considered to be until 50 years after the intake and for a member of the public it is taken to be up to age 70 years. The *committed equivalent dose* is the dose received by an organ or tissue over the lifespan. When summed over all tissues the quantity is the *committed effective dose*.

3.2.3 Cellular damage and repair following the primary radiation events

The mean energy dissipated per ionising event is approximately 33 eV. This is more than sufficient to break a strong chemical bond; for example, the energy associated with a C=C bond is 4.9 eV. This is referred to as a *direct effect*.

Alternatively, an ionising event may break the molecular bonds in a molecule, but the effect may be manifest elsewhere. This is referred to as an *indirect effect*. The latter is the predominant reaction after exposure of cells to low-LET radiation. Free hydroxyl and other highly reactive radicals are produced by ionising the abundant water molecules in cells and during their short existence of about a microsecond, these highly reactive radicals are capable of diffusing a few micrometres to reach and damage molecular bonds in nuclear deoxyribonucleic acid (DNA).

It is widely accepted that the most important cellular constituent to be damaged by radiation is DNA. The DNA molecule consists of a double helix formed from two complementary strands of nucleotides. Nucleotides are made up of deoxyribose molecules (sugars), phosphates, and nitrogenous bases. The sugar and phosphate molecules form the helical strands, while the bases form the cross-links between them. There are four bases, adenine and guanine (termed purines) and thymine and cytosine (pyrimidines). Adenine always bonds with thymine through two hydrogen bonds and guanine always bonds with cytosine through three hydrogen bonds. The unique pairing of the nucleotide bases provides DNA with its ability to replicate. The cell's genetic information is carried in a linear sequence of nucleotides that make up the organisms set of genes (its genome). Each gene controls a discrete hereditary characteristic corresponding to a segment of DNA coding for a single protein. Together with some binding protein, these genes make up the 23 pairs of chromosomes in the nuclei of all cells.

Just as cells inherit genes, they also inherit a set of instructions that tell the genes when to become active. These gene-regulatory proteins recognize short stretches of nucleotide sequences on the double helix and determine which of the genes in the cell will be transcribed. Genes provide instructions for cell division and for the synthesis of tens of the many proteins that provide the structural components of cells, as well as numerous enzymes promoting and controlling cellular activity. Ribonucleic acid (RNA) is the molecule that helps to transport, translate, and implement the coded instructions from the genes. All cell types contain the same genes, but encoding sets of genes is cell-specific. This uniqueness ensures that cells in each tissue produce their own proteins.

Maintaining stability in the genes is essential for cell survival. This stability requires not only extremely accurate mechanisms for DNA synthesis and replication but also precise mechanisms for repairing DNA damage before replication.

The most frequent changes during metabolic activity are DNA single-strand breaks, without base involvement.

This type of damage is effectively repaired by simple enzymatic ligation. *Base excision repair pathways* require other groups of enzymes whose roles are to identify and excise the damaged base site, make a complementary copy of the sequence of bases on the opposite undamaged strand, and seal the correct sequence of copied bases in the gap on the damaged strand. If nucleotide damage occurs, which involves strand breaks and bases, *nucleotide excision repair pathways* exist to repair the more extensive damage. The damaged nucleotides are removed and repair proceeds thereafter as for base damage.

DNA 'double-strand' damage, with or without base damage, occurs rarely during metabolism. *Recombination repair pathways* do exist, but they are not totally effective, mainly because there is no undamaged strand to act as a template for base or nucleotide replacement. When the repair processes fail, the resulting *misrepair* is referred to as a *mutation*. These chemical processes are mainly completed within a few tens of minutes.

Observations with proliferating cells *in vitro* indicate that DNA is subjected to only an occasional permanent base-pair or nucleotide change during metabolism, even though metabolic processes alter thousands of bases and nucleotides every day.

DNA damage due to radiation results in similar lesions to those occurring during metabolism, but double-strand breaks and more extensive expressions of damage (multiple gene losses and the translocation of gene sequences) occur more frequently and are considered the hallmark of radiation. The probability of misrepair is greater under these circumstances. Estimated yields of damage caused by low-LET radiation are shown in Table 3.2 [9].

Recent *in vitro* investigations have revealed that DNA repair pathways may work in conjunction with other cellular activities in order to minimize cell damage. These include delay in cell-cycling as a means of maximizing the chances of repair, and programmed cell death (apoptosis), whereby severely damaged cells are eliminated to stimulate cell proliferation.

3.2.4 Classification of radiation-induced damage in terms of cell survival

Radiation-induced cell damage can be classified in terms of survival or inherent damage in viable cells (deletions, translocations in gene structure–mutations) and oncogenic transformation (neoplasia). Dose–response relationships in terms of survival are considered in this section, and those in terms of damage to viable cells in §3.2.5.

Expressed graphically as the logarithm of the surviving fraction plotted against absorbed dose on a linear scale, the dose response for cell survival following acute exposure to low-LET radiation is initially linear followed by a quadratic response as the dose increases. A plausible explanation of the linear component is that the majority of DNA interactions are single-particle track events [6]. Under these circumstances, DNA damage can be effectively repaired before interaction with another single track, a process that is influenced by dose rate. As the dose (or dose rate) increases, multi-track events reflecting the quadratic component and associated with clustered DNA damage increasingly predominate with a consequent increase in the probability of misrepair and *lethal events*. After acute exposure to 1 Gy, for example, lethal events have a frequency of about 0.2 to 0.8 per cell (Table 3.2).

Table 3.2 Examples of damage in a mammalian cell nucleus from 1 Gy of low-LET radiation

Initial physical damage	
Ionisations in cell nucleus	~ 100 000
Ionisations directly in DNA	~ 2000
Excitations directly in DNA	~ 2000
Selected biochemical damage	
DNA single-strand breaks	1000
Base (8-hydroxyadenine) damage	700
Base (thymine) damage	250
DNA double-strand breaks	40
DNA–protein cross-links	150
Selected cellular effects	
Lethal events	~ 0.2–0.8
Chromosome aberrations	~ 0.4
Hprt gene mutations	0.6×10^{-5}
Translocation frequency (two loci)	1.2×10^{-4}

Table modified from Ward [9].

Protracted exposure to low-LET radiation results in less damage compared with acute exposure [3]. This is referred to as the *dose rate effect* and is due to the ability of cells to repair more *sublethal* damage as the dose rate is reduced. Below about 1 Gy min^{-1}, the slope on the exponential portion of the survival curve typically becomes progressively shallower as more and more sublethal damage is repaired, whereas below about 0.01 Gy min^{-1}, undamaged or repaired cells are able to proliferate at a sufficient rate to offset the reduction in cell numbers while further repair is progressing. These responses are illustrated diagrammatically in Figure 3.2. The dose–response relationship for high-LET radiation approximates to linearity and there is no dose-rate effect, suggesting little repair of sublethal damage.

3.2.5 Dose–response relationships expressed as damage to viable cells

Chromosome aberrations and gene mutations

A technique of culturing human lymphocytes *in vitro* and measuring the frequency of radiation damage to

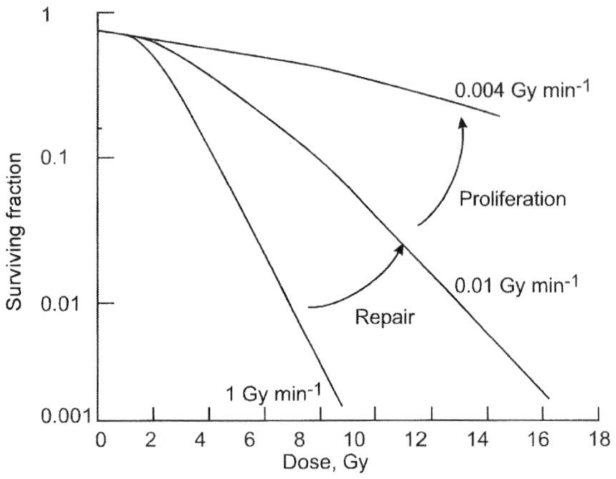

Figure 3.2 Dose-rate effect showing the influence of repair and repopulation on the dose–survival relationship for dose rates of 1, 0.01, and 0.004 Gy min^{-1}.

chromosomes has been available for many years. This frequency, expressed as dicentric aberrations (Box 3.2), increases from a base level of about 1 in 1000 cells to about 4 in 100 cells per gray after exposure to low-LET radiations. Dose–response relationships for X-rays and fission neutrons are shown in Figure 3.3 [10]. In general, high-LET radiations are more damaging than low-LET radiations. Measurement of dicentric chromosome aberrations has provided an important method for assessing doses in known or suspected cases of acute radiation exposure.

A number of mutation test systems using mouse, hamster, and human fibroblast cells have been developed. For acute exposure of human lymphoblastoid cells

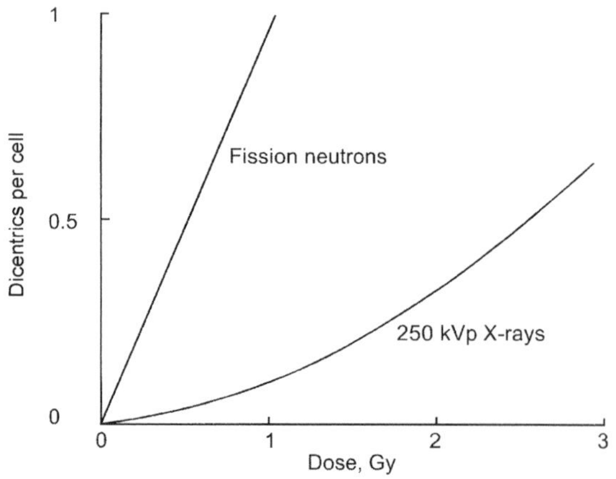

Figure 3.3 Dicentric yield in chromosomes per cultured human lymphocyte as a function of dose for selected radiations [10] (see §3.2.5). Reproduced with permission from Taylor & Francis, London.

to 100 kVp X-rays, a linear dose–response relationship for specific locus mutation induction has been observed [11]. For protracted exposure, a slight increase in mutation rate was observed, in contrast to a sparing effect seen using hamster cells. For continuous exposure to neutrons, there is a substantial increase in mutation rate compared to acute exposure. Unfortunately, different types of cultured cells and radiation modalities have produced different results, making it difficult to generalize on the value of mutation assays.

Cell transformation

An established technique for studying carcinogenic potential is that of culturing cells that can grow indefinitely. This is made possible by frequently transferring the growing cells to fresh media. Cells that have acquired this ability are said to be *immortalized*. A characteristic of these immortalized cells is that they stop dividing when they come into contact with similar cells in the culture medium (*contact inhibition*). They are not classified as malignant cells because they do not cause tumours when injected into immunologically suppressed animals. Occasionally, an immortalized cell undergoes a spontaneous change, whereby it loses its contact inhibition and continues to proliferate by spreading over adjacent immortalized cells to form a recognized foci of cells. Such cells are said to have undergone *transformation* and when they are injected into animals, they develop into tumours. Spontaneous transformation is a rare event, occurring at a rate of about 1 in 10 000 to 1 in 100 000 per surviving cell. The mechanism is not fully understood but it is thought to involve the mutation of two (or more) classes of genes. These are 'gain-of function' mutations of proto-oncogenes, whereby the mutated genes (oncogenes) stimulate cell proliferation in an uncontrolled manner; and 'loss-of function' tumour suppressor genes, whereby cells are no longer prevented from proliferating in defiance of normal controls. Exposure to radiation increases the rate of cell transformation as a dose-related response [12].

Estimated yields of chromosome aberrations, mutation frequency, and cell transformation are shown in Table 3.2 as typical responses to acute low-LET radiation.

Generalized dose–response relationships

Dose–response relationships for proliferating cells exposed to low-LET radiation can be expressed mathematically over a wide range of doses. The probability of an effect (E) occurring after dose (D) in each irradiated cell is

$$E = (\alpha_1 D + \beta_1 D^2) \exp - (\alpha_2 D + \beta_2 D^2) \qquad (3.5)$$

where α_1 and β_1 are coefficients for the linear and quadratic terms expressing the induction of aberrations,

Box 3.2 The formation of a dicentric

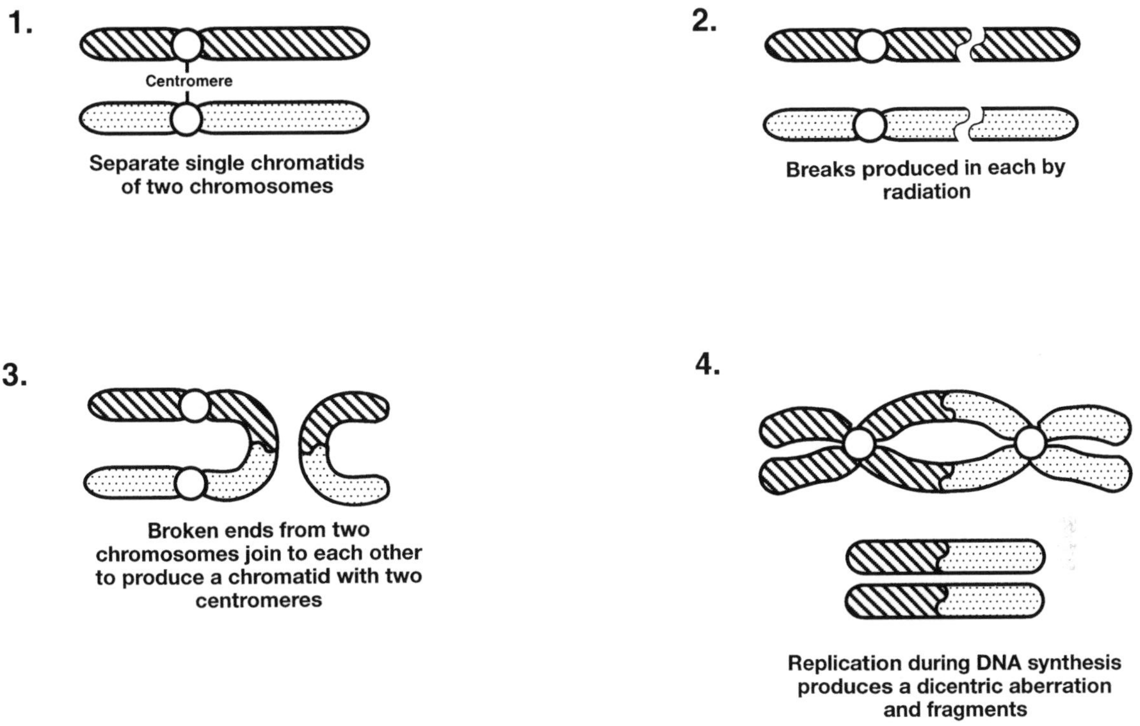
1.
Centromere
Separate single chromatids of two chromosomes
2.
Breaks produced in each by radiation
3.
Broken ends from two chromosomes join to each other to produce a chromatid with two centromeres
4.
Replication during DNA synthesis produces a dicentric aberration and fragments

mutations, or transformations, and α_2 and β_2 are coefficients for the linear and quadratic terms expressing cell killing.

Based on target theory, the linear component of the relationship for stochastic effects is interpreted as a region where only small numbers of cells are intersected by more than one particle track, the effect being independent of dose rate. The quadratic component is interpreted as reflecting multi-track events spread over time that are dose-rate dependent.

For high-LET radiations, it is generally accepted that the relationship approximates to linearity because of the intense clustering of ionisations along the particle track.

3.3 Deterministic effects

3.3.1 The role of stem cells in healthy tissues

In the space of a few weeks, a single fertilized human egg gives rise to a complex multicellular organism consisting of embryonic cells arranged in a precise pattern. In the subsequent period of fetal growth after the formation of organs and tissues, the cells continue to proliferate. Growth of many tissues and organs continues throughout childhood, but ceases in the adult when cell masses reach a predetermined size. The majority of cells in tissues and organs of the adult are *differentiated*, that is, they have developed specific morphology and function which is normally irreversible. These cells were programmed to die by the process of *apoptosis* during differentiation. In many, but not all, tissues, the rate of death of differentiated cells must be balanced by renewal from a reservoir of *stem cells* in order to maintain a healthy state. These cells have retained embryonic characteristics and are able to divide upon stimulation during the lifetime of the organism, yielding progeny that are destined to differentiate by a process of *clonal expansion*. Stem cells also retain the ability of *self-renewal*. These two characteristics are illustrated diagrammatically in Figure 3.4. The number of stem cells compared to differentiated cells varies according to the tissue, but they usually represent, at most, a few per cent of the total cell numbers. It is not known precisely how the balance between cell proliferation and cell death is achieved, but when differentiated cells die, a feedback mechanism has been shown to be activated to stimulate stem cells to divide. If sufficient numbers of cells are prevented from dividing at the appropriate rate, the tissue loses its ability to function effectively and may result in death of the individual.

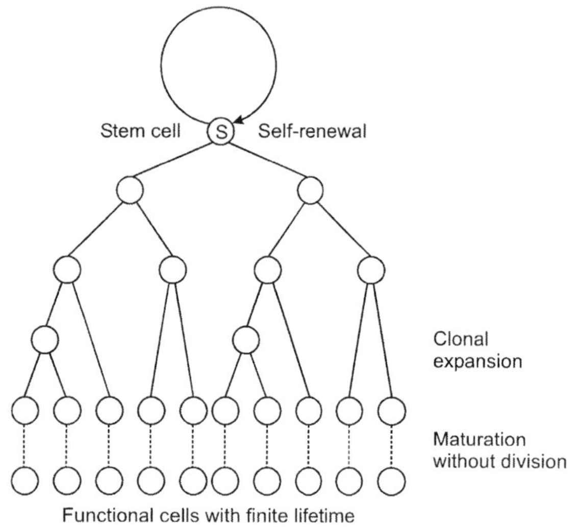

Figure 3.4 Derivation of differentiated cells from a self-renewing stem cell (see §3.3.1).

3.3.2 Dose–response relationships

The probability of loss of tissue or organ function following exposure to radiation increases steeply above a threshold dose up to a maximum. Expressed as a generalized dose–response relationship, the plot of the frequency of the effect versus absorbed dose expressed on linear axes is sigmoid (Figure 3.5, upper panel). Above the threshold dose, the severity of the effect also increases with dose (Figure 3.5, lower panel). Protracting the dose results in a lower frequency and less severe symptoms at a given dose compared with acute exposure, reflecting the importance of repair and stem cell repopulation.

There is individual variation in radiosensitivity in any exposed population which is influenced by the age and state of health of the individuals. This variation reflects differences in the ability of individuals to cope with radiation-induced cellular damage.

3.3.3 Effects following whole-body irradiation

Evidence of deterministic effects comes from several sources [2]. These include retrospective studies on radiotherapy patients, radiologists in the early part of this century who were inadequately protected, Japanese populations exposed to radiation from atom bombs, and individuals accidentally exposed to high doses following nuclear reactor accidents and unshielded radiographic sources. Deterministic effects following acute whole-body irradiation are summarized in Table 3.3. Understanding the syndromes associated with acute high doses is important as an aid to diagnosis and prognosis of accidental overexposure, and to ensure that deterministic effects are avoided in normal practices and minimized in accidents. The stages in the development of the various syndromes are summarized in Table 3.4.

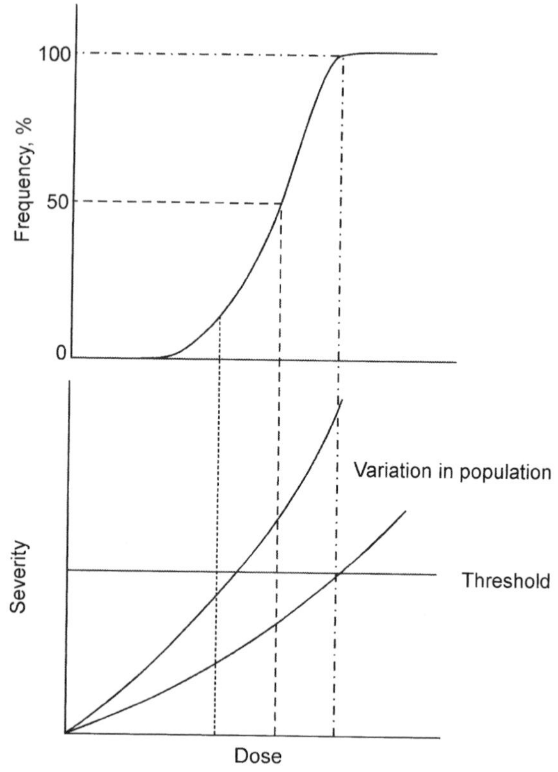

Figure 3.5 Dose–response relationship for deterministic effects. Variation in frequency and severity (see §3.3.2). Reproduced with permission from ICRP.

3.3.4 Effects following partial-body irradiation

Tolerance doses in adults after radiotherapy

Extensive experience in the treatment of patients undergoing radiotherapy has provided data upon which to determine the tolerability of healthy tissues and organs to radiation [13]. Called the *tolerance dose* by clinicians, it is defined as the amount of low-LET radiation received during conventional radiotherapy (typically, 20 to 30 fractions each of 2 to 6 Gy over several weeks) which is considered acceptable. The gonads, the lens of the eye, and the bone marrow contain the most radiosensitive tissues with tolerance doses after fractionated radiation below a few gray. For other tissues and organs, the tolerance doses are in the region of a few tens of a gray. In general, children are less tolerant to exposure.

Table 3.3 Range of doses associated with acute radiation syndromes in adults exposed to low-LET radiation

Whole-body absorbed dose (Gy)	Principal effect contributing to death	Time of death after exposure (days)
1–6	Damage to bone marrow[a]	30–60
5–15	Damage to the gastrointestinal tract and lungs[b]	10–20
> 15	Damage to nervous system and shock to the cardiovascular system	1–5

[a]Dose range considered to result in 50% of an exposed population dying (LD_{50} = 3–5 Gy).
[b]Damage to vasculature and cell membranes especially at high doses is an important factor in causing death.
Source: ICRP [1].

Table 3.4 Summary of acute radiation syndrome

	Syndrome		
	Cerebral	Intestinal	Bone marrow
Critical organ	Brain	Small intestine	Bone marrow
Latent period	20 min	3–5 days	2–3 weeks
Syndrome threshold (Gy)	20	3	1
Death threshold (Gy)	50	10	2
Death occurring within	2 days	2 weeks	3–8 weeks
Cause of death	Cerebral oedema, heart failure	Sloughing of gut, shock	Haemorrhage, infection
Prodromal vomiting	Minutes	1 hour	A few hours
Symptoms	Tremors, cramps, loss of coordination, lethargy, impaired vision, coma	Loss of appetite, vomiting, diarrhoea with bleeding, fever, electrolyte and fluid balance	Fever, breathlessness, internal bleeding, depletion of bone marrow leading to low blood counts
Treatment	Palliative	Barrier nursing, fluid and electrolyte replacement, transfusions of blood cells, bone marrow transplants	
Prognosis	Hopeless	Very poor	Dose-dependent and influenced by treatment

Threshold doses in radiological protection

The limitations of using data on tolerance doses to derive *threshold doses* for radiation protection purposes need to be recognized. In contrast to the precise fractionated exposure conditions of radiotherapy, accidental overexposure of workers is most likely to be from non-uniform fields and from mixed high- and low-LET radiations. The tolerance dose can therefore at best be used as a cautious approximation to a threshold dose.

The threshold doses recommended by the ICRP for the most radiosensitive tissues and organs are summarized in Table 3.5.

Skin irradiation

Based upon extensive experience in the use of fractionated X- and γ-radiation, various degrees of skin damage can be observed according to the area and depth of skin involved, the absorbed dose, and the duration and frequency of the exposure [14]. The types of damage after acute exposure are summarized in Box 3.3.

Quantifying the threshold doses for these effects is complicated, in practice, by the multiplicity of sensitive targets at different critical cell depths. This makes it difficult to select a single depth at which to specify the dose to the skin. The depths at which the most serious effects arise are estimated to be in the range of 300–500 μm. However, a conservative approach for protection purposes is to use shallower depths (in the range 20–100 μm, nominally 70 μm) for monitoring specifications.

The tolerance dose for skin damage increases as the radiation field is reduced. Thus, tolerance doses following a single treatment with orthovoltage X-rays was found to be 20 Gy for an area of 6 × 4 cm and 11 Gy for an area of 15 × 20 cm. Following fractionated treatment, exposure, the tolerance doses were estimated to be about 50 and 30 Gy, respectively, for the two field sizes.

In normal practices, the annual equivalent dose limit for occupational exposure recommended by the ICRP is

Table 3.5 Thresholds for deterministic effects recommended in radiological protection

Tissue and effect	Equivalent dose brief exposure (Sv)	Equivalent dose rate protracted exposure (Sv $year^{-1}$)
Testes		
Temporary sterility	0.15	0.4[a]
Permanent sterility	> 3.5	2.0
Ovaries		
Sterility	> 2.5	> 0.2
Lens		
Detectable opacities	> 0.5	> 1.0
Visual impairment (cataract)	> 0.1	> 0.15
Bone marrow		
Blood cell depletion	> 0.5	> 0.4[b]

[a]This dose is higher because differentiating cells are more radiosensitive than the stem cells so the latter can replenish the differentiating cells at an adequate rate.
[b]Supported by evidence of effects after chronic irradiation of beagle dogs.
Source: ICRP [1].

500 mSv averaged over any 1 cm^2, regardless of the area exposed. This becomes an important issue when considering the localized deposition of high-specific activity radioactive particulates which can give much higher doses in the immediate vicinity of the particles.

3.4 Radiation-induced cancer

3.4.1 The basic cellular process

The development of cancer is a major late effect resulting from exposure to radiation. The malignant changes occurring in cells (neoplasia) is a complex, multi-stage process that can be conveniently divided into four phases: initiation, promotion, conversion, and progression. The subdivisions are necessarily simplifications of the overall process but they do provide a basis from which to interpret the cellular and molecular changes [3].

Initiation encompasses the essentially irreversible DNA damage (§3.2.3), which provides the potential in cells for neoplastic development. *Promotion* is the stage where initiated cells receive an abnormal growth stimulus and begin to proliferate in a semi-independent manner. *Conversion* of these promoted cells to a form in which they are committed to become fully malignant is believed to be dependent upon further gene mutations The subsequent *progression* stage depends upon changes that involve invasion of adjacent tissues to other sites in the body. These secondary growths are referred to as *metastases* [3].

There is always a minimum period of time between irradiation and the appearance of a radiation-induced tumour. This period is termed the latent period and its length varies with age and from one tumour type to another. Some types of leukaemia and bone cancer have latent periods of only a few years but many solid tumours have latent periods of 10 years or more. For leukaemia and bone cancer there is fairly good evidence that the risk is complete expressed within about 30 years following exposure. For solid tumours of longer latency, such as those of the gastrointestinal tract and liver, it is not yet clear whether the incidence of tumours passes through a maximum and then declines with time or whether the risk

Box 3.3 Radiation-induced acute effects on skin

Dose (Gy)	Lesion	Time of appearance	Signs and symptoms
5	Initial erythema	1–3 days	Reddening
5	Dry desquamation	2–3 weeks	Scaling Pigmentation Itching Depilation
5	Erythema proper	3–4 weeks	Reddening
20	Moist desquamation	4–5 weeks	Blistering Oozing
50	Cell death	2–3 weeks	Necrosis

levels out or alternatively increases indefinitely through the rest of life.

To project the overall cancer risk for an exposed population, it is therefore necessary to use models that extrapolate over time data based on only a limited period of the lives of the individuals. Two such projection models have generally been used:

- the additive (absolute) risk model which postulates that radiation will induce cancer independently of the spontaneous rate after a period of latency, and variations in risk may occur due to sex and age at exposure;
- the multiplicative (relative) risk model in which the excess (after latency) is given by a constant or a time-varying factor applied to the age-dependent incidence of natural cancers in the population.

In most cases the spontaneous risk increases with age and therefore the multiplicatve model will predict an increasing incidence of radiation-induced cancer with increasing age. The relative risk model also gives different risks of radiation-induced cancer in different populations, depending upon the natural cancer incidence. Data now available from the Life Span Study (LSS) of the A-bomb survivors in Japan and from studies on uranium miners suggest that the multiplicative model gives a better fit to the data, at least for some of the most common cancer types. In some cases, however, there is evidence that the relative risk starts to decline a long time after exposure. This is the case, for example, for bone tumours and lung cancers.

3.4.2 Dose–response relationships for fatal cancers

The commonly-occurring cancers induced by radiation are indistinguishable from those occurring spontaneously and since cancer is the cause of death in about a quarter of the population in the developed countries, the problem of detecting a small radiation-induced excess is difficult. In general, large exposed compared with matched unexposed control populations are necessary to obtain statistically meaningful results. The chief sources of information on the occurrence of radiation-induced cancers are summarized in Box 3.4.

The continuing epidemiological study of the A-bomb survivors in Japan has provided the main source of risk estimates. A recent reassessment resulted in an increase in estimates of the risk of radiation-induced cancer from previous studies. This arose partly as a result of revised dosimetry and a longer follow-up of the population, but mainly it was attributed to the use of a multiplicative (relative) risk model (excess related by a constant factor applied to the age-dependent incidence of naturally-occurring cancers). Previously, an additive (absolute) risk model was used, where the excess was taken to be independent of the naturally-occurring rate [15,16].

UNSCEAR [2], in a report to the General Assembly, provided a total cancer risk at high doses and high-dose rates, estimated to be (7–11) $\times$ 10^{-2} Sv^{-1} using age-averaged and age-specific constant relative risk models. (A risk of 1 $\times$ 10^{-2} Sv^{-1} corresponds to a risk of cancer of 1 in 100 per Sv or 1 in 100 000 per mSv.) This compared with their 1977 assessment of 2.5 $\times$ 10^{-2} Sv^{-1} at high-dose rate using the additive model. Because

Box 3.4 Human populations available for risk estimation

Atomic bombs	Japanese survivors Marshall Islanders[a]
Medical diagnosis	Multiple fluoroscopies (breast) Prenatal irradiation Thorotrast injections[b]
Medical therapy	Pelvic radiotherapy (cervix) Spinal radiotherapy (ankylosing spondylitis) Neck and chest radiotherapy (thyroid) Scalp radiotherapy Radium treatment[b]
Occupational exposure	Uranium miners[b] Radium ingestion (dial painters)[b]

[a]Exposure to external radiation and β/γ-emitting radionuclides.
[b]Exposure to α-emitting radionuclides.

children and young persons are more sensitive to radiation than adults, the application of age-specific risk coefficients increases the predicted numbers of radiation-induced cancers in a population of all ages compared with that for a working population.

These risk estimates for whole-body radiation exposure were based on an extrapolation into the future which is somewhat uncertain for solid cancers because two-thirds of the Japanese survivors are still alive and the cancer risk has still to be expressed in these survivors. Up to 1985, about 80 excess leukaemias and 260 excess solid cancers had occurred in the LSS population out of a total of about 6000 cancer deaths [15].

In a more recent report on the LSS, Pierce *et al.* [17] reported on five more years of follow-up (1986–1990). Their analysis includes an additional 10500 survivors (86 572 in total). During 1950–1990 there have been 7827 cancer deaths, of which it is estimated that there are 85 excess leukaemias and 335 excess solid cancers. The mortality curve for all solid cancers combined shows essentially a linear dose–response in the range 0–3 Sv, whereas for leukaemia the trend in dose is non-linear with an upward curvature. A significant increase in the risk of solid cancers is now seen at doses down to 50 mSv.

3.4.3 Dose and dose-rate effectiveness factors (DDREFs)

Risk coefficients for radiological protection purposes are based mainly on population groups exposed at high doses and high-dose rates. Studies at the molecular, cellular, tissue, and whole-animal level have demonstrated that radiation damage increases with dose and that, at least for low-LET radiation, at high-dose rates it is often greater per unit of exposure than at low-dose rates. Thus, although the assumption normally made is that the dose–response relationship for cancer induction is linear, with the risk proportional to absorbed dose, in practice a dose and dose-rate effectiveness factor (DDREF) has been used to allow for a reduced effectiveness of radiation at low doses and low-dose rates. The choice of a suitable DDREF has caused considerable debate, with relevant data being available from cellular, animal, and human studies [3, 18] giving values within the range of 1 to 10. A value of 2 is recommended by the ICRP [1] for low-LET radiation. No DDREF is recommended for high-LET radiation.

3.4.4 Risk coefficients for protection

From these various sources, the ICRP have adopted a rounded value of 10×10^{-2} Sv^{-1} for the risk coefficient for fatal cancer at high doses and high-dose rate following exposure of a mixed population of all ages. Applying a DDREF of 2 gives a risk of 5×10^{-2} Sv^{-1} for radiation protection purposes. Risk coefficients for fatal cancer in named individual tissues and organs are given in Table 3.6. For workers the risk coefficient adopted for radiation protection purposes is 4×10^{-2} Sv^{-1}. These risk coefficients have been used by ICRP in developing the revised dose limits given in its 1990 Recommendations [1].

Table 3.6 Risk coefficients for fatal cancer adopted by ICRP and tissue weighting factors, w_T

Organ or tissue	w_T	Fatal cancer (10^{-2} Sv^{-1})	
		Population	Workers
Bladder	0.05	0.30	0.24
Red bone marrow	0.12	0.50	0.40
Bone surface	0.01	0.05	0.04
Breast	0.05	0.20	0.16
Colon	0.12	0.85	0.68
Liver	0.05	0.15	0.12
Lung	0.12	0.85	0.68
Oesophagus	0.05	0.30	0.24
Ovary	–	0.10	0.08
Skin	0.01	0.02	0.02
Stomach	0.12	1.10	0.88
Thyroid	0.05	0.08	0.06
Remainder	0.05	0.50	0.40
Gonads (hereditary disease)	0.20	–	–
Total	1.0	5.0	4.0

Source: ICRP [1].

Table 3.7 illustrates how the risk of cancer varies with age at exposure for the UK population. The results in the table have been calculated generally using a relative risk model and the spontaneous cancer rates for the UK [8]. The table shows that whereas the total cancer risk predicted over a lifetime increases monotonically with

Table 3.7 Estimates of radiation-induced fatal cancer in a UK population of both sexes according to age at exposure

Age at exposure (years)	Deaths (10^{-2} Sv^{-1})	
	Risk up to 40 years following exposure	Lifetime projection
0–9	1.2	11.1
10–19	1.8	9.9
20–29	1.9	6.6
30–39	2.8	4.5
40–49	3.8	4.2
50–59	4.0	4.0
60–69	3.1	3.1
70–79	1.6	1.6
80+	0.75	0.75
Total	2.4	5.9

Exposure to low doses or at low-dose rates [8].

decreasing age at exposure, the risk to 40 years following exposure is greatest for those irradiated at ages 50–59 years. Furthermore, the variation with age at exposure is not as great for the risk to 40 years as for the lifetime projected risk. These results demonstrate the importance of continued follow-up of groups such as the A-bomb survivors to improve estimates of lifetime risk for those in the younger age groups where only a small fraction of the risk has so far been expressed. The total cancer risk calculated for the UK population, 5.9×10^{-2} Sv^{-1}, is greater than the risk calculated for the world population, 5×10^{-2} Sv^{-1}, because of the higher spontaneous risk of cancer.

3.4.5 Low-dose studies

The majority of studies on which risk estimates for radiation-induced cancer are based are for populations exposed at high doses and high-dose rates. However, low dose and low-dose rate studies, although statistically weak, can provide a check on the upper bound of the risks derived by extrapolation from high-dose rate studies.

Several studies have been conducted of nuclear industry workers. In the USA, Gilbert *et al.* [19] performed a joint analysis of data for about 36 000 workers at the Hanford site, Oak Ridge National Laboratory and Rocky Flats weapons plant. Neither for the grouping of all cancers nor for leukaemia was there an indication of an increasing trend in risk with dose.

A study of just over 95 000 individuals on the UK's National Registry for Radiation Workers (NRRW) examined cancer mortality in relation to dose [20]. This study provided evidence of raised risks of leukaemia and multiple myeloma associated with occupational exposure to radiation, but, unlike the combined study of US workers, is consistent with the risk estimates derived by ICRP from the Japanese survivor data. Combining the NRRW and US results to strengthen the database produces central estimates for lifetime risk of 4.9×10^{-2} Sv^{-1} (90% CI < 0, 18) for all cancers and 0.30×10^{-2} Sv^{-1} (90% CI < 0, 1.04) for leukaemia, excluding chronic lymphatic leukaemia (CLL) [21].

A combined analysis of mortality among 95 673 workers (85.4% men) in the US, the UK, and Canada has also been published [22]. As with the NRRW, mortality from leukaemias, excluding CLL, was significantly associated with cumulative external radiation exposure. There was no evidence of an association between radiation dose and mortality from all cancers. It was concluded that the results of the study did not suggest that current radiation risk estimates for cancer at low levels of exposure, as recommended by ICRP [1], can be appreciably in error.

A second analysis of the NRRW published in 1999 provides more precise information on mortality in relation to occupational exposure. By including additional groups of workers the database now contains records for nearly 125 000 workers, of whom just under 13 000 had died. The analysis shows borderline evidence of an increasing trend with dose in the risk of leukaemia, the central estimate of risk is similar to that estimated for the Japanese A-bomb survivors, at low doses. For all cancers, other than leukaemia, the central estimate of the trend in risk with dose is closer to zero than in the first analysis but is compatible with the risks obtained from the A-bomb survivors [23].

Studies of exposure to natural radiation (other than radon) have generally involved looking for any geographical correlation with cancer rates. Such studies are difficult to interpret, however, because of the effect of confounding factors such as socio-demographic variables and other factors that vary geographically.

3.5 Radiation-induced hereditary disease

3.5.1 Naturally-occurring hereditary diseases

Hereditary diseases occur spontaneously. Examples of commonly-occurring diseases are given in Box 3.5. Radiation damage to the germinal cells in the gonads is assumed to result in an increase in hereditary disease in the offspring of irradiated parents. This assumption is based mainly on animal studies.

There are three main types of gene mutation: dominant, recessive, and X-linked. A dominant gene mutation in one set of genes in one parent (there is a set of genes from both parents in the fertilized egg cell) can express itself despite its counterpart from the other parent being normal. On the contrary, a recessive gene mutation cannot be expressed unless the genes from both parents carry the identical mutation. Females have two X chromosomes while males carry one X and one Y chromosome, the Y chromosome being almost inert apart from genes for maleness. An X-linked gene mutation can readily express itself in the male, whereas in the female the X-linked mutation is not expressed unless both X chromosomes carry the same mutation. There is at present no good evidence for the induction of diseases of chromosomal origin by radiation [25].

The genetics of some inherited diseases are more complicated because additional factors such as environment play a part in their expression. These are called the 'multifactorial' diseases.

Most live-born children with inherited chromosomal mutations exhibit mental and/or physical abnormalities. There is little or no chance of sufferers who reach adulthood reproducing and so passing these defects on to

Box 3.5 Examples of hereditary diseases

Dominant disorders
- congenital cataract
- cystic kidney disease
- Huntington's chorea
- (progressive mental retardation)

X-linked diseases
- haemophilia, albinism
- colour blindness
- heart valve defects

Autosomal recessive diseases
- Cretinism
- disorders of amino acid metabolism
- aplastic anaemia
- muscular dystrophy

Multifactorial diseases
- ankylosing spondylitis
- varicose veins
- cleft palate
- diabetes mellitus
- schizophrenia
- asthma

Chromosome anomalies
- Down's syndrome

Source: UNSCEAR [24].

their children. These conditions are therefore maintained in the population by new mutations either arising spontaneously or being induced by an environmental insult such as radiation. Dominant mutations show up in the first generation after exposure, as do X-linked mutations in males, and may occur in subsequent generations if they do not prevent childbearing. Recessive mutations, however, tend to occur in later generations. When assessing the risks of radiation it is therefore necessary to allow for hereditary effects which may not appear for several generations.

3.5.2 Risk coefficients for hereditary disease

No hereditary effects at levels that are statistically significant have been observed in human populations exposed to radiation [2]. Neel *et al.* [26] have reviewed all the genetic studies in Hiroshima and Nagasaki on the children born to irradiated survivors. No statistically significant effects were observed. Taken together, the data suggest a lower limit for the doubling dose (the radiation dose capable of doubling the spontaneous rate) for genetic damage following acute irradiation of approximately 1.4–1.8 Sv. This compares with a value of 0.3 Sv in the mouse for acute exposure and 1 Sv for chronic exposure.

For protection purposes, ICRP [1] recommend a risk factor of 1.0×10^{-2} Sv^{-1} for members of the public and 0.6×10^{-2} Sv^{-1} for workers.

3.6 Irradiation *in utero*

3.6.1 Fetal brain development

On the basis of results of animal studies, it is assumed that radiation-induced malformations in humans, following acute exposure *in utero*, may occur above a dose threshold of about 0.2 Gy in the later stages of pregnancy.

There is one type of low-dose effect in fetal brain tissue that is considered to be deterministic on biological grounds, although it may not be associated with a threshold. It was described in a study of about 1600 Japanese children who survived into adolescence after acute exposure to atomic bomb irradiation [3]. About 25

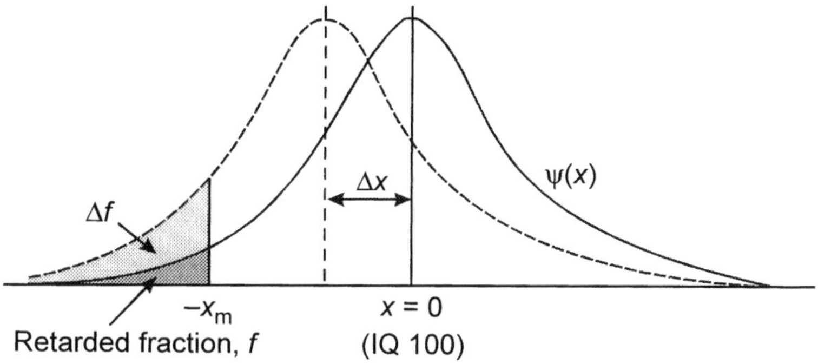

Figure 3.6 The shift to the left from $\psi(x)$ by Δx (30 IQ points) increases the background retarded fraction, f, by Δf. Δx_M denotes the number of standard deviations below IQ 100 to classify an individual as mentally retarded (see §3.6.1). Reproduced with permission from ICRP.

of these children who were exposed between 8 and 15 weeks after conception developed severe mental retardation (IQ < 70 points), on the assumption that their normal IQ would have been 100 points on the test system used. Other features observed were small head size and unprovoked seizures. The dose–response relationship was consistent with a frequency of 40% at 1 Gy and an IQ drop of about 30 points (Figure 3.6). At 0.05 Gy, the frequency was about 5% and the background frequency for comparison was 0.8%. Statistical analysis of the data could not prove or disprove the existence of a dose threshold. A period of less vulnerability was observed between 16 and 25 weeks after conception and there were no abnormalities before or after this 'window' of 8 to 25 weeks when critical neuron development is taking place. On this basis the ICRP recommended that once pregnancy was declared, the fetus should be adequately protected by ensuring that the methods of protection at work provided a standard of protection comparable with that recommended for members of the public. This advice is embodied in the European Directive [27] which states that 'the equivalent dose to the child to be born will be as low as reasonably achievable and that it is unlikely that the dose will exceed 1 mSv during at least the remainder of pregnancy after declaration of pregnancy'.

3.6.2 Risk of cancer

Estimates of cancer risk to age 15 years have been obtained by combining the excess risk observed in the Oxford Survey of Childhood Cancer with estimates of dose to the fetus from obstetric X-rays [8]. This yields an estimated risk of leukaemia of 2.5×10^{-2} Gy^{-1} and of other cancers of 3.5×10^{-2} Gy^{-1} (low-LET); about half of these cases are assumed to be fatal. These risk coefficients for cancer are directly applicable to low doses and low-dose rates. The lifetime risk of fatal cancer following exposure *in utero* may exceed that in the first 15 years of life by a factor of up to four. There are, however, considerable uncertainties in projecting lifetime risks from the current data and this factor may perhaps be about two. For hereditary risks it is assumed that the risks from *in utero* exposure are the same as after birth; 2.4×10^{-2} Sv^{-1} following irradiation of male or female germ cells.

3.7 Summary

This chapter provides a basic understanding of the biological basis upon which dose limits are derived in the System of Protection recommended by the ICRP in its 1990 Recommendations [1]. The nominal probability coefficients for stochastic effects are summarized in Table 3.8.

Since completion of this review UNSCEAR have issued two further reviews covering the health effects of exposure to ionising radiation. These are cited as references [28] and [29].

Table 3.8 Risk factors (10^{-2} Sv^{-1}) for protection

	ICRP 1977	ICRP 1991	
		Public	Workers
Fatal cancer	1.25	5.0	4.0
Hereditary defects	0.4[a]	1.0[b]	0.6[b]
Total	1.65	6.0	4.6
Total (weighted)[c]	–	7.3	5.6

[a]Two generations.
[b]All generations.
[c]To allow for non-fatal cancers and years of life lost for cancers and hereditary disease.
Source: ICRP [1].

3.8 References

1 International Commission on Radiological Protection (1991). 1990 Recommendations of the International Commission on Radiological Protection. ICRP Publication 60. *Ann. ICRP*, **21** (1–3).

2 United Nations Scientific Committee on the Effects of Radiation (1988). *Sources, effects and risks of ionising radiation.* 1988 Report to the General Assembly, with annexes.

3 United Nations Scientific Committee on the Effects of Radiation (1993). *Sources, effects and risks of ionising radiation.* 1993 Report to the General Assembly, with annexes.

4 United Nations Scientific Committee on the Effects of Radiation (1994). *Sources, effects and risks of ionising radiation.* 1994 Report to the General Assembly, with annexes.

5 International Commission on Radiation Units and Measurements (1993). *Quantities and units in radiation protection dosimetry.* ICRU Report 51. ICRU, Washington, DC.

6 Goodhead, D. T. (1994). Initial events in the cellular effects of ionising radiations: clustered damage in DNA. *Int. J. Radiat. Biol.*, **65** (1), 7–17.

7 National Council on Radiation Protection and Measurements (1990). *The relative biological effectiveness of radiations of different quality.* NCRP Report 104. NCRP, Bethesda, MD.

8 Muirhead, C. R., Cox, R., Stather, J. W., MacGibbon, B. H., Edwards, A. A., and Haylock, R. G. E. (1993). Estimates of late radiation risks to the UK population. *Doc. NRPB*, **4** (4).

9 Ward, F. (1988). DNA damage produced by ionising radiation in mammalian cells: identities, mechanisms of formation and reparability. *Prog. Nucleic Acid Res. Mol. Biol.*, **35**, 95–125.

10 Edwards, A. A., Lloyd, D. C., and Prosser, J. S. (1989). Chromosome aberrations in human lymphocytes – a radiobiological review. In: *Low dose radiation: biological bases of risk assessment* (ed. K. F. Baverstock and J. W. Stather), pp. 423–32. Taylor Francis, London.

11 Kronenberg, A. and Little, J. B. (1989). Mutagenic properties of low doses of X-rays, fast neutrons and selected heavy ions in human cells. In: *Low dose radiation: biological bases of risk assessment* (ed. K. F. Baverstock and J. W. Stather), pp. 554–9. Taylor Francis, London.

12 Mill, A. J., Frankenberg, D., Bettega, D., Hieber, L., Saran, A., Allen, L. A., *et al.* (1998). Transformation of C3H 10T1/2 cells by low doses of ionising radiation: a collaborative study by six European laboratories strongly supporting a linear dose–response relationship. *J. Radiol. Prot.*, **18** (2), 79–100.

13 Rubin, P. and Casarett, G. W. (1968). *Clinical radiation pathology.* Saunders, Philadelphia.

14 International Commission on Radiological Protection (1991). The biological basis for dose limitation in the skin. ICRP Publication 59. *Ann. ICRP*, **22** (2).

15 Preston, D. L. and Pierce, D. A. (1987). *The effects of changes in dosimetry on cancer mortality risk. Estimates in the atomic bomb survivors.* Radiation Effects Research Foundation, RERF TR 0-87, Hiroshima.

16 Shimizu, Y., Kato, H., and Schull, W. J. (1990). Studies of the mortality of A-bomb survivors. 9. Mortality 1950–1985. Part 2. Cancer mortality based on the recently revised doses (DS86). *Radiat. Res.*, **121**, 120–41.

17 Pierce, D. A., Shimizu, D. L., Preston, D. L., M. Vaeth and K. Mabuchi (1996). Studies of the mortality of A-bomb survivors. Report 12, Part I. Cancer: 1950–1990. *Radiat. Res.*, **146**, 1–27.

18 Pierce, D. A. and Vaeth, M. (1989). Cancer risk estimation from the A-bomb survivors: extrapolation to low doses, use of relative risk models and other uncertainties. In: *Low dose radiation: biological bases of risk assessment* (ed. K. F. Baverstock and J. W. Stather), pp. 54–75. Taylor & Francis, London.

19 Gilbert, E. S., Fry, S. A., Wiggs, L. D., Voelz, G. L., Cragle, D. L., and Petersen, G. R. (1989). Analyses of combined mortality data on workers at the Hanford site, Oak Ridge National Laboratory and Rocky Flats nuclear weapons plant. *Radiat. Res.*, **120**, 19–35.

20 Kendall, G. M., Muirhead, C. R., MacGibbon, B. H., O'Hagan, J. A., Conquest, A. J., Goodill, A. A., *et al.* (1992). Mortality and occupational exposure to radiation: first analysis of the National Registry for Radiation Workers. *Br. Med. J.*, **304**, 220–5.

21 Kendall, G. M., Muirhead, C. R., MacGibbon, B. H., O'Hagan, J. A., Conquest, A. J., Goodill, A. A., *et. al.* (1992). *First analysis of the National Registry for Radiation Workers: occupational exposure to ionising radiation and mortality.* NRPB-R251, Chilton. HMSO, London.

22 Cardis, E., Gilbert, E. S., Carpenter, L., *et al.* (1995). Effects of low doses and low dose rates of external ionising radiation: cancer mortality among nuclear industry workers in three countries. *Radiat. Res.*, **142**, 117–32.

23 Muirhead, C. R., Goodill, A. A., Haylock, R. G. E., *et al.* (1999). Occupational radiation exposure and mortality: second analysis of the National Registry for Radiation Workers. *J. Radiol. Prot.*, **19**, 3–26.

24 United Nations Scientific Committee on the Effects of Radiation (1977). *Sources and effects of ionising radiation.* 1977 Report to the General Assembly, with annexes.

25 United Nations Scientific Committee on the Effects of Radiation (1986). *Genetic and somatic effects of ionising radiation.* Report to the General Assembly, with annexes.

26 Neel, J. V., Schull, W. J., Awa, A. A., Satoh, C., Otake, M., Kato, H., *et al.* (1989). The genetic effects of the atomic bombs: problems in extrapolating from somatic cell findings to risk for children. In: *Low dose radiation: biological bases of risk assessment* (ed. K. F. Baverstock and J. W. Stather), pp 42–53. Taylor & Francis, London.

27 Euratom (1996). Basic safety standards for the protection of the health of workers and the general public against the dangers arising from ionising radiation. Council Directive 96/29/ Euratom at 13 May 1996. *Off. J. Eur. Commun.*, L159 39.

28 United Nations Scientific Committee on the Effects of Atomic Radiation (2000). Sources and effects of ionising radiation 2000. Report to the General Assembly, with scientific annexes. Volume II: Effects.

29 United Nations Scientific Committee on the Effects of Atomic Radiation (2001). Report to the General Assembly, with scientific annex.

Chapter 4
Radiation measurements

S. Green and R. G. Zamenhof

4.1 Scope

Radiation measurements are central to many areas of radiation-based medical physics. The ability to make accurate and reproducible measurements, which provides the subject matter for this chapter, requires a detailed knowledge of

- radiation detection mechanisms and the basis of practical detectors;
- quantities to be measured and the appropriate primary standard to which measurements should be traceable;
- basic measurement techniques and assessment of measurement uncertainties.

This chapter will attempt to cover these areas to a level of detail which should be sufficient for professionals working in radiation protection and includes examples drawn from the field of radiation protection.

4.2 Introduction

There are two basic types of radiation detector, those which operate as dosemeters, and those which operate as counters. The difference is almost self-explanatory. A dosemeter is designed such that its output is proportional to some dose-related quantity delivered to the detector and is usually scaled in μSv h^{-1} or μGy h^{-1}. Conversely, a counter gives an output which is a measure of the number of ionisation events which occur within the detector and is usually scaled in counts per second (cps).

In radiation protection applications, the measurements which are required have unique qualities which distinguish them from the kind of measurement made routinely in radiotherapy or nuclear medicine applications. Where ionisation chambers are used, they are generally not of the cavity design which predominates in megavoltage radiotherapy applications, but tend to be parallel-plate devices. Activity measurements are often required on samples with very low activity levels which are near the limit of detection of the measuring device and are often not of a standard geometry (the activity may be spread on contaminated clothing or flooring, for example). Hence, while the quantity to be measured may be the same, the measurement environments encountered in radiation protection can be such that purpose-built radiation detectors and specialized measurement techniques are required.

4.3 Quantities to be measured and traceability

Some of the quantities used in radiation protection measurement are obvious, but others are hidden within the chain of traceability to a primary standard. The concept of traceability refers to the way that a radiation measurement which is performed in any routine operational procedure is related, through a chain of measurements, to an appropriate primary standard. In the UK this falls within the overall remit of the National Measurement System (NMS) which is supported by the National Physical Laboratory (NPL). The NPL holds the majority of the UK primary standards. It is often assumed that the concept of traceability is simply a matter of ensuring that a field instrument is properly calibrated. However, the degree to which a particular measurement can be said to be traceable to a primary standard also depends on the way the instrument is used and the quantity to be measured. In radiation protection there are four principal primary standards which come into play:

- air kerma (§2.7.3) (Gy, or more usually mGy or μGy)
- surface emission rates for photon, β- and α-emission (s^{-1})
- activities for α-, β-, and γ-emitting radioactivity (Bq)
- neutron fluence (§2.7.1) (m^{-2}).

Generally, radiation protection measurements are not made in terms of surface emission rate. This quantity is hidden from the end-user who requires measurements of contamination levels in terms of activity per unit area. In addition, the operational dose quantities defined by the ICRU (Box 4.1) do not appear in the list.

Operational dose quantities are measurable quantities which provide a realistic assessment of the level of harm (in terms of effective dose) received by an individual from the radiation field. They are designed to include some safety margin to ensure that they are in fact an overestimate. The operational dose quantities will not generally equate with an available primary standard, so that some conversion factors are required. The ICRU provides such conversion factors, usually by reviewing the available scientific data.

The two operational dose quantities of interest are ambient dose equivalent and directional dose equivalent (Box 4.1). The use of operational quantities for external dosimetry dates back to 1985 [1]. However, the general philosophy has not yet been fully assimilated by detector manufacturers who still tend to optimise the response of many detectors in terms of air kerma (Box 4.3), an approach which stems from a historical focus on the quantity 'exposure' (§2.7.5). There are a number of radiation protection applications where the quantity air kerma is still in common use, including the measurement of leakage levels from diagnostic X-ray equipment and of attenuation by shielding.

4.4 Detector selection

General guidance on instrument selection for commonly encountered situations in radiation protection is provided in this section. Further guidance is given in an NRPB report published after the text of this chapter was prepared [3]. Readers may then go on to learn more about the theory and operating principles of instruments which may be suited to their application, in later sections.

4.4.1 Instruments for dosimetry

Requirement	Rugged instrument for field dosimetry measurements, approximate photon spectrum is known
Selection	Energy-compensated Geiger–Müller tube
Requirement	Rugged instrument for field dosimetry measurements, photon spectrum is not known and an accurate measure of ambient dose equivalent is required
Selection	Organic scintillator
Requirement	Instrument for field dosimetry measurements, photon spectrum is not known and an accurate measure of air kerma is required
Selection	Ionisation chamber
Requirement	Neutron component of a radiation field must be measured for ambient dose equivalent
Selection	Moderating neutron detector
Requirement	Measurement of dose or dose rate in a radiation field which is only present for a short period or is pulsed
Selection	There are many issues to consider here. Of all radiation detectors, organic scintillators tend to have the fastest response time. In fact, the charge pulse produced by a scintillator/photomultiplier combination must usually be integrated to a more slowly varying voltage pulse before further processing. Despite the intrinsic speed of the scintillator, the instrument as a whole might be quite slow due to the design of the pulse-processing electronics. The detector electronics are often designed to smooth out any fast transient signals, assuming that these will be from noise. It is therefore difficult to define firm rules if working in an environment where short pulsed radiation exposures are to be measured. If the pulse will be repeated many times in succession, then an ionisation chamber might work well; however, for a single shot, careful consideration of the instrument manual is required to ensure a faithful reading of dose rate. For measurements of dose, however, the integrating function on many ionisation chamber devices should give a reliable reading.

4.4.2 Instruments for contamination monitoring

It is possible to make high-sensitivity, reliable and accurate measurements in most situations with a range of detector types including scintillators, Geiger–Müller tubes, and proportional counters. However, the requirements below might be instructive:

Requirement	Rapid scanning of large surface for β/γ contamination
Selection	Large-area proportional counter (although inorganic scintillators are also available in large-area formats)
Requirement	Measurement of tritium contamination

Box 4.1 Operational dose quantities

Ambient dose equivalent, $H^*(d)$, equates to the dose delivered at a depth of d mm in the 300 mm diameter ICRU tissue-equivalent sphere under conditions of broad-field parallel-beam irradiation. $H^*(10)$ is the quantity used for characterization of what is termed 'strongly penetrating' radiation, and $H^*(0.07)$ for weakly penetrating radiation. $H^*(10)$ is therefore the dose equivalent at point A in Figure B4.1 when the variable angle α is zero.

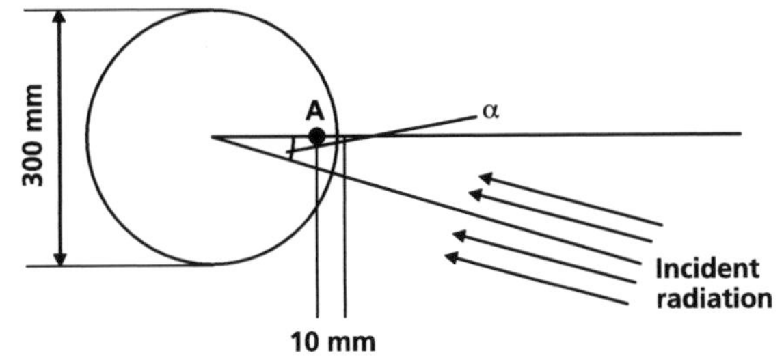

Figure B4.1 Geometry relating to the definition of ambient and directional dose equivalent.

The directional dose equivalent $H'(d, \alpha)$ relates to the general situation when the direction of the incident radiation field may be rotated by an angle α from the radius containing point A. It is also conventionally defined at depths of 10 and 0.07 mm, and from the definitions, $H'(10, 0)$ and $H^*(10)$ will be numerically identical.

The operational dose quantities are defined in such a way that they provide a measure of effective dose (E, §3.2.2), or at least a realistic overestimate of effective dose. Hence, a reference person standing in a uniform isotropic radiation field of 1 mSv h^{-1} in terms of ambient dose equivalent will receive an effective dose of approximately 1 mSv (or slightly less) in 1 hour. Without the sphere present, the ambient dose equivalent and directional dose equivalent for photons are related to the traceable quantity air kerma (K_{air}) through standard conversion factors such as those shown in Figure B4.2 [2].

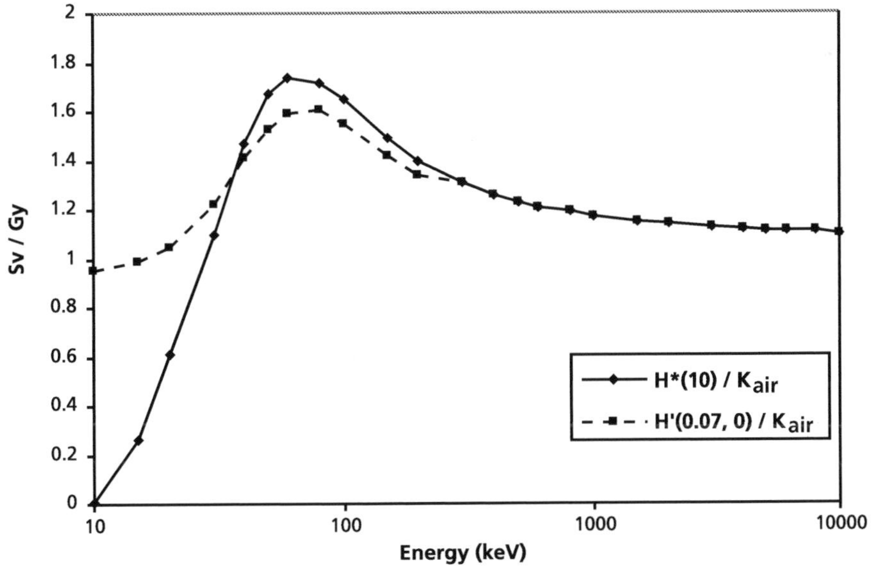

Figure B4.2 ICRU operational dose quantities.

The peak in the curve in this figure results from the increase in the incidence of large-angle Compton scattering at these energies, while the fall in the $H^*(10)$ curve at low energy is a result of photon attenuation in the 10 mm overlaying the reference point.

Ambient dose equivalent can also be related directly to the field quantities (fluence and fluence rate) (§2.7.1).

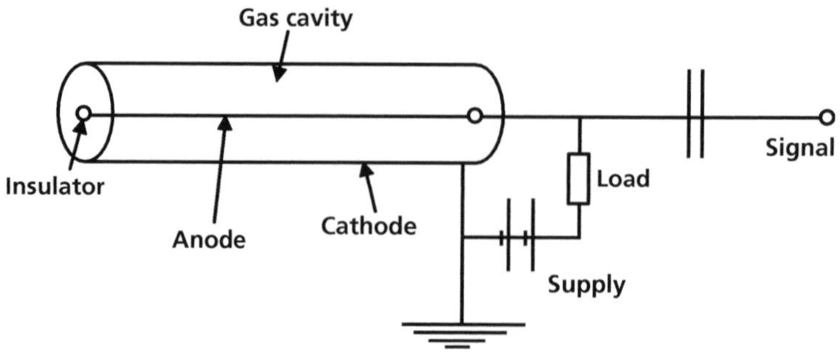

Figure 4.1 Schematic of a gas counter with cylindrical geometry.

Selection	Windowless proportional counter
Requirement	Inexpensive instrument for α-particle detection, where other radiations are not present
Selection	Geiger counter with mylar end window
Requirement	α/β discrimination
Selection	Dual phosphor scintillator. Note that this task can also be achieved using a general-purpose detector and a piece of paper as a filter to absorb αs and transmit βs
Requirement	Location of very low-activity photon sources
Selection	Large-volume inorganic scintillator or Geiger counter
Requirement	Measurement of β or low-energy photon contamination
Selection	Inorganic scintillator with thin entrance window

There are some situations where there are practical advantages to having a single instrument which can monitor both dose and contamination level. The availability of such instruments is increasing. They are generally based on Geiger–Müller tube technology, with an energy compensation shield which can be manually moved into place when dosimetric measurements are required.

The utility of a range of detection systems and the factors which impact on their performance have been reviewed by the US Nuclear Regulatory Commission [4]. The majority of the major instrument manufacturers now have information, including detector selection guides, available on their websites.

Once selected as appropriate for a particular measurement task, the instrument will go into routine service and must be subject to regular quality assurance measurements to ensure consistent performance. It is good practice to maintain a calibration record for any instrument in routine use, in which any variations in selected results from regular calibration measurements are tracked with time [5].

4.5 Gas detectors

4.5.1 Theory of operation

The basic theory of operation of all gas counters, whether they are ionisation chambers, proportional counters, or Geiger–Müller (GM) tubes has much common ground. Operation involves the application of a high voltage across a gas-filled cavity. Ionising radiation induces ionisation in the gas and the electron-ion pairs are separated by the applied electric field. The movement of charges within the electric field results in a measurable electrical current. A gas detector can be represented by the simple geometry shown in Figure 4.1.

A gas counter can function in a number of voltage domains as determined by the relationship between the applied high voltage and the measured signal height. This is represented schematically by Figure 4.2.

4.5.2 Recombination region

In this low collection-voltage region, ion drift velocities are small and significant recombination of positive ions and electrons occurs. Field instruments are never used in this region.

4.5.3 Ion saturation region (ionisation chamber)

All ions created by the initial ionising radiation are swept to the electrodes. Signals are small and there is a need for amplification. A typical ionisation current would be of the order of 10^{-12} A (1 picoamp) so that leakage currents in the circuit need to be inhibited by the use of high-quality components. Choice of suitable electronic circuitry will allow an ionisation chamber to be run in 'pulse' mode. All the charges created by individual

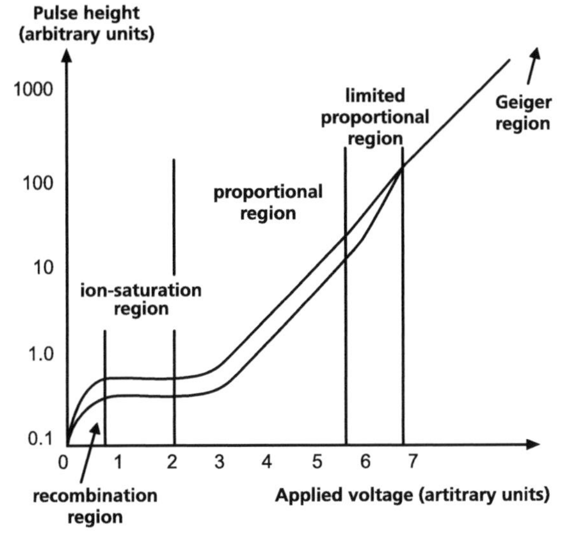

Figure 4.2 Pulse height/voltage characteristics of an idealized gas counter.

ionising events or radiation interactions are recorded to give a measurement which can be related to dose. In many radiation protection applications a chamber is operated in 'DC' or 'current mode' with the overall ionisation current produced by a summation of many individual ionising events being measured to provide an assessment related to dose rate.

4.5.4 Proportional region (proportional counter)

Gas multiplication occurs in the region close to the anode wire (i.e. electrons gain sufficient energy to cause further ionisation). The amplification process produces larger and more easily measurable pulses, which are proportional in amplitude to the energy of the initial ionising event. Gains in signal amplitude ranging up to five orders of magnitude can be achieved. These detectors are almost always operated in pulse mode, the individual pulses being counted by appropriate electronic circuitry.

The anode of a proportional counter is usually a wire, the diameter of which is typically much smaller than those found in ionisation chambers, being perhaps as low as 10 μm. For the same applied voltage, this results in a much more intense electric field around the wire. Pulse height is therefore a strong function of applied voltage and so proportional counters require a much more stable supply voltage than either ionisation chambers or GM tubes.

4.5.5 Geiger region (Geiger counter)

Very large pulses are produced in which the whole chamber is driven into discharge for a short time. The output pulse size is independent of the energy of the initial ionising event. The discharge is prompted by the production of light and ultraviolet photons which are produced by electron excitation of the gas molecules inside the tube. (The electrons are produced by the interaction of ionising radiation within the tube.)

The progression of the discharge from anode to cathode results in a short period of time in which the tube is not able to respond to further incident ionising radiation. GM tubes contain an electronegative quench gas which mops up excess electrons and therefore 'quenches' each new discharge shortly after its initiation. The rate with which this quenching process occurs places a limit on the count rate, because there is a 'dead-time' when a GM tube will not register another pulse, which is effectively the time taken for each pulse to be processed. The rate meter which is attached to the tube must be set up to allow for this tube 'dead-time' or corrections can be applied to measured pulse rates as

$$n' = n/(1 - n\tau)$$

where n' is the corrected count rate, n is the measured count rate, and τ is the tube dead-time.

Dead-times vary from around 10 µs up to as much as 1 ms, limiting the count-rate capability of Geiger counters to between 1000 and 100 000 cps. The resultant pulses are so large that further amplification is unnecessary.

When configured as surface contamination monitors, GM tubes have thin entrance windows. These are generally designed to allow β- and α-particles to enter the gas cavity and their attenuation properties affect the response of the meter. The window may be located at the end or to the side of the counter chamber.

General comments on the setting up and domains of use of each type of gas detector are given in the following sections. However, the details of operation of a particular detector may differ from the general guidelines described below and there is no substitute for a thorough review of the manufacturer's instructions. In all cases, however, the instrument will fail to hazard if the battery fails. It is therefore essential to check the battery voltage before embarking on measurements.

4.6 Ionisation chambers

4.6.1 Set-up instructions

Setting up an ionisation chamber involves measuring the current/voltage characteristic at voltages up to the upper limit of the ion-saturation region. This would typically be obtained by providing a constant and high-intensity irradiation (usually obtained by fixing the detector at a specified distance from a source of constant radiation output) and then increasing the applied voltage in steps, recording the ionisation current (or instrument reading) at each step. When the whole extent of the plateau region has been defined, the appropriate operating voltage for the instrument is selected at the approximate midpoint of the plateau.

4.6.2 Areas of use

Ionisation chambers are standard instruments used for routine dosimetry in radiation therapy and diagnostic radiology. They generally have a very low variation in energy response in terms of instrument reading per unit incident air kerma. Any variation that there is will probably be within 10% in the photon energy interval from 20 keV to a few MeV. However, measurements of photon ambient dose equivalent are not readily achievable with ionisation chambers unless the incident photon spectrum is well known. In this case the conversions shown in Box 4.1 can be employed. The measurement of low-energy photons, β- or α-particles can be facilitated by using a detector with a thin entrance window made with a low atomic number material such as mylar.

4.6.3 Limitations of performance

Historically, ionisation chambers have been less robust than alternative detector types, but more recent advances in fabrication techniques have led to lower detector leakage currents and to electronic circuits which can reliably detect the very low ionisation currents that may be produced. As a result, these types of detectors are becoming more common.

4.7 Proportional counters

4.7.1 Set-up instructions

Setting up a proportional counter will usually involve following the manufacturer's guidelines to set an applied voltage which is high enough to produce gas multiplication and hence a good signal-to-noise ratio but insufficient to cause Geiger discharge within the detector.

Experimentally it may be possible to make measurements in pulse mode of the detector pulse height spectrum as a function of applied voltage for a fixed detector–source configuration. Before the onset of discharge pulses or electrical breakdown, the gas multiplication region grows and is no longer constrained to be close to the anode wire. As the multiplication region extends out into the detector cavity, the height of a detector pulse becomes dependent on the location within the detector at which the original ionising event occurred. As a result a reduction in detector pulse-height resolution can be expected as the bias voltage increases.

4.7.2 Areas of use

Proportional counters form the basis of many large-area contamination monitors for use with all radiations including (for thin window or windowless designs) α-emitters and very low-energy β-emitters such as tritium. They are also the most common type of neutron detector in the form of BF_3 and ^3He detectors (Box 4.2). In addition, they form the basis of some of the most sophisticated radiation measurement devices to be found in radiation protection. These are tissue equivalent proportional counters configured as microdosimetric detectors for photon and neutron dose determination in mixed neutron and photon radiation fields [6].

4.7.3 Limitations of performance

Proportional counters are sensitive instruments and are not suited to rough handling or robust demands. Large-area contamination monitors may require charging with a suitable gas filling before use (e.g. butane), and so will need to be prepared in advance of a measurement, typically some 30 minutes to 1 hour beforehand. For very low-energy particle detection, windowless detectors are available but these require a gas-flow system which adds considerably to the complexity of the measurement device.

4.7.4 Practical example

A proportional counter which is commonly encountered in hospitals is the large-area contamination monitor manufactured by EG&G Berthold. The detector element of this instrument is often the BZ100XEP which is a xenon-filled proportional counter. Such detectors find general utility for photon and β contamination monitoring in nuclear medicine departments. Large-area detectors such as this provide an excellent method of rapidly scanning a worksurface to identify the presence of contamination.

Analysis of the responses exhibited by 11 instruments tested by the Regional Radiation Physics and Protection Service (RRPPS) during 1997 show a standard deviation in response to ^{129}I of 11% (^{129}I has a mean emitted photon energy of 31.5 keV). Such a high degree of consistency means that it is a relatively simple process to identify instruments which are not performing in a satisfactory manner. The variation in response of this batch of instruments to ^{36}Cl (maximum β energy = 710 keV) is similarly low but the actual response figure is very much greater. For ^{36}Cl the mean detector response is 22 cps (Bq cm^{-2})$^{-1}$ compared with just over 3 cps (Bq cm^{-2})$^{-1}$ for ^{129}I.

Box 4.2 Moderating neutron detectors

It is possible to design a neutron detection system with a reasonably uniform energy dependence, which consists of a thermal neutron detector at the centre of a specially designed moderator. In many ways this is analogous to the design of the shield on an energy-compensated Geiger detector for determination of photon dose rates (Box 4.3). The most commonly used detection mechanisms for such instruments are the ^{10}B and ^{3}He neutron capture reactions:

$$^{10}\text{B} + \text{n} \longrightarrow {}^{7}\text{Li} + {}^{4}\text{He} + 2.79\ \text{MeV} \qquad (6\%)$$
$$\longrightarrow {}^{7}\text{Li}^{*} + {}^{4}\text{He} + 2.31\ \text{MeV} \qquad (94\%)$$

$$^{3}\text{He} + \text{n} \longrightarrow {}^{3}\text{H} + {}^{1}\text{p} + 0.764\ \text{MeV}$$

Both of these reactions occur predominantly with neutrons at what are termed thermal energies, the initial neutron energy having been degraded by scattering interactions until the neutrons are in thermal equilibrium with the detector material. In this case their characteristic energy equals kT (where k is the Boltzmann constant and T the temperature in Kelvin) and is typically 0.025 eV. In addition, both reactions have a relatively high positive Q value which means that the reaction products carry kinetic energy which is much greater than that of the incoming thermal neutron. This is deposited within the detector and means that the detector signals are easily distinguishable from any photon-induced signals and background electronic noise.

In order to ensure that the instrument as a whole provides a measure of an appropriate dose quantification (usually ambient dose equivalent), the detector must be surrounded by a moderator. This moderator will be designed to ensure that neutrons reach the central detector roughly in proportion to their weighting in the fluence to dose equivalent conversion curve shown in Figure B4.3. This is obviously not a trivial task as the conversion factor shown in this figure varies by more than a factor of 50 across the neutron energy range of interest.

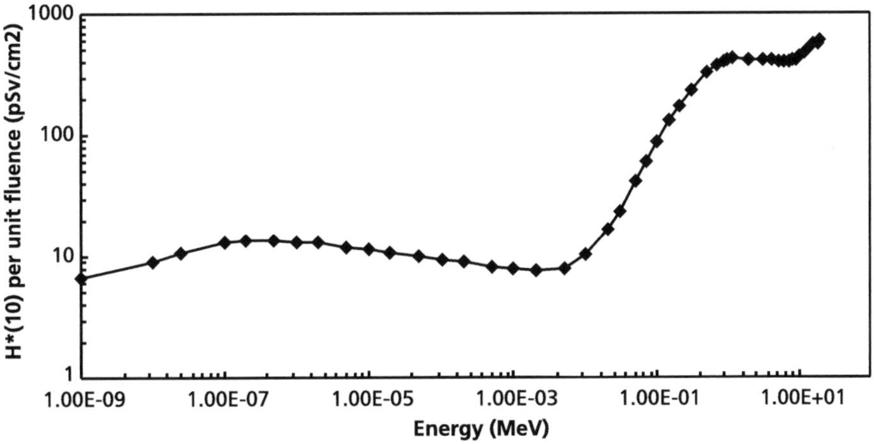

Figure B4.3 Neutron conversion coefficients.

One such instrument in common use is the NM2 marketed in the UK by Bicron/NE. The NM2 has a polythene moderator which produces an instrument energy response which is within –40% and +100% of the desired response across a very broad range of energy from thermal to 15 MeV. Hence, such an instrument can function as a device for measuring operational dose quantities, even though the neutron interaction in the sensitive volume of the detector contains no explicit information on the energy of the neutron.

4.8 Geiger–Müller tubes

4.8.1 Set-up instructions

For a GM tube connected to a rate meter with a fixed lower-level discriminator setting, the curve shown in Figure 4.3 will be obtained when increasing the applied voltage under conditions of constant irradiation.

The threshold voltage defines the point at which the applied voltage is large enough to drive the tube into Geiger discharge for some of the radiation interactions.

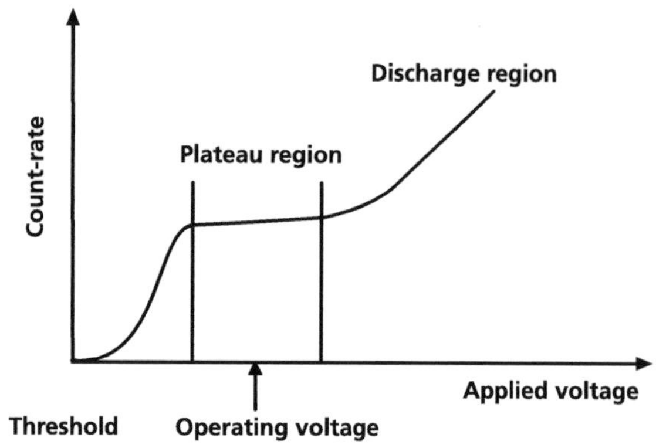

Figure 4.3 Characteristic count rate–voltage curve for a Geiger–Müller tube.

The number of counts recorded increases rapidly above the threshold voltage until the plateau is reached. Above this point the number of counts recorded increases slowly over a range of applied voltages. The operating voltage should be chosen on this plateau, and it is usually at the centre of the plateau where the detector operation is least affected by variations in the supply voltage. Typically the operating voltage will be in the range from 500 to 1000 V. As the tube ages, the quench gas will be used up gradually and the plateau will become shorter. It may then become necessary to decrease the operating voltage towards the lower third of the plateau. This has the effect of achieving stable operation with the minimum discharge size, and therefore the minimum use of quench gas. These factors will tend to extend the life of the detector. Under no circumstances should a GM tube be subjected to prolonged operation at voltages beyond the plateau. This will produce a continuous discharge which would almost certainly destroy the device.

The usual filling gas for a GM tube would be a high atomic number gas such as neon or argon with a suitable quench gas such as chlorine or bromine. The high atomic number of the filling gas and the metallic nature of the tube cathode give significant opportunity for interaction via the photoelectric effect and, as a result, the energy response of a GM tube tends to peak at low energies of around 60–80 keV. An overresponse is desirable in certain circumstances, such as in the construction of a sensitive contamination monitor for location and measurement of ^{125}I spillage. For application in contamination detectors, thin entrance windows are required to allow entry of poorly penetrating radiations. Such a configuration may also be suitable for the measurement of α contamination. For use as a dosemeter, an overresponse is undesirable and techniques are required to balance the response of the tube across its energy range. These techniques are referred to as energy compensation (Box 4.3) and are in many ways analogous to the design of the moderator around a moderating neutron detector (Box 4.2).

4.8.2 Areas of use

These detectors can be used in areas where more sensitive instruments might easily become damaged. Their robust construction and large signal size make them suitable for use with very basic pulse-counting circuitry, making them amongst the cheapest of radiation survey instruments.

4.8.3 Limitations of performance

Uncompensated GM tubes are only suitable for monitoring medium- to low-energy β-emissions if they have a very thin entrance window. Such instruments are fragile and puncturing the window will destroy the detector. The very lowest energy β-emissions encountered in laboratory situations, such as those from ^{3}H, cannot be monitored with windowed Geiger detectors. The energy response of compensated devices is generally such that photons below around 50 keV are not measured in the correct proportion for dosimetry.

4.8.4 Practical example

A detector based on an energy-compensated GM tube is the type D probe supplied by Mini Instruments. This instrument features a Centronic ZP1490 GM tube which has a gas filling of neon and argon with a halogen quenching agent. It is configured as a dosemeter and is scaled in terms of ambient dose equivalent (in μSv).

Analysis of instrument response data from calibrations of 13 instruments (RRPPS) with a range of ages and previous usage histories gave a spread of only 6% in results from ^{137}Cs (660 keV) and a spread of 20% in results for ^{241}Am (60 keV). Any differences in tube characteristics are more likely to show up at the lower photon energy where complete tube discharge may not be initiated by the lower energy of the incident radiation. The 60 keV photon energy of ^{241}Am is towards the lower end of the energy range for a type D probe (quoted as 30 keV by the manufacturer).

On the issue of optimisation of tube energy compensation in terms of air kerma (Box 4.3), the actual response figures for air kerma derived for a Mini Instruments Type D probe at 660 and 60 keV are very similar. However, the ambient dose equivalent figure would be around 40% higher for 60 keV. Hence, in terms of ambient dose equivalent such probes end up under-responding at lower photon energies.

Box 4.3 Energy compensation for Geiger-Mueller detectors

The main constituent of the filling gas for a Geiger tube is generally a high atomic number material such as neon or argon. This fact, combined with the metallic nature of the tube cathode, gives a high probability of interaction via the photoelectric effect and so the energy response of a Geiger tube tends to peak at photon energies of 60–80 keV Energy compensation involves the construction of a detector shield which balances the increased response of the detector at low energies, with an increased attenuation of incident photons in the shield. It is usual to use material such as lead and tin, and to cover only part of the tube surface, leaving a proportion unshielded. The general practice is to design energy compensation such that the relative air-kerma response of the detector becomes flat. Figure B4.4 shows the relative air-kerma response of a Centronic ZP1300 tube (solid line) [7], that is the number of counts in the detector per unit delivered air kerma as a function of photon energy. At energies below 60 keV, the attenuation in the tube materials is seen to have a significant impact, reducing the relative air-kerma response of the detector. The ZP1301 is the energy-compensated version of the ZP1300 and the response data for both shown in the figure have been normalized to unity for 660 keV γ-rays from ^{137}Cs. Inevitably, this leads to a restriction of the energy range of the detector; increasing the minimum photon energy which can be detected. Care must also be taken to maintain a reasonably uniform detector response with the direction of the incident radiation since the design of the compensating shield will affect this property.

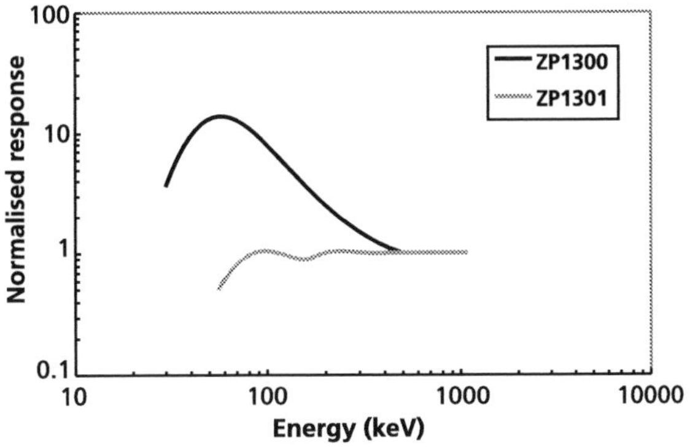

Figure B4.4 Relative response data for compensated and uncompensated Geiger tubes.

The practice of optimising the detector response in terms of air kerma, which is in fact based on a historical focus on measurements in terms of exposure, does not fit with the ICRU recommendations regarding the use of the operational dose quantity, ambient dose equivalent [1]. Ideally, this practice will change in time to one of optimisation in terms of the recommended quantity following current IEC guidance [8].

4.9 Scintillation detectors

4.9.1 Fundamentals

A scintillator is a material which produces light when it is exposed to ionising radiation. It must have a high degree of transparency to the light that it emits, so that the light can leave the scintillator, travel through the light guide (if present), and fall onto the sensitive region of the photocathode. The scintillator and light guide/photomultiplier assembly are generally housed together in a light-tight case and a complete detector would also include a power supply and some pulse- or current-counting circuitry. The scintillation medium itself may be an inorganic crystal such as thallium-activated sodium iodide [NaI(Tl)] or zinc sulphide (ZnS), or an organic plastic which might be referred to by the manufacturer's code, such as NE-102 (now BC400) from Bicron/NE. Liquid scintillators are used where low-level α- or β-activity sources are mixed with the liquid (Box 4.4). Such systems provide high-efficiency 4π counting configurations, enabling the majority of emitted radiations to be detected.

In order to tune the optical properties of a scintillator to ensure maximal light output per unit radiation energy deposited it is often necessary during its formation to incorporate trace elements. These will be incorporated into the crystal structure and modify its optical characteristics. An example of this is the introduction of thallium in a standard NaI(Tl) crystal

Box 4.4 Internal liquid scintillation counting

It is possible to determine the activity of a sample by dissolving or distributing the sample within a liquid scintillator. This is termed internal liquid scintillation counting and provides a high efficiency (close to 100%) counting configuration. A typical configuration for internal liquid scintillation counting would include a vial containing the scintillator and sample. These are placed in a light-tight enclosure where the emitted light is viewed by a photomultiplier tube with the appropriate pulse-counting electronics.

While the technique is not without problems of its own, it does remove many of the difficulties inherent in using hand-held detectors such as those described so far in this chapter for measuring β- and α-emissions. There is no detector entrance widow through which the radiation must pass, no air gap between the sample and the detector, particle absorption within the sample is avoided, and the sample geometry is forced to be highly reproducible.

Of the measurement problems created by this technique, perhaps the most significant is the effect that the dissolved sample has on the optical properties of the scintillator. This can lead to a reduction (or quenching) of the light output. Quenching also occurs with insoluble samples which are not dissolved but are distributed as a fine particulate suspension within the scintillator material. The magnitude of these problems is difficult to predict and is therefore usually accounted for by use of an internal standard. A known activity of a reference radionuclide is introduced into the sample. Its determined activity is then used to provide a normalization signal for other activity estimates from the sample.

scintillator, which modifies the optical properties of the resultant crystal and makes it transparent to the emitted light. Scintillation materials have a characteristic efficiency with which the initial radiation energy is converted to light. This is referred to as the scintillation efficiency and it is usually desirable to maximize this quantity. However, in certain circumstances the difference in scintillation efficiency of two scintillator materials can be used to great effect to create a detector which can discriminate between different radiations (Box 4.5).

The photomultiplier converts the incident light pulse into a measurable electrical pulse by first using a converter screen referred to as the photocathode to produce electrons when illuminated by light photons, and then by a staged amplification process to produce a measurable electrical pulse. The photocathode should be matched to the scintillator to ensure that it is sensitive to the wavelength of the light that the scintillator emits, and the scintillator/light-guide/photomultiplier assembly is usually coupled with some form of 'optical coupling grease' to ensure good optical contact between the components.

Scintillation detectors may be operated in either 'pulse' or 'current' mode. The monitoring circuit can be sensitive either to the number of pulses which are produced by the detector or to the overall magnitude of the current produced by the detector, where the current will be representative of the average rate of production of pulses in the detector. It is also possible to use these sorts of detectors for spectrometry purposes, in which case the sensing circuitry must be able to distinguish between voltage pulses on the basis of amplitude.

There are basic differences between the types of photon interactions which occur in inorganic and organic scintillators [9]. In order to maximize photon interaction probability and hence detection efficiency, inorganic scintillators tend to be made of medium to high atomic number materials. This inevitably means that there is a high probability of photoelectric interactions occurring within the detector. This is usually not the case in organic scintillators where interactions are dominated by Compton scatter.

4.9.2 Set-up instructions

The size of the signal produced by the photomultiplier, under conditions of constant irradiation, will increase very rapidly with applied voltage. The characteristic curve derived for constant irradiation conditions will show a similar shape to the curve for GM detectors (Figure 4.3). At low voltage, the pulses are too small to register above the internal discriminators of the pulse-counting circuit, while at high voltage, background noise signals generated within the photomultiplier may also be sufficiently large to register. Between these two extremes there may be a fairly wide 'plateau' region where the detector will operate in a satisfactory manner. The operating voltage should be set sufficiently high to ensure that any low-energy radiation fields will be properly measured. If accurate measurements of low-energy radiation sources are desired, it is sensible to derive the detector count rate versus voltage curve (and thereby set the operating voltage) using a similar low-energy calibration source.

4.9.3 Areas of use

Scintillation detectors are used widely in photon dose-rate meters, and in β and photon contamination monitors.

Box 4.5 The design and operation of a dual phosphor detector

Different scintillator materials have different scintillation efficiencies which means that they are able to convert different proportions of the incident radiation energy into light. Conventionally, figures for scintillation efficiency are presented in relative terms. For inorganic materials, figures are relative to NaI(Tl) which is 100%, whereas for organic materials, figures are quoted relative to anthracene at 100%. Anthracene has a scintillation efficiency of approximately 43% of NaI(Tl) and so further scaling is required in order to compare organic and inorganic scintillators.

Consider, as a practical example, the discriminating probe DP2R manufactured by Bicron/NE. This has a thin layer of ZnS powder deposited onto an NE-102A plastic scintillator. The scintillation efficiencies are:

ZnS	130% of NaI
NE-102A	65% of anthracene, 28% of NaI, 21.5% of ZnS

Hence ZnS has around 500% of the scintillation efficiency of NE-102A and would therefore have around 500% of the light output for the same energy deposition. In the DP2R the scintillator materials are arranged so that incident radiation must pass through the thin ZnS layer to reach the NE-102A plastic. α-particles are unable to penetrate the ZnS layer and therefore deposit all of their energy in the ZnS. Low-energy β-particles may also be stopped in the ZnS layer but their low energy (and hence low light output) will only give small detector pulses. Higher energy βs and photons will be more penetrating and will deposit the majority of their energy in the NE-102A layer. It is perhaps worth remembering that a typical α-emitter will have an energy of around 5 MeV whereas β-emissions tend to have maximum energies substantially lower than this, generally lower than 3 MeV.

By coupling such a probe to a rate-meter unit which can also provide some pulse height discrimination it is possible to discriminate the generally smaller β and photon pulses from the much larger α pulses. A DP2R/rate-meter combination is usually set up for optimum α discrimination by monitoring the counts in the β channel of the rate-meter while exposing the detector to a constant α-irradiation, varying the voltage (see plot) and selecting the minimum in the response. As an additional check it is sensible to perform sequential measurements on a β-source using first the β and then the α channel. The count-rate in the α channel should be less than 0.1% of that in the β channel. In this way an operating voltage which gives good α/β discrimination will be obtained. However, in environments where it is important to ensure that low-energy α-particle emissions are not overlooked, an alternative set-up procedure might be more appropriate.

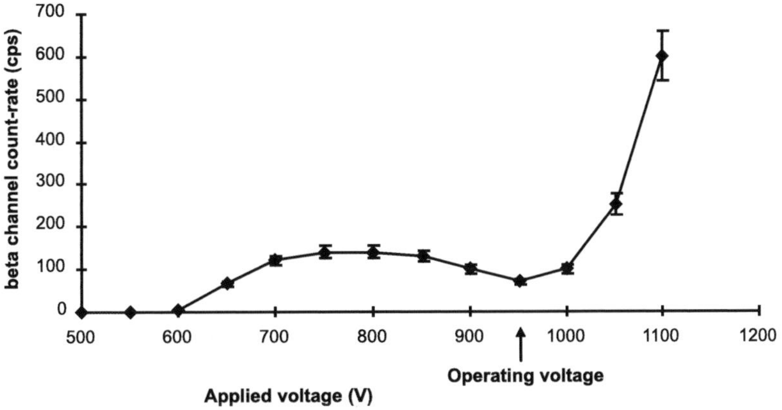

Figure B4.5 β-channel count rate vs. operating voltage.

When incorporated into a detector with a thin entrance window, they can be used for monitoring levels of less penetrating radiations including α-particles. The use of organic scintillators opens up the possibility for building detectors which closely mimic the dosimetric properties of tissue. For example, the 'microSv' instrument manufactured by Bicron/NE uses an organic scintillator with a thin entrance window (5.4 mg cm^{-2} mylar) to achieve a detector response in terms of signal measured per unit ambient dose equivalent, $H^*(10)$, which varies by only around $\pm10\%$ from 15 keV to over 1 MeV photon energy.

4.9.4 Limitations of performance

The outer casing of a scintillation detector must not transmit light since the photocathode in the photomultiplier is very sensitive to light and if the case were not sealed correctly it would lead to the detector dramatically overreading. The cases of these detectors therefore need to be robust, which also has the advantage of providing a secure and vibration-free housing for the photomultiplier tube. This in turn tends to reduce the sensitivity of the detector to low-energy photons and β- and α-radiations. This is often compensated by using a thin entrance window made of a material such as aluminized mylar. This will allow scintillation detectors to be used to detect low-energy photons, β- and α-radiations, provided these are incident on the thin window rather than on to the side walls of the detector. Unlike the case for GM tubes, puncture of the window should not destroy the detector and temporary repairs can often be performed in the field.

4.9.5 Practical example

A detector based on a scintillator with a thin entrance window is the type 44A probe supplied by Mini Instruments and in widespread use in nuclear medicine departments for routine monitoring of surface contamination levels. This instrument features an NaI(Tl) scintillator of diameter 32 mm and thickness 2.5 mm, with a 14 mg cm^{-2} aluminium entrance window and an outer lead shield to give the probe a highly directional response. Analysis of the performance of 20 such instruments in annual calibrations (RRPPS) show variations in response of 5% for ^{129}I and 8% for ^{36}Cl. For ^{129}I the response of this detector is similar to that of the large-area proportional counter described above at around 3 cps (Bq cm^{-2})$^{-1}$ but it exhibits a lower response of slightly below 2 cps (Bq cm^{-2})$^{-1}$ for the βs emitted by ^{36}Cl.

4.10 Semiconductor detectors

4.10.1 Fundamentals

Semiconductor detectors rely on the production and movement of electron-hole pairs within the electronic band structure of the material, in a way which has much in common with the dependence of gas detectors on electron-ion pair movement. The elements of semiconductor band theory which are useful for understanding semiconductor detectors are outlined in Box 4.6.

The most common semiconductor radiation detectors encountered in radiation protection are based either on silicon diodes, such as those found in many personal monitoring devices, e.g. the Siemens EPD, or on very pure (Hyper-pure) crystals of germanium.

Hyper-pure (or intrinsic) germanium (HpGe) detectors for photon spectroscopy applications contain impurity levels which are typically of the order of 1 part in 10^{12}. Such low impurity levels are necessary to ensure that a substantial charge depletion region can be created within the crystal to form the sensitive volume of the radiation detector. Even with these very low impurity levels, there will still be an excess of either donor or acceptor impurities, leaving either n-type or p-type HpGe. These detectors take advantage of the low average energy to produce an electron-hole pair (3 eV in germanium) to create a detector with excellent energy resolution (§4.11). However, this low-energy value means that at room temperature, there is a significant probability that electron-hole pairs will be thermally generated rather than produced only by the action of ionising radiation. For this reason HpGe detectors must be cooled to liquid nitrogen temperatures for satisfactory operation.

One semiconductor detector which has found application in charged particle spectroscopy applications is the silicon surface barrier detector. The fabrication process for these detectors ensures that the active detector volume is formed on the surface of the silicon crystal, and so incident radiation does not have to penetrate an intervening 'dead-layer' before detection. These detectors are sensitive to optical radiation and so must be operated in a darkened environment.

4.10.2 Areas of use

Silicon diode detectors are finding increasing use in active devices for personal monitoring, while the more established silicon surface barrier detectors have an established role in α and β spectrometry applications. Lithium-drifted silicon [Si(Li)] and HpGe detectors are highly stable, high-resolution devices for photon spectrometry. HpGe detectors are widely used for environmental sample counting, while Si(Li) detectors are generally confined to low-energy X-ray spectrometry.

4.10.3 Limitations of performance

Si(Li) and HpGe detectors are generally confined to laboratory use in closely controlled metrological conditions and with a highly reliable liquid nitrogen and mains electrical supply. The higher atomic number of germanium gives HpGe better efficiency at higher photon energies, but the lower efficiency of Si(Li) is an advantage in low-energy spectrometry where unwanted signals resulting from interactions of high-energy photons are much reduced. Detectors can be provided with thin (usually beryllium) entrance windows for the measurement of low-energy photons but are not generally used for β or α spectroscopy. Silicon diode detectors are robust field devices requiring only low-voltage supplies and operating at room temperature.

Box 4.6 Theory of semiconductor detectors

The electrical properties of semiconductors have their origins in the restricted energy levels which are available to electrons within the crystal. This electronic *band* structure has two regions: the valence band, populated by electrons in specific lattice sites within the crystal, and the conduction band, populated by free electrons. The energy difference between the top of the valence band and the bottom of the conduction band is know as the band-gap. Electrons can be promoted across the band-gap by thermal excitation. Hence, as the temperature of the crystal rises the number of electrons in the conduction band increases with a corresponding change in the conductivity of the material. Adding other (impurity) elements to the crystal can change its energy structure by creating intermediate energy levels which dramatically alter the electrical properties of the material.

In p-type material, added impurities have one less valence electron than silicon, and therefore leave a vacancy which has much in common with one left by an electron which has moved to the conduction band. However, electrons which are captured by this 'hole' will be slightly less tightly bound than those captured by normal silicon atoms since the impurity (normally having fewer valence electrons) does not really need the additional electron. The result is an available energy level, the acceptor level, which sits just above the valence band, and a silicon region which is p-type since the positive charge carriers (holes) now have increased mobility. By an entirely analogous process, n-type silicon regions are created by addition of impurities which have one more valence electron than silicon.

To detect the effects of radiation it is necessary to create a volume where charges liberated as a result of radiation interactions can be efficiently collected and in which leakage currents are small. Collection of such charges obviously requires external electrical contacts which are normally designed to minimize leakage currents by *blocking*. That is, when a charge carrier is collected at one electrode it is not replaced by injection of a similar carrier at the other electrode.

Semiconductor diode detectors generally consist of a junction between two regions of silicon with different types of doping, one p-type and one n-type. Diode radiation detectors are operated in a reverse-bias configuration which means that the applied electric field is acting to impede the flow of thermally generated current across the diode. Essentially the applied voltage serves to increase the energy that an electron needs to remain in the conduction band while migrating across the junction. It can therefore be seen as a distortion of the normal electronic band structure [9] and serves multiple functions in a practical detector. It extends the depletion region between the two types of semiconductor, therefore increasing the volume of the radiation-sensitive region; it affects the injection of carriers into the depletion region from elsewhere; it ensures that electron-hole pairs generated in the depletion region do not recombine and that they move rapidly through the crystal.

It is possible to separate the p- and n-type regions at a junction, with a layer of intrinsic (undoped) material to provide a p–i–n configuration. With appropriate contacts, this configuration will be fully depleted with the application of only a small applied voltage. Hence it is ideal for situations where the maximum detection efficiency is required at minimum power consumption.

They are generally light sensitive and therefore require robust encapsulation.

4.10.4 Practical examples

HpGe systems for low-level γ-emitting activity counting in soil and foods

It is often desirable to quantify low-activity levels in environmental samples for radiation protection purposes. One example is the monitoring of foodstuffs, which has become a matter of routine for many local authorities. Other applications include the monitoring of potentially contaminated ash from incinerators and soil/rock deposits from mineral extraction plants. Furthermore, the water and gas industries have a need for low-level radioactivity monitoring since both industries have to deal with the carriage of the natural decay series of radionuclides from underground to the surface (§10.2.1).

These kinds of measurements often rely on large-volume semiconductor (usually HpGe) or scintillation (usually NaI(Tl)) detectors. They are usually placed within thick shields to reduce the intensity of background radiation reaching the detector. Such shields are made of low-activity lead or steel. The shields should be of sufficient size that the detector does not see significant backscattered radiation from the shield and are often lined with a material of medium atomic number, such as copper, to attenuate any fluorescence photons produced in the outer shield (sometimes referred to as the 'step-down' shield). The detector signals are amplified and then fed into sophisticated pulse height analysis systems to ensure that the full details of the detector response function are available for further off-line analysis.

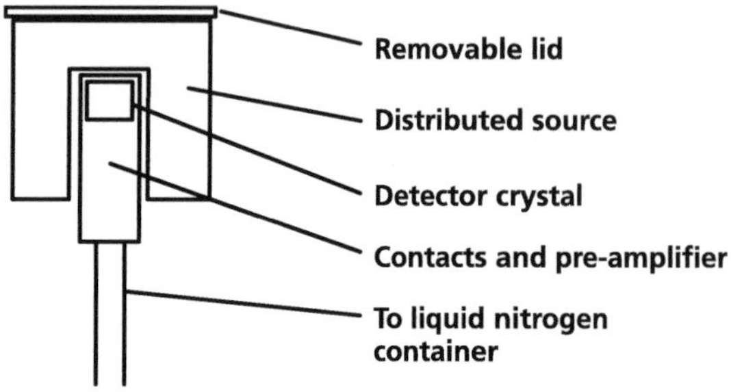

Figure 4.4 HpGe detector with Marinelli Beaker insert.

One of the key requirements for making accurate measurements of any kind is a high degree of consistency between the calibration and measurement conditions. In order to maximize detection efficiency and ensure a reproducible sample geometry, Marinelli beakers (Figure 4.4), which surround the sensitive detector element with the sample, are widely used for measurements of low activities. These are available in a number of sizes to fit a wide range of detectors.

Calibration of a detector system such as this type involves a number of steps:

- Determination of the relationship between pulse height and photon energy
- Determination of the efficiency function for the detector, i.e. detector counts per source emitted photon as a function of energy
- Determination of the resolution function for the detector
- Assessment of the impact of the sample matrix on the detection efficiency function.

In practice, the first three of these can be achieved using a suitably diluted calibration source which can be obtained from a standards laboratory. These are issued in a range of activities and include a number of photon-emitting radionuclides to span the energy range of interest. They are usually delivered in a sealed glass ampoule and need to be appropriately diluted into a volume sufficient for use with the required Marinelli container. The issue of the sample matrix can be addressed with either measurement-based techniques, using a range of practical matrices and calibrated sources, or with Monte Carlo simulation techniques.

The Siemens EPD, a silicon diode-based measuring instrument

The Siemens electronic personal dosemeter (EPD) [10] is widely used for personal monitoring. It uses silicon diode technology and combines many of the advantages of active and passive radiation-monitoring devices. It consists of three diodes with appropriate filter materials to provide some energy selectivity and an array of internal discriminators and counters to provide instantaneous measures of $H_p(10)$ and $H_p(0.07)$ (§8.1.1). The three diodes are used as follows. The first is positioned under a thin window for enhanced β sensitivity, the second under a nickel–aluminium shield for β compensation and detection of soft γ-radiation, and the third under a tin shield for hard γ-ray detection. Each signal is separately amplified and individually counted.

4.11 General detector resolution issues for active detector systems

In radiation protection, it might seem that the pulse height resolution of a detector is of little importance, except for the more obvious cases where full spectrum information is being collected for analysis (§4.10.1). However, the pulse height resolution has a direct effect on the general performance of various instruments. It determines the slope of the plateau on a GM tube (Figure 4.3) and therefore determines the ease with which one can set the operating voltage. It determines the degree to which the true signal is separated from electronic noise in a whole range of detectors and therefore is intimately related to performance at low pulse rates (corresponding to low dose rates or low levels of surface contamination).

There are a range of factors which affect the pulse–height resolution of radiation detectors operated in pulse mode. These are described briefly for each major instrument category. Statistical processes tend to dominate the achievable detector resolution in many situations. However, in the case of both gas and semiconductor detectors, the statistical processes are modified during the initial stages of pulse formation in the detector. These modifications mean that the predicted statistical variance in, for example, the number of ion-pairs produced in a proportional counter is much larger than that which is observed experimentally. The extent of the difference from pure Poisson statistical behaviour involves complex issues and is different for each detector type. This is quantified in the Fano factor for that detector. The Fano factor relates the experimentally observed variance in the number of charge carriers produced in the detector to the variance that is predicted on the basis of pure Poisson statistics. The Poisson statistics themselves are the dominant process in scintillators and Fano factors are close to unity.

The size of the Fano factor varies but guideline values [9] are:

Proportional counters	F 0.05 to 0.2
Semiconductor detectors	F 0.14
Scintillation detectors	F approx. 1.0

The principal factors which determine resolution for different types of detector are as follows:

Gas counters
- statistics of ion-pair formation (*w*-value typically 30 eV)
- charge collection characteristics of detector
- electronic properties of amplification circuits

Scintillators
- statistics of photostimulation
- light transport properties of scintillator and light guide
- statistics of electron production in the photocathode
- statistics of pulse amplification in the photomultiplier
- electronic properties of amplification circuits

Semiconductors
- statistics of electron-hole pair formation
- charge collection characteristics of detectors and impact of leakage currents
- electronic properties of amplification circuits

It is interesting to note the similarities of the items listed for each detector category, and in particular for the gas and semiconductor detectors. The principal reason for the significant difference in resolution for these two kinds of detectors is the energy required to produce a signal. In a gas detector this is principally determined by the energy to produce an electron-ion pair, or the *w*-value for the gas, which is typically of the order of 30 eV. In a semiconductor it is determined by the energy to produce an electron-hole pair in the electronic structure of the detector material which is typically 3–4 eV. (Note that this energy is significantly greater than the band-gap energy between the highest energy of the valence band and the lowest energy of the conduction band.) Since a very significant component of the detector resolution is derived from the statistics of charge formation, the fact that a typical semiconductor detector is able to produce roughly 10 times as many electron-hole pairs as the same radiation energy would produce electron-ion pairs in an ionisation chamber leads to a dramatically improved pulse height resolution.

4.12 Passive measurement systems (film and thermoluminescent dosimetry)

It is impossible to prepare a comprehensive text on radiation measurement systems without some mention of passive detection systems. In this chapter, the fundamentals of film and thermoluminescence (TL) techniques are described and practical examples are given in §8.3.

4.12.1 Film-based dosimetry

Film is an emulsion of gelatine with suspended particles of silver halide (usually AgBr) located on a backing material. When an X-ray falls on the film, a photoelectron or Compton electron is ejected from the atoms in the AgBr. This first-degree process produces second-degree ionisation upon collision with other atoms from the AgBr. The electrons freed by the ionisation process preferentially move into vacancies/imperfect sites in the lattice of the AgBr grains. Here a silver ion is reduced to a silver atom by the process $Ag^+ + e^- \rightarrow Ag$. When at least four neighbouring silver atoms have been formed, there is a 'latent image'. These silver specks catalyse the conversion of the whole AgBr crystal when Ag is subjected to a suitable developer solution. The image is 'fixed' by dissolving the nonionised AgBr grains in a weakly acidic solution of sodium thiosulphate.

The image produced after processing has a variable optical density which is determined by the quantity of converted Ag grains and is therefore dependent on the quantity of radiation which was incident. At low radiation exposures, too few grains of metallic Ag are produced to significantly affect the film density and thus the emulsion is underexposed. Such regions appear white on the developed film. If the radiation exposure is high, the result is a dense concentration of developed grains and a black region is produced on the developed film. Intermediate exposures result in a density that varies approximately linearly with exposure over the normal region of operation.

Radiation dosimetry with film as the sensitive element requires some additional information on the type and energy of radiation which was incident on the film. This can be obtained by placing selected filter materials between the radiation source and the film. In practice, different thicknesses of plastic can be used to provide information on β-particle energy and to discriminate β-particles from low-energy photons, while aluminium, tin, and lead filters in various combinations are often used to provide energy information for incident X- and γ-rays. A common feature of film dosemeters is also the presence of a filter with a high cross-section for (n, γ) reactions at thermal neutron energies. Such filters, often made of cadmium or gadolinium, give the dosemeter the ability for very approximate measurements of the irradiating thermal neutron fluence.

4.12.2 Thermoluminescent dosimetry

Thermoluminscent dosimetry (TLD) is a passive technique which relies on radiation energy being trapped in material which can later be released as visible light by a controlled heating cycle [11]. The electronic band structure model of valence and conduction bands separated by a forbidden energy interval or band gap (Box 4.6) is again necessary for the understanding of thermoluminescence. In the case of TL materials, the forbidden energy interval contains a number of available energy levels provided by trapping centres within the

Box 4.7 TLD: annealing, reading, calibrating

Before TLD materials can be used in dosimetry, they must be annealed to empty the traps of any residual signal. The annealing process has a direct effect on the sensitivity of the material. It should be tightly controlled to keep precision at acceptable levels and be performed in a programmable oven. Before the chips are exposed to radiation, it can be worthwhile stabilizing their behaviour by putting them through the read cycle three times.

The read cycle for TLD materials consists of two or possibly three stages.

- *Preheat phase* designed to depopulate those traps which are not wanted in the glow curve (generally because they are unstable).
- *Read phase* ensures that the material is heated to a temperature above that of all of the desired glow peaks, but not high enough to either destroy the thermoluminescent characteristics of the material or include information from unwanted peaks.
- *Anneal phase* may be incorporated into the read cycle. This is commonly done when TLD-100 is used as a dosimeter in diagnostic radiology. A 400°C post read anneal lasting some 20 seconds is applied and no other anneal performed. This approach will result in reduced precision and accuracy and is not recommended.

The area under the resulting composite glow curve (see Figure 4.5) can be integrated and the radiation dose obtained via a calibration factor. In this case, the influence of background (which is a function of time) should not be ignored, especially at low radiation doses. Alternatively, individual glow curves can be stripped out from the composite curves. This latter approach will result in a lowering of the minimum detectable dose.

The following are recommended anneal and read parameters for TLD-100:

- *Anneal cycle:* Heat from room temperature to 400°C at about ~8°C/min. Maintain at 400°C for 1 h followed by a slow (about ~12°C/min) cool to 75°C which is maintained for 18 h. Run through the read cycle three times to stabilize the response.
- *Read cycle:* Preheat for 20 s at 140°C. Read for 20 s at 250°C.

Calibration

TLDs used for personnel dosimetry are usually calibrated free in air in the field from a suitable γ-ray source (e.g. ^{137}Cs) or, for staff working in diagnostic radiology, an X-ray field. Points to be considered when performing calibrations are:

- The calibration will usually be in terms of air kerma, which should be measured with a standard ionisation chamber that has a calibration traceable to a primary standard.
- The TLDs should be supported in a manner that will minimize scatter, such as on a membrane.
- The TLDs should be located as far as practicable from other objects in the radiation field which might give rise to scatter.
- A standard geometry and configuration is recommended to ensure that the required accuracy is achieved.
- If a large number of TLDs are to be irradiated at the same time, the source to dosimeter distance should be large enough to reduce the variation in dose to the required level.

Factors are available to convert from air kerma to personal dose equivalent, $H_p(d)$, at different tissue depths d (§8.1.1) [2, 12].

For TLD measurements of patient dose in radiology, information on levels of accuracy required can be found in the UK national protocol [13]. For this application, the calibration may be performed either 'free in air' as already described or on top of a tissue-equivalent scatter medium. The method using a phantom will include backscatter and here the TLD readout should be compared with a measurement of phantom entrance dose made with the ionisation chamber placed in the beam in contact with the phantom to include backscatter. Calibrations for patient dosimetry should be performed:

- by placing the TLDs at the centre of an X-ray field, which is at least 100 mm × 100 mm
- using a radiation dose similar in magnitude to the doses to be measured
- using a representative kVp and beam quality
- if a phantom is used, this should be at least 100 mm thick and have an area larger than the X-ray field.

Box 4.7 *(continued)*

The TLD response varies over the diagnostic X-ray energy range (e.g. Figure 2.10), but because of the broad spectrum of photon energies within an X-ray beam, the difference between energy absorbed in TLD and that in air or tissue over the diagnostic X-ray energy range 60 to 120 kV is only 8–10%. Thus a broad-brush approach to X-ray calibration with a representative kVp and beam quality is sufficiently accurate for most purposes. However, average ratios for the mass energy absorption coefficients for LiF, air, and tissue are given in Table 2.1, which may be used to correct calibration data if greater accuracy for varying X-ray spectra is required.

Type	Materials	Dosimetry applications	Zeff	Sensitivity at ^{60}Co relative to LiF	Energy response 30 keV/^{60}Co
TLD-100	Lithium fluoride LiF:Mg,Ti	Health and medical physics	8.2	1.0	1.25
TLD-100H	Lithium fluoride LiF:Mg,Cu,P	Environmental, Personnel, Extremity	8.2	15	0.98
TLD-200	Calcium fluoride Dysprosium CaF_2:Dy	Environmental	16.3	30 at 5765 Å	~12.5
TLD-800	Lithium borate Manganese $Li_2B_4O_7$:Mn	High-range dosimetry	7.4	0.15	0.9
TLD-900	Calcium sulphate	Environmental	15.5	20	12.5

Type	Useful range	Fading	Temperature of main TL glow peak
TLD-100	50 μGy–10^3 Gy	5%/year at 20°C corrected	195°C
TLD-100H	1 μGy–10 Gy	Negligible	225°C
TLD-200	0.1 μGy–10 Gy	10% in first 24 h 16% total in 2 weeks	180°C
TLD-800	0.5 mGy–10^5 Gy	< 5% in 3 months	210°C
TLD-900	1 μGy–100 Gy	2% in 1 month	

The lower limit for TLD-100 can be reduced to between 10 and 20 μGy if stringent annealing procedures are used in conjunction with glow curve deconvolution techniques (Burke and Sutton, 1997). [14]

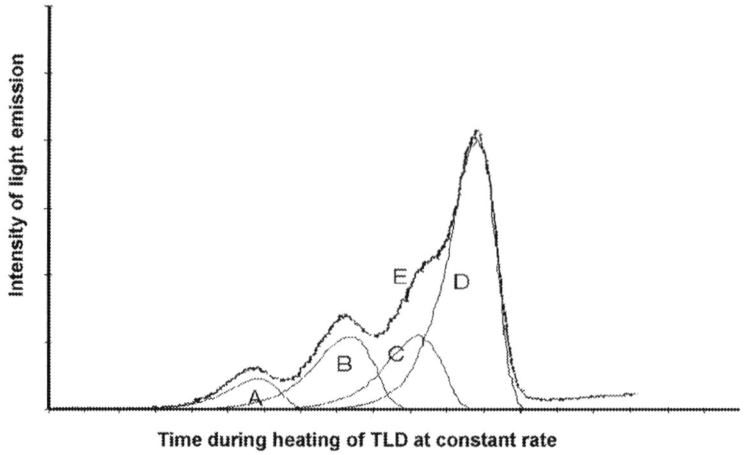

Figure 4.5 Composite glow curve for TLD (LiF: Mg, Ti). The four glow peaks at 386 K (A), 426 K (B), 458 K (C), and 481 K (D) combine to form the composite curve E. Curve E is a measured curve obtained by heating using a temperature profile that varies linearly with time. The heating rate will affect the resolution of the individual peaks. A, B, C, and D were obtained using glow curve deconvolution techniques.

material. These trapping centres may be provided by the addition of impurities (termed activators) or may result from the naturally occurring impurity levels and defects in the crystal.

The radiation sensitivity of a TL material varies with both the atomic number (due to increased photon interactions) and the energy of the trapping centres. For materials with relatively shallow traps, a large number will be populated by only a small radiation exposure leading to high radiation sensitivity and low minimum detectable dose. However, there will be an increased possibility of thermally induced depopulation of the traps, and therefore 'fading' of the radiation-induced signal.

The characteristic 'glow curve' of a TL material is produced by a controlled increase in temperature across a range which is determined by the trap-depths within the material. As the temperature increases, traps of different depths may be depopulated by providing sufficient energy for the electrons to jump back into the conduction band. From here they de-excite by emission of a visible photon which can be measured using a photomultiplier tube (PMT) system. The number of glow peaks and their properties depend on the material being used; for example, TLD-100 has seven glow peaks under 300°C, all of which have different half-lives. A typical glow curve for TLD-100 is shown in Figure 4.5. The complete TL readout system consists of the following parts: a heater, a light measurement system (a PMT) in a light-tight enclosure, a mechanism for introducing the TL dosemeter into the reader, and computer hardware and software to control the readout process and calculate the resultant doses.

To gain consistent and reliable results, the heating cycle that the dosemeter experiences must be reproducible (Box 4.7). Various methods of heating are available.

- *Contact heating*. This is the most common method. The dosemeter is mounted in a tray or holder and a large current is passed through a small strip of metal which is brought into contact with the tray. This method is simple and can be accurately controlled by using a thermocouple but it is dependent on reproducible thermal contact between the heater and the tray. Alternatively, a large block of material maintained at a set temperature can be brought into contact with the dosemeter.
- *Hot gas heating*. The dosemeter is removed from any holder/card and held by a vacuum needle or other support in a flow of hot nitrogen gas (or another inert gas). Heating by this method is more rapid than contact heating thus enabling faster readout times.
- *Optical heating*. It is possible to use lasers or a focused infrared bulb to heat the dosemeter. The various stages of the readout cycle (preheat, read, and anneal) are obtained by pulsing the light beam. Very high heating rates can be achieved using lasers but the system is more expensive and bulkier.

The sensitivity of the PMT will vary as the voltage applied to it varies. A consistent response is maintained by measuring the light from an internal stable light source at regular intervals (e.g. after each complete readout cycle). The light reading is used to automatically adjust the PMT supply voltage as required.

Box 4.8 Calibration of contamination monitors

In order to define a test for contamination monitors which is reproducible from year to year, it is necessary to use radiation sources which can be well characterized; that is for which maintenance of a stable radiation emission over time has been considered by the manufacturer and which can be monitored by regular calibration of the sources themselves. The construction of such sources is a highly specialized process, involving the deposition of a uniform active source layer over a large area (usually at least 100 cm^2) onto a rigid substrate and then sealing under an impermeable membrane and in some cases an additional filter [17] to ensure that only the radiation of interest impinges the detector. It is therefore not sufficient to use the known activity deposited on the source as a measure of the radiation that the source will emit from its surface, since this will not allow for any attenuation in the source layer itself or the membrane/filter, or any additional scatter from the substrate. This 'surface emission rate' must be measured directly, usually making use of a gas-flow proportional counter into which the source can be placed. This task is generally within the sphere of expertise of primary standards laboratories which are also able to make a proper estimate of the measurement uncertainties associated with the final measurement on each source.

Using a variety of suitably calibrated large-area sources for probes which are smaller than the source area, a calibration can be fairly easily achieved at a range of incident energies and radiation types [16]. There are additional requirements for calibration of larger-area probes [18]. The annual instrument test would also include a test of the linearity of the instrument reading to changes in incident radiation intensity throughout the working range, a light leakage test (for scintillation probes), and for the first use of large-area detectors, some assessment of the spatial uniformity of the detector response.

The calibration factors derived by such 'surface emission rate' calibrations are not directly useful for the routine operation of the instrument. Their purpose is to ensure that the instrument is performing as intended by the manufacturer. Once this has been established, the calibration factors for commonly encountered radionuclides are generally available from the manual of the instrument. However, it is also possible to use the surface emission rate calibration data to derive more useful figures such as the instrument response for a particular radionuclide (in terms of instrument counts per second [cps] per Bq cm^{-2}). In this respect, one calibration which is commonly undertaken does tend to cause confusion. This involves the use of a filtered ^{129}I source as a 'mock' ^{125}I source. The use of the term 'mock' in this case does not mean that response figures derived at calibration are directly applicable to use for ^{125}I. In fact the process is as follows.

Ignoring any changes in spectrum of the photons emitted by the source as a result of the presence of the filter [17]:

1. At the annual calibration, derive a calibration factor for ^{129}I in terms of surface emission rate. For a Mini 44A (§4.9.5) probe this would typically be 0.12 emissions s^{-1} cm^{-2} per instrument reading.
2. Convert this to a response in terms of instrument reading (Bq $cm^{-2})^{-1}$ for either ^{129}I or ^{125}I.

For ^{129}I, the figure for total photon emissions per Bq (branching ratio) is approximately 78%, while for ^{125}I the corresponding figure is 144%.

If R = instrument response (in cps (Bq $cm^{-2})^{-1}$)
S = calibration factor (in emissions s^{-1} cm^{-2} cps^{-1})
P = geometrical factor (taken to be 2 here)
BR = branching ratio (conversion from emissions to Bq)

Then $$R = \frac{BR}{S \times P}$$

Hence for ^{129}I, $R = 3.25$ cps (Bq $cm^{-2})^{-1}$, while for ^{125}I, $R = 6$ cps (Bq $cm^{-2})^{-1}$. Hence it is clear that while the calibration factor which relates the instrument reading to emissions from the source is assumed to be the same, the instrument response per unit activity is quite different for these two radionuclides.

In addition, there are factors related to the surface on which activity has been spilled which should also be considered before making an estimate of activity from the readings of hand-held surface contamination monitors. These relate principally to the absorption characteristics of the surface, the type and energy of the emissions from the source, and the energy response characteristics of the monitor. These factors are discussed in greater detail in [19].

4.13 Issues in practical measurements

There are a few simple rules which govern the making of reliable radiation measurements. Although most appear to be obvious, they are worth stating since failure to follow one or more of these basic guidelines often compromises the utility of field radiation measurements.

- Understand the measuring device (principally in terms of its energy and count-rate response).
- Check that the measuring device is stable (over time).
- Make sure any calibration factors apply in the field. If they do not, derive some which do apply, and understand the uncertainties involved in doing so.
- Make sure that critical influence quantities are identified and controlled where possible.
- Make repeat measurements where possible.
- Vary the measurement conditions in a controlled way to see how the measured result is affected.
- Make a statement of the measured result with an unambiguous statement of uncertainty.

All of the above steps can also contribute to the estimation of uncertainties in the measurement. The estimation of uncertainty should be followed through rigorously if a proper understanding of the measurement is to be obtained. Standard guidance on how uncertainty components should be combined has been issued by the UK Accreditation Service [15].

4.14 Annual instrument tests

One of the situations where a full uncertainty analysis is necessary is during the annual test or calibration of a radiation protection instrument. This activity is usually performed by a recognized calibration laboratory which, under UK regulations, must come under the direction of a 'qualified person'. Measurements for calibration require a high degree of metrological accuracy which must sometimes be achieved at the expense of providing an accurate simulation of the field conditions under which the instrument may be routinely used.

The purpose of an annual instrument test, as required by UK regulations for certain categories of instrument, is to ensure that the instrument is performing in the manner intended by the manufacturer and that its performance is stable from year to year. The complementary task of ensuring that what the manufacturer intends is sensible in the context of the measurements to be made in the field generally requires the involvement of a radiation protection adviser, who may examine the results of annual instrument tests and the data contained in the 'Type Test' report for the instrument model.

For the UK, the latest guidance on good practice for laboratories undertaking calibrations of instruments for measuring both dose rate and contamination levels is described by NPL [16]. Perhaps the most confusion arises in the annual testing of contamination monitors, where sources are characterized by their 'surface emission rate' rather than the activity of the radionuclide which they contain. This quantity, as well as the application of calibration factors derived during the annual test to everyday measurement situations, is discussed in Box 4.8.

4.15 References

1 International Commission on Radiological Units and Measurements (1985). *Determination of dose equivalents resulting from external radiation sources.* ICRU Report 39. ICRU, Bethesda, MD.

2 International Commission on Radiological Protection (1996). Conversion coefficients for use in radiological protection against external radiation. ICRP Report 74. *Ann. ICRP*, **26**.

3 Burgess, P. (2001). *Guidance on the choice, use and maintenance of hand-held radiation monitoring equipment.* NRPB Report R326. NRPB, Chilton.

4 US Nuclear Regulatory Commission (NUREG-1507). www.nrc.gov.

5 International Organization for Standardization (1993). *Quality assurance requirements for measuring equipment–Part 1: Metrological conformation system for measuring equipment.* ISO-10012-1.

6 Rossi, H. H. and Zaider, M. (1996). *Microdosimetry and its applications.* Springer-Verlag, Heidelberg.

7 Centronic Ltd. (1997) *Geiger Mueller tubes data book.* Centronic Ltd, King Henry's Drive, New Addinton, Croydon CR9 OBG, UK.

8 International Electrotechnical Commission. (Original 1989, Edition 2.0 in preparation) *Radiation protection instrumentation–ambient and/or directional dose equivalent (rate) meters and/or monitors for β-, X- and γ-radiation.* IEC 60846. (In preparation.)

9 Knoll, G. F. (1989). *Radiation detection and measurement* (2nd edn). Wiley.

10 Siemens, E. P. D. (1995). Improvements in or relating to personal radiation dose indicators. UK Patent GB 2 255 177 B.

11 McKinlay, A. F. (1981). *Thermoluminescence dosimetry.* Medical Physics Handbook 5. Adam Hilger, Bristol.

12 International Organization for Standardization (1999). *X- and γ-reference radiation for calibrating dosemeters and dose rate meters and for determining their response as a function of photon energy–Part 3: Calibration of area and personal dosemeters and the measurement of their response as a function of energy and angle of incidence.* ISO 4037-3.

13 Institute of Physical Scientists in Medicine/National Radiological Protection Board/College of Radiographers (1992). *National protocol for patient dose measurements in diagnostic radiology.* NRPB, Chilton.

14 Burke, K. and Sutton, D. G. (1997) Optimisation and deconvolution of lithium fluoride TLD-100 in diagnostic radiology. *Br. J. Radiol.* **70**, 261–71.

15 National Physical Laboratory (1995). NIS3003. *The expression of uncertainty and confidence in measurement for calibrations.* NAMAS Executive, NPL, Teddington, Middlesex, UK.

16 National Physical Laboratory (1999). GPG 14. *The examination, testing and calibration of portable radiation protection instruments.* Measurement Good Practice Guide 14. NPL, Teddington, UK.

17 International Organization for Standardization (1996). *Reference sources for the calibration of surface contamination monitors–Part 2: electrons of energy less than 0.15 MeV and photons of energy less than 1.5 MeV.* ISO 8769-2.

18 Scott, C. J., Woods, M. J., and Keightley, J. D. (1997). *The use of relatively small sources for the calibration of area survey meters.* NPL Report CIRM 6.

19 Green, S., Peach, D., Palethorpe, J., Anderson, P., Nightingale, A., and Bradley, D. A. (1999). The monitoring of contaminated impervious planar surfaces. *J. Radiol. Prot.*, **19**, 45–9.

4.16 Useful websites

Standards laboratories

National Physical Laboratory, NPL	www.npl.co.uk
National Institute of Standards and Technology, NIST	www.nist.gov
Physikalish-Technische Budesanstalt, PTB	www.ptb.de
Bureau International des Poids et Mesures (BIPM)	www.bipm.fr
National organizations US Nuclear Regulatory Commission	www.nrc.gov
National Radiological Protection Board	www.nrpb.org.uk

Part II

Protection against ionising radiations

The principles of radiation protection practice have evolved gradually with time. Standards have been developed through international organizations, which have then been incorporated into national legislation. Chapter 5 examines aspects of this process and outlines how radiation protection practices and legislation have been implemented in different parts of the world. The principles of current radiation protection thinking are outlined in Chapter 6 and their implementation is discussed in Chapter 7, together with practical principles for dealing with different types of hazard. The next two chapters deal with specialist aspects of radiation protection, namely techniques for monitoring the radiation exposure of personnel (Chapter 8) and methods applied to control the use, disposal, and transport of radioactive materials (Chapter 9). Radiation protection practitioners in healthcare may also be called upon to deal with radiation exposures from sources outside hospitals in the event of an incident, and the range of sources, both natural and man-made, and practical methods for dealing with emergencies are covered in Chapter 10.

Symbols

absorbed dose rate from external radiation	D_{ext} (Gy h^{-1})
absorbed external dose rate from cloud	D_{cloud} [Gy h^{-1} year^{-1})
air kerma rate	K_{air} (dK_{air}/dt) (mGy h^{-1})
air kerma rate constant	Γ(mGy h^{-1} MBq^{-1} m^2)
annual consumption of food, e.g. fish	M_{food}, M_{fish} (kg year^{-1})
annual consumption of water	M_{water} (m^3 year^{-1})
atomic number	Z
atomic number (effective value for mixture of atoms)	Z_{eff}
build-up factor	B
committed effective dose	$E(50)$ (Sv)
committed effective dose (ingestion/inhalation)	E_{ing}/E_{inh} (Sv)
committed effective dose coefficient	$e(50)$ (Sv Bq^{-1})
committed effective dose coefficient from ingestion	D_{ing} (Sv Bq^{-1})
committed effective dose coefficient from inhalation	D_{inh} (Sv Bq^{-1})
committed equivalent dose to tissue T (ICRP)	$H_T(50)$ (Sv)
concentration factor for radioactivity in medium	k_{medium} [Bq kg^{-1} (Bq m^{-3})$^{-1}$]
concentration of radioactivity in liquid	C_{vol} (Bq m^{-3})
concentration of radioactivity in solid	C_{wt} (Bq kg^{-1})
concentration of radioactivity along pipe	C_L (Bq m^{-1})
concentration of radioactivity in plume	C_{plume} (Bq m^{-3})
cumulative activity (with/without excretion)	A_s/A_n (Bq h)
decay constants (physical/ biological/effective)	$\lambda_{phys}/\lambda_{biol}/\lambda_{eff}$ (time^{-1})
density	ρ (kg m^{-3})
diameter of source	$2h$ (m)
discharge rate of gaseous radionuclide	R (Bq s^{-1})
distance from source	r (m)
distance/depth travelled through medium	d (m)
effective atomic number	Z_{eff}
effective dose	E (Sv)
effective dose from external radiation	E_{ext} (Sv)
energy	E (eV)

energy of β-particles (maximum for transition)	E_β (eV)
energies of photons weighted sum from radionuclide	E_{output} (eV)
equivalent dose to tissue T (ICRP)	H_T (Sv)
equivalent dose (true) (other positions)	H_t (H_N, H_W) (Sv)
fluence	φ (m^{-2})
food transfer factor (air deposition to food)	T [Bq kg^{-1} (Bq m^{-2} $s^{-1})^{-1}$]
food concentration factor (air) for ^{14}C and ^{3}H	T^* (Bq kg^{-1} {Bq m^{-2} $s^{-1}\}^{-1}$)
fraction of disintegrations emitting radiation	F
half-life (biological excretion)	T_{biol} (years, days, h)
half-life (effective)	T_{eff} (year, days, h)
half-life (radioactive decay)	$T_{1/2}$ (year, days, h)
half-thickness for βs	$D_{1/2}$ (mg cm^{-2})
intake of radioactivity	I (Bq)
intake rate for liquid release (ingestion/inhalation)	I_{ing} (kg h^{-1})/I_{inh} (m^3 $year^{-1}$)
intake rate by inhalation for gaseous release	I_{atmos} (m^3 $year^{-1}$)
internal bremsstrahlung factor	I
mass attenuation coefficient	μ/ρ (kg^{-1} m^2)
mass energy absorption coefficient	μ_{en}/ρ (kg^{-1} m^2)
occupancy	O (h $year^{-1}$)
personal dose equivalent (depth d) (ICRU)	$H_p(d)$
proportion of activity excreted	p_1, p_2
radionuclide activity/administered activity	A (Bq)/A_o (Bq)
radionuclide activity in body at time t	m(t) (Bq per Bq intake)
radionuclide activity in body (measured)	M (Bq)
range of particle in medium	R (mm) or (mg cm^{-2})
time	t (h)
tissue weighting factor	w_T, $w_{remainder}$
transmission	B
volume flow rates	V (m^3 d^{-1})

Chapter 5
Ionising radiation legislation

P. Allisy-Roberts and C. J. Martin

5.1 International basis for legislation

5.1.1 Historical background

Following the discoveries of X-rays (1895) by Wilhelm C. Roentgen and radioactivity (1896) by Henri Becquerel, radiation protection at the beginning of the twentieth century was based on the experience of individual practitioners. Those who had already suffered erythema or had produced burns on their patients took extra care to protect themselves and others with the basic tenets of shielding, distance, and time embodied in 'local rules'. However, it was not until the advent of international agreement on radiation units through the establishment of the International Commission on Radiation Units and Measurements (ICRU) in 1925 (http://www.icru.org/) that radiation protection had a foundation in dosimetry. Since that time, radiation dose limits have been reduced gradually and if the original units are converted to the SI system and the doses extrapolated from a week to one year, one finds that the 'tolerance dose' in 1925 was effectively 600 mSv, 30 times the present limit (Table 5.1).

The International Commission for Radiological Protection (ICRP), sister commission to the ICRU, can be traced back to 1928, having been set up by the International Congress of Radiology at its meeting in Stockholm (http://www.icrp.org). The task given to the ICRP was to advise on the measures deemed necessary for protection against the damaging effects of the use of X-rays and radium. The original recommendations of this body and the consequent regulations on dose limitation issued by various countries were based on the three principles of shielding, distance, and time to minimize the dose, together with an upper limit of dose to avoid somatic effects in the individuals exposed. Although the recommended dose limits have reduced with time (Table 5.1), the basic principles of radiation protection are still valid. The basis of the dose limits has changed with time, the original limits being based on avoiding erythema doses whereas modern limits are based on minimizing the risk of cancer induction. The ICRP recommendations have evolved throughout its history but have, since the early 1970s, based the concept of dose limitation on a risk-based analysis [1].

The ICRP developed the concepts of

- justification of the use of any radiation which results in exposures
- optimisation of exposures (the ALARA principle, 'as low as reasonably achievable')
- and limitation of exposures

in their recommendations made in 1977 (ICRP 26) [1]. These concepts are already familiar in litigation over medical radiation incidents and the ideas are more fully exploited in ICRP 60 [2], in which risked-based limits are developed. The system of protection for 'practices',

Table 5.1 Recommended whole-body dose limits throughout the years

Year	Limit	Equivalent value in mSv	Recommended for the reduction of
1925	Tolerance	600	erythema
1934	ICRP	500	immediate effects (individual)
1950 (post-war)	ICRP	150	somatic effects
1977	ICRP	50	genetic effects (population risk)
1990	ICRP	20	stochastic effects (cancer risk)
2005	ICRP	20?	individual risk (cancer)

including justification, optimisation, and dose limitation, has been extended to include 'medical exposures' and 'potential exposures'. The concept of 'interventions' has been introduced concerning not only accidents but also situations such as those where exposure to radiation from natural sources, e.g. radon (§10.3), is enhanced. These now form the recommendations on which almost all countries base their legislation. The ideas of the ICRP continue to evolve and discussion currently concerns a possible simplification of the overall system of protection to make it all-embracing rather than selective.

ICRP has working committees in addition to the main Commission and it is the committees which produce the scientific and philosophical reports from which the main Commission chooses its recommendations. There are four committees which deal with different areas (see http://www.icrp.org):

- Committee 1—the biological and other effects of ionising radiation
- Committee 2—the doses from radiation exposures
- Committee 3—radiation protection needs in medicine
- Committee 4—occupational exposures and the general application of ICRP recommendations.

5.1.2 International cooperation on basic safety standards

Implementing safety standards internationally is not a simple process. The International Atomic Energy Agency (IAEA) (http://www.iaea.org/worldatom/) with 130 member states has a major interest in having common standards worldwide. Indeed it is in all our interests that radiation protection is maintained at the same high standard everywhere. Unfortunately this is not yet the case, but six major international organizations (FAO, IAEA, ILO, OECD/NEA, PAHO, and WHO) have collaborated very effectively to produce the International Basic Safety Standards (BSS) [3] on which every country can base its national radiation protection legislation.

The BSS draw heavily on the recommendations of ICRP 60 [2] and are being implemented in many countries worldwide. They cover basic radiation protection for workers and the public, safety of radioactive sources and some radiation protection concerning the patient, including diagnostic reference levels. Although the member states which are signatories to the IAEA statute have no legal obligation to comply with the International BSS, failure to implement appropriate radiation protection legislation can result in the IAEA withdrawing support for projects concerning the peaceful use of radiation, such as for medical diagnosis and treatment facilities, being supplied in the member state concerned. Indeed many members states have specific agreements with the IAEA concerning support projects and the necessary radiation protection for these.

The IAEA also produces recommendations in the form of Safety Series of which the Regulations for the Safe Transport of Radioactive Materials [4] are followed almost worldwide. The IAEA General Conference in 2000 adopted a resolution that encouraged all member states to bring their national regulatory documents into conformity with these regulations. The IAEA also intends to review its regulations every two years and to revise its standards as appropriate.

Working in close collaboration with the IAEA is the Organization for Economic Development (OECD) within which the semi-autonomous body, the Nuclear Energy Agency (NEA) (http://nea.net.fr) established in 1958 and now consisting of 27 OECD member countries, has the particular interest regarding nuclear energy and safety. The mission of the NEA includes assisting its member countries in developing and maintaining the legal basis for the safe and environmentally friendly use of nuclear energy for peaceful purposes. In particular, they advise on safety and regulation of nuclear activities, maintain a databank of nuclear data and computer programs, and publish a journal of *Nuclear Law*. In this way, each country can identify how international recommendations are being incorporated into their national legislation with case law examples.

It is worth noting that according to the World Health Organization (WHO), more than two-thirds of the world's population have no access to radiation medicine services. Accessibility and quality of radiation medicine need to be substantially improved worldwide because they are an important part of successful medical treatment. The WHO programme in radiation medicine (RAD) aims to improve access to diagnostic imaging and therapeutic radiological services while maintaining quality and safety through support to countries by:

- development of guidelines and standards
- giving advice on adequate and safe use of radiation medicine technology
- giving advice on training and education
- giving advice on quality assurance and safety
- giving advice on further development of radiation medicine services.

5.1.3 International Radiation Protection Association

The International Radiation Protection Association (IRPA) is a worldwide organization with membership comprising individuals who themselves are members of an affiliated national or regional associate society. Only one associate society is accepted per country and IRPA currently has members in 48 countries (http://www.irpa.net/).

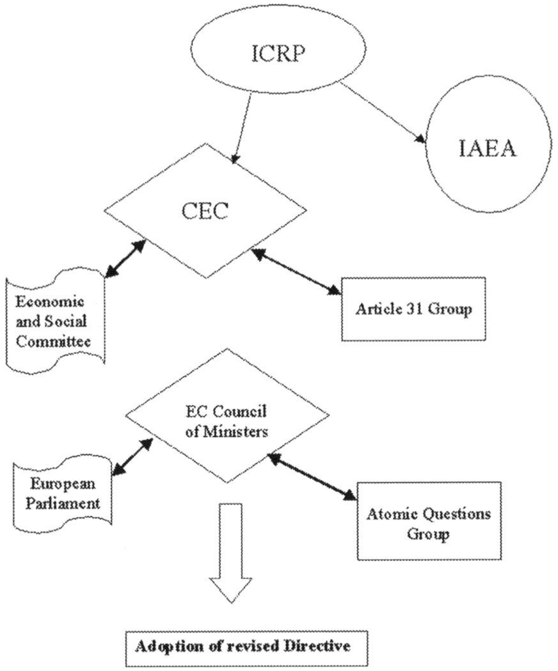

Figure 5.1 European framework for radiation protection legislation.

The primary purpose of IRPA is to provide a medium whereby those engaged in radiation protection activities in all countries may communicate more readily with each other and through this process advance radiation protection in many parts of the world. This includes relevant aspects of such branches of knowledge as science, medicine, engineering, technology and law, to provide for the protection of man and his environment from the hazards caused by radiation, and thereby to facilitate the safe use of medical, scientific, and industrial radiological practices for the benefit of mankind.

5.2 Foundation for European legislation

5.2.1 The formulation of Euratom directives

New recommendations of the ICRP produce a strong impetus for the European Commission to revise its legislation on radiation protection. Revisions are enacted through Euratom directives under the auspices of the Euratom Treaty.

In 1991, the ICRP published general recommendations in ICRP 60 [2], updating their previous general recommendations ICRP 26 of 1977 [1]. Since its publication, ICRP 60 has been considered within the European frame and new directives have been negotiated to include the latest concepts. There are two fundamental directives in force currently in Europe concerning radiation protection. Staff and public (environmental) protection is covered by a BSS directive, 96/29/Euratom [5], the previous version of which was enacted in 1980 [6, 7] and followed the recommendations in ICRP 26 [1], while the adequate protection of patients and others undergoing medical exposures is covered by the Medical Exposures Directive, 97/43/Euratom [8], which replaced the first such European directive dating from 1984 [9].

The amendment of European radiation protection legislation can be a long and complex process involving a number of defined stages (Figure 5.1). Reasons to change legislation are usually based on external influences, principally the ICRP recommendations. Changes also occur on other international levels; for example, the International BSS mentioned earlier [3] were in fact published before these European directives and several of the participants in the discussions were the same which helped to have some commonality internationally.

Any new international recommendations are considered by a group of experts (under Article 31 of the Euratom Treaty) who advise the European Commission as to whether amendments to European legislation are necessary to comply with the recommendations. The aim of any such changes should of course be to improve occupational, public, and patient protection during the medical diagnostic and therapeutic uses of ionising radiation.

Article 31 Group and European directives

The group of scientific experts in public health referred to in Article 31 of the Euratom Treaty (Article 31 Group) and appointed by the member states of the European Union (EU) advises the European Commission on matters concerning radiation protection within the EU. In 1993, the Article 31 Group proposed revisions to the 1980 BSS directive to take into account the recommendations of ICRP 60. Their proposal was amended on its journey through the European legal process and was finally approved in 1997. The corresponding UK legislation was enacted in 1999. To understand the general legislative process, one can take as an example the adoption of the Medical Exposures Directive.

5.2.2 The Medical Exposures Directive

In 1994, the Article 31 Group set up a working party on medical exposures which had as its members, radiation physicists and medical practitioners from radiotherapy, nuclear medicine, and radiology. They were asked to review the previous directive on patient protection and the

Box 5.1 The content of the Medical Exposures Directive

Although the general recommendations of ICRP 60, where they relate to medical exposures, had been taken into account during the discussions by the Article 31 Group, other ICRP publications relating to medical exposures have obviously influenced the outcome of the proposals for revision which produced the new Medical Exposures Directive (MED). One consequence of this is that the MED has been enlarged in scope since previous legislation to include both volunteers in research and individuals, such as close family or friends, helping voluntarily in the support and comfort of patients (often referred to as comforters and carers).

The earlier 1984 directive [9] had already incorporated the principles of justification and optimisation as they relate to medical exposures. The new MED has several specific requirements which reinforce these concepts, such as referral criteria and the use of reference levels for medical diagnostic exposures. There is published evidence that by applying the principles of justification and optimisation, exposures can be reduced in a cost-effective manner without losing the efficacy of the related practice [12,13].

The concept of potential exposures to patients, together with the requirement of keeping their probability and magnitude as low as reasonably achievable, is specifically included in the MED.

An important requirement of the previous directive is that any use of ionising radiation in medical procedures is effected under the responsibility of a practitioner (this term being clearly defined within the directive as relating to medical, dental, or other health professional entitled to take clinical responsibility within their member state). The current MED requires that the overall responsibility remains with the practitioner but to provide support to the practitioner, practical aspects of the medical procedure can be delegated to other individuals as authorized by the competent national authorities. Interestingly, in member states other than the UK, the 'practitioner' is interpreted as being medically qualified. The requirements for the training of practitioners and these other individuals (interpreted in UK law as 'operators') are now explicit, including continuing education and training, which should lead to improvements in practice.

The MED expands the existing requirements on quality control of radiological installations and supplements them by requiring the establishment of quality assurance programmes which also include assessment of doses received by patients. Such programmes [13] have been demonstrated to reduce individual exposures [14]. Health and safety requirements that include radiation protection aspects regarding the design, manufacture, and placing on the market of the medical devices used are in fact covered by another council directive: 93/42/EEC concerning medical devices [15].

Special requirements have been included for subsets of individuals who are deemed to be at particular risk from radiation exposure. These include paediatric patients, asymptomatic individuals entering health screening programmes, patients undergoing interventional radiology or high exposure studies such as computed tomography, pregnant patients, breastfeeding patients (and their infants), and comforters and carers.

In the last part of the MED, to monitor progress, member states are requested to ensure the establishment of processes for auditing the implementation of the requirements of the directive, and to make estimates of individual and collective doses from the various medical practices.

experience gained in its implementation in the member states. The working party considered the developments in the medical uses of ionising radiation, the progress in radiation protection epitomized by the recommendations of ICRP, and relevant aspects of the then proposed BSS directive. The outcome of this work was a revised patient protection directive which was then discussed and revised by the full Article 31 Group (see Box 5.1).

The final opinion of the Article 31 Group supporting this revision of the previous patient protection directive was reached at a meeting on 31 May 1995. This revised directive on 'health protection of individuals against the dangers of ionising radiation in relation to medical exposures' (hereafter referred to as the Medical Exposures Directive or MED) was submitted in Autumn 1996 to the European Commission for adoption. The MED then went to the Economic and Social Committee of the EU (which is the procedure laid down by Article 31) in April 1996. The following summer it was introduced to the European Council who then sought the opinion of the European Parliament in the winter of 1996. The new directive was finally adopted by the European Council the following summer in July 1997.

Each member state in the EU then has a given period, of for example two years, to produce enacting legislation to implement the directive. In the UK this required revision to the regulations on patient protection [10] which were enacted in 2000 [11].

The protection of workers, including medical and paramedical staff, and of members of the public such as visitors to medical centres, is not affected by the directive on medical exposures but is ensured by the BSS directive [8].

It is perhaps not surprising that the recommendations of the ICRP were incorporated into European legislation comparatively quickly. On the Article 31 Group at the time, there were three members of ICRP Committee 3 (all of whom were members of the medical exposures working party), members of the three other ICRP committees, and the chairman of the main Commission. All the members of the Article 31 Group either work directly with radiation (necessarily not just in the medical field) or have a role in radiation protection in their member state.

ICRP Committee 3 (medical radiation) is currently producing reports on the practical aspects of implementing the ICRP recommendations. These are being designed to help, not just the legislators and practitioners within European member states but also those in every country worldwide, to apply the principles of radiation protection every day as a natural extension of their medical radiation practices.

The objective of the 1984 Euratom directive [9] on patient protection was to reduce medical radiation exposures to the population without jeopardizing the benefits, whether these were early recognition of disease, diagnosis, or therapy. With the continuing expansion of medical practices using ionising radiation, measures need to be taken to reduce individual exposures so that collective effective dose is limited. The 1997 MED [8] maintains the previous objective and provides further detail, founded on practical experience and ICRP reports, as a base for European member states to develop their own legislation. This should result in improved use of radiological practices so that the population can continue to receive the benefits of medical exposures while the collective effective dose is better controlled.

5.3 UK legislation in practice

5.3.1 Development of UK legislation

Before radiation protection legislation in the UK covered medical practices, a voluntary code of practice, first published in 1957, was used in hospitals. This voluntary code was revised, still as a voluntary code, in 1972 and was finally replaced in 1988 with Guidance Notes after new, all-embracing legislation was enacted in 1985 and 1988. With this evolution from a voluntary code to compulsory regulations has grown a continuing awareness of radiation protection needs and a growing desire to be involved with the legislative process so that it is 'user-friendly'.

The Health and Safety Executive (HSE), which is responsible for drawing up the appropriate legislation for the UK government, formed an Advisory Committee in 1995, the Ionising Radiations Advisory Committee (IRAC) which grew out of a working group on ionising radiation which it had previously set up in 1986 to consider the implementation of the regulations. The HSE uses IRAC (which has members from the Confederation of British Industry (CBI), the Trades Union Congress (TUC), various governments departments, six 'independent' scientists, and a 'member of the public') to test draft regulations and guidance before issuing them formally for public consultation.

Consequently, the UK legislation which has been developed as a result of the Euratom directives subsequent to ICRP 60 was the subject of open discussion and debate to ensure its practicability before being enacted by parliament in 1999. Other government departments such as health, environment, and transport, which are responsible for different aspects of radiation protection legislation, are also 'open' to comment during the drafting process. As a result of such open practices, legislation in the UK is often used as an example in other countries of how to proceed and the guidance produced by professional groups is often cited as 'good practice'.

5.3.2 UK regulations

UK national regulations are produced under the auspices of the HSE, the Environment Agency and the government departments responsible for the environment, transport, and health (Box 5.2). Each of these bodies has a different interest and, even with some overlap of committee membership and the use of open consultation processes, national consistency is not always easy to achieve across the different sectors. However, to implement the various European Council (Euratom) directives (http://europa.eu.int/comm/environment/radprot/), the UK has enacted the regulations listed in Box 5.2, all of which concern work in clinical areas, under various Acts of Parliament.

The BSS directive 96/29/Euratom [5] is implemented in the main by the Ionising Radiations Regulations. This covers the radiation protection and dose limitation of people who are occupationally exposed to radiation, in whatever 'industry' they work, the radiation protection of members of the public who are exposed by the 'industry', the safe use of radioactive materials, and the general requirements regarding transport and disposal of radioactive materials. These latter aspects are covered in detail in other regulations, those regarding transport being in compliance with the IAEA transport codes.

The MED 97/43/Euratom [8] is implemented by the Ionising Radiation (Medical Exposure) Regulations [11] except for the special group of persons designated as voluntary 'comforters and carers' of those undergoing medical exposures. This group of persons is covered by the Ionising Radiations Regulations, although no legal dose limits apply to this group.

5.4 European legislation in practice

5.4.1 European Union

In 2000, the European Commission reassigned responsibilities for nuclear safety from the Directorate General (DG) for the Environment to the DG for Transport and Energy, except for the new independent states which come under the DG for External Relations. Although each of the member states of the EU is obliged to implement the European Council directives, the national legislation to achieve this is extremely varied, partly

Box 5.2 UK regulations and guidance

Acts of the UK parliament set out the framework of principles and objectives, under which regulations or orders are made by statutory instrument. Thus the acts of parliament are the primary legislation and the regulations secondary or subordinate. Acts are accepted following a series of parliamentary readings, but regulations have only to be laid before parliament.

Various government bodies and agencies are concerned with enforcement of legislation covering different aspects of radiation safety and information on some of the acts and regulations is given here. The regulations are listed beneath the acts under which they became law.
(www.legislation.hmso.gov.uk/si/si2000/20001059.htm)

Regulatory body—Health and Safety Executive (HSE) (www.hse.gov.uk)

The HSE has responsibility for drawing up and enforcement of legislation concerned with the safety of individuals both at work and members of the public.

Health and Safety at Work etc. Act 1974 and European Communities Act 1972 (ECA 1972)

Ionising Radiations Regulations 1999

Control of Substances Hazardous to Health (COSHH) Regulations 1999

Management of Health and Safety at Work Regulations 1999

Health and Safety at Work etc. Act 1974

Personal Protective Equipment at Work Regulations 1992

Health and Safety (Safety Signs and Signals) Regulations 1996

Carriage of Dangerous Goods (Classification, Packaging and Labelling) and Use of Transportable Pressure Receptacles Regulations 1996

Carriage of Dangerous Goods by Road (Driver Training) Regulations 1996

Packaging, Labelling and Carriage of Radioactive Material by Rail Regulations 1996

The Transport of Dangerous Goods (Safety Advisers) Regulations 1999

Consumer Protection Act 1987 and ECA 1972

Medical Devices Regulations 1994

Radiation (Emergency Preparedness and Public Information) Regulations 2001

Regulatory body—Department of Health (DoH) (www.doh.gov.uk)

The DoH prepares legislation relating to medical administration of radioactive substances and medical exposures. It also enforces this legislation in England, but in other countries in the UK it is enforced by the appropriate National Executive.

Medicines Act 1968 and ECA 1972

Medicines (Administration of Radioactive Substances) Regulations 1978

Medicines (Administration of Radioactive Substances) Amendment Regulations 1995 (ECA 1972 only)

The Ionising Radiation (Medical Exposure) Regulations 2000 (ECA 1972 only)

related to whether there are nuclear power installations in a given country. At the time of going to press, although each member state has legislation covering earlier directives, the situation regarding the new directives is not uniform and is summarized in this section.

BSS Directive 96/29/Euratom

- Eight member states have incorporated legislation to cover the directive, namely Austria, Finland, Greece, Ireland, Italy, Luxembourg, Sweden, and the UK (except for Gibraltar).

Box 5.2 (continued)

Regulatory body—Department of Transport

The government department responsible for transport enforces regulations relating to transportation of radioactive materials. Currently this is the Department of Transport, Local Government and the Regions, but was formerly the Department of the Environment, Transport and the Regions (DETR).

Radioactive Material (Road Transport) Act 1991

Radioactive Material (Road Transport) (Great Britain) Regulations 1996

Enforcing agency—Environment Agency (EA)

(www.environment-agency.gov.uk)
The EA and equivalent national organizations SEPA for Scotland and EHSNI for Northern Ireland (Chapter 9) are quasi-autonomous government agencies with responsibility for enforcement of environmental legislation. The legislation is drawn up by the government department responsible for the environment, this is currently the Department of the Environment, Food and Rural Affairs (DEFRA), but was formerly the DETR.

Radioactive Substances Act 1993

The Radioactive Substances (Basic Safety Standards) Regulations 2000

Exemption Orders

Control of Pollution Act 1974, Environmental Protection Act 1990, and ECA 1972

Special Waste Regulations 1996

Codes of Practice and Regulatory Guidance (produced by regulatory bodies)

Work with ionising radiation: Approved Code of Practice and practical guidance on the Ionising Radiations Regulations 1999. HSE Books, HMSO, London

Regulatory Guidance to support the Ionising Radiation (Medical Exposure) Regulations 2000

Management of health and safety at work: Appro.ved Code of Practice, HSC, 2000

Fitness of equipment used for medical exposure to ionising radiation. Guidance Note PM77, HSE 1998

Health and Safety (Safety Signs and Signals) Guidance 1996

Guidance Notes (produced by professional bodies and NRPB)

Medical and Dental Guidance Notes (in publication http://www.ipem.org.uk/)

Guidance Notes for Dental Practitioners on the Safe Use of X-ray Equipment

http://www.nrpb.org.uk/Dentalgn.htm

AURPO Guidance Notes on Working with Ionising Radiations in Research and Teaching 2001 http://www.shef.ac.uk/uni/projects/aurpo/publns.html

Notes for Guidance on the Clinical Administration of Radiopharmaceuticals and Use of Sealed Radioactive Sources 1998 (ARSAC)

- Four member states have incorporated legislation to cover some but not yet all aspects: Denmark, Germany, the Netherlands, and Spain.
- Three member states, Belgium, France, and Portugal, have not produced their implementing legislation, although there are drafts in evidence.

Medical Exposures Directive 97/43/Euratom

- Seven member states have incorporated legislation to cover the directive, namely Austria, Denmark, Finland, Greece, Italy, Sweden, and the UK (except for Gibraltar).
- Three member states have incorporated legislation to cover some but not yet all aspects: Germany, the Netherlands, and Spain.
- Five member states, Belgium, France, Ireland, Luxembourg, and Portugal, have not yet produced their implementing legislation.

Detailed examples of procedures for some individual countries are given below.

Ireland

EC (Radiological and Nuclear Medicine Installations) Regulations 1998 implement the 1984 Euratom directive on patient protection. The Radiological Protection Act 1991 (Ionising Radiation) Order (2000) implements 96/29/Euratom. The major changes introduced include work activities involving exposure to natural sources of radiation, the stricter application of existing radiation protection principles through the use of lower dose limits and constraints, the extension of justification and the use of intervention in cases of radiological emergencies or lasting exposures.

Italy

Serious delays have occurred in implementing EU directives in the past. For example, implementation of the 1984 EU directive on patient protection was made by an Italian decree in 1995 which was mostly concerned with BSS and amended in 1997 to take into account the 1997 directive and so include quality control issues, staff training, and equipment acceptance criteria regarding medical exposures.

Community law No. 25 (1999) aimed to implement several EU directives into Italian legislation as a method of speeding up the process of incorporating Community regulations into national legislation. Both directives 96/29/Euratom and 97/43/Euratom were covered in this way until the Italian Parliamentary Decrees 187 (on medical exposures) and 241 (on the BSS) were adopted (2000). Decree 187 now replaces the earlier decree 230/95 with regard to medical exposures and 241/2000 amends 230/95 to incorporate, among other items, natural radiation sources, intervention, and potential exposures.

Netherlands

The Nuclear Safety Department was transferred to the Ministry for Housing, Regional Development and the Environment in 2000. The Ministry is currently drawing up legislation to implement the Euratom directives.

General information concerning radiation protection within the EU can be obtained from http://europa.eu.int/comm/environment/radprot/index.htm#activities from which many guidance documents can be downloaded.

5.4.2 *Rest of Europe*

An overview of nuclear legislation in central and eastern Europe and the new independent states can be obtained from the OECD-NEA. Legislation is mostly focused on safety in nuclear installations, rather than radiation protection in hospitals. In Lithuania, a law governing radiation protection was implemented in 1999 which follows ICRP 60 recommendations and establishes a 'Radiation Protection Centre' which has similar functions to the NRPB in the UK, but is also responsible for drafting laws related to radiation protection. The Ukraine has legislation governing the licensing of activities in the field of nuclear energy, which aims to control national security interests (observing the non-proliferation of nuclear weapons), to protect individuals from overexposure, and to protect the environment from contamination. In Romania, Order No. 14 on the Basic Standards for Radiological Safety (2000) incorporates 96/29 Euratom and takes into account IAEA Safety Series 115-1996 and ICRP 60, while in the Slovak Republic, a series of decrees and regulations implemented in 1998 cover emergency planning for nuclear accidents, control of nuclear materials, and radioactive waste management. The impact of the Chernobyl accident (Box 10.10) and the need for tighter controls relating to radioactive contamination and movement of radioactive materials have influenced legislation in Eastern Europe, for example in Belarus legislation was enacted on radiation protection of the public, decontamination controls, and border export controls in 1998. Switzerland implemented an Ordinance on Radiological Installations for Medical Use (Ordinance on X-rays) in 1998, but few controls covering medical exposures have so far been introduced in Eastern Europe.

5.5 Legislation in the Americas

5.5.1 *The United States of America*

The USA was involved in setting radiation protection standards at an early stage. The National Council for

Box 5.3 US regulations and guidance

A number of government agencies are involved in regulation of the use of ionising radiation. Requirements are embodied in Codes of Federal Regulation (CFR) with 10CFR20 being the 'gold' standard, and these are enforced by the organizations listed below.

Nuclear Regulatory Commission (NRC)
The NRC provides regulations for NRC licence holders, including power generation, hospitals, and universities: Standards for protection against ionising radiation (1991) (10CFR 0-199)

Food and Drug Administration (FDA)
The FDA regulates the design and manufacture of X-ray and other radiation equipment. It sets standards and carries out inspections to determine compliance (21CFR part 1000)

Department of Transportation
The Department of Transportation regulates the shipment of radioactive materials under 49CFR (parts 170–175)

Department of Energy (DOE)
The DOE provides regulations for DOE National Laboratories and test facilities under 10CFR (parts 200–1000)

Occupational Safety and Health Agency (OHSA)
OHSA regulates the control of radioactive materials in the workplace that are not controlled by the NRC and DOE. The OSHA regulates overall safety in the workplace, including that concerning ionising radiations. Ionising Radiation Protection Standards (1971). 29CFR (parts 1910, 1926)

Environment Protection Agency (EPA)
The EPA is concerned with the regulation of releases of radioactive materials under 40CFR (parts 61, 141, 190, 192, 220–229, and 440)

Federal Guidance
Federal guidance on occupational radiation exposures (1987)
Federal guidance on diagnostic X-ray exposures (1978)

Radiological Protection (NCRP) was founded in 1928 and produces recommendations which are enacted in the USA. ICRP 26 has been implemented but despite representation on the group which drew up the International BSS, the USA has not yet implemented ICRP 60. Several agencies in the USA have responsibilities for enforcing standards and more information on this is given in Box 5.3. On a national level, Congress has designated the Nuclear Regulatory Commission (NRC) to regulate safety concerning reactor products. This relates to possession, transport, and use, as well as safety of the worker. Aspects of the regulation may be covered by state rather than national legislation and this is the approach adopted in most states. The NRC enters into an agreement with the state government allowing them to enforce state regulations, but must determine that the state radiation safety programme is at least as stringent as that of the NRC. Likewise, a state may enter into an agreement with one of its cities along similar lines. Agencies involved in overseeing different aspects of radiation safety are outlined in Box 5.3. Mammography is the only 'controlled' diagnostic medical exposure requiring quality assurance programmes and patient dose limitation.

5.5.2 Canada

On 31 May 2000, the Atomic Energy Control Board became the Canadian Nuclear Safety Commission (CNSC) (www.nuclearsafety.gc.ca) and has subsequently implemented the Nuclear Safety and Control Act (2000) after three years of drafting and consultation. As part of the package of 10 different regulations, the Radiation Protection Regulations implement ICRP 60 principles for occupational and public exposures.

The CNSC has no regulations concerning patient doses resulting from medical exposures, which are specifically exempted by section 2 of the Radiation Protection Regulations. The regulations do require that any radioactive material or associated radiation is only used in or on a patient under the direction of a qualified medical practitioner and that nuclear medicine patients are informed about how to reduce the dose to other persons from their medical exposure.

As in the USA, X-rays are regulated by a different organization from radioactive materials, in this case the federal department of health (Health Canada) and the provinces. Particular emphasis is placed on quality assurance (http://www.hc-sc.gc.ca/ehp/ehd/rpb/).

5.6 Legislation in some other parts of the world

Brief accounts of legislation in a selection of countries are given. This is not intended to give a complete picture, but simply snapshots of the approach adopted in different parts of the world.

5.6.1 Australasia

Australia

Radiation protection in Australia is governed by the Radiation Safety (general) Amendment Regulations. Practices follow ICRP60, but legislation is complicated in that radiation protection is the legal responsibility of the states and each state has its own legislation. Recommendations for limiting exposure to ionising radiation (1995) (Guidance note [NOHSC:3022(1995)]) have been published jointly by the National Health and Medical Research Council (NHMRC) and the National Occupational Health and Safety Commission Worksafe Australia. These national recommendations are adopted by the Australian states in their regulations.

The Australian Radiation Protection and Nuclear Safety Act recently set up the Australian Radiation Protection and Nuclear Safety Agency ARPANSA, which covers the activities of the Federal bodies on Commonwealth properties. The ARPANSA regulations are based on the IAEA BSS. The functions of the Radiation Health Committee of the NHMRC are being taken on by a Radiation Health Committee of ARPANSA (http://www.arl.gov.au/arps/ANZ_Regs.htm).

The NHMRC has prepared codes of practice on issues such as waste, discharge of radioactive patients from hospitals, and disposal of radioactive corpses. These have legal standing only if explicitly specified by the states in their regulations. Many patient related protection issues, such as reference doses, are not included directly in the regulations, but are considered in guidelines which are issued by the states. The NHMRC recommendations listed above give dose limits for volunteers in medical research, and reference doses for mammography.

New Zealand

The Radiation Protection Act 1965 and Radiation Protection Regulations 1982 govern radiation safety in New Zealand. The act sets up the regulatory structure via licensing individual users of irradiating apparatus and radioactive materials, and the regulations set out general requirements for safety. The act allows conditions to be placed on licences, and this mechanism is used to make compliance with the relevant code of safe practice mandatory. Specific radiation protection requirements are laid down in the Codes of Safe Practice.

The National Radiation Laboratory, Ministry of Health, is New Zealand's regulatory authority, issuing licences, writing codes of safe practice, performing compliance monitoring audits, maintaining national primary standards in radiation, and providing advice. In addition, the National Radiation Laboratory has official observer status on the Australian Radiation Health Committee and is a member of the (Australian) National Uniformity Panel with a view to trans-Tasman uniformity.

Recommendations of the ICRP, the IAEA, and other international bodies are incorporated in the various codes of safe practice. There are specific codes for the use of X-rays in medical diagnosis, the use of unsealed radioactive materials in medical diagnosis and therapy, the use of irradiating apparatus in medical therapy, and the use of sealed radioactive material in brachytherapy.

5.6.2 Asia and the Middle East

South-East Asia

Most countries have specific ionising radiation legislation, but there are large variations in the degree of enforcement. Traditionally, legislation relating to radiation safety has been enforced by the government department responsible for health: the Department of Health in Thailand and the Philippines and the Ministry of Health in Malaysia and Singapore. In Malaysia and Singapore the Ministry of Health also controls the use of radioactive substances, but in the Philippines this is under the jurisdiction of the department dealing with atomic energy. All legislation follows ICRP 26, but most countries are in the process of revision to meet standards set out in ICRP 60 and IAEA BSS. There is no legislation relating to medical exposures at the present time.

Japan

The structure of the Japanese government was reorganized in 2001 with respect to the nuclear sector. A new Ministry of Education, Culture, Sports, Science, and Technology is now responsible for the science and technology aspects of nuclear energy, including safety regulations for research reactors, protection against radiation hazards, use and transport of nuclear materials, use, storage, transport of radionuclides, and peaceful uses of nuclear energy (safeguards).

Central Asia

Countries in central Asia have legislation relating to nuclear safety and radioactive materials, for example Pakistan has regulations made by the Directorate of Nuclear Safety and Radiation Protection (DNSRP) of the Pakistan Atomic Energy Commission, while Kazakhstan has regulations on Safe Transport of Radioactive Materials (1999) which is based on the IAEA BSS. However, there is little legislation relating to radiological protection in healthcare.

Middle East

In Saudi Arabia some legislation has been developed by the King Abdulaziz City for Science and Technology (KACST) relating to the use of ionising radiation and implementing ICRP 60. In Oman the use of radioactive materials is governed by Regulations for the Control and Management of Radioactive Materials (1997), which is enforced by the Ministry of Regional Municipalities and the Environment. The current Omani regulations do not follow either ICRP 26 or ICRP 60, but revisions are expected within the next few years. The regulations cover radioactive materials, with an emphasis on industrial applications rather than medical uses.

5.7 Conclusions

The aim of this chapter has been to provide some background to how international recommendations on ionising radiation safety are developed and look at their implementation in a selection of countries. Whether or not legislation governing the use of radiation has been produced, as well as the extent to which such legislation is implemented, varies substantially in different parts of the world. National culture, priorities, resources, and education are so diverse that the variation seen is not surprising. However, the fact that international bodies have developed a recommended approach to radiological protection for most applications provides standards which legislators and workers in all countries can use as a guide. The amount of legislation that has so far been implemented explicitly to cover medical applications and exposure of the patient is limited. Europe has been at the forefront in these developments. In some countries, which have little apparent national radiation protection legislation, physicists and others have developed radiation protection protocols for their own institutions, usually based on ICRP recommendations or regulations from other countries such as the UK, which they have implemented as a voluntary code of practice. The aim of this book is to provide a practical guide to radiation protection in healthcare. This is, by necessity, related to the approach and standards that are implemented. The text follows methods required to implement ICRP recommendations and is written with particular reference to UK legislation. However, guidance is generally applicable and can be used by radiation protection practitioners in other countries with only minor modification.

5.8 References

1 International Commission on Radiological Protection (1977). Recommendations of the International Commission on Radiological Protection. ICRP Publication 26. *Ann. ICRP*, **1** (3).

2 International Commission on Radiological Protection (1991). Recommendations of the International Commission on Radiological Protection. ICRP Publication 60. *Ann. ICRP*, **21** (1–3).

3 International Atomic Energy Agency (1996). *International basic safety standards for protection against ionising radiation and for the safety of radiation sources.* IAEA Safety Series No. 115. IAEA, Vienna.

4 International Atomic Energy Agency (1996). *Regulations for the safe transport of radioactive materials.* IAEA Safety Series No. 6 (1996 Revision). IAEA, Vienna.

5 European Commission (1996). Council directive (96/29/Euratom) laying down BSS for the protection of the health of workers and the general public against the dangers arising from ionising radiation. *Off. J. Eur. Communities*, No. L159.

6 European Commission (1980). Euratom (80/836) directive laying down the BSS for the health protection of the general public and workers against the dangers of ionising radiation. *Off. J. Eur. Communities*, **23**, No. L246.

7 European Commission (1984). Euratom (84/467) directive amending directive 80/836/Euratom. *Off. J. Eur. Communities*, **27**, No. L265/4.

8 European Commission (1997). Council directive (97/43/Euratom) laying down measures on health protection of individuals against the dangers of ionising radiation in relation to medical exposure. *Off. J. Eur. Communities*, No. L180.

9 European Commission (1984). Euratom (84/466) directive laying down basic measures for the radiation protection of persons undergoing medical examination or treatment. *Off. J. Eur. Communities*, **27**, No. L265/1.

10 *The Ionising Radiation (Protection of Persons Undergoing Medical Examination or Treatment) Regulations* (1988). SI (1988)778. HMSO, London.

11 *The Ionising Radiation (Medical Exposure) Regulations (2000).* SI (2000) 1059. HMSO, London.

12 National Radiological Protection Board (1990). Patient dose reduction in diagnostic radiology. *Doc. NRPB*, **1** (3).

13 Institution of Physical Scientists in Medicine/National Radiological Protection Board/College of Radiographers (1992). *National protocol for patient dose measurements in diagnostic radiology.* Chilton, NRPB.

14 International Atomic Energy Agency (1995). *Radiation doses in diagnostic radiology and methods for dose reduction.* IAEA-TEC-DOC-796. IAEA, Vienna.

15 European Commission (1993). Council directive on medical devices. 93/42/EEC. *Off. J. Eur. Communities*, No. L169.

Chapter 6
Principles and control methods

K. E. Goldstone

6.1 Introduction

The three important principles which are the foundation of radiation protection are justification, optimisation, and limitation. The principles of justification and optimisation apply to all exposed individuals, while dose limitation is applicable to employees and the public, but not to patients. The concepts were first proposed by the ICRP in 1977 [1] and developed in later recommendations [2]. It is the purpose of this chapter to explore the three concepts and to demonstrate how they are applied in practical everyday radiation protection.

It should be remembered that in the context of radiation protection, some terms have particular meanings. Thus a 'practice' means an activity which increases overall exposure to radiation, either to individuals or groups of individuals; for example the medical use of ionising radiation. A 'potential exposure' takes into account that not all exposures happen as predicted, for example there may be changes in the environment after disposal of radioactive waste or equipment designed to prevent exposures may fail. A probability of occurrence can be estimated for this type of event and risk limits used instead of dose limits. Risk limits take into account the probability of incurring a dose and the detriment associated with that dose.

6.2 Justification

Justification of a practice: No practice involving exposures to radiation should be adopted unless it produces sufficient benefit to the exposed individuals or to society to offset the radiation detriment it causes.

Justification can be considered at two levels:

(1) the generic level—whether it is justified to use ionising radiation or radioactive materials at all for the practice;

(2) the individual case level.

The question that has to be answered at both levels is whether the practice does more good than harm. The radiation detriment is only one aspect of justifying a practice; others may be cost, inconvenience, or inaccuracy. For example, in many laboratories the use of radioactive materials has declined and alternative methods have been adopted. In justifying these changes consideration will have be given as to whether results can be obtained as quickly and accurately, whether the costs are reasonable, and whether radiation hazards are going to be replaced by other ones. In the world at large, questions of justification have to be addressed in, for example, the use of radioactive sources in fire detectors or exit signs. In the medical field one of the main ways of reducing radiation dose to the population is to take fewer X-rays. The Royal College of Radiologists has published guidelines [3] for medical practitioners setting out criteria stipulating when X-ray procedures are justified. In addition to following the general guidance given, the individual patient's X-ray has to be justified. The process may be affected by factors such as the age of the patient or whether they are or may be pregnant. If the result of an X-ray procedure will not alter the patient's management the X-ray is unjustified. The principle of justification also applies to research projects involving humans, where the researcher will have to consider whether the information can be obtained as effectively without using ionising radiation and, if not, whether the value of the expected outcome is sufficient to justify the radiation dose [4].

In all these situations, from the most trivial to the most complex, good decisions can only be made on the basis of comprehensive information of which the radiation physicist can supply only a small part of the total.

Even after the process of justification has taken place, reviews will be required to determine whether the practice is still justified. One example where such a review has been undertaken is the use of scintigraphy of the placenta to diagnose placenta praevia. This was

Table 6.1 Basic dose limits in millisieverts for a calendar year

Limit	Employees of 18 years and above	Trainees aged under 18 years	Other persons
Effective dose	20	6	1
Equivalent dose to lens of eye	150	50	15
Equivalent dose to skin (averaged over 1 cm^2 regardless of area exposed)	500	150	50
Equivalent dose to hands, forearms, feet, and ankles	500	150	50

common practice 25 years ago, but has been replaced by ultrasound scanning and is no longer considered justified.

6.3 Optimisation

Optimisation of protection: In relation to any particular source within a practice, the magnitude of individual doses, the number of people exposed, and the likelihood of incurring exposures should all be kept as low as reasonably achievable, economic and social factors being taken into account. This procedure should be constrained by restrictions on the doses to individuals (dose constraints), or the risks to individuals in the case of potential exposures (risk constraints), so as to limit the inequity likely to result from the inherent economic and social judgements.

Once a practice has been justified then efforts must be made to reduce radiation risks to the individual and the population. This means reducing doses and minimizing the possibility of accidents and incidents where doses might be raised. This dose reduction should be to a level which is 'as low as reasonably achievable' (ALARA), economic and social factors being taken into account.

Much effort in the medical field has concentrated on reducing doses to patients while not compromising image quality for diagnostic procedures or reducing doses to healthy tissue of patients undergoing therapeutic procedures . Usually any reduction in doses to patients will decrease doses to the associated staff (and the public), but this is not always the case and the correct balance of effort must be put towards minimizing patient, staff, and public doses. Optimisation is closely linked to the process of risk assessment (§6.8).

6.4 Limitation

Individual dose and risk limits: The exposure of individuals resulting from the combination of all relevant practices should be subject to dose limits or to some control of risk in the case of potential exposures. The aim is to ensure that no individual is exposed under normal circumstances to unacceptable risks from practices using radiation. It is not possible to exercise direct control over exposure from all sources and it is necessary to specify the sources to be included as relevant before selecting a dose limit.

This is perhaps the easiest principle to understand. Doses to employees and the public must not exceed certain dose levels known as dose limits. The dose limits are set at a level such that a dose above the limit and the consequences for an individual would be regarded as unacceptable [2]. The dose limit should not be seen as demarcation between safe and dangerous conditions since for ionising radiation the dose–risk relationship for stochastic effects is assumed to be continuous and linear (§3.4 and §3.5). There are circumstances in which the limits may be exceeded, for example in emergencies (§10.6) or particular operations of importance where specially planned limits may be employed. However, these are rare occurrences and, in general, if the processes of justification and optimisation are applied correctly the principle of limitation will rarely come into play.

6.5 Dose limits

Dose limits apply to those who are occupationally exposed to ionising radiation and to members of the public. They do not apply to potential exposures where risk limits are more appropriate. Over the years as epidemiological data have continued to be analysed and reassessed, dose limits have been reduced (Table 5.1). A summary of dose limits in normal use in the UK is given in Table 6.1. In special circumstances the employee dose limit may be averaged over 5 years.

The dose limits are set such that regular and continued exposure above the dose limits would be regarded as unacceptable (Box 6.1). In recommending levels for dose

Box 6.1 Acceptable risk and dose limits

Limits on radiation dose must be set at a level such that the risk to the individual is acceptable. The matter of acceptability was addressed in a report by the British Royal Society [5], which concluded that a continuing annual probability of death of 1 in 100 would be clearly unacceptable, but one of 1 in 1000 could hardly be called unacceptable provided that the individual at risk knew of the situation. The UK Health and Safety Executive (HSE) examined its approach to risk following the Hinkley Point inquiry [6] and concluded that an annual risk of death of 1 in 1000 was the most that is ordinarily accepted for a worker in the UK. An annual risk of death of 1 in 1000 has been adopted as the boundary between tolerable and unacceptable for occupational risk [7]. An occupational dose limit of 20 mSv per year would carry with it a 4% lifetime risk of induced fatal cancer and a 5% lifetime attributable risk, which is comparable to an annual risk of 1 in 1000. It should be remembered that the risk of death from radiation-induced cancer tends to follow the natural probability of death from cancer, which increases with age (§3.4). Thus for any worker who receives regular doses of radiation, the risk of death from radiation-induced cancer is low below the age of 50 years and peaks later in life (Figure B6.1). For a worker receiving 20 mSv per year the risk would only be of the order of 1 in 1000 between the ages of 70 and 90 years.

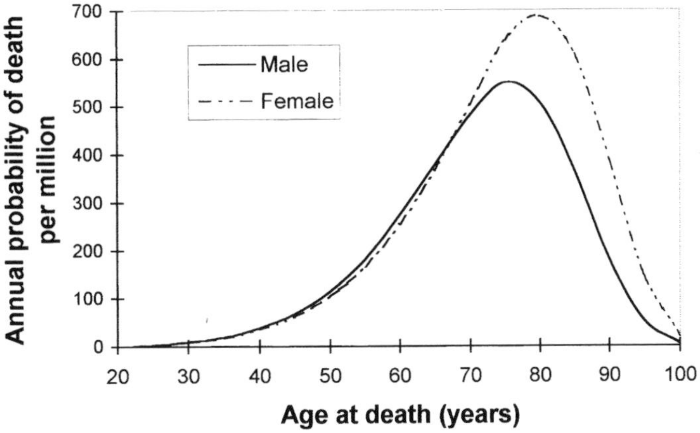

Figure B6.1 Annual probability of death from radiation-induced cancer for males and females per million of the initial population, following an annual exposure of 10 mSv per year from the age of 18 to 65 years. Results were derived using the multiplicative model (§3.4.1).

Views on the level of risk that it is acceptable to impose on members of the public have varied, but a risk of 1 in 100 000 of death is now regarded as the maximum acceptable involuntary risk from any single source [6,7]. Exposure at the public dose limit of 1 mSv per year over a lifetime is estimated to have a 0.4% risk of fatal cancer. The application of a dose constraint of 0.3 mSv to a single radiation source has an associated annual risk of similar order to that regarded as acceptable.

limits, the ICRP take into account not only the probability of fatal cancer and severe hereditary effects but also the total health detriment [2]. The limitation on effective dose is used to keep risks of stochastic effects (§3.4 and §3.5) at an acceptable level and is sufficient to ensure the avoidance of deterministic effects (§3.3) except in the eye lens and in the skin, which may be subject to high localized doses. Separate dose limits are applied to the eye and the skin which for category A radiation workers in Europe are 150 and 500 mSv, respectively. The dose to the skin is averaged over any 1 cm^2 area and in practice can prove difficult to measure (§8.4). Separate dose limits are applied to members of the public, which should include employees not normally exposed in the course of their work (Table 6.1).

Dose limits are not applied to certain individuals involved in medical exposures. They do *not* apply to patients undergoing medical exposures where the exposure usually is of direct benefit to the individual; if the exposure has been justified and optimised the dose to the patient should be as low as compatible with the required diagnostic or therapeutic purpose. Dose limits do *not* apply to 'comforters and carers', that is individuals who knowingly and willingly incur an exposure to ionising radiation as a result of providing comfort and support to another undergoing a medical exposure [8]. In this latter case a dose constraint (§6.7) may be more appropriate. A special dose limit of 5 mSv in five consecutive calendar years applies to any person other than a comforter or carer or employee who may be exposed due to the medical exposure of another. This could apply to a patient in an adjacent room to a brachytherapy patient, but such a dose limit may be difficult to apply in practice because of tracking effectively the 5-year period.

6.6 ALARA—as low as reasonably achievable

ALARA or ALARP (as low as reasonably practicable) as it appears in legislation [8] is the concept central to optimisation. Employers have a responsibility to ensure that radiation doses to their employees and the public, who may be affected by their work activity, are kept as low as reasonably practicable. This may be achieved with a hierarchy of methods, examples of which are given below. The methods adopted will depend on the outcome of a prior risk assessment (see §6.8).

6.6.1 Engineering controls

Example design features

- Lead shielding that surrounds X-ray tubes
- Shielded source enclosures
- Air extract systems in areas where volatile radioactive substances are used
- Methods of containment where unsealed sources are used.

Example safety features

- Key locks to prevent unauthorized exposures
- Shutter mechanisms and door interlocks on X-ray installations: such interlocks should always be fail-safe, that is if they fail emission of radiation is prevented. Interlocks tend to be less effective than design features for ensuring dose reduction because they can be overridden and in some circumstances, e. g. during maintenance, have to be overridden.

Example warning devices

- Warning lights and audible warnings
- Permanently sited radiation monitors triggered to alarm at a certain dose level. These may fail, so need to be checked regularly (with records being kept) to confirm their correct operation. The disadvantage of warning devices is that they may be ignored.

6.6.2 Systems of work and written procedures

Systems of work and procedures are likely to include the application of distance, shielding, and time to reduce exposure. Box 6.2 shows an example system of work for radionuclide work which also emphasizes containment and use of sources with the lowest activity to achieve the desired result. Procedures must always reflect local practice. Practically speaking, the disadvantage of procedures is that they may be ignored and it can be difficult to bring them effectively to the relevant individual's attention in the first place.

If the area to which the system of work applies is one in which the exposure to an individual may potentially exceed the relevant dose limit in a short time, then more complex procedures should apply. For example, local

Box 6.2 A system of work for an area where unsealed radioactive sources are in use

1. Do not eat, drink, apply make-up, or smoke in this room
2. Wear a laboratory coat done up to the neck
3. Wear protective gloves
4. Wear the personal dosimeters provided
5. Ensure radionuclides are placed behind appropriate shielding whenever practicable
6. Do not leave radioactive materials unattended on the bench—lock them away
7. Work over trays lined with absorbent material
8. Clear up a spill as soon as you are aware one has occurred
9. Monitor yourself before leaving the work area—decontaminate yourself if required
10. Thoroughly monitor the area when you have completed your experiment and decontaminate if required
11. Dispose of radioactive waste in the correct bin and down the appropriate drain

Box 6.3 Example of permit to work

Permit to work on the roof of the Radiotherapy Department

This permit is issued to: ____________________________

This permit allows access to the roof of the radiotherapy department HR 03.
Access to the area marked with yellow lines is restricted. Entry is permitted as detailed below (physicist to complete).

Area	A	Permitted/forbidden	above simulator
Area	B	Permitted/forbidden	above accelerator 1
Area	C	Permitted/forbidden	above accelerators 2 and 3
Area	D	Permitted/forbidden	above orthovoltage unit

I have checked that the above-mentioned will not enter the other areas.
I have asked (radiographer) to place the restriction notice.

Signed: ____________________________; Date: ______________
For the Medical Physics Department

I have placed prohibition notices on the ____________________________(state machines)

Signed: ____________________________ (physicist/technician/radiographer)

This permit will expire at: ______________; on ______________.

I have had explained to me and understand the conditions relating to this permit to work and I agree to them.

Signed: ____________________________; Date: ______________

Return this permit to Medical Physics immediately on completion of work.

arrangements may indicate that a 'permit to work' is required, as demonstrated in Box 6.3.

6.6.3 Personal protective equipment

Exposures may be restricted by the provision of adequate and suitable personal protective equipment, such as lead rubber aprons to reduce external radiation or protective clothing to reduce the risk of contamination. The employer should provide appropriate protective equipment, as indicated by a prior risk assessment.

6.6.4 Medical exposure

Employers responsible for medical exposures whether to patients, volunteers, those undergoing medico-legal exposures or health screening must ensure that doses to their patients are optimised and kept as low as reasonably practicable. It is a legal requirement in the UK and elsewhere in Europe (§5.2.2) that there should be diagnostic reference levels for diagnostic imaging procedures [9, 10] (§11.5.2). For nuclear medicine procedures, maximum activities to be administered are recommended [11]. These levels should be sufficient to ensure that an adequate image can be obtained in an acceptable time.

6.7 Dose constraints

Dose constraints [2] are intimately linked to the principle of optimisation. The methodology relates to benefits and detriment to society as a whole, rather than individuals, although the benefits and detriments are unlikely to be evenly distributed. For example, at a nuclear power station the population as a whole receives the benefits, but the employees and public living near the installation receive the detriment. Therefore, a source-related dose constraint is introduced to limit the detriment to any individual. Dose constraints are used in different ways depending on the context—whether occupational, public, or medical exposure. They are applied at the planning stage in order to exclude options which would give an unacceptably high radiation dose to an individual. It is important to appreciate that dose constraints are not synonymous with dose limits.

6.7.1 Dose constraints for occupational exposures

A dose constraint for occupational exposure should represent a level of dose that can be achieved in a well-managed practice. The need for, and value of, a dose constraint should be determined as part of the prior risk assessment for that practice. Advice from the radiation protection adviser and relevant professional associations should be sought in determining the value of the constraint. As far as occupational exposure is concerned, it is considered that constraints are only applicable where individual doses from a single type of radiation source are a significant fraction of the dose limit. Constraints would not normally be needed for employees in healthcare, except perhaps for interventional radiology or radiopharmacy work where doses may be more than a few millisieverts per year. The National Radiological Protection Board (NRPB) recommended 15 mSv as a maximum value for a dose constraint [12], with the expectation that it would be much lower than this.

Dose constraints may sometimes be confused with investigation levels. The main conceptual difference is that a dose constraint is applied prospectively and an investigation level retrospectively, although in fact they may be the same numerically. This is illustrated by the inclusion of a 15 mSv (or lower if so specified by the employer) investigation level in UK regulations [8].

6.7.2 Dose constraints for public exposures

The dose limit for members of the public is 1 mSv per year, but the dose constraint for any particular source must be set lower to ensure that the limit is not exceeded. The NRPB has recommended [12] a maximum dose constraint of 0.3 mSv per year. When using a dose constraint the critical group most irradiated by the source in question should be considered. For example, in considering liquid radioactive discharges from a site, the sewerage workers may be the critical group, whereas for gaseous disposals the group will be the nearest inhabitants.

In the medical context one may need to apply a dose constraint to members of the public who enter the hospital, when accompanying or visiting patients, or to individuals in an office adjacent to a radiation area (§13.3.1). So, for example, in the case of planning shielding for a linear accelerator, the time spent in areas close to a radiation source during the year, together with the dose rates and the beam-on time, should be taken into account.

6.7.3 Dose constraints and medical exposures for research

Where an individual is undergoing a medical exposure for research from which they personally expect to derive some benefit, dose constraints do not apply, although the use of target doses is required (§11.5.2). However, in research studies involving the irradiation of a volunteer, who may or may not be a patient but who will derive no benefit, a dose constraint must be set down as part of the procedure and adhered to. The dose constraint would be set by the researcher in agreement with the local research ethics committee. The radiation protection adviser should have input into setting the dose constraint and the level will be influenced by the expected benefit to society arising from the study. ICRP 62 [4] provides information on the use of dose constraints in medical and biomedical research.

6.8 Risk assessment

Before starting any work with ionising radiation, whether with unsealed or closed sources or machines producing radiation, the employer must undertake a prior risk assessment [13]. The purpose is to identify control measures that need to be put in place to restrict exposures to employees and others (see Box 6.4) . The risk assessment should identify all hazards with a potential to cause a radiation accident and evaluate the risks arising from them. It should:

- identify the risks from the work
- ensure that risks to all persons who might be affected are considered
- take account of existing precautionary measures
- identify measures which need to be put in place to control the risk and ensure compliance with relevant legislation.

The information required for the risk assessment includes:

- the source of radiation
- estimates of dose rates to which persons may be exposed
- the possibility, in the case of an unsealed source, of contamination and its spread
- results of personal dosimetry or monitoring for similar activities
- relevant instructions from the manufacturer or supplier about safe use and maintenance of equipment
- engineering and other control measures already in place and what happens if they fail
- planned systems of work
- options for shielding and use of personal protective equipment

Box 6.4 Risk assessment

Performance of a risk assessment involves defining the hazard and identifying the risks associated with the hazard. It is commonly acknowledged that there are five steps involved in the risk assessment process [11]:

- Step 1: Identify the hazard
- Step 2: Identify who might be harmed and how
- Step 3: Evaluate the risk and decide whether the proposed and/or existing precautions are adequate or whether more should be done
- Step 4: Record the findings of the evaluation
- Step 5: Review the assessment and revise if necessary.

In terms of radiation safety, the hazard involves the potential for exposure to radiation employees, members of the public, and patients. The details involved in Step 2 depend on the individual circumstance; for example, when calculating the effect of radionuclide discharge, the critical group might be hypothetical sewage workers, while when considering radiation shielding, occupancy of surrounding areas have to be taken into consideration.

In Step 3 of the risk assessment process the proposed control methods should be scrutinized in terms of:

- Do they enable compliance with legal requirements?
- Do they represent good practice?
- Do they reduce the risk to levels which are ALARP?

As part of this phase of the process, the assessor should determine whether the proposals allow for the distribution of appropriate information to whichever groups are concerned and whether provision has been made for adequate staff training.

The next stage of the risk assessment process involves the formal documentation of the outcome of the assessment, together with any proposals developed to ensure that the proposed operations reduce the risk to levels which are ALARP. In this context, it should be noted that practices which result in effective doses or committed effective doses to members of the public of 20 μSv or less are considered by some commentators to represent a trivial risk. This represents a risk of death of the order of 1 in a million.

The final phase of the assessment process requires that a commitment be made to visit the work area once the proposed work has started and review the risk assessment in the light of actual working practices.

A typical risk assessment form may have the following format:

- Location of work
- Date of commencement
- Description of work
- Source of radiation
- Staff involved
- Other persons involved
- Exposed groups and dose constraints
- Assessment
- Control measures
- Action to be taken

Signature	Date:
Designation: RPA	Date of review:

Box 6.5 Essential features of local rules

1. Specification of dose investigation level
2. Contingency plan
3. The name of the radiation protection supervisor
4. Description of controlled or supervised area to which rules apply
5. Arrangements whereby non-classified persons can enter or remain in the controlled area
6. Key working instructions to restrict exposure

- options for control of access to areas of significant dose rate or contamination
- available advice on good practice
- whether pregnant or breastfeeding women are likely to be involved.

The doses to which persons may be exposed can be estimated and an indication of the level of risk obtained. A form which could be used for risk assessment is shown in Box 6.4.

The assessment should indicate whether additional measures are required to keep doses as low as reasonably practicable. These may include:

- shielding and personal protective equipment
- personal and environmental dose monitoring
- training
- local rules and procedures
- whether dose constraints are indicated
- need to limit access to certain areas
- action needed if a female member of staff becomes pregnant
- maintenance and testing schedules for various safety devices.

6.9 Designation of areas

An important way in which doses to employees and others may be controlled is through the designation of areas where doses may be higher or there is a possibility of significant contamination. A controlled area is defined in UK legislation [8] as an area in which it is necessary for an individual to follow special procedures to restrict their exposure or to prevent or minimize the chance of a radiation accident. An area where a person is likely to receive an effective dose greater than 6 mSv (or an equivalent dose greater than three-tenths of any dose limit) must be designated as a controlled area. Other areas where radiation is used may need to be kept under review to determine whether, at some later stage, they should be controlled, and these are designated as supervised areas in the UK. An area should be supervised if a person is likely to exceed an effective dose of 1 mSv, a dose to the eye of 15 mSv, or a skin dose of 50 mSv.

The employer must indicate the extent of any controlled areas. This is usually done with physical barriers, but for cases such as the use of mobile X-ray equipment where a physical barrier is not usually used, the operator must be able to control the boundary of the area. It is not necessary to delineate the boundaries of supervised areas. Warning signs are required for fixed controlled areas and for supervised areas.

Once controlled areas have been identified the employer must prepare written local rules (Box 6.5), appropriate to the risk and the work activity in the area to ensure the work is carried out in accordance with the regulations. Local rules may also be required for supervised areas depending on the nature of the hazard, such as for an area where open sources are used and a spill could create a significant hazard. Local rules set out key arrangements for restricting the exposure in the area. They should cover the work in normal circumstances and anticipate possible accident situations. Local rules must be brought to the attention of those who need to know about them and one way in which this can be achieved is to display them at the entrance to the area.

6.10 Classification of employees

Risk assessments will quantify the radiation doses that may be received by staff in the course of their work. If, with the control measures in place, an employee is likely to exceed an effective dose of 6 mSv or an equivalent dose exceeding three-tenths of a dose limit, e.g. 150 mSv to the skin, then the employer must designate that person as a category A worker or a classified worker in the UK. Those under 18 years of age cannot be classified workers. The majority of employees in healthcare do not need to be classified workers, but a few will on the grounds of equivalent dose; for example a radiopharmacist may require classification because of the dose to the hands. When classification is considered, the employer must take into account the potential for an exposure to occur, including exposure as a result of an accident. This is particularly relevant where unsealed sources are involved. Classification is also required if an employee works with a high dose-rate source capable of giving a dose in excess of a dose limit within several minutes. Classified workers must be subject to comprehensive personal radiation monitoring by an approved dosimetry service (§8.2). Extensive dose records are required (§8.2.3) and medical surveillance must be carried out by an approved medical practitioner with an entry in the health records being made at least every 12 months. In general, an employer can only 'declassify' an employee at the end of a calendar year.

6.11 Special staff groups

Risk assessment should highlight whether there are any staff groups for whom special precautions are required. Staff coming into this category are those who are pregnant and, for situations involving unsealed sources, those who are breastfeeding. These groups are singled out for special treatment because of the greater radio-sensitivity of the fetus than the adult (§3.6, Box 11.4, §16.5.1). In the UK, the employee is required to notify her employer in writing that she is pregnant or breastfeeding and the employer must then take measures to ensure that the fetus is unlikely to receive a dose exceeding 1 mSv during the remainder of the pregnancy. In practice, where external radiation is concerned, this is equivalent to a dose of about 2 mSv to the surface of the abdomen for X-rays, but a lower surface dose for higher energy γ-rays (§16.7.3). Where an employee is breast-feeding, significant bodily contamination must be avoided.

Where unsealed sources are used, the question of an accident leading to significant ingestion of radioactive material should be considered.

6.12 Outside workers

Another group of workers that need to be considered are classified workers who carry out work in the controlled area of an employer other than their own, so-called outside workers. An example is a service engineer for radiation-generating equipment. The employer of an outside worker must issue the worker with a radiation passbook, obtainable from an approved dosimetry service, which has a personal identification and is not transferable to another worker. Although it is the responsibility of the outside worker's employer to ensure the passbook is kept up to date, it is the employer in whose controlled area the individual is working who is responsible for estimating the dose received in that area and entering it into the passbook. The simplest way of making this dose estimate is to issue the outside worker, upon arrival at the site, with a direct-reading personal dosemeter. The HSE have published a useful information sheet setting out the detailed procedures relating to outside workers [14].

6.13 References

1 International Commission on Radiological Protection (1977). Recommendations of the International Commission on Radiological Protection. ICRP Publication 26. *Ann. ICRP*, **1** (3).

2 International Commission on Radiological Protection (1991). 1990 Recommendations of the International Commission on Radiological Protection. ICRP Publication 60. *Ann. ICRP*, **21** (1–3).

3 The Royal College of Radiologists (1998). *Making the best use of a department of clinical radiology* (4th edn). The Royal College of Radiologists, London.

4 International Commission on Radiological Protection (1991). Radiological protection in biomedical research. ICRP Publication 62. *Ann. ICRP*, **22** (3).

5 Royal Society (1983). *Risk assessment: a study group report.* Royal Society, London.

6 Barnes, M. (1990). *The Hinkley Point public inquiry*, vol. 4, paragraphs 35 and 36. HMSO, London.

7 National Radiological Protection Board (1993). Board statement on the 1990 recommendations of the ICRP. *Doc. NRPB*, **4** (1).

8 *The Ionising Radiations Regulations* (1999). HMSO, London.

9 National Radiological Protection Board (1999). Guidelines on patient dose to promote the optimisation of protection for diagnostic medical exposures. *Doc. NRPB*, **10** (1).

10 *The Ionising Radiation (Medical Exposures) Regulations* (2000). HMSO, London.

11 Administration of Radioactive Substances Advisory Committee (1998). *Notes for guidance on the clinical administration of radiopharmaceuticals and use of sealed radioactive sources.* NRPB, Chilton, Didcot, Oxon.

12 National Radiological Protection Board (1993). Occupational, public and medical exposure. *Doc. NRPB*, **4** (2), 7–9, 32–3.

13 *The Management of Health and Safety at Work Regulations* (1992). HMSO, London.

14 Health and Safety Executive (1999). *Ionising Radiation Regulations 1999. Procedures relating to outside workers.* HSE information sheet. HSE, London.

Chapter 7
Operational radiation protection

D. G. Sutton

7.1 Introduction

Efficient day-to-day radiation protection requires the protection physicist to apply radiation protection theory, techniques, and procedures to every operation being undertaken. Hence the term operational radiation protection. This chapter covers the framework required to manage radiation protection and the practical techniques important in restricting exposure. As has been discussed in Chapter 6, the three main principles of radiation protection–justification, optimisation, and limitation–apply at every level. All three have their place in operational protection. However, the justification process plays only a small part at the operational level since, in broad terms, the operation forms part of a practice which is already in existence. Undoubtedly, decisions will need to be taken as to whether a particular type of procedure is justified; for example, use of a radiopharmaceutical which will deliver a relatively high effective dose to a young cohort of patients in a research study may well not be considered to be appropriate. Individual decisions on justification will be taken when deciding whether particular requests for procedures involving irradiation of patients produce a net benefit. Much more effort, in radiation protection terms, is placed on the optimisation process; that is, on ensuring that radiation doses to critical groups are kept as low as reasonably achievable (ALARA), bearing in mind economic and social factors. What this means is that protection measures should be taken to reduce the detriment resulting from any practice or operation as long as the effort required to bring about the reduction is less than the significance of the reduction (i.e. a pragmatic approach). Provided a radiation protection programme is properly managed and optimised, then all work involving significant exposure will be planned so that the probability of inadvertent exposure in excess of any relevant dose limit will be a very low [1]. Thus, in operational terms, limitation results from appropriate optimisation.

Operational radiation protection therefore revolves around application of the ALARA principle and can be thought of as applying protection principles to ensure that radiation doses to staff, patients, and members of the public are kept to levels which are as low as reasonably practicable (ALARP). This seemingly simple statement covers a broad range of principles and has implications for all those involved in the use of radiation at both a managerial and a practical level. A point to be borne in mind is that the ALARA principle is qualitative rather than quantitative and as such is open to different interpretation by different people. There is no right answer and the ALARA principle should be seen merely as an aid to decision making. The making of the decision itself remains the responsibility of the decision maker [2]. It is therefore of fundamental importance to know (a) who the decision maker is and (b) who it is that should give that person advice to aid in their decision-making processes.

Successful operational radiation protection relies on the provision of a sound management framework supporting a robust practical approach to optimisation.

7.2 Establishing a framework for radiation protection

In terms of management and organizational response, radiation protection does not differ significantly from other health and safety operations. The fundamental building-block of a sound operational health and safety programme is a firm management framework underpinning the programme. Without such a framework, the programme cannot succeed. There has to be an explicit commitment by senior management to the aim of restricting exposure of staff, patients, and members of the public to levels which are ALARP. This commitment must be translated into practice with the aid of documentation, organization, review, and reporting.

7.2.1 Radiation safety policies

Probably the most important element of the required documentation is a written overall policy clearly enunciating the commitment to ALARA. Such a policy defines the attitude of the entire organization and demonstrates the direction in which management wish to go. It represents a firm documented pledge by the organization to honour its obligations. The policy should ensure that appropriate senior managers are given responsibility for implementation and review of the programme and should define the structure and organizational relationships which must be in place to ensure that it is delivered. The policy must demonstrate that hazards have been identified and provide a commitment to risk assessment. It is vital that the health and safety structure is both completely transparent and workable, so it is important that the policy is laid only following consultation with appropriate groups within the organization. It is imperative that staff groups are aware of its existence; communication is of paramount importance.

There may be more than one policy concerned with different aspects of the optimisation process; for example, one policy might be concerned with restriction of occupational exposure and another with ensuring that the appropriate exposures are delivered to patients undergoing medical examination or treatment and that all patient exposures are justified. These policies should, however, be made under the auspices of the overall policy; that is, there must be a hierarchical approach so that overall control and direction are clearly understood. In fact, it may well be that the commitment to the ALARA/ALARP principle is made in the general health and safety policy of the organization and that further policies are made to cover different areas of use of ionising and non-ionising radiation.

7.2.2 Organization of radiation protection

Associated with the radiation safety policy should be a clear definition of the manner in which protection is organized. This can take many forms; it could be by way of an organizational diagram or written instruction and might be reinforced in individual job descriptions.

In general, the organization will have to appoint one or more Radiation Protection Advisers (RPAs) who will have the responsibility of informing management of their responsibilities under appropriate legislation. There will also need to be a Medical Physics Expert (MPE) who will have the function of advising on matters regarding restriction of patient exposure. The RPA and the MPE may or may not be the same person, depending on local circumstances. It is important that a person be appointed to supervise the radiation work in each department where either X-rays or radionuclides are used. However, this Radiation Protection Supervisor (RPS) should not be considered as being responsible in management terms. That responsibility must lie with the head of the department concerned and be seen as being consequent to the line management structure defined in the appropriate radiation safety policy.

There may well be radiation protection support staff such as health physicists, radiation physicists, and technical staff involved in the overall protection effort and their role should be recognized in organizational diagrams and their job descriptions. Where staff have more than one role (for example a nuclear medicine physicist may also have radiation protection responsibilities), then the distinct roles should be defined explicitly.

It is important that both senior management and management at departmental level are aware of the radiation safety hierarchy and of the personnel involved. Line managers should be made aware of the need to cooperate in the implementation of the radiation safety programme. Where appropriate, there should be provision for out-of-hours advice and practical input to be obtained. Emergency planning groups should take into account the potential for any radiation incidents occurring within their sphere of influence.

The end user should also have a place in the organizational arrangements; in many ways it is they who act as the linchpins of an optimised radiation programme. They have responsibilities to themselves, to the public, and to any patients with whom they are involved. The management framework must be capable of identifying the end user; that is, all users of radiation should be registered, since the employer has to be able to demonstrate that their radiation doses do not exceed the prescribed dose limits. There must be appropriate channels of communication to, and training for, the end user, be they clinician, nurse, radiographer, or technical officer, and they should have representation at development and review forums such as the radiation safety committee.

The radiation safety committee will be the focal point of the organization of radiation protection and should meet regularly to review elements of the radiation safety programme. This committee should be made up of representatives of the major groups involved; i.e. RPA, MPE, representative RPSs, senior management, staff members, and so on. In large organizations, such as multi-hospital trusts, it may prove more effective to constitute a radiation safety committee at each hospital. The radiation safety committee should itself report to the general health and safety committee.

7.2.3 Establishment of controls and limits

The radiation safety policy should make clear that compliance with all legislative elements relating to radiation safety of staff, patients, and members of the

Box 7.1 Application of controls and procedures

- Acceptance testing/commissioning
- Arrangements for pregnancy and breastfeeding
- Compliance with dose limits
- Definition of controlled areas
- Environmental impact assessments
- Equipment calibration
- Equipment quality assurance
- Identification of persons entitled to refer patients for diagnostic and therapeutic radiation exposures
- Identification of persons responsible for diagnostic and therapeutic radiological procedures
- Incident reporting procedures
- Local rules/manuals of good practice
- Patient dosimetry programmes
- Personnel monitoring
- Radioactive substances (keeping, using, disposal, transporting)
- Radiological facility (design criteria/dose constraints—staff and members of public)
- Requirements for personnel monitoring—routine use and investigation levels
- Requirements for record keeping
- Research involving ionising radiation
- Specification of protection aspects of radiology equipment
- Training

public is seen as obligatory. The policy should indicate that advice on the establishment of the controls and procedures will be obtained from the RPA and MPE, although it must be stressed that any organizational framework must allow for input from others. For example, rules and codes of practice are unlikely to be workable unless they are drawn up with input from the RPS and other end users. Similarly, advice on patient dose reduction techniques can only be given in the context of practicality and resulting diagnostic quality, both of which require input from radiology professionals. The establishment of controls must be seen as a multidisciplinary matter. Box 7.1 shows some areas which will require the establishment of controls and procedures.

7.2.4 Communication and training

Communication is important in any management structure. In the context of radiation protection it ensures that management can explain their perspectives, priorities, and proposed methods of implementation of the ALARP principle. Similarly, an effective communication strategy ensures that staff can provide feedback on implementation and play a positive role in any review of radiation protection practice. Unfortunately, effective communication is one of the most difficult aspects of any operation to effect or guarantee.

One of the main channels of communication will be local rules and manuals of good practice which should be available to members of staff who should regularly reappraise themselves of their content. It may be that a procedure is put in place whereby staff record that they have read the rules or manuals. The rules should themselves be subject to regular review to reflect any changes in the legal framework, day-to-day working practices and organizational structure. A fundamental communication route is provided by the radiation safety committee which ensures that a bidirectional exchange of information between management and staff representatives is possible. To ensure that appropriate levels of communication are achieved, the radiation safety committee should meet regularly and not just 'when something comes up'.

Other routes of communication should be considered. Local intranets and hospital/university-wide information networks provide, in theory, excellent methods for at least the unidirectional dissemination of information from management and radiation safety professionals to staff groups. Such systems are especially useful in times of change, such as, for example, when new legislation is being implemented and working groups or committees have been convened to aid in the implementation. Drafts and discussion documents can then be circulated to a wider audience than might previously have been possible. Once change has been effected, all relevant documentation can be made readily available without incurring significant administrative overheads and, potentially, without the document control problems encountered with the traditional paper route. For example, it is possible to incorporate a hypertext linked set of radiology referral guidelines on any hospital intranet. These guidelines are then available to any qualified practitioner wishing to request a procedure, and yet only one update is required should the referral criteria change.

Management have an obligation to provide adequate and appropriate training for their employees. The provision for such training should be firmly enshrined within the organizational framework for radiation safety. Some training may be statutory and may well have been provided prior to the staff member taking up post. The provision of some training may even be contingent on the staff member being allowed to take up post since some members of staff will have received no radiation safety training prior to their employment. Whatever the case, there will always be the need for staff training to be provided, either in-house or outsourced, and this must be reflected in the radiation protection infrastructure. Training might be either practical or theoretical and can be concerned with basic or more complex issues. It should, however, take place on a continuing basis and refresher and update training should be provided at regular intervals.

7.2.5 Planning and risk assessment

Work with radiation should always be planned. It is not possible to apply the optimisation principle without due consideration being given, in advance, to the engineering and/or procedural controls which may be necessary. As discussed in §6.8, the first part of the planning cycle should be a risk assessment (see also Box 6.3). Arrangements should be in place to ensure that all proposals for the use of radiation are subject to such an assessment, the results of which can be used to define appropriate controls. For example, one proposed use of radiation might be the use of mobile radiography on hospital wards, while another may involve the use of a similar X-ray set as a fixed installation in a radiographic room. A risk assessment could well show that engineering controls, such as the use of lead sheet in the construction of the walls, are necessary in the case of the fixed installation. However, it is quite likely that the assessment would reveal that only procedural controls such as the establishment of a 2-m-radius exclusion zone would be required for mobile radiography. Another proposed use of radiation might involve the use of ^{35}S in a laboratory. A risk assessment might demonstrate that the area does not need to be controlled in terms of the legislation but will allow in-house control procedures to be specified.

The organizational structure and communication pathways must be such that the RPA has input to the risk assessment; without such input it is possible that inappropriate control measures will be adopted. There must be a mechanism in place for ensuring that the outcome of the risk assessment and any control measures resulting from its implementation are incorporated into the overall design.

In any project, it is essential that the radiation safety risk assessment takes place at an early stage and that the RPA, MPE, or both have a role within the project team. Depending on the scale of the project, this role may well extend to providing more than input to the risk assessment. The advice and skills of the radiation safety professionals will be needed when engineering controls are being considered and when specifications are being drawn up. Input will also be required when proposals from outside contractors and suppliers are being considered. At the end of the project, radiation safety personnel will be needed to assess the effectiveness of the control measures adopted, whether they be aimed at the reduction of exposure to occupationally exposed staff members, members of the public, or patients.

To summarize, organizational arrangements must be such that the project coordinator is aware that there are issues surrounding radiation safety (and patient protection where appropriate) and that radiation safety issues are incorporated into the project cycle.

7.2.6 Local rules and manuals of good practice

The provision of local rules is a legal requirement in certain areas where radiation is used and the framework underlying radiation protection should facilitate their production. However, the commitment to radiation protection should extend beyond that which is done merely to satisfy regulatory requirements and it is desirable that local rules and/or manuals of good practice be made available to all users of radiation whether their particular application comes under the legal framework or not. They should always be available to staff and should act both as a reminder of the elements of good practice and to emphasize those elements of the relevant legislation that might be applicable. Their overall purpose is to reinforce the culture of radiation safety. The essential contents of local rules can be found in Box 6.4, although the actual content of the rules will depend on the circumstances surrounding the work involved and should be drawn up in consultation with the users of radiation. Manuals of good practice can be more generic and may cover an entire field of endeavour. For example, all of the laboratories that use radionuclides in a medical school might be issued with a single code of practice covering use of a wide range of radionuclides and containing general information on such diverse aspects as arrangements for waste disposal and spill containment. Similarly, a radiology department may have a radiation protection folder, containing, as well as the local rules, information on patient protection legislation and quality control.

7.2.7 Audit and review

The protection framework should include arrangements for reviews of work involving the use of radiation to be carried out from time to time. It should also allow for the systematic appraisal of the radiation protection programme itself. The purpose of any such review or audit is simple; it is to ensure that the optimisation process is working and to effect remedial action to address shortcomings. A review itself does not serve to optimise radiation protection, it is merely a tool designed to collect data which can then be assessed in the context of the aims of the radiation protection programme [2]. Reviews can be carried out in-house, in which case they are performed on behalf of the management, or by and on behalf of the regulatory authorities, when they may well be called inspections.

The results of any review or audit of radiation protection should be documented and appropriate actions highlighted when required. It is essential that the loop can be closed and that the recommendations resulting from any review are acted upon; this can only be achieved by incorporating the concept of reviews within the organizational framework for radiation protection. The results of reviews should be considered by the radiation safety committee.

Reviews should be scheduled to take place at regular intervals, not just as a response to some external trigger such as a dose limit being exceeded or as the result of an incident occurring. There are several reasons for initiating regular reviews, some of which are:

- The initial design parameters and control procedures may not have been optimised.
- The local rules may not work.
- Working practice may have become careless.
- Working practices may have changed.
- Workload may have increased.
- Communication pathways may be ineffective.

The review can be based on a simple checklist or can be performed using an analytical tree [2]. The specifics of the review depend, of course, on what it is that is being reviewed. The aim, however, is always the same—to demonstrate that the ALARA principle is being adhered to. The reviews of individual work areas can be used as the basis for a review of the protection programme as a whole.

7.3 Protection against external radiation

The degree of protection required depends on the type of radiation involved and the risk associated with that radiation. The radiation can comprise α-particles, β-particles, γ-rays, neutrons, X-rays, or a composite of these. The sources may vary–accelerators, X-ray sets, radionuclides, or even reactors. All sources and types of radiation present their own particular practical problems in terms of radiation protection and these are discussed in depth in the chapters that follow. There are, however, fundamental practical principles which do not differ and which are applied to any radiation protection problem. In all cases, a robust operational approach to radiation protection can only be developed by taking into account the requirements of the management framework discussed above. The radiation hazard itself can be subcategorized into that arising from external radiation, the external hazard, and that resulting from internal deposition, the internal hazard.

7.3.1 Risk assessment

The risk from external radiation exists in all the major areas where ionising radiation is used in medicine and research: in laboratories, radiotherapy departments, nuclear medicine departments, and diagnostic radiology departments. There may also be a hazard on wards (mobile radiography, radionuclide injections, and radiation therapies) and in other areas where circumstances might require its use, for example clinics where radionuclide therapies are administered. In each case an assessment of the risk will be required to evaluate the hazard and recommend protection measures that should be implemented.

The five steps to risk assessment outlined in Box 6.3 should be applied to any use of radiation which results in an external hazard. Identification of the hazard is straightforward but it is important to consider the differing groups to whom the radiation might be considered as constituting a hazard. There will be at least two groups to consider: occupationally exposed members of staff (registered radiation workers) and members of the public. For both of these groups, the optimisation problem will be defined around dose limits. In most hospital uses of radiation, there will be a third group who are not subject to dose limit, namely patients. In this group, the protection issues revolve around optimisation of the radiation exposure, which is discussed in §11.5.

7.3.2 Compliance with dose limits

Dose limits form the upper limit when decisions are being made about what is as low as reasonably achievable, while dose constraints provide a mechanism for structuring the optimisation problem (§6.7). Dose limits and constraints form a central pillar of the protection framework so it is essential that the protection physicist is able to demonstrate compliance. In most cases the easiest way to do this is by measurement. The appropriate measurement steps will have been identified in the risk assessment.

Occasional radiation surveys can demonstrate that radiation doses both inside and outside a facility comply with design parameters and legal requirements. However, in most cases it will be necessary to perform such surveys at regular intervals for much the same reasons as regular reviews of the protection programme are required (§7.2.7). Contamination monitoring is important in the control of the external and internal hazards and should be performed at planned and regular intervals. For both dose and contamination surveys, the choice of monitor is very important and time should be invested in selecting the appropriate instrument (§4.4) It is also important to have an understanding of what the measured quantity represents, that is whether it is a simple count rate, a measure of kerma, an operational quantity such as ambient or directional dose equivalent or even an indication of exposure. Equally important is the requirement that all monitors be calibrated, either according to local protocol or against an external standard, depending on the resources available and their projected use.

Monitoring compliance with individual occupational dose limits is most easily achieved with a personnel monitoring programme (Chapter 8) which should be structured according to the outcome of the risk assessment. For example, it might be that the risk to a particular group of radionuclide users has been identified as being to their fingers. It might be inappropriate and not at all cost-effective to issue them with body dosemeters but it may well prove advisable to ensure that they wear finger-stalls while performing procedures. On the other hand it might be decided that all radiography staff are issued with film badges as a matter of policy irrespective of their potential for exposure. An appropriate and effective monitoring policy can only be effected by taking local considerations into account; there is no blanket approach which will result in an optimised solution. Staff perception should be taken into account and the reasons for any decisions should be communicated appropriately. This is especially important when the decision is made not to provide personnel monitoring to any group. Special attention should be paid to the monitoring requirements of pregnant staff since the dose limits are lower than those for other staff and the issue of risk perception may be more important.

7.3.3 Patient protection

Dose limits do not apply to patients exposed to radiation for therapeutic or diagnostic purposes, but the principle of justification certainly does. There must be a sound basis for deciding to expose patients to radiation and the benefit of the procedure must exceed the potential risk. In many respects the process of justification is clinical and is not the role of the protection physicist. However, the physicist should be in a position to advise on the adoption and application of techniques and practices from the point of view of patient dose.

The optimisation principle also applies to the area of patient radiation protection. In imaging procedures, the patient radiation dose should be appropriately balanced against the quality of the resulting image so that neither too much nor too little information is provided to answer the clinical question being asked. The issue in therapeutic procedures is to ensure that the patient receives neither too little nor too much radiation and in many cases the concerns of radiation protection are inextricably linked with those of radiotherapy physics. The issues of justification and optimisation relating to medical exposures are dealt with in more depth in Chapter 11.

To achieve the above, a programme centred around patient radiation protection against external hazards should concern itself with relevant practical aspects of

- equipment specification, selection, acceptance, and commissioning
- equipment quality assurance and performance programmes
- staff training and technique
- patient dosimetry programmes
- incident investigation.

There will also be issues surrounding the irradiation of particular subgroups of patients, for example children and pregnant women. The operational programme should also concern itself with the groups of people who do not receive any benefit from exposure to radiation and are not classed as patients, i.e. research volunteers.

It is important that any patient programme is multidisciplinary in nature since no one staff group is likely to have the appropriate levels of expertise. It is therefore equally important that appropriate communication routes have been established and defined in the management framework.

7.4 Practical control measures for external radiation

In general terms the three overriding principles which ensure that the hazard from external radiation exposure will be minimized are:

Box 7.2 Handling P-32: time and distance

1 MBq P-32 in a 1.5 ml Eppendorf tube.

Possible operation

1. Hold the Eppendorf at its base. The dose rate to the finger is approximately 1.2 mSv/min.
2. Hold the Eppendorf at the top. The dose rate to the finger is approximately 30 μSv/min.
3. Use a 10-cm-long remote handling tool. The dose rate to the finger is approximately 4.7 μSv/min.
4. Use a 20-cm-long remote handling tool. The dose rate to the finger is approximately 1.2 μSv/min.

If one assumes that a researcher performs the operation five times a day and that each time it takes only 1 min, then the annual dose rate to his or her fingers, assuming a 200-day working year, for P-32 will be:

Method	*Annual finger dose (mSv)*
1	1200
2	30
3	4.7
4	1.2

A 2-min handling time will double these doses and a 30-s handling time will decrease it by a factor of two.

1200 mSv is in excess of the UK upper limit on exposure to the fingers of an occupationally exposed worker. 30 mSv represents the same radiation dose as 300 X-rays of a finger. The effect of even a 10 cm air gap is immediately apparent.
Source: [11].

1. Restrict the time during which a person may be exposed to the radiation as much as possible.
2. Ensure that the distance between a person and the source of radiation is kept as large as practicable.
3. Employ appropriate measures to ensure that the person is shielded from the source of radiation.

These three principles are collectively described by the phrase 'Time, Distance, and Shielding'. It will not always be necessary or possible to apply all three principles at the same time. There will be occasions when only one or two should be considered as an option, either because of operational demands or because of the nature of the hazard. However, there will also be occasions when all three should be used to ensure that doses are kept as low as reasonably practicable.

7.4.1 Time

Minimization of the time spent exposed to any source of radiation is to a large extent a matter of planning, organization, and training. Examples of how time might affect exposure are somewhat trivial, given that the product of dose rate and time is dose, but the example in Box 7.2 provides an illustration of the application of the principles of time and distance for dose reduction.

7.4.2 Distance

If one assumes no interaction with the surrounding medium, then the fluence of ionising radiation will decrease with distance from the source. The manner in which the fluence decreases with distance depends on the source geometry.

If the origin of the radiation is a point source, then since the fluence is homogeneously distributed and is irradiating a sphere with surface area $4\pi r^2$—where r is the distance from the source—the fluence at any point will be inversely proportional to r^2. Therefore, the dose rate will be inversely proportional to the square of the distance from a point source.

In the case of X-rays, it is usual to assume that the $1/r^2$ rule applies when considering machine output. For radionuclides, the air kerma rate constant Γ(μGy $h^{-1}MBq^{-1}m^2$) enables absolute determinations of air kerma with distance using the inverse square law:

$$K_{air} = A\Gamma/r^2$$

where K_{air} is the air kerma rate at a distance resulting from a source with activity A and rate constant Γ. Table 7.1 gives values of Γ for some common radionuclides and Figure 7.1 is a plot of Γ versus energy, assuming emission of 1 photon per disintegration. Knowledge of the decay scheme for any radionuclide will allow calculation of Γ. Further values of Γ are tabulated in the literature but the reader should be wary of the fact that they are sometimes presented as the exposure rate constant, which has the units of R h^{-1} mCi^{-1} cm^2. A rule of thumb for dose rate at distance r from a point source of S MBq is given by $K_{air} = SEF/6r^2$, where E is the emission energy in MeV and F is the fraction of disintegrations emitting a γ-ray.

Table 7.1 Γ for some common radionuclides

Radionuclide	Γ 1 MBq at 1 m ($\mu Gy\ h^{-1}$)
^{18}F	0.134
^{22}Na	0.28
^{24}Na	0.43
^{42}K	0.033
^{43}K	0.13
^{51}Cr	0.004
^{59}Fe	0.15
^{57}Co	0.02
^{58}Co	0.13
^{60}Co	0.32
^{65}Zn	0.07
^{67}Ga	0.02
^{75}Se	0.15
^{86}Rb	0.012
^{99}Mo	0.041
^{99m}Tc	0.017
^{111}In	0.084
^{123}I	0.04
^{125}I	0.034
^{131}I	0.052
^{127}Xe	0.058
^{133}Xe	0.012
^{137}Cs	0.078
^{192}Ir	0.113
^{201}Tl	0.12

The case of a line source is somewhat more complex. As an approximation one can assume that when the distance (r) from the source to the measuring point is of the same order as the length of the line (l), then the dose rate falls off as $1/r$, while when $r > 10l$, then the inverse square law can be assumed to hold.

The dose rate from a plane large-area source is invariant with distance provided that the monitor to source distance is small compared to the area of the source. This property is useful in the case of large-area contamination monitoring or when contamination monitors are to be calibrated. As the distance between the source and the monitor increases, initially the dose rate falls with distance as $1/r$ and as distance increases further, the relationship tends to $1/r^2$(see Box 7.3).

The above discussion *only* applies in cases where there is no appreciable attenuation of the radiation by the medium through which it travels. It is therefore applicable for estimates made of γ- and X-radiation in air but not for β- and α-particles which are attenuated considerably by air. The inverse square law will overestimate the dose rate from both of these types of radiation and, in fact, the variation of dose rate with distance in air can be considered as an example of the use of shielding. The attenuation of α-particles is completely dominated by the fact that they have extremely high values of linear energy transfer (LET) and consequently the stopping power of air is also high. The range of an α-particle in air is typically less than 75 mm (Box 7.4). α-particles with energies less than 7.5 MeV cannot penetrate the outer layer of the skin and do not present an external hazard.

The situation with β-particles is different although the concept of range applies here as well. The degree of variance from an inverse square law behaviour will depend on the energy and spectral distribution of the β-particles, as will their maximum ranges (Box 7.5). For example, the maximum range of a ^{32}P β-particle (1.7 MeV) is approximately 6 m while that of a ^{33}P β-particle (0.249 MeV) is 0.46 m. A rule of thumb for β-particles with energies between 0.5 MeV and 40 MeV is that the range in air is 3.6 m per MeV. β-particles can represent a significant hazard to the skin. For instance, the dose rate at 1 cm from a β-particle source is about 80 mGy h^{-1} per MBq, and a radionuclide deposited on a surface with a

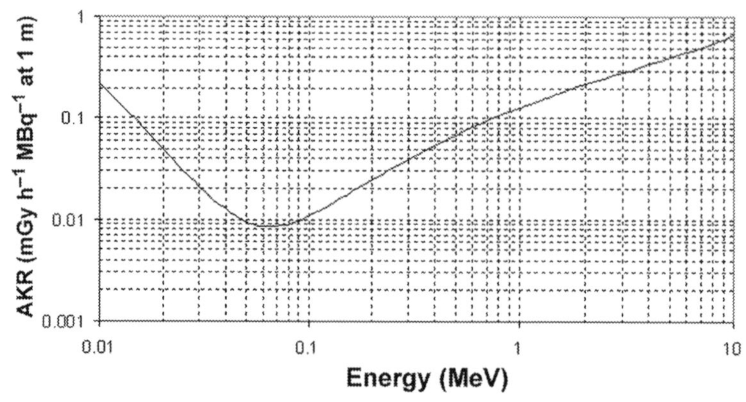

Figure 7.1 AKR constant: variation with energy in MeV.

Box 7.3 Variation of fluence with distance from a plane source

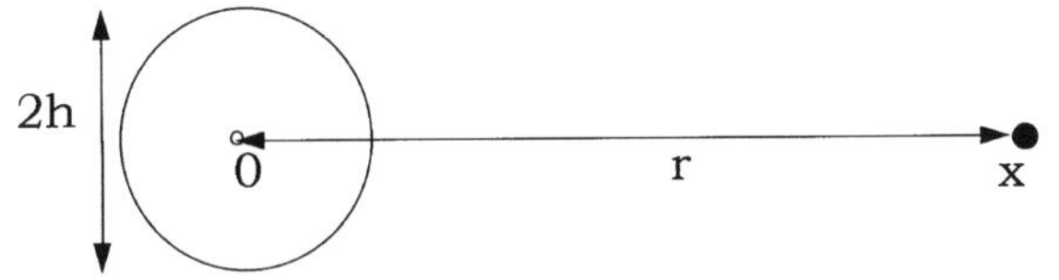

Figure B7.1 A plane source of uniform activity.

It can be shown that for a plane source of uniform activity as shown in Figure B7.1, the measured fluence at any position x is proportional to $\ln[(r^2 + h^2)/r^2]$, where h is the radius of the plane source and r is the distance from the source.

The function $\ln[r^2 + h^2)/r^2]$ is plotted in Figure B7.2 as a function of h/r. From the point at which h is equal to r, analysis of this function shows that the inverse square law becomes the dominant influence.

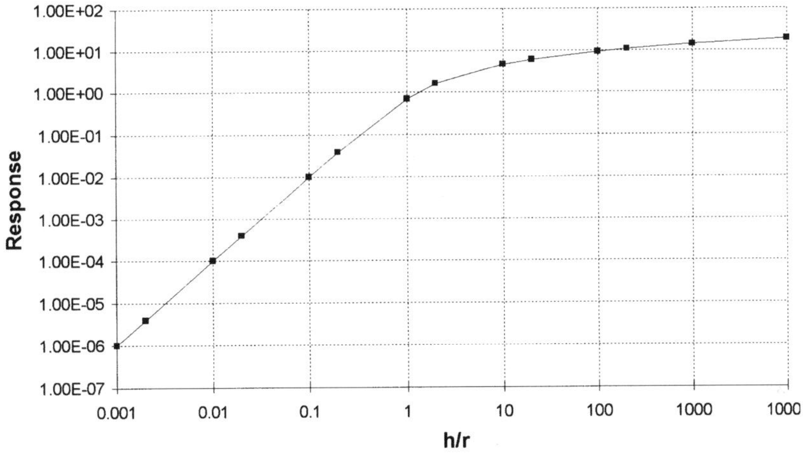

Figure B7.2 Variation in dose rate with *h/r*.

Box 7.4 Range of α-particles in air and other media

The range (in mm) of an α-particle in air can be estimated with the following equations [3]:

1. Range (mm) = 5.6 × (energy in MeV) for particles of energy up to 4 MeV.
2. Range (mm) = 12.4 × (energy in MeV – 26.2) for particles with energy greater than 4 MeV and less than 8 MeV.

Consider a 6 MeV α-particle arising from $^{241}Am/^{238}Pu$ cell irradiator. The range, from equation (2) above, is 48.2 mm.

The range in any other medium R_{med} can be obtained from the range in air R_{air} using the Bragg–Kleeman rule: $R_{med} = R_{air} \times 0.32 \times A^{1/2}/\rho$ where ρ is the density (kg/m^3) and A is the atomic number.

Box 7.5 Range of β-particles in a medium

The range (in units of density thickness) of β-particles with maximum energy E can be determined for any medium using the following empirical equations [3]:

$$R\ (\text{mg cm}^{-2}) = 412E^{(1.265\ -\ 0.0954\ \ln E)} \qquad 0.01 < E\ 2.5\ \text{MeV}$$
$$R\ (\text{mg cm}^{-2}) = 530E - 106 \qquad E > 2.5\ \text{MeV}$$

The attenuation of β-particles in air can be considered in the same way as the attenuation in any other medium. The stopping power of β-particles in air is 0.367 MeV/kg/m^2. Figure B7.3 shows how the range of β-particles varies with the thickness of air (density 1.29 kg/m^3).

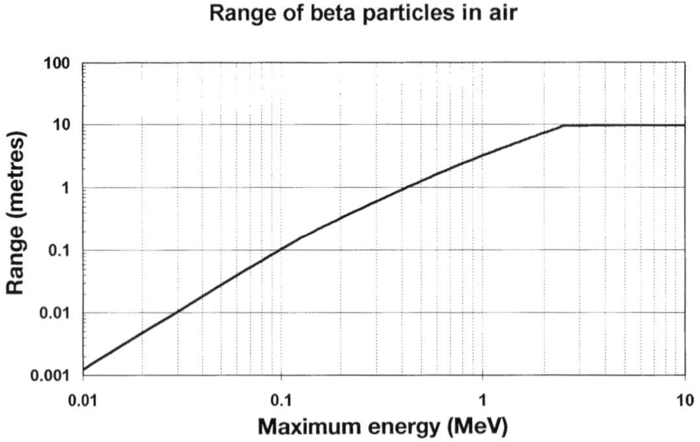

Figure B7.3 Range of β-particles in air.

The maximum β-particle energies from some commonly used nuclides are given in the following table.

Nuclide	Energy (MeV)
C-14	0.156
Ca-45	0.25
C-36	0.710
H-3	0.0186
K-42	3.52
Ni-63	0.067
P-32	1.7
P-33	0.249
S-35	0.167

concentration of 100 Bq cm^{-2} (1 MBq m^{-2}), emitting β-particles with energies over 0.6 MeV, will give a dose rate of over 200 μGy h^{-1} through the protective layer of the skin.

7.4.3 Shielding

Charged particles

As stated above, the distinction between what constitutes an example of protection using distance and what constitutes an example of shielding is somewhat blurred in the case of charged particles. The range of an α-particle in any medium can be obtained from the range in air following the application of a simple equation (Box 7.4). It is generally accepted that α-particles do not present a shielding problem and can be stopped by one or two sheets of paper.

β radiation

The transmission curves for continuous β-ray spectra are similar to those for monoenergetic electrons and are in fact very nearly exponential over almost the entire range

Table 7.2 Z and I bremsstrahlung factors for various absorbers [4]

Material	Effective atomic number Z_{eff}	I factor for ^{32}P	$(Z + I)$
Water	6.6	5.4	12.0
Perspex	5.9	5.4	11.3
Pyrex glass	10	4	14
Steel	26	4.5	30
Lead	82	4	86

of the β-particles. The mass attenuation coefficient for β-particles is almost independent of the atomic number of the absorber, and is for the most part determined by E_{max}. Evans [3] has given a rule of thumb for the half-thickness (in mg cm^{-2} of any material): $D_{1/2} = 40\ E_{\beta}^{1.14}$.

The transmission of β-particles through any material is given by the equation

$$\varphi/\varphi_0 = \exp(-\{-0.693d/D_{\frac{1}{2}}\})$$

where d is the distance travelled through the medium. It is only when the range is almost reached that this equation is not followed.

One complication brought about by the passage of β radiations through a medium is the production of bremsstrahlung radiation (§2.3.1). The relevance of the bremsstrahlung radiation to the protection question will effectively depend on the energy of the β radiation. Two types of bremsstrahlung radiation result from the passage of β-particles through any medium: internal and external. The theory is well documented elsewhere (e.g. [3]).

The continuous spectrum resulting from interaction between the β radiation and the absorber (external bremsstrahlung) is normally the dominant process but the relative contribution will diminish with the atomic number of the absorber [4].

The fraction of the incident β energy converted into external bremsstrahlung radiation is approximately $3 \times 10^{-3}ZE_{\beta}$, where E_{β} is the maximum energy of the β spectrum. The total bremsstrahlung dose rate from a point source of β radiation is given by the equation

$$K_{air} = 6AE_{\beta}^{2}/d^{2}\ [(Z_{eff} + I)\mu_{en}/\rho]\ \mu\text{Gy h}^{-1}$$

where A is the activity in MBq, I takes account of the internal bremsstrahlung, and Z_{eff} is the effective atomic number. This latter quantity can be shown to be equal to

$$Z_{eff} = \sum_{i} N_i Z_i^2 / N_i Z_i$$

where N_i is the fraction of atoms having atomic number Z_i.

The highest energy β emitters likely to be encountered in the medical or laboratory environments are ^{32}P, ^{90}Sr, and ^{90}Y. Of these, ^{32}P is probably the most common. Conventional wisdom has it that such high-energy β-particles should be shielded with low atomic number absorbers such as perspex in order to minimize the bremsstrahlung yield within the absorber. The rationale behind this can be seen directly from Table 7.2 which gives values of Z_{eff} and I for various absorbers of ^{32}P β radiation.

Suppliers often warn against the use of leaded perspex because of the supposed increased hazard produced by bremsstrahlung production in the higher atomic number lead. However, in separate studies, Comben [5] and McLintock [4] have shown that this warning is unwarranted and that in all situations leaded perspex will reduce the bremsstrahlung dose rate from ^{32}P, ^{90}Y, and ^{90}Sr rather than increase it since the lead will attenuate the X-rays. They do, however, conclude that use of leaded perspex is unjustified in laboratories using ^{32}P on cost grounds, although it might be justified if ^{125}I is being used in the same laboratory.

γ- and X-radiation

The major interaction processes that X- and γ-radiation undergo with matter at the energies relevant to this discussion are the photoelectric effect, the Compton effect, and the pair production process (§2.4). The shielding problem is primarily energy specific and is dealt with in depth in Chapters 13 and 17. It is, however, worthwhile to review one or two concepts which are general in nature.

The transmission curve for a monoenergetic gamma ray in 'narrow beam geometry' is exponential and has the form $\varphi = \varphi_0 \exp[(-\mu/\rho)x]$ where φ and φ_0 are the attenuated and unattenuated fluences, respectively, μ/ρ is the mass attenuation coefficient, and x is the thickness traversed in units of density thickness. In the real world, there is no such thing as narrow beam geometry and the implicit assumption that single or multiple Compton events do not make a contribution to the beam becomes invalid. A shield constructed against gamma radiation using the assumption of monoenergetic behaviour will be less effective than envisaged because of the build up of scattered photons. A more appropriate form of the attenuation equation is therefore $\varphi = B\varphi_0 \exp[(-\mu/\rho)x]$, where B is known as the build-up factor. B is dependent on the energy of the radiation,

Table 7.3 Transmission coefficients for ^{131}I, ^{137}Cs, ^{192}Ir, and ^{22}Na

	α	β	γ	Limiting HVL (mm)
^{131}I				
Lead	0.0946	0.1755	0.549	7.3
Concrete	0.0148	7.54e–05	0.203	47
^{137}Cs				
Lead	0.105	–0.002	7.98	6.6
Concrete	0.0144	–0.007	0.9	48.2
^{192}Ir				
Lead	0.118	0.15	0.525	5.9
Concrete	0.0166	–0.008	0.774	42
^{22}Na				
Lead	0.0522	0.0271	0.72	13.3
^{99m}Tc				
Lead	0.24	–0.72	9.51	2.88

the atomic number, and thickness of the absorber. Calculations of B are complex and experimental determination is difficult to achieve.

The shielding problem is different in the case of bremsstrahlung radiation where there is a spectrum of radiation present and the analytical approach produces the equation $\varphi = \sum_{E} \varphi_E = \sum_{E} \varphi_{0E}\, B_E \exp[(-\mu/\rho)x]$ which sums the exponential attenuation over all the energies of the spectrum. There is no mathematically simple descriptor of the attenuation properties of the spectrum. Bremsstrahlung radiation is often described in terms of its 'quality', which is a term that loosely refers to the relative amounts of higher and lower energy radiations present in the spectrum. Thus a beam of 'harder' quality will have relatively more high-energy photons than one of a lower quality produced at the same accelerating potential and will consequently demonstrate lower attenuation. For this reason, such radiation tends to be characterized by its half-value layer (HVL) or tenth-value layer (TVL). As the name suggests, the HVL represents the quantity of a material which reduces the intensity of a beam by a factor of 2. A TVL will reduce the intensity of the radiation by a factor of 10. It is important to note that since the lower energy radiation in the spectrum is attenuated to a greater degree than the higher energy radiation, the first HVL will not be the same as the second, which will not be the same as the third, and so on. Therefore, 3.32 HVLs will not equal one TVL. However, the half-value thickness will tend to a limiting value. To all intents and purposes, the second, third, and ensuing TVLs will be identical.

In 1983, Archer *et al.* [6] developed an empirical model to describe the broad-beam transmission B of X-rays through a material of thickness x provided that the parameters α, β, and γ could be determined for the particular medium:

$$B = [(1 + \beta/\alpha)\ \exp(\alpha\gamma x) - \beta/\alpha]^{-1/\gamma}$$

Hence

$$x = 1/\alpha\gamma\ \ln\,[(B^{-\gamma} + \beta/\alpha)/(1 + \beta/\alpha)].$$

These equations are conventionally used to design shielding for diagnostic radiology applications; if the desired transmission is known then the thickness of any material required to provide that degree of shielding can be evaluated and vice versa. Values for α, β, and γ for a variety of materials at differing accelerating potentials can be found in Chapter 13 and in Sutton and Williams [7] and Simpkin [8]. However, use of the equation is not restricted to diagnostic radiology applications. It is applicable to any broad-beam geometry and can be used for any shielding problem, although in some cases, particularly those involving transmission through heavy elements such as lead, the dominant factor will be α. Table 7.3 gives values for α, β, and γ to describe the broad-beam transmission of ^{131}I, ^{137}Cs, ^{192}Ir, and ^{22}Na through lead and concrete. Analysis of the Archer equation shows that at large values of x the second β/α becomes insignificant and the transmission tends to a simple exponential with a constant equal to α [7]. Thus the final column of Table 7.3 shows the limiting HVL given by $(\ln 2)/\alpha$ which represents the transmission of heavily filtered radiation.

Shielding against neutrons

Radiotherapy is the only mainstream application in medicine where neutrons may be produced and where neutron protection needs to be considered. Neutron production and interactions have been discussed in §2.6. Since the accelerator head does not shield the neutrons in any meaningful way, the neutron fluence in a therapy room will consist of fast neutrons arising from the accelerator head, fast neutrons scattered in the room, and thermal neutrons arising from capture interactions within the room. There will also be prompt γ-rays arising from the capture process.

Reference to equation (2.11) shows that the problem of shielding for neutrons is very different to that for shielding electromagnetic radiation since the most efficient elastic interaction in terms of neutron energy loss is an interaction with the lightest element, hydrogen. In terms of shielding a therapy room, the implication is that any heavy elements incorporated into the fabric of the shielding material, for example steel reinforcing bars in the concrete or iron filings in the wall, which may improve the attenuation of electromagnetic radiation and perhaps reduce the footprint of the bunker, will have the opposite effect for the neutron component. Concrete itself is relatively efficient at attenuating neutrons and the TVL for neutrons in concrete is considerably less than that for any γ radiation; as a result any concrete shielding designed for γ radiation will be enough to absorb any neutrons present.

The remaining problem is that of protection against neutrons scattered down the maze which is a complex process. Concrete lintels are often added to reduce the neutron fluence and it can be advisable to line the inner end of the maze with boron-loaded polythene which has the effect of providing increased shielding against low-energy neutrons (see Chapter 17).

7.5 Protection against internal radiation

Radioactive material can find its way into the body in three ways: ingestion, inhalation, and absorption. The main thrust of the radiation protection effort is to minimize individual exposures by minimizing the intake of radioactive materials into the body. As in the external case this aim can only be achieved by the application of appropriate procedural and operational controls. The same dose limits apply and it can be argued that the principles of shielding, distance, and time are as effective in internal protection as in external protection. Some type of shielding is undoubtedly important since appropriate containment of the radionuclide is the primary method of ensuring that the risk of personal contamination is minimized. The wearing of appropriate clothing and masks can also reduce the possibility of inadvertent contamination. Keeping one's distance is again a sensible precaution as the risk of contamination will be reduced by the use of remote handling equipment where appropriate and the risk of contamination is reduced by minimizing the time of potential exposure to the hazard.

However, the radiation hazard is different from that of external radiation since it does not cease once the exposed person has left the environs of the radiation source, and the radiation dose is delivered over a period of time determined by the residence of the nuclide in the body, the metabolic pathway of the nuclide, the characteristics of the radiation and the target organ or organs. For this reason, the concept of committed effective dose $E(50)$ is used to indicate the dose which will be delivered in the 50 years following the deposition of the radionuclide in the body. The committed effective dose is given by

$$E(50) = \sum_{\mathrm{T}} w_{\mathrm{T}} H_{\mathrm{T}}(50) + w_{\mathrm{remainder}} H_{\mathrm{remainder}}(50)$$

where w_T is the weighting factor applied to the tissue T with committed equivalent dose $H_T(50)$, $w_{\mathrm{remainder}}$ is the weighting factor applied to the remainder tissues, and $H_{\mathrm{remainder}}(50)$ is the committed equivalent dose to the remainder. (For examples of effective dose calculations see Boxes 11.1 and 16.1.)

ICRP 68 [9] publishes values of the dose coefficient $e(50)$ which correspond to the committed effective dose resulting from the intake of 1 Bq of any particular radionuclide. The coefficients are presented for exposure resulting from both ingestion and inhalation and values for some common radionuclides are given in Table 9.5. The ingestion model is relatively straightforward and one value of $e(50)$ is given for each radionuclide. For example, ingestion of 1 Bq ^{131}I results in a committed effective dose of 2.2×10^{-8} Sv. The respiratory tract model is more complex and values of $e(50)$ depend on whether the absorption process is considered to be fast (class F, 100% in 10 min), medium (class M, 10% in 10 min), or slow (class S, 0.1% in 10 min). Further complexity is added by these classes being themselves subdivided according to the average mean aerodynamic diameter (AMAD) of the aerosol in question; values of $e(50)$ are presented for 1 and 5 μm AMAD. In the context of practical modelling, it should be noted that for estimates of occupational exposure use of the 5 μm AMAD value for $e(50)$ is recommended. By way of example, inhalation of a 5 μm aerosol of ^{131}I, which will be treated as being in class F, results in a committed effective dose of 1.1×10^{-8} Sv. For completeness, values of $e(50)$ are also given for both reactive gases, such as $^{14}CO_2$, and for inert gases, for example ^{85m}Kr.

Control of occupational exposure is exercised by the application of a quantity termed the annual limit on intake (ALI) which is directly related to the existing 20 mSv limit on effective dose. ALI is a derived quantity and represents the amount of a radionuclide which, when ingested or inhaled, would result in a committed effective dose of 20 mSv. It is treated as a secondary radiation limit and the ALI (in Bq) for any radionuclide can easily be derived by dividing the annual dose limit of 20 mSv by $e(50)$ thus:

$$\text{ALI} = 0.02/e(50).$$

It should be noted that the definition of ALI changed with the publication of ICRP 60 [10]. The previous definition of ALI as introduced in ICRP 30 and based on the framework introduced by ICRP 26 used the occupational dose limit for effective dose of 50 mSv and included the additional inequality that committed equivalent dose to any one organ should not exceed 500 mSv. This extra requirement has now been dropped, the implication being that while ALIs based on the recommendations of ICRP 60 will in general be more restrictive than those based on the previous framework, there is the possibility that individual committed equivalent doses to specific organs might well be higher than was previously permitted. The ICRP justify this change on the basis that the long-term nature of the radiation exposure from many internally deposited radionuclides makes it extremely unlikely that deterministic effects will occur.

7.5.1 Operational aspects

As stated above, the principal aim of radiation protection against internal sources of radiation is to ensure that the potential for intake into the body is as low as possible. It should be remembered that it is necessary to think beyond the environment where the work is being carried out and consider the eventual fate of the radionuclide, that is the disposal route should be taken into account. There is no substitute for the adoption of good working practices and techniques, coupled with the application of strict regulation.

No new technique or method should be allowed to start without some type of risk assessment being carried out. Before considering what practical steps are necessary to minimize the risk of contamination, it will always be necessary to consider the results of the risk assessment which will take into account both the activity and the radiotoxicity of the nuclide being used. The same risk assessment should take into account whether the eventual disposal will result in non-trivial committed doses to members of the public (i.e. whether it is within the limits allowable for the overall site authorization to dispose of radioactive waste; see §9.3).

It is always a good idea to segregate areas within laboratories or departments where work with radionuclides will be performed, irrespective of the nuclide or activity. There are several advantages to this approach even when low levels of activity are being used. For example, staff always know that particular precautions need to be taken in the designated area, contamination monitoring and decontamination can be carried out according to a fixed protocol, any bench surfaces can be covered appropriately, and records of usage and disposal are much easier to maintain. (For detail on the practicalities involved in the above procedures, see Chapter 15.) As levels of activity increase, it becomes imperative to allocate particular areas for radionuclide work alone, if only to comply with legislative requirements.

7.5.2 Containment of radionuclides

Within any area set aside for use with radionuclides, it is important that steps should be taken to ensure that appropriate procedures and techniques for containing the radionuclide are adopted. The degree of containment required will depend on the particular radionuclide and activity, as identified in the risk assessment performed prior to using the radionuclide. In the simplest case, it may be appropriate to carry out the procedure in a tray, so that any spills are contained easily. In some cases, for example where there is a risk of aerosol production or a volatile substance is being used, it may be necessary to work in a fume cupboard. In others, a negative-pressure remote-handling cabinet may be needed. Special conditions will apply if the work is being carried out in an aseptic environment (see Chapter 15). When not being used, radionuclides must be contained appropriately. At the simplest level appropriate containment will be provided by placing the radionuclide in a lead pot in a cupboard or refrigerator, which must be lockable if it is in an area with open access. Increasing activity and/or radiotoxicity will require increased, but not necessarily more sophisticated, containment.

7.5.3 Technique and training

Irrespective of the quantity or nature of the radionuclide being used, it is imperative that all users be appropriately trained in terms of both technique and radiation protection. The training should cover both theoretical and practical considerations; there is no acceptable substitute for 'hands on' practical training. The type and level of training required will depend on the application and also on whether the use of radionuclides involves the irradiation of patients or not.

If the use of radionuclides is clinical and results in the irradiation of a patient, then the degree of training required will be specified in the applicable legislation; for example, the Ionising Radiation (Medical Exposure) Regulations 2000 and the ARSAC (Administration of Radioactive Substances Committee) notes for guidance laid down under the Medicines (Administration of Medical Substances) Regulations 1978. In most cases the training will need to have been formally completed before the user can work in an unsupervised manner. However, before being allowed to work, the user should be made familiar with the local rules and practices in the area in which they are employed.

If radionuclides are not being used in the clinical sense described above, then there will not be the same level of prescription. However, some generalizations can be made. New users of radionuclides should attend a centrally organized radiation training course. Since it is unreasonable to expect a course to be organized for individual members of staff, arrangements will need to be made for basic protection training to be delivered at local (i.e. departmental) level. This training can, for example, be delivered via a computerized distance-learning package or training video. The user should read the local rules applying to his or her laboratory and be aware of the properties of the radionuclides being used. If such training cannot be organized, then the potential user should not start work. Practical training regarding techniques used in the laboratory will be given by the user's supervisor, line manager, or departmental trainer. The role of the centrally organized course is to reinforce the messages already delivered and familiarize the user with the radiation protection framework and personnel involved.

Advanced training will be required for personnel who are given a supervisory role over radiation work in their area. Although such training can be organized in-house, given the generally low turnover of such staff, it may prove to be more cost-effective to use an external course.

The training process is continual and refresher courses should be organized from time to time. Such courses can serve both to remind staff of some of the more important aspects such as the use and choice of contamination monitors and to bring users up to date with any new developments in the field such as changes in the applicable legislation.

7.5.4 Protective equipment

The degree of personal protection required will depend on the work being carried out. In laboratories and nuclear medicine departments, the contamination hazard will be reduced for the most part by the use of appropriate techniques and methods. However, to further minimize the risk of contamination, and as a minimum, laboratory coats and gloves should always be worn when radionuclides are being used or injected. Contamination monitoring of work areas and personnel should be carried out when work on a particular operation has finished. Some areas of work will require increased levels of protection. For example:

- Staff involved with lung ventilation scanning may be advised to wear face masks to reduce the risk of inhalation.
- Staff preparing radiopharmaceuticals in an aseptic suite may be advised to wear a suit which covers the whole body as well as a face mask and a hair cover.
- Staff involved with iodination work should wear two pairs of gloves because of the ability of iodine-labelled compounds to penetrate gloves and be absorbed firmly onto the skin.
- Staff performing multiple operations might wear two pairs of gloves and change the outer pair frequently, to reduce contamination levels.
- Where appropriate, work should be carried out behind a splash guard.

The above list is by no means exhaustive but is designed to demonstrate the types of protection required and the different scenarios involved. The actual personal protection requirements and practices must be tailored to the application. They will be determined when the work is first considered and, like all other elements of the protection programme, should be reviewed from time to time.

7.5.5 Record keeping

Record keeping is an important part of operational radiation protection against the internal radiation hazard. It serves the dual purpose of ensuring that users employ good practice and giving a firm focus to audit.

- To ensure that proper operational control be maintained, all users of radionuclides should be registered, as should all areas in which the nuclides are used.
- The use to which the radionuclides are put should be known.
- Each area or department where radionuclides are used should be allocated a maximum amount of any particular radionuclide based upon the global site limits for disposal and retention.
- There should be records which enable any delivery of radioactivity to be traced from receipt on the premises to eventual disposal. (For example, in the laboratory environment, it should be possible to trace a disposal to drain back to the stock solution and thence to the original order.)
- Records of contamination monitoring should be maintained for inspection, as should records of disposal via all routes.

All of the above records, which are discussed in greater detail in Chapter 9, can be used as part of the audit process (ALARA review) to ensure that the ALARA principle is being adhered to.

7.6 References

1 International Atomic Energy Agency (1990). *Operational Radiation Protection: a guide to optimisation.* Safety Series No. 101. IAEA, Vienna.

2 EUR 13796 (1992). *ALARA—from theory towards practice.* CEC, Luxembourg.
3 Evans, R. D. (1955). *The atomic nucleus.* McGraw-Hill, New York.
4 McLintock, I. S. (1994). *Bremsstrahlung from radionuclides.* HHSC Handbook No. 15. HHSC, Leeds.
5 Comben, J. Y. (1991). Perspex shields. *J. Radiol. Prot.*, **11**, 139.
6 Archer, B. R., Thornby, J. I., and Bushong, S. C. (1983) Diagnostic X-ray shielding design based on an empirical model of photon attenuation. *Health Phys.*, **44**, 507–17.
7 Sutton, D. G. and Williams, J. R. (2000). *Radiation shielding for diagnostic X-rays.* BIR, London.
8 Simpkin, D. J. (1995). Transmission data for shielding diagnostic X-ray facilities. *Health Phys.*, **70**, 238–44.
9 International Commission for Radiological Protection (1994). Dose coefficients for intakes of radionuclides by workers. ICRP 68. *Ann. ICRP*, **24**, 4.
10 International Commission for Radiological Protection (1991). 1990 Recommendations of the International Commission on Radiological Protection. ICRP 60. *Ann. ICRP*, **21**, 1–3.
11 Delacroix, D., Guerre, J. P., Leblanc, P., and Hickman, C. (1998). Radionuclide and radiation protection data handbook. *Radiat. Prot. Dosim.*, **76**, 1–126.

Chapter 8
Personal monitoring

D. H. Temperton and S. Green

8.1 Theory and units

The concept of effective dose [1] was discussed in Chapter 3 as a limiting quantity in radiological protection. Calculating the effective dose, E, requires the determination of equivalent doses to various individual tissues or organs (H_T) in the body which have to be multiplied by the appropriate tissue weighting factor (w_T) and then summed according to equation (3.3). Effective dose includes exposures from both external and internal (or committed) exposures. Effective dose is therefore difficult to assess and impossible to measure directly. In order to monitor occupational doses a simpler approach is necessary. The simplest solution for external irradiation would be to use a primary physical quantity such as air kerma. However, such a simple approach can lead to a significant *underestimation* of the effective dose [2]. To overcome these problems the International Commission on Radiation Units (ICRU) has recommended operational dose equivalent quantities for practical use in radiological protection where external sources are concerned [3]. The quantity which is relevant to external personal monitoring is personal dose equivalent, $H_p(d)$. (ICRU also define two other quantities, ambient dose equivalent and directional dose equivalent, which are relevant for area monitoring but which will not be discussed further in this chapter.) Dose quantities for protection against external radiations are discussed in detail by NRPB [4].

For assessments of committed effective dose the operational quantity is the intake of radioactive material in becquerels. In particular, the annual limit on intake (ALI) is the activity of a particular radionuclide which will give a committed effective dose of 20 mSv. Internal dosimetry is discussed further in §8.5.

8.1.1 Personal dose equivalent, $H_p(d)$

The personal dose equivalent, $H_p(d)$, is the dose equivalent in soft tissue below a specified point on the body at an appropriate depth, d. Soft tissue is ICRU 4-element tissue. The unit of personal dose equivalent is joules per kilogram (J kg^{-1}) with the special name sievert (Sv). When quoting personal dose equivalent it is important to specify the reference depth, d, which should be in millimetres. It is important to note that ICRU still uses dose equivalent and not equivalent dose. These two quantities are different. Equivalent dose is the absorbed dose averaged over a tissue or organ and weighted for the type of radiation *incident* on the body (§3.2.2), whereas dose equivalent is a *point* quantity in an organ, obtained by multiplying absorbed dose by a quality factor which depends on the radiation type and energy at that point. For penetrating radiations this difference is not significant but this is not the case for low-energy photons or neutrons.

A depth of 10 mm is usually employed for monitoring of effective dose or other organs deep in the body and the personal dose equivalent is denoted by $H_p(10)$. Depths of 0.07 mm and 3 mm are employed (and denoted as $H_p(0.07)$ and $H_p(3)$) when controlling doses to superficial organs like the skin and eye respectively. For a comparison of effective dose and personal dose equivalent, see Box 8.1.

$H_p(d)$ is defined *in the body* and is therefore still not measurable. The value of $H_p(d)$ will vary from person to person and with the location on the body at which it is measured. However, in practice, $H_p(d)$ can be assessed with a detector which is worn at the surface of the body and covered with an appropriate thickness of tissue-equivalent material [3]. To make the quantity single-valued, a particular location on the human body needs to be specified, together with a particular phantom of the body for calibration. 'Surrogate' quantities for $H_p(10)$ have been introduced with respect to the phantom that is used for calibration to overcome this difficulty, e.g. $H_{p,slab}(d)$ when using a slab phantom [5]. The true quantity is obtained through calculation, utilizing Monte Carlo simulation of radiation interactions within mathematical models of the relevant phantoms.

Box 8.1 Comparison of effective dose and personal dose equivalent

NRPB [4] concluded that for photon radiations 'the operational dose quantities $H_p(10)$ and $H_p(0.07)$ should provide a good measure of effective dose without any underestimation'. However, for neutron irradiations they concluded that 'there is a potential for both overestimation and underestimation, but practical field measurements show that overestimates are more likely to occur'.

Zankl [6] evaluated the ratio $E/H_p(10)$ for external irradiation by monoenergetic photons for a dosemeter worn in a typical position 14.4 cm below the thyroid and 4 cm from the midline using a voxel model of the human trunk. For most energies and irradiation geometries $H_p(10)$ is a conservative or close approximation of E. The major exceptions are lateral irradiation by photons below 20 keV, posterior anterior (PA) irradiation and lateral irradiation by photons of all energies from the side away from the dosemeter. The underestimation for PA irradiation corresponds to the practical situation where a dosemeter is worn on the front of the body but is primarily irradiated through the back. Zankl concluded that the underestimation for lateral irradiations is caused partly by the definition of $H_p(10)$ at a depth *in the body*. If $H_p(10)$ was evaluated at specific locations on the *surface of the trunk*, there would be reduced shielding by overlying tissue. This altered definition would reflect the way that personal dosemeters are used in practice.

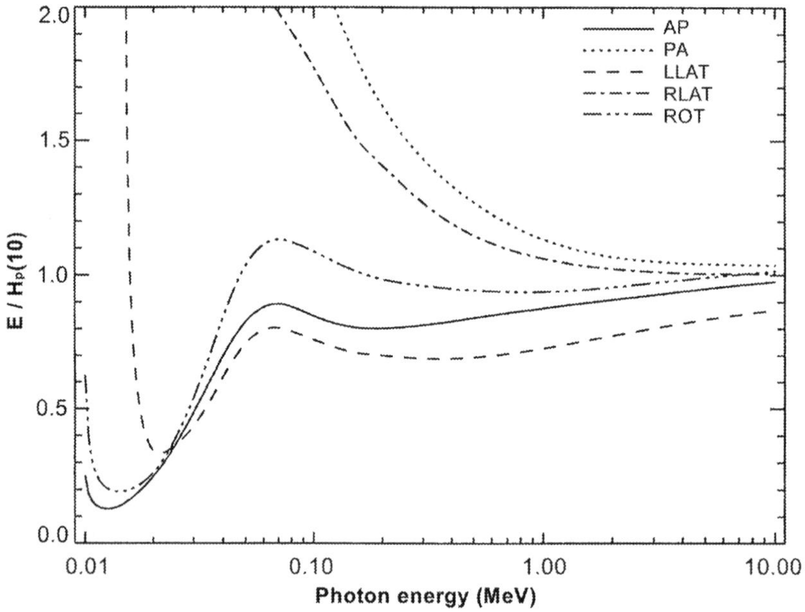

Figure B8.1 Ratio of effective dose, E, to personal dose equivalent, $H_p(10)$, for a typical dosimeter position on the left side of the trunk for monoenergetic photons incident in various irradiation geometries. The directions of the beam were antero-posterior (AP), postero-anterior (PA), left lateral (LLAT), right lateral (RLAT), full 360° rotation of beam around longitudinal axis of body (ROT). Reproduced from the journal *Health Physics* [6] with permission from the Health Physics Society.

8.1.2 Calibration of dosimeters

Type tests

A type test is designed to evaluate the performance of a dosemeter over a range of energies and angles of incidence, and would normally be performed by a specialized calibration laboratory.

The calibration of the dosemeters used for individual or personal monitoring needs to be carried out on a phantom which will mimic the backscatter properties of the part of the body on which it is worn. ISO has recommended that a water-filled phantom of dimensions 30 cm × 30 cm × 15 cm depth and made of PMMA (perspex) walls is used for dosemeters worn on the body [7]. A PMMA cylinder phantom 19 mm in diameter and with a length of 300 mm is recommended for dosemeters worn on the fingers. Full secondary charged-particle equilibrium has to be achieved [8]. The radiation type and energy is selected from the series of ISO reference radiations.

Table 8.1 Selected conversion coefficients from air kerma to $H_p(10)$ in the ICRU slab phantom for monoenergetic and parallel radiation

Photon energy (keV)	Conversion coefficient (Sv/Gy) for different angles of incidence			
	0°	20°	45°	80°
15	0.26	0.25	0.15	0.00
20	0.61	0.59	0.47	0.04
30	1.11	1.09	0.96	0.28
40	1.49	1.46	1.33	0.50
50	1.77	1.74	1.57	0.67
80	1.90	1.88	1.75	0.86
100	1.81	1.79	1.68	0.87
150	1.61	1.60	1.52	0.86
400	1.30	1.30	1.29	0.89
600	1.23	1.23	1.23	0.92
1250	1.15	1.15	1.16	0.96

Source: ISO [7].

Calculation of the true value of $H_p(10)$ and $H_p(0.07)$ is achieved by using published conversion coefficients. The ISO standard contains factors to convert air kerma to personal dose equivalent in the relevant phantoms for different standard radiation qualities or monoenergetic energies and for different angles of incidence [7]. Table 8.1 gives examples of these for the ICRU slab phantom.

Routine calibrations

Routine calibrations are carried out to determine the calibration factors for individual dosemeters or batches of dosemeters. Provided the performance of the dosemeters, as determined by the type test, is constant, routine calibrations can be carried out free in air and in calibration rooms where there may be a significant amount of room scatter. However, the true calibration of a dosemeter in terms of $H_p(d)$ needs to be established either by using the dosemeter as a transfer instrument or by using a radiation instrument whose energy response in terms of air kerma is similar to the dosemeter [8].

8.2 Requirements for personal dosimetry services

As was described in Chapter 6, radiation workers who are likely to be exposed to significant doses of radiation (more than three-tenths of the dose limit) must be identified. Within the European Basic Safety Standard they are termed category A workers; within UK legislation they are designated as classified persons. Individual (or personal) monitoring on these workers must be systematic. The required standards for dosimetry services carrying out monitoring are specified in the country of operation. For example, in the USA, the National Voluntary Laboratory Accreditation Programme (NVLAP) and the Department of Energy Laboratory Accreditation Programme (DOELAP) accredit monitoring services. In the UK, services are approved by the Health and Safety Executive (HSE)—a clear distinction is made between external dose assessments, internal dose assessments, and record keeping. The standards specified by HSE include the facilities, general arrangements necessary for dose assessment, including calibration and traceability, and the calibre of staff engaged in the work. Key requirements for approval as an external dosimetry service in the UK are:

1. Dose assessment methods must normally comply with published data.
2. Individually identifiable personal dosemeters must be used.
3. The dosemeter used must have the required accuracy, reliability, and suitability for the environment in which it will be used and over an appropriate dose range (§8.2.1). A whole-body dosemeter must be able to cover the dose range 0.2 mSv–1 Sv (gamma radiation) and 0.2 mSv to at least 50 mSv (neutrons).
4. The calibration system must be traceable to National Standards.
5. Re-evaluation of doses must be possible for up to 2 years after receipt of the dosemeter. For TLD systems (§8.3.3), this requirement is satisfied by retaining the glow curve.
6. Assessed doses must be transferred to a record-keeping service within 14 days.
7. Periodic performance tests must be carried out (§8.2.2).
8. Advice must be provided about the handling, storage, issue, and use of dosemeters.

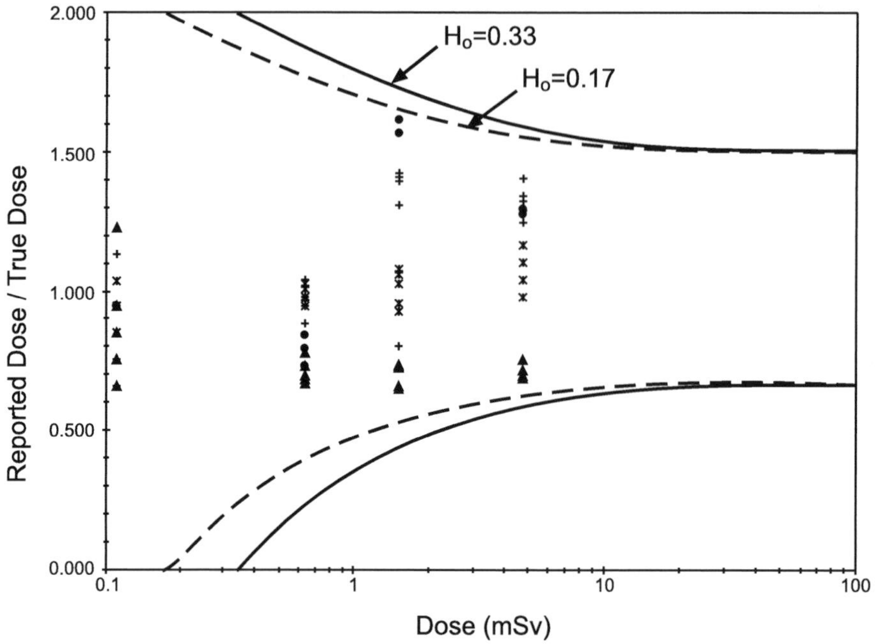

Figure 8.1 Sample results from an intercomparison carried out by the Personal Radiation Monitoring Group (PRMG) within the UK using ISO wide-series X-ray spectrum at 80 kVp using trumpet curves (see §8.2.1) with an H_o value of 0.17 mSv (monthly) and 0.33 mSv (2 monthly). For clarity, results are only shown for two centres using TLD and two centres using film with 5 dose points per centre. The results for all PRMG members fell within the curves.

9. Written quality assurance procedures must exist for monitoring performance.

8.2.1 Accuracy

The overall accuracy required in personal monitoring has been stated by ICRP [1, 9, 10]. Christensen and Griffith [11] summarized the requirements for external photon monitoring by smoothing the allowable accuracy interval as a function of dose resulting in the so-called trumpet curves (see Figure 8.1). These curves define upper and lower levels between which 19 out of 20 dose assessments made by a monitoring service should lie, i. e. 95% confidence intervals. The upper accuracy level, H_{ul}, is given by the equation:

$$H_{ul} = 1.5[1 + H_o/(2H_o + H_t)]$$

and the lower level, H_{ll}, is given by

$$H_{ll} = 0 \qquad \text{for } H_t < Ho$$

$$H_{ll} = (1/1.5)[1 - 2H_o/(H_o + H_t)] \qquad \text{for } H_t = H_o$$

where H_t is the conventional true dose and H_o is the lowest dose required to be measured. H_o is set to one-tenth of the fraction of the annual dose limit, corresponding to the issuing period, i.e. 0.17 mSv (20 mSv ÷10 ÷ 12) for monthly monitoring of $H_p(10)$. The interval between the upper and lower levels increases as the monitoring period increases, particularly at low doses. Examples of the use of these curves are given in Figure 8.1 which shows the results of intercomparisons organized between monitoring services in the UK. The confidence limits allow for errors due to variations in the dosemeter sensitivity with incident energy and direction of incidence as well as intrinsic errors in the dosemeter and its calibration. They do not allow for uncertainties in deriving tissue or organ dose equivalents from the dosemeter results.

ICRP noted that the uncertainty may be substantially greater for neutrons of uncertain energy and electrons compared with photons without quantifying this greater uncertainty [10].

The overall accuracy that can be achieved when assessing the dose from internal exposures is likely to be lower than external exposure. In particular, the time distribution of the intake of radionuclide is rarely known for routine monitoring. Sampling frequencies recommended by ICRP are chosen to avoid errors due to this cause of more than a factor of 3 [12]. For simple monitoring (e.g. for ^{131}I), this may be the predominant factor. For more complex assessments (e.g. for insoluble plutonium), the overall uncertainty may be about one order of magnitude [12].

8.2.2 Performance tests

The bodies accrediting or approving dosimetry services require some kind of performance test. The service sends dosemeters to a recognized irradiation laboratory which gives them a known dose and they are then sent back to the service for evaluation. The exact requirements vary from country to country. For example, in Germany, the Physikalisch-Technische Bundesanstalt (PTB) carries out unannounced tests once a year. The service has to evaluate the doses on previously irradiated dosemeters within a day in the presence of an official. Failure to achieve a satisfactory result can lead to removal of the service's approval or accreditation. Results from these performance tests demonstrate that the difference between film and TL dosemeters is minimal [13].

Within the UK performance tests must be undertaken at least once every 18 months. The performance tests are designed to relate the test results to the *expected* values for the dosemeter. In effect they are testing the quality of the service being provided (e.g. calibration, consistency, etc.) rather than the performance of the dosemeter itself (i.e. energy and angular dependence).

8.2.3 Requirements for coordination and record keeping

An individual radiation worker may be monitored for whole-body external photon and neutron irradiation and internal radiation. All these exposures will contribute towards the limiting quantity, effective dose. In addition, the wearer may have worn dosemeters to check doses to the hands or eyes. All these dose assessments may be carried out by a variety of approved dosimetry services. In order for an employer to have an accurate indication of the total radiation exposure of his/her radiation workers and check compliance with legal dose limits, it is important that the results of all these measurements are collated in secure and clear records. The requirements for record keeping and coordination in the UK are expressed more clearly than in other countries such as the USA and are summarized below.

1. Have clear records which contain a very comprehensive list of specified items.
2. Have a system which prevents corruption or degradation of data.
3. Ensure dose information is transferred into the records within 14 days.
4. Exchange information to the Central Index of Dose Information (CIDI).
5. Inform the employer when an estimated dose is required because, for example, a dosemeter has been lost or damaged.
6. Flag and notify the employer regarding doses above specified action levels.
7. Alter the dose record only in authorized circumstances.
8. Maintain the records until the wearer reaches the age of 75 and for 50 years.
9. Provide the employer with regular clear written dose summaries and whenever an employee leaves their employment. An example of a personal dose summary is given in Figure 8.2.

8.3 Whole-body (external) monitoring

8.3.1 Introduction

Any staff who have to regularly enter a controlled radiation area should definitely be monitored for external whole-body irradiation. ICRP concluded that 'individual monitoring for external radiation is fairly simple and does not require a heavy commitment of resources' [1]. Radiation Protection Advisers often advise that other staff regularly working with radiation but not necessarily in controlled areas, e.g. laboratory workers, should also be individually monitored to demonstrate that dose reduction techniques are effective. Receptionist staff and others who work in departments such as imaging and radiotherapy but do not have to enter controlled areas do not normally need monitoring. Occasionally, however, monitoring is necessary purely for reassurance purposes even though there is not a significant risk of exposure. In these cases monitoring can usually be for a restricted period (e.g. 3–4 months). If a large number of staff intermittently perform a task with a relatively low risk of significant exposure (for example escort nurses in X-ray departments) it is acceptable to issue a single dosemeter which is shared between staff. Provided this dosemeter records no doses it is a valid demonstration that staff are not being exposed. If, however, doses are recorded, further investigations are required. The use of an electronic dosemeter with an immediate readout (§8.3.5) is then particularly useful.

Conversion coefficients per air kerma free-in-air for $H_p(10)$ vary with dosemeter position [6]. In other words the position in which a whole-body dosemeter is worn will influence the value of the assessed dose. In the UK, guidance states that the dosemeter should be 'worn on the trunk at chest or waist height' [14].

Staff involved with fluoroscopic X-ray examinations wear lead aprons to shield various organs in the trunk region (§13.5.2) and therefore will be receiving non-uniform irradiation. Faulkner and Marshall [15] concluded that a single whole-body dosemeter worn above the apron (at the neck or forehead) will always significantly overestimate the effective dose, but if worn

PS/12/01/01/002

Employer
MIDLANDS NHS TRUST
BIRMINGHAM, WEST MIDLANDS

RRPPS Approved Dosimetry Service
P.O.Box 803, Edgbaston, BIRMINGHAM B15 2TB
Tel. 0121 627 2091, Fax 0121 472 0393

12/01/2001

PERSONAL DOSE SUMMARY

for DIANA MAY MORGAN (396)
MIDLANDS NHS TRUST

For the attention of: MIDLANDS NHS TRUST

Personal details
Name: MORGAN,DIANA MAY
Sex: F
Date of birth: 04/03/1958
NI number: WE 45 68 74 D

Employment details
Work category: Cycl. and X-ray
Commenced as classified worker: 01/06/1988
Terminated as classified worker:
CIDI occupation code: 341

Current employer details
SIC code: N/A
CIDI employer code: N/A
Current Passbook: **000004**

PERSONAL DOSE SUMMARY

YEAR	DOSE TYPE	POSITION	MONTH DOSES in mSv Jan	Feb	Mar	Apr	May	Jun	Jul	Aug	Sep	Oct	Nov	Dec	TOTAL	ANNUAL DOSES in mSv E_{ext}	E	LIMIT
2000	xbg	Whole Body	0.4	P	0.6	0.3	*			*	0.4				1.7	1.7	1.7	20.0
1999	xbg	Whole Body	2.2	1.4	P	0.3	0.4[ZE]								4.3	4.3	4.3	50.0
	Organ H_T	Right Hand			6.8	12.2	8.6								27.6			500.0
1998	xbg	Whole Body	*	0.3	0.4	P	P	*[C]	0.3	*	0.5	*	0.2[QE]	*[$]	1.7	3.6	4.3	50.0
	Non-th. neutron	Whole Body	0.3[500]	*[500]	0.5[500]									0.5[500]	1.3			
	Skin beta	Skin		2.4	1.3				5.6		2.2				11.5			
	Entered E_{int}	Whole Body		0.6[190]	0.1[190]	*[190]									0.7			
	Entered CED	Bone Surface		0.8[190]	0.2[190]	0.2[190]									1.2			
	Organ H_T	Right Hand	0.6	0.5	0.3	0.4	0.6								2.4			500.0
	Organ H_T	Left Hand	0.3	0.2	0.3	0.2	0.2								1.2			500.0
	Organ H_T	Thyroid						18.4[160]							18.4			

Notes
P: Meter un-used Z: Dose assessment impossible E: Estimated reading given C: Contaminated meter/holder Q: Meter lost $: Non-standard dates

Dosimetry services providing information
500 : NRPB,Chilton Didcot Oxon OX11 0RQ
190 : AWE,Atomic Weapons Research Est Approved Dosimetry Service Building A6.1 Aldermaston Reading RG7 4PR
160 : JET Joint Undertaking,JET Personnel Dosimetry Service Building k2 Room 1/09 Culham Labortory Abingdon Oxon OX14 3GA

Prior to 1st January 2000, E, E_{ext}, E_{int} and H_T were measured as effective dose equivalent, effective dose equivalent from external radiation, committed effective dose equivalent, and dose equivalent respectively.
Where a meter was worn for non-standard dates, rounding may mean that the annual total does not equal the sum of the period doses. The annual total is correct.
E_{ext}: Effective dose equivalent E_{int}: Committed Effective dose equivalent H_T: Equivalent dose CED: Committed equivalent dose
* = below recording level (0.2 mSv for RRPPS). Record allocated 0.2mSv before 1986, 0.0mSv afterwards An Entered E_{ext} or E_{int} supersedes other contributions to E_{ext} or E_{int} in the same period.
Dose limit to abdomen of woman of reproductive capacity = 13mSv in three months xbg: Penetrating dose from x-rays, betas and gammas

Figure 8.2 Example of coordinated dose record for an individual wearer.

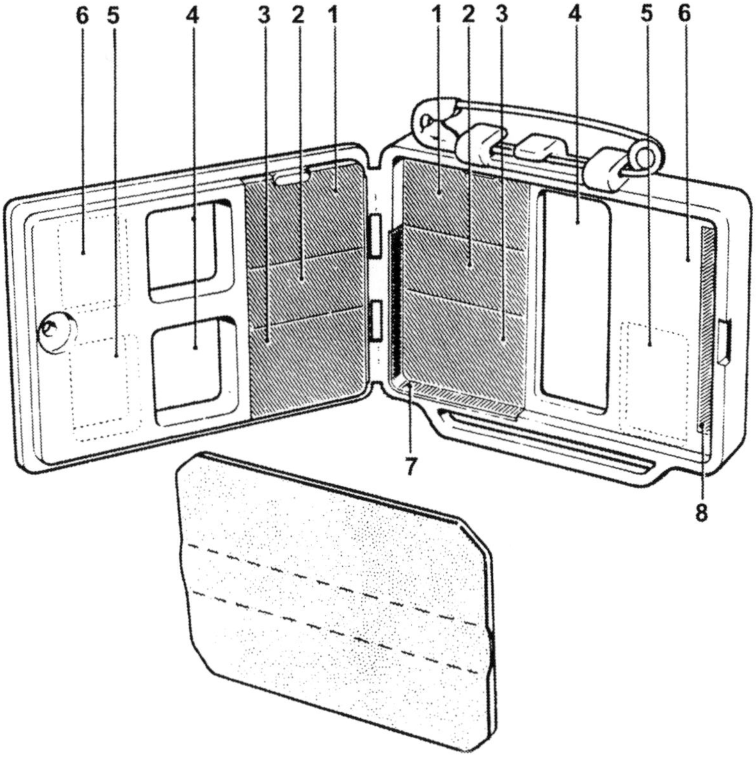

1	0.040" Dural	5	50 mg cm^{-2} plastics
2	0.028" Cd+0.012" Pb	6	300 mg cm^{-2} plastics
3	0.028" Sn+0.012" Pb	7	0.012" Pb edge shielding
4	Open Window	8	0.40 gm indium

Figure 8.3 NRPB/AERE film badge holder. Reproduced from Iles *et al.* [17] with permission from the National Radiological Protection Board.

under the lead apron it will provide a closer estimate of the effective dose, although it may underestimate the true value in many cases. In the UK, it is normal practice for staff wearing only one dosemeter to wear this under the lead apron. Staff carrying out high-interventional radiology workloads are sometimes issued with additional dosemeters that are worn outside and above the apron at the neck. Various empirical combinations of the two values have been proposed to give a better estimate of the effective dose. NCRP [16] recommended the formula

$$E(\text{estimate}) = 0.5\ H_w + 0.025\ H_N$$

where H_W is the $H_p(10)$ value for the dosemeter worn at the waist or on the chest under the apron and H_N is the $H_p(10)$ value for the dosemeter worn outside the apron. The resulting value of E(estimate) will be in the range 1.06 to 2.03 E. There is no obligation for dosimetry services within the UK to apply such a formula.

8.3.2 Film dosemeters

Various systems using film as the detector are available (e.g. ICN, California; NRPB/AERE). They consist of a film sandwiched within a film holder which has several different filter areas. Figure 8.3 shows the construction of the NRPB/AERE holder. These filters are necessary because of the large inherent photon energy dependence of the film. This high-energy dependence also requires the use of two emulsions to extend the useful dose range of the dosemeter—a fast emulsion on one side and a slow emulsion on the other. The energy-dependent information below the filters can be combined to give a response which is substantially independent of energy over a large energy range. However, because the optical density of the film after exposure to radiation does not vary linearly with dose, the *densities* cannot be simply combined. Instead, it is necessary to convert the measured densities to a radiation quantity. Recent calibrations of the

NRPB/AERE system use the 'apparent gamma air kerma'. Algorithms have been derived for combining these apparent gamma air kermas to optimise the energy response of the dosemeter [17]. The type of radiation and, in some cases, the energy range determine the filtered areas used. Beta doses in terms of $H_p(0.07)$ can be evaluated using apparent gamma air kermas under the open window and plastic filter areas, and thermal neutron dose evaluation uses the cadmium and tin/lead filter areas. Thermal neutrons interact with cadmium via an (n, γ) reaction to produce additional film blackening.

The dose range covered varies, depending on the radiation type and energy, but is typically: 0.1 mSv to 10 Sv (hard gamma radiation); 0.1 mSv to about 300 mSv (diagnostic energy X-rays at the peak response of the film); 0.1 mSv to about 1 Sv (beta radiation); and 0.1 mSv to about 5 Sv (thermal neutrons).

Film has the advantage of giving a permanent visual record of the exposure which can be used for reassessment. Ratios of the optical densities under different filter areas can be used to give an estimate of the radiation energy. It is also possible to see the circumstances of the exposure. For example, a sharp edge to the shadows of filter edges indicates a single exposure; a blurred edge indicates an exposure to scattered radiation or that the wearer has been moving about in a radiation field. It is possible to see whether the film has been contaminated with radioactive material. If the contamination is very localized it is often possible to still read the film by measuring areas away from the contamination. Green and Palethorpe [18] have reported that the NRPB/AERE film dosemeter meets the requirements of ICRP [19] for personal monitoring.

8.3.3 Thermoluminescence dosemeters (TLDs)

The physics of thermoluminescence (TL) dosimetry was discussed in §4.12.2. TLD personal monitoring is carried out by a variety of commercial systems and different TL materials. The most common TL material used for personal monitoring is LiF:Mg,Ti but $Li_2B_4O_7$:Mn and CaF_2 are also used. The properties of these materials are summarized in Table 8.2. LiF:Mg,Ti is popular because

- it is nearly tissue equivalent
- it emits light at 400 nm which matches the peak spectral response of common photomultiplier tubes
- its main TL peak occurs at 200°C which is high enough to minimize fading of the stored signal at room temperature but not so high as to generate infrared emissions from the dosemeter during readout
- its glow curve enables easy separation of low-temperature peaks
- it is not adversely affected by ambient conditions except for ultraviolet light.

Whole-body TL dosemeters or badges consist of a holder with different filter areas and a robust card, made of aluminium for example, to which multiple TLDs are fixed. The performance of each system will depend on which particular TL materials are used, the size (particularly thickness) and form of the TLD (e.g. whether chips or PTFE discs), the filter holder and the readout process. The dosemeter card has at least two dosemeters. One TLD is positioned below a very thin filter (essentially just protecting the TLD) so that it can measure $H_p(0.07)$. The second TLD is below a thicker filter designed to enable it to measure $H_p(10)$. The card may contain additional dosemeters, for example:

- another TLD below a different filter to provide information on the energy of the incident radiation, in a similar fashion to the film badge holder described above. A TL material with a larger energy response than LiF:Mg,Ti can be selected to increase the ability

Table 8.2 Characteristics of some thermoluminescent materials

Phosphor characteristics	LiF:Mg,Ti	$Li_2B_4O_7$	CaF_2:nat
Density (g cm^{-3})	2.64	2.3	3.18
Chemical stability	Good	Hygroscopic	Good
Effective atomic number	8.2	7.4	16.3
Main glow peak temperature (°C) (at heating rate of 100°C/min)	210	200	270
Spectral emission peak (nm)	400	605	380
Fading of dosimetry peak at normal ambient temperature	5% in 3 months	10% in 2 months	<3% in 9 months
Ratio of TL response at 30 keV/1.25 MeV	1.3	0.9	13
Useful dose range (Gy)	5×10^{-5}–10^{3}	10^{-4}–10^{4}	10^{-5}–10^{2}

Adapted from McKinlay [20].

to distinguish between different radiation energies. Algorithms within the computer software compare the ratios of the responses from the different TL materials to evaluate the energy and can then apply any necessary corrections for the energy responses of the material to provide a more accurate assessment of the dose.

- a pair of TLDs to give thermal neutron doses or even a non-TL fast neutron dosemeter.

The dosemeter card contains a unique identifier such as a barcode which enables the system to be automated. Multiple cards can be preloaded in a holding device which is placed in the reader. The reader will then process all the dosemeters automatically. By reading the barcode, the system knows the wearer to whom an individual card was issued and can automatically allocate the assessed dose to that wearer. The card can be reused many times—often more than 500 times if it has not been damaged or lost. A full history of that card can also be kept, including individual calibration factors for the TLDs on the card, the date of the last calibration, the number of times it has been used, whether it has received exceptionally large doses, etc. Each TLD is calibrated, usually annually. Some readers include an inbuilt irradiator to facilitate this calibration.

Individual performance figures for the various TLD systems are quoted by the manufacturers. TL dosimetry typically provides a linear response over a very large dose range (typically 0.01 mSv to 1 Sv) with a supralinear response between 1 Sv to 20 Sv. Its energy range is similar to film. By applying corrections for fading (§4.12.2), the assessed dose will be constant within 5% for 3 months using LiF:Mg,Ti. Compared with the film dosemeter, the initial cost of TL dosemeter cards are very expensive but the cost per issue decreases the more times they are reused. Evaluation of thermal neutron response and detailed information regarding the energy and type of the radiation is only possible with extra TLDs within the card which increases the cost even further. Unlike film, TL dosimeters cannot differentiate between contamination and normal external exposure. Finally, no permanent record is available after the dosemeter has been read except for the glow curve. Although it is not possible to routinely reread TLDs, information on dosimetry stored in high-temperature traps (320–360°C) that are not included in the normal glow curve can be released by exposing the TLD to ultraviolet light (at elevated temperatures) before rereading. The UV light raises electrons to the excited state which then become retrapped in the normal dosimetry peaks. If the high-temperature peaks are not removed by annealing, the total dose the TLD has received during its lifetime will be recorded, so the full history of the dosemeter is required when rereading using this technique.

8.3.4 Optically stimulated luminescence (OSL)

Optically stimulated luminescence (OSL) has been used for archaeological studies for many years. It is also now used in computed radiography. Its application to personal monitoring has been restricted because of the lack of a good luminescence material with the required properties. One commercial application has been radiophotoluminescence (RPL) from glasses. A fully automated system, Toshiba FBD-10, began operation in Germany for routine monitoring in 1991. It now consists of flat-glass dosemeters (40 mm × 30 mm × 0.9 mm) encapsulated with energy-compensation filters of tin and plastic on both sides [21]. Irradiation of the detector results in stable radiation-induced defects. A pulsed UV laser is used to excite electrons from the defect ground state to the defect excited state. Relaxation back to the ground state yields luminescence which is read by a photomultiplier tube. The intensity of the luminescence is proportional to the absorbed dose. The dose can be read multiple times without destroying the signal. The system allows measurement of $H_p(10)$ with a coefficient of variation of about 1% at 1 mSv and 3% at 0.1 mSv. The energy response of the dosemeter is within ±15% in the energy range 10 keV–10 MeV and the angular response investigated up to 90° increases this to about 25%. The dose range is 0.03 mSv to 8 Sv.

A more recent modification of OSL methods, which relies on the ionisation of radiation-induced defects, uses crystalline Al_2O_3:C as the luminescent material and is called pulsed optically stimulated luminescence (POSL) [22]. Irradiated Al_2O_3:C is exposed to a pulsed light source and the emitted light is detected between pulses. POSL differs from earlier techniques of 'delayed' OSL and 'cooled' OSL by detecting the *prompt* luminescence which increases sensitivity and decreases temperature dependence. The technique has been optimised by carefully choosing the laser pulse width, the peak laser power, and the timing sequence for signal collection [22]. A stream of laser pulses with a full width at half maximum of T_1 excites the material. Acquisition of the emitted luminescence is switched off for a dead time period, T_2, from shortly before the pulse until shortly after the pulse. The emitted luminescence is acquired for a period T_3 between each pulse (Figure 8.4). For Al_2O_3:C, T_1 = 300 ns, T_2 =15 μs, and T_3 = 235 μs.

The apparatus used in a POSL system is shown in Figure 8.5. The laser beam is split into 'weak' (0.01 W) and 'strong' (1.2 W) beams. Samples of unknown dose are excited by the weak beam. If the resultant POSL signal is below a pre-programmed threshold (corresponding to a dose of 30 mGy in Al_2O_3:C powder), the main measurement is made with the strong beam. The POSL is integrated over a stimulation period of 1 s. The minimum detectable dose is estimated as less than 1 μGy with a

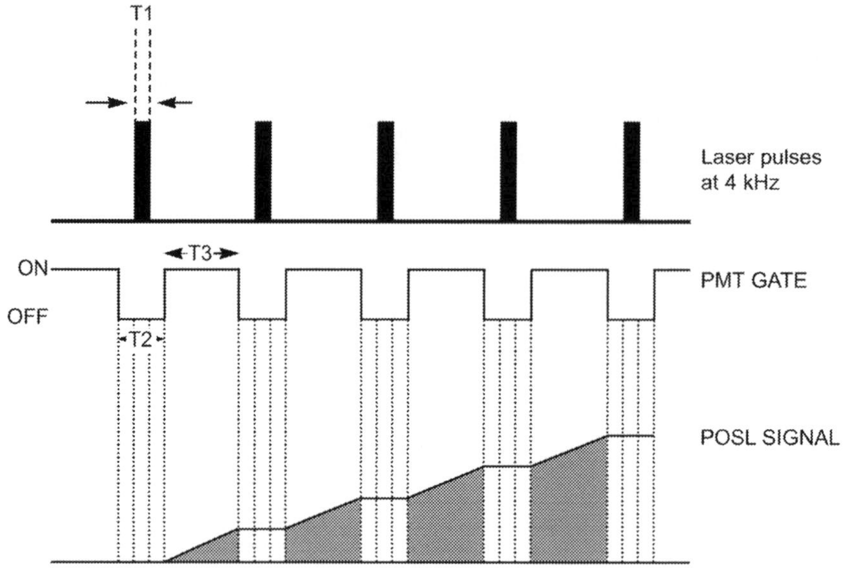

Figure 8.4 Schematic diagram of the timing of POSL measurement with laser pulses. Data acquisition only occurs during period T3 when the PMT or photon counter is gated on (235 μs in every 250 μs cycle). There is a dead time T2 when the PMT is gated off (15 μs in every cycle). Time period T1 is the full-width half-maximum of the laser pulse (0.3 μs). Modified from Akselrod and McKeever [22] with permission from Nuclear Technology Publishing.

linear response over almost seven orders of magnitude. A typical standard deviation between repeated measurement is ±1.5%.

This type of POSL system is now being supplied commercially (Landauer, Inc., USA). The Al_2O_3:C is supplied as a powder of grain size 40–60 μm between plastic layers. The dosemeter is placed between a three-element filter pack that is heat sealed. The manufacturer's data state that the system measures, with an accuracy of ±15% at the 95% confidence level, $H_p(10)$ for photons

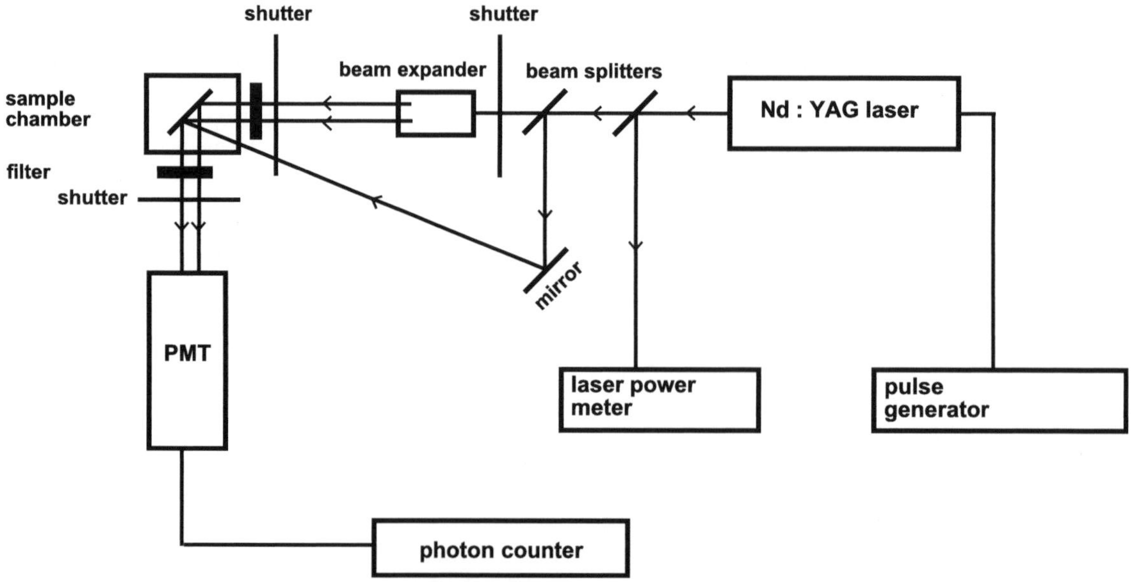

Figure 8.5 Simplified diagram of the apparatus used by Akselrod and McKeever [22] for POSL measurements. Reproduced with permission from Nuclear Technology Publishing.

above 20 keV, and $H_p(0.07)$ for photons above 20 keV, and β-particles above 200 keV. The dose measurement range is 0.01 mSv to 10 Sv for photons and 0.1 mSv to 10 Sv for electrons. Only a fraction of the charge trapped in a sample is depleted during a normal POSL measurement. The POSL signal can therefore be remeasured provided the fraction depleted by previous measurements is known. The image produced under a special filter area can be analysed to identify static, dynamic irradiations, or contamination (like the film dosemeter) but this is only available for beta and low-energy photon measurements yielding doses in excess of 5 mSv. The signal is stable for up to a year.

8.3.5 Electronic personal dosemeters

The obvious advantages of electronic personal dosemeters are instantaneous digital readout of accumulated dose and dose rate and user-programmable features ranging from simple dose and dose-rate alarm levels to dose histograms. Electronic dosemeters are therefore very useful for staff who are working in environments with variable but potentially high dose rates—the instrument can warn the wearer when the dose rate or cumulative dose exceeds a certain value. The instantaneous reading can be used to identify which procedures in a whole work process are making the most significant contributions to a wearer's dose. For example, someone working in a nuclear medicine department could identify whether they are receiving doses from the radiopharmaceutical preparation, administration of the radiopharmceutical or during the imaging of the patient. There are several electronic dosemeters on the market—the majority of these consist of energy-compensated Geiger–Müller tubes (see Box 4.3). These instruments will typically measure $H_p(10)$ between 1 μSv to 1 Sv or higher with an energy response of ±25% between 50 keV to a few MeV. They are stable, accurate (e.g. within ±10%), reasonably rugged, and relatively insensitive to environmental changes in humidity, temperature, and pressure. Dosemeters using ionisation chambers are available which extend the energy response down to 10 keV but with a resultant reduced sensitivity, so that the minimum detectable dose increases to about 0.1 mSv.

At first sight an electronic dosemeter seems to be an ideal instrument. However, for many employers, like the NHS, whose employees receive very little radiation dose, the relatively high cost of electronic dosemeters preclude their use as routine dosemeters. In addition, although energy-compensated Geiger–Müller tube dosemeters will be satisfactory for most radiotherapy and nuclear medicine applications, their insensitivity to low-energy photons may result in significant underestimation of doses from scattered diagnostic X-rays or work with, for example, ^{125}I. If the battery fails, the dose reading might be lost and individuals are usually able to erase any dose they may have received (either deliberately or accidentally). The instrument may also be sensitive to electromagnetic interference. It is for these reasons that, until recently, no electronic dosemeter was offered as an approved dosemeter. Any wearer who was issued with an electronic dosemeter would also have to wear a passive dosemeter (film badge, TLD, RPL, etc.) to satisfy legal requirements.

Siemens Environmental Systems (Poole, UK), in conjunction with NRPB, have developed an electronic personal dosemeter or EPD which uses three silicon diode detectors which are sensitive to different types and energies of radiation. Their outputs are combined to measure $H_p(10)$ and $H_p(0.07)$ for photons between 20 keV and 6 MeV and $H_p(0.07)$ for electrons between 250 keV and 1.5 MeV with an energy response of ±30% down to doses of 1 μSv.

Another development is electronic dosemeters which do not have a direct display. This approach has the advantage of reducing their weight, size, and cost. The user can get dose readout at will with electronic readers at strategic locations, perhaps even operating with a wireless link. At present, the passive so-called MOS dosemeters used are not sufficiently sensitive for personnel monitoring. A new technology under development is direct ion storage (DIS) [23]. These devices offer the wearer the choice of using the dosemeter either as a passive device without a direct display or as a conventional direct reading type.

8.3.6 Neutron detectors

Healthcare workers have potential for neutron exposures if they are working in and around megavoltage radiotherapy facilities or positron emission tomography (PET) cyclotrons. For dosimetry purposes, neutron fields tend to be divided into two energy intervals described as 'fast' and 'slow' neutrons. A fast neutron exposure would usually result from exposure to the unshielded source of neutrons, the head of the linac, or the target/beam tube of the cyclotron for example. A slow neutron exposure would be the result of exposure to a scattered neutron field in which the source energy had been reduced by scattering collisions in some shielding or moderating material. The assessment of whole-body doses from neutron radiation fields can be achieved by a number of measurement systems, some of which have been mentioned in the preceding sections.

Nuclear emulsions are some of the most widely used dosemeter types in which neutron interactions produce a number of distinct tracks which may be viewed (and counted) through a microscope when the emulsion is developed. The emulsions are used in holders which have some features in common with those used for photon dosimetry. There is usually shielding to attenuate any incident photons, and often some kind of energy-discriminating filter to provide neutron energy selectivity. In the later versions of the NRPB nuclear emulsion dosemeter, the need for neutron energy discrimination (via filters) has been removed by incorporation of a boron-loaded plastic into the holder. This has the effect of providing a uniform dosemeter sensitivity regardless of neutron energy and is placed at the back of the holder only, to absorb any albedo thermal neutrons from the body of the wearer. The dosemeter response has been shown to vary by only around 50% from thermal to 14.9 MeV neutron energy. Although such variation is deemed to be acceptable for neutron personal monitoring, such dosemeters are gradually being superseded. For example, within the UK, NRPB withdrew the dosemeter service in 2001 in favour of the PADC dosemeter (see below).

The use of TLDs for monitoring radiation exposures from photons has been discussed previously. The naturally occurring isotopes of lithium (^{6}Li and ^{7}Li) have similar photon interaction properties, but their neutron interaction characteristics are quite different. ^{6}Li has a strong affinity for neutrons, particularly thermal neutrons, whereas ^{7}Li only has a significant neutron interaction cross-section at high neutron energies (above about 4 MeV) and it therefore has a low probability of interaction with neutrons of energies typical in shielded and/or highly scattering environments. It is therefore possible to introduce ^{6}Li and ^{7}Li TL chips into TLD monitoring systems to provide some neutron/photon discrimination, and also to produce a neutron personal dosimeter. Such a detector will usually comprise at least two ^{6}Li chips, one 'bare' and one filtered with cadmium or boron, and sufficient ^{7}Li chips under different filters to provide accurate photon dosimetry and for subtraction from the measured ^{6}Li chip responses. The KfK dosimeter, which is widely used in Germany, is a TL-based albedo dosemeter—with a useful dose range from 0.1 mSv to 2 Sv.

The two neutron dosimetry systems described above have much in common with photon dosimetry systems described previously in this chapter. There are a number of other systems which also draw heavily on experience in photon dosimetry, including systems based on silicon PIN diodes. For a review of the status of electronic neutron dosimetry, see Barthe *et al.* [24]. There are two neutron detection systems which are quite different in nature to any used for photon dosimetry. These are the bubble detector and the solid-state nuclear track detector (SSNTD), both of which have the advantage of excellent photon discrimination.

SSNTDs provide a very commonly used neutron personal dosemeter that is based on the realization by chemical or electrochemical etching of the latent damage in a suitable material caused by a neutron interaction. The most widely used material is polyallyl diglycol carbonate (PADC or Columbia Resin 39 (CR-39) or Tastrak). Developments in plastic curing cycles, etch conditions, and automatic microscope viewing and counting of recorded tracks have meant that dosimetry based on PADC detectors has become an integral part of the service offered by organizations such as the NRPB in the UK and Landauer and ICN in the USA. It is common to introduce materials to act as sources of charged particles, which are more easily detected in the track detector. Such materials, often termed 'radiators', are usually used to enhance the response of the dosemeter to thermal neutrons and include materials such as lithium-loaded polyethylene. The dosemeters offered by the NRPB have a nylon holder which, through its nitrogen content, enhances the low-energy response of the system through detection of protons from the ^{14}N(n,p) reactions in the holder. The response of this detector per unit H_p (10) appears now to vary by only around a factor of two from thermal energies to 10 MeV although there is an intermediate energy interval where sensitivity is poor. It is perhaps fortuitous that this energy interval tends not to provide a significant contribution to effective dose in typical working environments. The latest versions of the NRPB track-etch dosimetry service can measure $H_p(10)$ down to 0.2 mSv. A typical upper dose measurement limit for an automatic read system would be 50 mSv although higher doses can be read using a manual microscope system.

Bubble detectors rely on the ability of radiation interactions to provide a nucleation site for bubble formation in a superheated suspension of halocarbon droplets. These are both active devices based on acoustic measurements of bubble formation and passive devices based on optical counting of bubbles [25]. The active devices are generally used for area monitoring while passive devices are available for personal monitoring. Apfel [26] reported tests on direct reading (i.e. no processing required) personal bubble dosemeters which had different dose ranges, one from 5 μSv to 8 mSv and the other from 0.5 mSv to 50 mSv.

8.4 Extremity and eye monitoring

The European Basic Safety Standard and UK legislation stipulate separate dose limits for the equivalent dose (H_T) to the lens of the eye and H_T for the extremities (hands, forearms, feet, and ankles). In most practical radiation fields the true equivalent dose to the extremity will be less than the equivalent dose to the skin of the extremity. The relevant dose quantity for extremity measurement is therefore usually $H_p(0.07)$. Assessment of $H_p(d)$ using other values for d may be appropriate in other circumstances: for example, where the extremity dose may exceed the skin dose (if there is significant build-up) or protective clothing is always worn. The quantity $H_p(3)$ should be used for the eye.

Certain staff groups, in particular some clinicians undertaking interventional radiological procedures (radiologists, cardiologists, and neuroradiologists), radiopharmacists or other staff handling large quantities of unsealed radioactive materials, and staff handling brachytherapy sources for patients, where afterloading facilities are not available, may receive large hand doses. These staff should certainly be monitored.

Extremity and eye dose assessments are carried out using TLDs because of their convenient size. Two commonly used materials are LiF and $Li_2B_4O_7$. To accurately measure $H_p(0.07)$ for the localized doses from weakly penetrating radiations such as low-energy beta radiations, the dosemeter must be physically thin to avoid significant attenuation of the radiation within the dosemeter. The dosemeter also needs to be robust because it may be placed on the hands carrying out manual work, etc. Commercially available extremity dosemeters may therefore consist of a thin uniform layer of phosphor (5–10 mg cm^{-2}) sandwiched between a backing substance and a thin covering material (e.g. 3–4 mg cm^{-2}). The covering layer has to be peeled off during readout and therefore the dosemeter can only be used once. The dosemeter can be placed in finger-stalls which enable doses at the tip of the finger to be measured [27]. The manufacture of these thin powders increases the variability in sensitivity between dosemeters. Obviously it is not possible to sort dosemeters into batches of similar sensitivity or evaluate dosemeter sensitivity correction factors when the dosemeters can only be used once. More recently, small reusable thin-chip or disc dosemeters have become available that can be inserted into protective pouches or finger rings. These dosemeters have the disadvantage for some applications that they cannot measure the dose at the tip of the finger where the largest dose might occur. An alternative approach is to use carbon-loaded dosemeters [28] which enable thicker and therefore more robust pellets to be used. The carbon effectively absorbs all the thermoluminescent light emitted within the pellet except for surface light. The thick dosemeter therefore only has a thin sensitive layer. For assessment of eye doses and extremity doses from higher energy photons (e.g. above 20 keV), thicker TLDs of the order of 200 mg cm^{-2} or more can be used. More recently, electronic gamma extremity monitoring systems (GEMS and AEGIS) have been developed to give a continuous readout of dose rate from a small probe attached to the finger (Box 8.2).

The position on the hand at which a dosemeter is worn and the choice of hand on which it is placed can both have a large influence on the value of the dose assessed, especially when working with localized sources. The skin dose limit applies to the dose averaged over any area of 1 cm^2, regardless of the area exposed. It is therefore necessary to identify, as accurately as possible, the location of the highest dose. This might vary from person to person depending on how they carry out a specific task. In a study of vascular/interventional radiologists, the fingers received approximately 30% lower dose than the palm of the hand and the left hand received 28% more dose than the right hand [30]. However, during radiopharmaceutical dispensing the dose to the tip of the finger can be twice that at the base of the finger [31]. Extremity doses to staff carrying out nuclear medicine procedures are discussed further in §15.7.1.

8.5 Monitoring for internal exposure

Individual monitoring for intakes of radioactive material is usually much more difficult than external monitoring. The ICRP [1] therefore recommended that monitoring for internal exposure (from now on referred to as internal monitoring), 'should be used routinely only for workers who are employed in areas that are designated as controlled areas specifically in relation to the control of contamination and in which there are grounds for suspecting significant exposures.' The Commission consider it is generally inappropriate to formally assess doses when they are lower than 1 mSv in a year [12]. Apart from radon monitoring (§10.3), the only likely application of internal monitoring for healthcare workers is for checking intakes of radioactive iodine. The topic will be discussed briefly with specific reference to monitoring for iodine. Airborne contamination levels resulting from leakage from the ^{99m}Tc nebulizers used for nuclear medicine lung ventilation studies are not normally sufficient to result in doses more than 0.3 mSv per year [32] and probably significantly smaller still [33].

Evaluation of committed effective dose, E_{int}, (§3.2.2) from intakes of radionuclides requires

- individual monitoring measurements to determine the activity in Bq in a particular body organ or component at a particular time
- knowledge of the temporal pattern and mode of intake
- assessment of intake (Bq) from the above measurement using various models which describe the route of intakes of radionuclides into the body and subsequent transfers within the body for different physicochemical forms of the radionuclide
- assessment of E_{int} from the intake.

8.5.1 Methods for individual monitoring

Individual monitoring can be achieved by body activity measurements, excreta monitoring, or air sampling with personal air samplers. The choice of method depends on several factors: the type of radiation emitted; the biokinetic behaviour of the radionuclide and its biologi-

Box 8.2 Electronic extremity dosemeters

Dosimetry systems with small semiconductor probes which can be attached to the side of a finger can provide a continuous record of dose rate at the fingertip [29]. Data are fed via a preamplifier to a data-logger which can be interrogated after use to view patterns of exposure (Figure B8.2). Since doses from individual actions can be observed, these instruments can be used to identify manipulations which make significant contributions to finger doses. This allows dose reductions from implementation of new techniques to be evaluated and facilitates optimisation of finger doses.

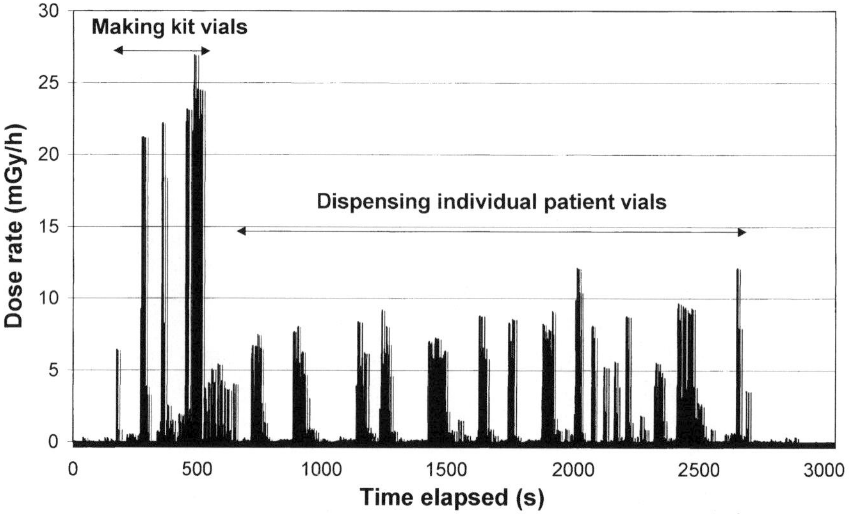

Figure B8.2 Variation in dose rate at the tip of the index finger for a radiopharmacy technician during a session dispensing methylene diphosphonate labelled with ^{99m}Tc. The dose rate is measured using an electronic extremity dosemeter (AEGIS), which records the dose at one second intervals. During the first part of the session kit vials are prepared from which radiopharmaceutical is sub-dispensed into patient vials during the remainder of the session. Each period where the dose rate is raised for tens of seconds is made up from several peaks each representing dispensing to an individual vial.

cal clearance and half-life; and the required frequency of measurement. Nose-blow samples or nasal smears can give a preliminary indication of the seriousness of an incident (§10.6.4).

In vivo measurements

Direct measurement of a body or organ content is only feasible for radionuclides which emit radiation that can escape from the body. The most obvious application is for X- or γ-radiation but positrons can be detected by their annihilation radiation and energetic beta particles by their associated bremsstahlung [34]. For radiation protection purposes, commonly encountered fission products such as ^{131}I, ^{137}Cs, and ^{60}Co can be detected by comparatively simple equipment such as a single detector viewing the whole body or, for iodine, a smaller detector placed close to the thyroid. Most systems have traditionally used thallium-activated sodium iodide detectors which have a high sensitivity for detecting γ-rays. These detectors work well for simple γ-spectra but the analysis of the spectrum obtained from a mixture of radionuclides becomes difficult. Germanium detectors have a superior energy-resolving power which simplifies the interpretation of the spectra and now have sufficiently high efficiency to be used (§4.10).

The detection of ^{125}I, ^{129}I, and ^{131}I presents no problems. The threshold detection limit for photon spectrometry of the thyroid *in vivo* is 100 Bq [12]. Allowance for the attenuation of the low-energy (27–35.5 keV) photons from ^{125}I both within the thyroid and by varying thicknesses of overlying tissues is particularly beneficial.

Analysis of excreta and other biological materials

Excreta monitoring may be the only technique possible for radionuclides with no gamma emission. Routine programmes usually involve analysis of urine or faeces.

Radionuclides emitting γ-rays can be determined by direct measurement but analysis of β- and α-emitters requires chemical separation before the appropriate measurement technique.

Urine monitoring can be used to detect ^{125}I (liquid scintillation counting), ^{129}I (radiochemical separation and counting), and ^{131}I (γ-spectrometry) with a typical detection limit of 1 Bq l^{-1} [12]. This method is required if thyroid uptake has been blocked by issuing stable iodine as a blocking agent, e.g. after a known accident. As the urinary excretion rate decreases rapidly with time following intake, thyroid monitoring is preferred unless the time of intake is known.

Air sampling

Air sampling of airborne particulate materials can be carried out by drawing air through a filter using a calibrated air pump. A static air sampler (SAS) or a personal air sampler (PAS) may be used. The activity deposited on the filter, or a collection of filters, can be determined by radiochemical separation and high-sensitivity measurement techniques. Some method of distinguishing between natural radioactivity in air and the radionuclides(s) under investigation will often be required. Available pumps for the PAS only sample the air at rates of about one-tenth of the typical breathing rate (1.2 m^3 h^{-1}). The sampling head should be close to the normal breathing zone of the worker. The PAS therefore gives an indication of the time-integrated concentration of activity in the sampled air. The activity breathed by the worker is obtained by multiplying the measured integrated air concentration by the volume breathed.

The adequacy of air-sampling measurements in providing a realistic assessment of intake of radioactivity by an individual in a particular working environment should be evaluated by correlating the air-sampling results with either *in vivo* and excreta measurements or workplace monitoring. At very low levels of exposure (very much less than one-tenth of the annual limit of intake), an SAS system can demonstrate that more systematic assessment is not required. For larger levels of exposure a PAS system is required unless results can demonstrate the validity and reliability of an SAS system.

PASs were used to confirm the likely doses from ^{99m}Tc nebulizers used in nuclear medicine departments [32, 33].

8.5.2 Models to represent the intake, transfer, and excretion of radioactive material

An overview of the models, with references to original reports, used to describe intake, internal transfers, and routes of excretion is given by ICRP [12]. These models provide data for a large number of radionuclides including ^{125}I, ^{129}I, and ^{131}I. The data presented include

- fractional absorption (f_1 value) in the gastrointestinal tract for different compounds and classification of the radionuclide/chemical form into either fast (F), moderate (M), or slow (S) absorption rates from the respiratory tract;
- possible methods of monitoring with typical detection limits;
- effective dose coefficients, $e(50)$, for inhalation and ingestion;
- tables and graphs of $m(t)$—i.e. the predicted value of activity (body content, organ content, or daily excretion) as a function of time, t, for single intakes by inhalation, ingestion, or injection. Values of $m(t)$ are given in Bq per Bq intake;
- table of recommended routine monitoring intervals;
- tables of equilibrium values of activity (body content, organ content, or daily excretion) for continuous intake.

Some data values associated with ^{131}I are given in Table 8.3 as examples. The biokinetic model for iodine assumes that, of the iodine reaching the blood, a fraction of 0.3 is accumulated in the thyroid and 0.7 is excreted directly in urine. The biological half-life in blood is taken to be 0.25 days. These parameters will vary between individuals especially for thyroid dysfunctions. When such cases are suspected, individual values should be used.

8.5.3 Estimation of intake and dose

When the time of intake is known, the intake can be estimated from the measured values using the data from 'special monitoring' (Table 8.3). If only a single measurement is made, the intake (I) is calculated as:

$$I = \text{measured activity}, M/m(t).$$

For routine monitoring, it is assumed that intake took place in the middle of the monitoring interval of T days so

$$I = M/m(T/2).$$

An intake in the previous monitoring interval can influence the result obtained. ICRP recommend that a correction should be applied (from the retention graphs given) if more than 10% of the measured activity may be

Table 8.3 Sample data for monitoring for internal exposure following inhalation of ^{131}I vapour by workers

(a) Dose coefficient, $e(50) = 2.0 \times 10^{-8}$ Sv Bq^{-1}

(b) $m(t)$ = predicted value of activity in thyroid and urine after intake of 1 Bq ^{131}I

Days	$m(t)$ (Bq per Bq intake)	
	Thyroid	Daily urinary excretion
Special monitoring		
Time after intake		
1	0.23	5.3×10^{-1}
3	0.20	2.5×10^{-3}
5	0.17	1.7×10^{-4}
7	0.14	1.9×10^{-4}
9	0.12	2.1×10^{-4}
Routine monitoring		
Monitoring interval		
14	0.14	1.9×10^{-4}
7	0.19	2.7×10^{-4}

(c) Continuous intake

	Thyroid	Daily urinary excretion
Equilibrium activity (Bq) for chronic inhalation at 1 Bq year^{-1}	7.6×10^{-3}	1.6×10^{-3}
Time to equilibrium	2 months	4 days
Inhalation rate (Bq) to give 20 mSv year^{-1}	7.6×10^{3}	1.6×10^{3}

Source: ICRP [12].

attributed to intakes in previous periods [12]. The estimated intake can then be compared directly with the ALI or E_{int} can be calculated using the appropriate effective dose coefficients, $e(50)$.

8.6 Results

Doses to UK classified workers for the period 1990–6 and the distribution of doses for different occupational groups are reported by HSE [35]. In addition, many of the major employers with radiation workers send dose information on all their workers to a National Registry for Radiation Workers (NRRW) which is used for epidemiological studies into the effects of humans exposed to chronic low-dose radiation [36]. However, staff in the health service are rarely classified and information on their doses are not sent to the NRRW. Approved dosimetry services do, however, contribute information on whole-body doses to the reviews of doses to the UK population [37] which provide a breakdown of doses to different staff groups in the healthcare professions. Only 16 out of a total of nearly 18 000 wearers received effective doses above 5 mSv (Table 8.4). Thus very few workers in the medical sector need to be classified persons on the basis of their whole-body doses. Occasionally, however, their hand doses may exceed 150 mSv per year (§8.4) and therefore these staff need to be classified. Although doses to the lens of the eye of staff involved in interventional procedures are sometimes assessed, doses greater than 45 mSv are rarely measured and so classification is not required on this basis.

8.7 References

1 International Commission on Radiological Protection (1991). Recommendations of the International Commission on Radiological Protection. ICRP Publication 60. *Ann. ICRP*, **21** (1–3).

2 Kim, C. H., Reece, W. D., and Poston, J. W. (1999). Calculation of effective dose for broad parallel photon beams. *Health Phys.*, **76** (2), 156–61.

3 International Commission on Radiation Units and Measurements (1993). *Quantities and units in radiation protection dosimetry*. ICRU Report 51. ICRU, Bethesda, MD.

4 National Radiological Protection Board (1993). Dose quantities for protection against external radiations. *Doc. NRPB*, **4** (3).

5 International Commission on Radiation Units and Measure-

Table 8.4 Annual whole-body doses to healthcare workers (from data mostly for 1996 and some for 1995) [37]

Occupational group	Number of workers in annual dose range (mSv)						Total number of workers	Annual collective dose (man Sv)	Average annual dose (mSv)
	0–1	1–5	5–10	10–15	15–20	>20			
Diagnostic radiology									
Radiographers	4962	62	1	0	0	0	5025	0.243	0.05
Radiologists	946	53	2	0	0	1	1002	0.192	0.19
Cardiologists	432	26	1	1	1	0	461	0.120	0.26
Other clinicians	649	7	0	0	0	0	656	0.026	0.04
Nurses	2238	38	0	0	0	1	2277	0.163	0.07
Scientist and technicians	627	4	0	1	1	0	633	0.042	0.07
Other staff	567	8	0	0	0	0	575	0.021	0.04
Radiotherapy									
Beam radiographers	861	3	0	0	0	1	865	0.052	0.06
Radiotherapists	239	3	0	0	0	1	243	0.055	0.23
Sources technicians	16	0	0	0	0	0	16	0.002	0.15
Theatre nurses	476	5	0	0	0	0	481	0.024	0.05
Ward nurses	645	1	1	0	0	1	648	0.067	0.10
Other nurses	63	1	0	0	0	0	64	0.007	0.10
Scientists and technicians	250	1	2	0	0	0	253	0.025	0.10
Other staff	352	0	0	0	0	0	352	0.002	0.01
Nuclear medicine									
Pharmacists	148	20	0	0	0	0	168	0.059	0.35
Radiographers	207	55	0	0	0	0	262	0.140	0.53
Scientists and technicians	75	11	0	0	0	0	86	0.025	0.29
Clinicians	51	3	0	0	0	0	54	0.010	0.18
Nurses	54	19	0	0	0	0	73	0.045	0.61
Other staff	106	3	0	0	0	0	109	0.006	0.06
Research workers	129	2	0	0	0	0	131	0.010	0.07
Survey total	**14093**	**325**	**7**	**2**	**2**	**5***	**14434**	**1.335**	**0.09**
Extrapolated UK totals	39100	850	< 50	< 10	< 10	< 20	40000	4000	0.1

*Four of these were in the 20–30 mSv band and one in the 30–40 mSv band.

ments (1998). *Conversion coefficients for use in radiological protection against external irradiation external photon and electron radiations*. ICRU Report 57. ICRU, Bethesda, MD.

6 Zankl, M. (1999). Personal dose equivalent for photons and its variation with dosemeter position. *Health Phys.*, **76** (2), 162–70.

7 International Organization for Standardization (1996). *X and gamma reference radiation for calibrating dosemeters and dose rate meters and for determining their response as a function of energy–Part 3: Area and personal dosemeters*. ISO/DIS 4037-3. British Standards Institution, London.

8 Bartlett, D. T. and Iles, W. J. (1994). *Calibration of personal dosemeters*. Report NRPB-M520. NRPB, Chilton.

9 International Commission on Radiological Protection (1982). General principles of monitoring for radiation workers. *Ann. ICRP*, **9** (4).

10 International Commission on Radiological Protection (1997). General principles for the radiation protection of workers. ICRP Publication 75. *Ann. ICRP*, **27** (1).

11 Christensen, P. and Griffith, R. V. (1994). Required accuracy and dose thresholds in individual monitoring. *Radiat. Prot. Dosim.*, **54**, 279–85.

12 International Commission on Radiological Protection (1997). Individual monitoring for internal exposure of workers. ICRP Publication 78. *Ann. ICRP*, **27** (3/4).

13 Ambrosi, P. and Bartlett, D. (1998). Dosimeter characteristics/dosimeter and service performance requirements. Physikalisch-Technische Bundesanstalt, Report PTB-Bericht Dos-27. Braunschweig, Germany.

14 Institute of Physics and Engineering in Medicine (2002). Medical and dental guidance notes: A good practice guide to implementing ionising radiation protection legislation in the clinical environment. IPEM, York.

15 Faulkner, K. and Marshall, N. W. (1993). The relationship of effective dose to personnel and monitor reading for stimulated fluoroscopic irradiation conditions. *Health Phys.*, **64** (5), 502–8.

16 National Council on Radiation Protection and Measurements (1995). *Use of personal monitors to estimate effective dose equivalent and effective dose to workers for external exposure to low-LET radiation*. NCRP Report 122. NCRP, Bethesda, MD.

17 Iles, W. J., Milton, M. I. L., Bartlett, D. T., Burgess, P. H., and Hill, C. E. (1990). *Type testing of the NRPB/AERE film badge dosemeter in terms of the new ICRU secondary quantities–Part*

1: Photons over the energy range 10 keV–1250 keV. Report NRPB-R236. NRPB, Chilton.

18 Green, S. and Palethorpe, J. (1999). Blowing the trumpet for the film dosemeter. Institute of Physics and Engineering in Medicine. *Scope*, **8** (1), 15–17.

19 International Commission on Radiological Protection (1990). Radiological protection of the worker in medicine and dentistry. ICRP Publication 57. *Ann. ICRP*, **20** (3).

20 McKinlay, A. F. (1981). *Thermoluminescence dosimetry*. Medical Physics Handbook 5. Adam Hilger, Bristol.

21 Piesch, E., Burghart, B., and Vilgis, M. (1993). Progress in phosphate glass dosimetry: experiences and routine monitoring with a modern dosimetry system. *Radiat. Prot. Dosim.*, **47**, 407–14.

22 Akselrod, M. S. and McKeever, S. W. S. (1999). A radiation dosimetry method using pulsed optically stimulated luminescence. *Radiat. Prot. Dosim.*, **81**, 167–76.

23 Kahilainen, J. (1996). The direct ion storage dosemeter. *Radiat. Prot. Dosim.*, **66**, 459–62.

24 Barthe, J., Bordy, J. M., and Lahaye, T. (1997). Electronic neutron dosemeters: history and state of the art. *Radiat. Prot. Dosim.*, **70** (1–4), 59–66.

25 d'Errico, F., Alberts, W. G., and Matzke, M. (1997). Advances in superheated drop (bubble) detector techniques. *Radiat. Prot. Dosim.*, **70** (1–4), 103–8.

26 Apfel, R. E. (1992). Characterisation of new passive superheated drop (bubble) dosemeters. *Radiat. Prot. Dosim.*, **44** (1–4), 343–6.

27 Dutt, J. C., Iles, W. J., and Bartlett, D. T. (1990). Characteristics of a new type of Vinten dosemeter for skin/extremity monitoring. *Radiat. Prot. Dosim.*, **33**, 303–6.

28 Zha, Z, Wang, S., Shen, W., and Cai, G. (1993). Preparation and characteristics of LiF: Mg, Cu, P thermoluminescent material. *Radiat. Prot. Dosim.*, **47** (1–4), 111–18.

29 Montgomery, A., Martin, C. J., Anstee, D., and Hilditch, T. (1997). Application of a gamma extremity monitoring system in a radiopharmaceutical dispensary. *Nucl. Med. Commun.*, **18**, 673–9.

30 Anderson, N. E., King, S. H., and Miller, K. L. (1999). Variations in dose to the extremities of vascular/interventional radiologists. *Health Phys.*, **76** (Suppl.), S39–S40.

31 Dhanse, S., Martin, C. J., Hilditch, T., and Elliott, A. T. (2000). A study of doses to the hands during dispensing of radiopharmaceuticals. *Nucl. Med. Commun.*, **21**, 511–19.

32 MacKie, A., Hart, G. C., Ibbett, D. A., and Whitehead, R. J. S. (1994). Airborne radioactive contamination following aerosol ventilation studies. *Nucl. Med. Commun.*, **15**, 161–7.

33 Greaves, C. D., Sanderson, R., and Tindale, W. B. (1995). Air contamination following aerosol ventilation in the gamma camera room. *Nucl. Med. Commun.*, **16**, 901–4.

34 International Atomic Energy Agency (1996). *Direct methods for measuring radionuclides in man*. Safety Series 114. IAEA, Vienna, Austria.

35 Health and Safety Executive (1998). *Occupational exposure to ionising radiation 1990–1996*. Analysis of doses reported to the Health and Safety Executive's Central Index of Dose Information. HSE, London.

36 Muirhead, C. R., Goodhill, A. A., Haylock, R. G. E., Vokes, J., Little, M. P., and Jackson, D. A. (1999). Occupational radiation exposure and mortality: second analysis of the national registry for radiation workers. *J. Radiol. Prot.*, **19**, 3–26.

37 Hughes, J. S. (1999). *Ionising radiation exposure of the UK population–1999 review*. National Radiological Protection Board Report, NRPB-R311. NRPB, Chilton.

Chapter 9
Control of radioactive substances

C. J. Martin and E. M. Pitcher

9.1 Introduction

Regulation of the possession, use, transport, and disposal of radioactive materials is necessary to safeguard society from the potentially harmful effects of radiation. Major radiation exposure accidents have occurred where control has been inadequate (e.g. Box 10.7). Minimization of the amount of radioactive waste produced and regulation of disposal of waste are also essential components in the overall strategy to protect the environment. The regulatory approach to control of radioactive substances is exercised through a system of notification and licensing, which is based upon recommendations from the IAEA and ICRP [1–3]. Through this system, a competent authority is empowered to permit an organization to hold, use, or dispose of any radionuclide provided certain conditions are met. The conditions take the form of limits on the type and quantities of radioactive materials held, requirements for security and protection, and evaluation of the impact of waste disposal. An organization obtains one type of licence or registration before it is allowed to keep and use radioactive materials and another type of licence or authorization before it can accumulate and dispose of radioactive waste. In European countries all controls are implemented through national legislation, whereas in the United States, use of reactor-produced radionuclides is licensed through the Federal Government under the Atomic Energy Act 1954, but control over other radionuclides is exercised by state or local governments. The authorities given responsibility for controlling radioactive materials in the UK are the Environment Agency in England and Wales, the Scottish Environment Protection Agency in Scotland, and the Environment and Heritage Service in Northern Ireland. For simplicity, regulatory bodies with responsibility for control of radioactive substances will be referred to here as Environment Agencies. In this chapter, the processes involved in control of radioactive substances are described and specific reference is made to UK legislation for which controls are embodied in the Radioactive Substances Act 1993 [4]. In the later part of the chapter, controls over the transport of radioactive materials and medical administrations to patients are discussed.

9.2 Registration of sources

9.2.1 Regulatory requirements

Registrations are licences for the keeping and use of radioactive materials at one premise or for 'mobile sources', which may be moved from one location to another [4]. Radioactive sources are divided into two categories, closed and open.

- *Closed sources* are those in which the radioactive substance is firmly incorporated or sealed within a solid inactive material so as to prevent the dispersion of any radioactive material. These would include sources where the radioactive material is bonded into the matrix, sources electrodeposited onto a metal substrate (often used for calibration), laminated sources where the active material is sandwiched between inactive layers, and sources where the radioactive substance is sealed within a robust capsule of inactive material. It is appropriate for most sealed sources to be tested at least every 2 years to confirm there has been no leakage of radioactivity (Box 18.1).
- *Open sources* are ones where the radioactive material is dispersible and not firmly incorporated. In the hospital environment, radiopharmaceuticals in liquid form for administration to patients are open sources or unsealed radionuclides. Others are in the form of gases, such as ^{133}Xe and ^{81m}Kr, which are inhaled for certain procedures, and solids such as ^{131}I therapy capsules. Wire made from ^{192}Ir which is used for therapy is also classed as an open source, since the ^{192}Ir is not sealed in an inactive medium and pieces

may be cut from the wire. Open sources require specialized handling techniques which are described in Chapters 15 and 18.

When applying for a registration, the user must provide detailed information on the radionuclides, the purpose for which they are to be used, for example *in vivo* or *in vitro* medical diagnosis, and the method of storage and security. Applications for closed-source registrations must list activities for individual sources or groups of sources, while for open registrations, the maximum activities of the radionuclides, which may be held on site at any one time, are required, together with a justification for these amounts. Groups of radionuclides may be acceptable for those only used occasionally. A general group of beta/gamma-emitting radionuclides is useful for hospital and medical research environments where the introduction of new radionuclides for clinical trials would otherwise entail expensive and time-consuming variations to a registration.

Any apparatus which incorporates a radioactive source and is constructed or adapted for being transported from place to place is regarded as a mobile source and requires a 'mobile' registration. This definition includes ^{241}Am or ^{137}Cs sources used by some medical physics departments to measure the transmission of radiation protection barriers.

9.2.2 Exemption orders

Some sources with limited activities or practices involving limited radiation exposure do not need to be subject to such stringent regulatory control because they present such a low level of risk [5]. In these cases exemption orders are applied which allow a user to hold a source without the need for registration, provided that the radionuclide activity is below specified limits and the source is held in accordance with specified conditions. Exemption orders take account of the detriment associated with the source and its use, and the probability and possible consequences of any accidents. Exemption from registration does not mean exemption from regulation or from proper accounting and record-keeping. Adequate records must be kept to prove that the relevant limits are not exceeded. The application of exemption orders to sources and practices involving use of sources will be considered here and implications for the disposal of very low-level radioactive waste are discussed in §9.3.1.

Many materials are radioactive because they contain low levels of natural radionuclides and control of these would be impossible. Therefore, radioactive substances in the form in which they occur in nature are excluded from the basic safety standards. However, practices which result in inadvertent mobilization and/or concentration of radionuclides are not excluded from regulation. This includes concentration of radium in scale deposits in drilling pipes used for oil exploration and production.

Exemption orders are applied to the use of consumer products containing low-level sources, such as smoke detectors containing ^{241}Am. However, if an exemption order is utilized, it is important to ensure that it is still current. Examples of some UK exemption orders that are relevant to hospitals and medical research laboratories are as follows:

- *The Testing Instruments Exemption Order* [6] covers low-activity sources which are incorporated within apparatus or used for testing and measurement, such as calibration of contamination monitors. It applies, in general, to sources of activity less than 4 MBq, although higher limits apply in certain cases depending on the source construction and radionuclide involved (e.g. 600 MBq for ^{63}Ni foil source).
- *The Hospitals Exemption Order* [7] allows hospitals, nursing homes, and clinics to hold 1 GBq of ^{99m}Tc and 100 MBq of other β/γ-emitting radionuclides, with a limit of 20 MBq on ^{131}I, without a registration.
- *The Substances of Low Activity Exemption Order* [8] allows insoluble solids with concentrations of radioactivity less than 0.4 Bq g^{-1} to be held or disposed of.

Note: Depleted uranium (over 2 kg in mass), which is used as shielding in some linear accelerators and ^{99m}Tc generators, must be registered and is quantified in terms of mass.

9.2.3 Record keeping

The keeping and use of radioactive materials should always be supervised by a competent person. This will usually be the same person who acts as Radiation Protection Supervisor (RPS) for the area under Ionising Radiations Regulations. A qualified expert who has the relevant expertise, training, and knowledge must be employed to advise on requirements to fulfil radioactive substances legislation. In many cases, this will be the person appointed as the radiation protection adviser under Ionising Radiations Regulations.

Radioactive substances legislation requires the location of all radioactive sources and the total activity on site at any time to be known to ensure that sources or radioactive materials are not lost and that the registered activity limits are not exceeded. This is not a simple task in hospitals or laboratories where a number of workers use different short-lived radionuclides. Larger establishments with many users may find it easier to divide up the registration limits and to give each laboratory or department its own sub-limit. The RPS is then responsible for ensuring that these 'laboratory' limits are not exceeded. In order that staff are aware of the limits on holdings and disposals, copies of the department's certificates of registration and waste authorizations should be displayed in a location where they are readily accessible.

The information required for each source, be it a long-lived sealed source or a vial containing a radiopharmaceutical labelled with a short half-life radionuclide should include:

- the radionuclide
- a means of identification, usually a unique number
- the date received on site
- the activity at a specified reference date
- the storage location
- the date of disposal or transfer to another site
- the site to which it is transferred.

If the source is a stock vial from which small quantities of the radiopharmaceutical are sub-dispensed, the records should also include:

- the activity and date of each removal of material
- the assay or process for which the vial is used.

Written records are often adequate for users with limited numbers of radionuclides for well-defined processes. Examples would be a haematology department which received a monthly standing order of kits for carrying out Schilling tests or a nuclear medicine department receiving daily deliveries of ^{99m}Tc-labelled radiopharmaceuticals. Larger establishments may find a purpose-designed computer database, either a commercial package or developed in-house, more useful. This can allow calculation of the activity for each radionuclide on site at any one time. If records of each assay or process are entered, the database can be employed to calculate the waste generated. The accounting record for unsealed radionuclides should be supported by documentation relating to ordering, receipt, holding, and disposal. Periodic checks of these records, together with a full annual audit, are advisable.

Regular checks of sealed-source inventories showing the location of all longer-lived sources should be carried out to ensure that the records are correct. The frequency will depend on the number of source movements and the restriction of access. Sealed sources need to be tested for any leak of radioactivity at least every 2 years (Box 18.1) or if damage is suspected and this can be combined with carrying out the check of the inventory.

9.2.4 Requirements for safe-keeping

The facilities required in a laboratory will depend on the radionuclides used, their activities, and the processes to be carried out, and these are covered in detailed in Chapter 15. As a general principle, the total activity on the premises should be kept to the minimum and radionuclides no longer required should be disposed of as radioactive waste. Radiopharmaceuticals for administration to patients will normally have a useful lifetime of only one or two days, while radiochemicals used in the laboratory will have a longer lifetime, but radiation damage or chemical degradation will often render solutions unusable after a few weeks or months.

Radioactive materials should be stored in a container which is constructed:

- to prevent the loss or escape of the radioactive material
- to provide protection against damage from foreseeable use/misuse and accidents
- to provide adequate shielding.

Each vial or source must be stored in an appropriately shielded and labelled non-flammable container. γ-emitting sources would normally be stored within lead pots to reduce the dose rate to an acceptable level. The thickness of lead required would depend on the radionuclide used and the activity. As a general rule the external dose rate should be less than 2.5 μSv h^{-1}. Containers for β-emitting radionuclides should have walls (glass/plastic) of thickness greater than or equal to the maximum β-particle range, and at energies above 1 MeV lead shielding may be required to attenuate bremsstrahlung (§7.4). Any vessels containing radioactive liquids which could leak or break should be placed within a secondary, unbreakable container lined with an absorbent material, large enough to hold the whole contents in the event of a spillage. Particular care should be taken in dealing with containers which have been stored for several months, as there may be a risk of bursting or frothing. Such containers should be opened over a drip tray and in a fume cupboard.

Source containers should be kept in a suitable store. Kits containing small quantities (a few kBq) of low-energy beta-emitters may simply be stored on a designated shelf in a refrigerator or freezer. If the room is not locked or is left unattended, the refrigerator should be lockable to prevent unauthorized removal. A locked cupboard in the working area is suitable for short-term storage of radiopharmaceuticals or small marker sources which are in regular use, while a specially designed shielded store will be required for long-term storage of radiotherapy sources (§18.6). The store should be marked with the radiation trefoil.

In addition to radioactive substances legislation [4], the statutory body enforcing ionising radiation regulations [9] (the Health and Safety Executive (HSE) in the UK) must be notified of the holding and use of radioactive materials. A significant spillage or release of radioactive material outside a normal working area or loss of a radioactive source must also be reported to the

Table 9.1 Activity levels for radionuclides used in hospitals at which occurrences need to be notified to the HSE in the UK [9] and for those determining the type of transport package from UK legislation at the time of publication [19, 21]. Values from the new European agreement are given in brackets where these are different [31].

Radionuclide	Notification of use (MBq)	Notification of spillage (MBq)	Notification of loss (MBq)	Transport of sealed source A_1 (TBq)		Transport of unsealed source A_2 (TBq)	
^{241}Am	10^{-2}	1	0.1	2	(10)	2×10^{-4}	(1×10^{-3})
^{198}Au	1	10^5	10	3	(1)	0.5	(0.6)
^{133}Ba	1	10^5	10	3	(20)	3	(0.6)
^{14}C	10	10^5	100	40		2	(3)
^{57}Co	1	10^5	10	8	(10)	8	(10)
^{58}Co	1	10^4	10	1		1	
^{60}Co	0.1	10^4	1	0.4		0.4	
^{51}Cr	10	10^6	10^2	30		30	
^{137}Cs	10^{-2}	10^4	0.1	2		0.5	(0.6)
^{59}Fe	1	10^4	10	0.8	(0.9)	0.8	(0.9)
^{67}Ga	1	10^5	10	6	(7)	6	(3)
^{153}Gd	10	10^4	10^2	10		5	(9)
^{3}H	10^3	10^6	10^4	40		40	
^{123}I	10	10^6	10^2	6		6	(3)
^{125}I	1	10^4	10	20		2	(3)
^{131}I	1	10^4	10	3		0.5	(0.7)
^{111}In	1	10^5	10	2	(3)	2	(3)
^{192}Ir	10^{-2}	10^4	0.1	1		0.5	(0.6)
^{99}Mo	1	10^5	10	0.6	(1)	0.5	(0.6)
^{22}Na	1	10^4	10	0.5		0.5	
^{24}Na	0.1	10^5	1	0.2		0.2	
^{32}P	0.1	10^4	1	0.3	(0.5)	0.3	(0.5)
^{33}P	10^2	10^5	10^3	40		0.9	(1)
^{226}Ra	10^{-2}	10	0.1	0.3	(0.2)	2×10^{-2}	(3×10^{-3})
^{106}Ru	0.1	10^3	1	0.2		0.2	
^{81}Rb	1	10^6	10	2		0.9	(0.8)
^{35}S	10^2	10^5	10^3	40		2	(3)
^{75}Se	1	10^5	10	3		3	
^{89}Sr	1	10^4	10	0.6		0.5	(0.6)
^{90}Sr	10^{-2}	10^3	0.1	0.2	(0.3)	0.1	(0.3)
^{99m}Tc	10	10^7	10^2	8	(10)	8	(4)
^{201}Tl	1	10^5	10	10		10	(4)
^{133}Xe	10^{-2}	10^5	-	20		20	(10)
^{90}Y	0.1	10^5	1	0.2	(0.3)	0.2	(0.3)
^{65}Zn	1	10^4	10	2		2	

statutory body and the Environment Agency. Activity levels for which notification of various occurrences to the HSE is required in the UK [9] are given in Table 9.1.

9.3 Radioactive waste

Radioactive waste is an inevitable by-product from the use of unsealed radioactive materials. As public awareness of consequences of pollution has been raised, the need for the social and environmental effects of radioactive waste disposal to be taken into account has increased. Radioactive waste may be in liquid, solid, or gaseous form and this will determine the methods available for disposal. There are two strategies for waste disposal:

- concentrate and retain
- dilute and disperse.

The second strategy will eventually be used for disposal of the majority of waste from unsealed radionuclides used in medicine and research. For example, disposal of aqueous liquid waste through the drainage system minimizes the radiation doses to hospital personnel. However, for items contaminated with unsealed radionuclides making up solid waste, the first approach might be adopted in the initial management of the waste through segregation and storage to allow decay, followed by the second in the form of incineration, where much of the activity is released as gas from the incinerator stack. Disposal to an older landfill site from where radioactive material may be leached into

Box 9.1 Disposal routes and potential disposal options for radioactive waste

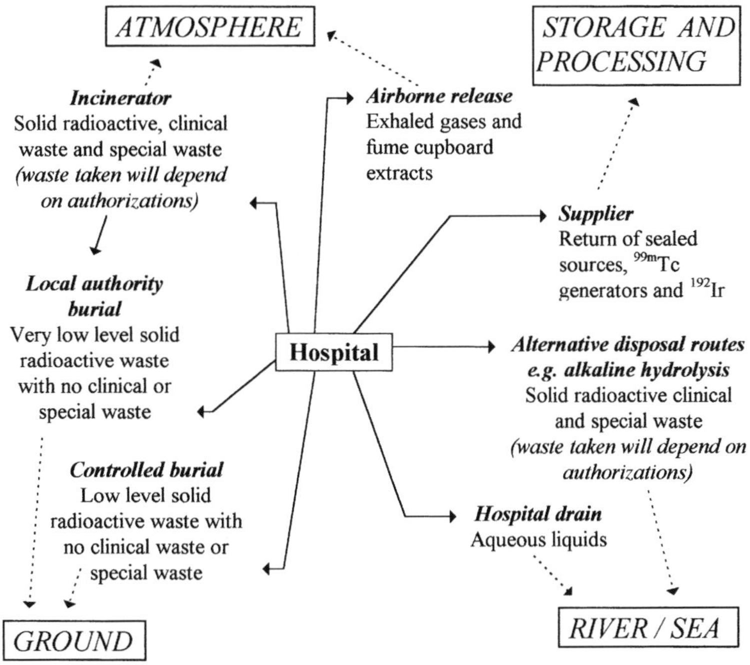

groundwater is also a dilute-and-disperse strategy. However, modern landfill sites are built to a concentrate-and-retain strategy for which the design objective is not to release leachate into groundwater. Return of sources to the supplier is one route where the concentrate-and-retain approach may be followed.

Radioactive waste must be managed from the time at which it is declared waste, through any period of storage until its eventual disposal. The location and the activity should be recorded and accounted for at each stage. Decisions on the routes and methods adopted should be based on an assessment of the occupational risks, the environmental risks, the costs, and the social implications of each route. This is often referred to as the 'best practicable means' (BPM). The possible routes that may be available are summarized in Box 9.1.

9.3.1 Regulation of waste disposal

Hospitals or medical research establishments which generate radioactive waste require a licence or authorization to allow the accumulation of radioactive waste and its disposal under relevant radioactive substances legislation [4]. No person may dispose of radioactive waste unless it is in accordance with such an authorization or exempted from provision of the radioactive substances legislation by an exemption order (§9.2.2). The principal aims of regulation are that:

- radioactive wastes are not created unnecessarily
- all radioactive wastes are managed safely and appropriately
- wastes are safely disposed of at appropriate times and in appropriate ways.

The application for an authorization will require details of how the waste is to be managed and a radiological assessment to determine the environmental impact of the disposals in terms of the doses to members of the public (§9.4). An authorization will only be granted if various conditions are met, including provision of adequate facilities and appropriately trained staff and a satisfactory outcome of the radiological assessment.

When issued, an authorization for the disposal of radioactive waste will give activity limits for each category of waste for each radionuclide or group of radionuclides. Limits for liquid and gaseous waste will be specified for a given time period, which may be a day, a week, a month, or a year depending on circumstances. Limits may be specified for single radionuclides, where large quantities are to be disposed of, but it is usual to group radionuclides together where amounts are smaller.

Exemption orders

If a hospital only disposes of small quantities of radioactivity, it may be able to do this under an exemption order. In this case, it will not require an

Table 9.2 Percentages of radionuclides administered discharged as liquid waste

Radio-pharmaceutical	Medical purpose	Patient management	% of activity administered used to derive activity to waste in the UK[a]	Calc. % of activity administered going to waste[b]
^{131}I	Ablation therapy	In-patients	100	80–100
^{131}I	Thyrotoxicosis treatment	In-patients	50	40–60
^{131}I	Thyrotoxicosis treatment	Out-patients	30	10–20
^{99m}Tc	Typical range of tests	Administering hospital	30	25–30
^{99m}Tc		Hospital to which patient returns	10	5–10
^{32}P	All tests	Administering hospital	30	2–6
^{67}Ga	All tests	Administering hospital	30	0.5–2
^{201}Tl	All tests	Administering hospital	30	0.5–2
^{123}I	As MIBG		60	8–22
^{123}I	As any other compound		100	
Others (e.g. ^{111}In, ^{75}Se, ^{51}Cr)			100	

[a]Percentages agreed by the IPEM Special Interest Group and adopted by the Environment Agency.
[b]Calculation of p_2 using method described in Box 9.3 for comparison with data in previous column.

authorization, but the organization must keep the Environment Agency informed of the application of the exemption order. In the UK, hospitals and nursing homes are allowed to dispose of up to 1 GBq ^{99m}Tc and 500 MBq of any other radionuclides per month to the drainage system in human excreta [7]. This enables patients to return to the hospital or nursing home in which they were being treated after radionuclide examinations performed elsewhere or following ^{131}I therapy. Records must be kept to show that the exemption limits are not exceeded. Percentages which are applied to the activities administered to determine the quantities of liquid waste in the UK are given in Table 9.2.

An exemption for substances of low activity allows some radioactive waste of low-level activity which is solid and insoluble in water to be classed as non-radioactive [8], although this is not normally useful for hospitals and laboratories. In addition, gaseous waste containing only radionuclides with half-lives less than 100 seconds may be released without the need for an authorization and this can be applied to the disposal of ^{81m}Kr ($T_{\frac{1}{2}} = 13$ s). Sources formerly used for testing instruments which have activities less than 200 kBq may also be disposed of to landfill sites (§9.3.5) [6].

Enforcement

If an organization does not comply with a registration or authorization, the Environment Agency may serve an enforcement notice which specifies steps that must be undertaken to achieve compliance within a certain time period [4]. If it is considered that continuation of the practice involves a significant risk of pollution of the environment or harm to human health, a prohibition notice may be issued withdrawing permission granted in the registration or authorization until the matter of concern has been rectified.

9.3.2 Aqueous liquid waste

Radioactive waste in an aqueous solution or solid matter in suspension in water may be discharged to the drainage system. Most of the liquid waste from hospitals will be urine and faeces from patients undergoing nuclear medicine procedures and will include large quantities of ^{99m}Tc. Nuclear medicine departments should provide patient toilets near the waiting area, although there is usually no necessity for strict segregation and diagnostic patients may be allowed to use toilet facilities elsewhere in the hospital. Separate toilet facilities should be allocated for in-patients undergoing therapy with radio-iodine and some other radiopharmaceuticals. Smaller amounts of waste will arise from preparation of radiopharmaceuticals, *in vitro* procedures, or unused patient administrations, which are usually discharged into sinks designated for this purpose (§15.3.2). Radioactive waste should be poured directly into the sink outlet and particular care taken to avoid splashing. Simultaneously, large amounts of water should be poured down the drain from the sink to reduce the radionuclide concentration to below 1 MBq l^{-1}. Designated sinks should be connected directly to the sewer system, wherever possible, and use of traps avoided. The route through which the radioactive waste

Table 9.3 Guide to authorization conditions commonly used for solid radioactive waste

Category of waste or disposal route	Concentrations of ^{14}C and ^{3}H	Maximum activity of ^{14}C or ^{3}H in one item	Concentrations of other radionuclides	Maximum activity of other radionuclide in one item	Other exclusions
Exempt waste	0.4 Bq g^{-1}	0.4 Bq g^{-1}	0.4 Bq g^{-1}	0.4 Bq g^{-1}	
Disposal with domestic refuse	4 MBq in 0.1 m^3	0.4 MBq	0.4 MBq in 0.1 m^3	0.04 MBq	No α-emitters
Controlled burial (special precautions)	200 MBq in 0.1 m^3	–	4 MBq in 0.1 m^3 (HL > 1 year) 40 MBq in 0.1 m^3 (HL < 1 year)	0.4 MBq	
Intermediate level waste	> 12 GBq ton^{-1}	–	β/γ > 12 GBq ton^{-1} α > 4 GBq ton^{-1}	–	

HL Half-life

reaches the sewer should be mapped and both the sink and pipework should be labelled to reduce the potential risk of exposure to plumbers working on the system. This is particularly important for higher activities of relatively long-lived radionuclides such as ^{125}I. If significant quantities of γ-emitting radioactive materials are to be disposed of, it is important to ensure that there are no lengths of poorly drained pipework that lie near to working areas where others could be irradiated. This may be checked by releasing a bolus of activity into the sink or toilet, measuring count rates at positions lower down the pipes with a suitable contamination monitor, and checking the speed of clearance as more water is released.

9.3.3 Gaseous waste

Releases into the atmosphere of radioactive gas or vapour may result from patient investigations in nuclear medicine departments using radioactive gases such as ^{133}Xe and ^{81m}Kr, aerosols such as ^{99m}Tc DTPA, or exhaling of $^{14}CO_2$ from breath tests. Xenon will need to be vented to the outside through an exhaust pipe, which may lead out through a window or other suitable outlet located to avoid gas re-entry to occupied areas, but this is not usually considered necessary for ^{81m}Kr as the half-life is less than 100 s [8]. Normally, most of the ^{99m}Tc aerosol and ^{133}Xe released from the lungs is trapped by the dispensing equipment and the amount released to the atmosphere is small enough to be considered radiologically insignificant. Radioactive gases may be produced during laboratory chemical procedures such as the volatilization of ^{125}I during the iodination of proteins or production of gases during work with ^{14}C bicarbonates or ^{3}H borohydrides. These operations would normally be performed in a fume cupboard so that the radioactive gas was not recirculated into the laboratory but discharged from an external exhaust stack. Outlet stacks must be at a height and position to minimize the risk of any released gas entering a building before adequate dilution has taken place. It is good practice to check fume cupboard exhaust systems using a smoke candle at installation. Appropriate precautions must be taken beforehand to disable relevant fire-alarm systems to avoid the repercussions of an unintended triggering of a smoke detector.

9.3.4 Solid waste

General categories which are used to describe solid radioactive waste, based on the radiations emitted and the activity concentrations, are given in Table 9.3. These apply to the whole range of wastes generated by all users of radioactivity including the nuclear industry. Hospital wastes only fall into the lowest three categories.

Clinical waste

The bulk of solid radioactive waste from hospitals and research laboratories is made up of articles which have been contaminated with liquid radiopharmaceuticals. This includes syringes, needles, paper tissues, disposable gloves, etc., used in laboratories and nuclear medicine departments and materials contaminated from being used by patients treated in hospital following radionuclide therapy. Clinical waste will also include biological materials, such as human and animal tissues, blood samples, contaminated swabs and dressings, and sharps (i.e. discarded syringe needles, broken glass, disposable instruments, and empty vials), which should be collected in purpose-designed containers (e.g. Cinbins). This type of waste would normally be regarded as clinical waste but some may fall into the category of special waste.

Special waste

Some of the radioactive clinical waste that is generated in healthcare may possess other properties which will require it to be treated as special waste as defined in Special Waste Regulations [10]. If this is the case, both the radioactive content and special waste properties must be taken into account in determining the method for disposal. Substances which are highly flammable, toxic, carcinogenic, corrosive, or irritant must be treated as special waste. Biological samples that contain viable microorganisms believed to cause disease or materials having other hazardous properties are also included in certain cases [10].

Some liquid scintillants used for counting low-energy beta-emitters such as tritium or ^{14}C contain one or more organic chemical compounds and these fall into the category of special waste. Vials containing small volumes of liquid scintillant can be classed as solid waste. Larger quantities must be disposed of as organic liquid. There are alternative biodegradable versions of scintillants which may be disposed of down the drains with permission from the local water authority. Radiopharmaceuticals, because they are administered to patients as prescription only medicines (POMs), are regarded as special waste in the UK at the time of publication.

Decayed sources

Closed or sealed sources will eventually become waste when they are no longer usable. This may be because the activity has decayed to a level such that the source is no longer suitable for the application or because the design lifetime of the source has been exceeded and the potential consequences of failure mean that it is no longer safe to use. It may also be because the source has been damaged, rendering it no longer suitable for use. Radionuclide generators also become waste when the activity has fallen below the useful level.

9.3.5 Disposal routes for solid waste

The most important characteristics of waste relating to its management and ultimate disposal are:

- volume of waste
- radionuclide content (in particular, half-lives)
- special waste content.

The radionuclide concentration in much of the solid waste generated by hospitals may be such that it falls into the category that would allow its disposal with domestic refuse (Table 9.3). However, it is necessary to take account of the chemical and biological components as well as the radioactive content in determining the possible disposal routes. Radiopharmaceuticals and radiochemicals may be regarded as special waste and these will need to be treated at a plant licensed to dispose of special waste. The Environment Agency may agree to avoid unnecessary duplication of paperwork for radioactive substances and special waste legislation if levels of hazardous material in the waste are small, but suitable disposal routes must be used. The various options for disposal route are summarized in Box 9.1 and those for solid waste are discussed here in turn. Apart from disposal under the Substances of Low Activity Exemption Order [8], all require specific authorization.

Incineration

Incineration is an appropriate means for disposal of all clinical wastes including radioactive waste. The incinerator must meet strict design and emission standards, relating to the temperature and completeness of combustion, before disposal of special waste may be allowed. Limits will be placed on radionuclide activities disposed of within defined time intervals (e.g. daily and monthly) and radionuclide concentration in the waste. Incineration will disperse most radionuclides into the atmosphere. European legislation imposes strict requirements on combustion and particulate matter must be scrubbed out. Some activity may be concentrated in the fly ash when the bulk of the material has been removed and monitoring of the residual ash will be required. The ash can be disposed of with ordinary refuse if the activity is below the appropriate limit (Table 9.3). However, it may in some circumstances be necessary to have an authorization for disposal of the ash via an alternative route, such as controlled burial.

Landfill with ordinary refuse

Large volumes of conventional waste are disposed of in landfill sites usually run by the local authority. However, control over the sites after they have been filled is only for a few years. If radioactive waste is disposed of in this way, human exposure could occur through movement of radionuclides in groundwater or accidental intrusion by man. Waste that comes under the exemption order (Table 9.3), which does not contain any of the components that must be regarded as clinical or special waste, can be disposed of with domestic refuse to these sites for shallow burial. All labels and markings referring to the radioactive nature of the material must be removed to avoid misinterpretation of the status of the waste, as this could trigger a radiation incident procedure. This route may be appropriate for disposal of decayed check or marker sources, which, because of the construction, may be less suitable for disposal by incineration. Single small sources with activities less than 200 kBq used for testing instruments may be disposed of to a waste collection authority under an exemption order (§9.3.1).

Controlled burial

Disposal of radionuclides to a trench within a landfill site is used for disposal of some low-level waste (Table 9.3).

The trench will be filled in immediately after a disposal has been made and its location recorded so that further disturbance can be avoided. Radionuclides in the wastes will be immediately accessible to leaching and dispersion, so stricter limits must be applied to long half-life wastes. It may be possible to dispose of some small closed sources through a controlled burial site within the terms of the authorization.

Burial within specialized facilities with watertight barriers to contain the waste provides a method for disposal or storage for waste of greater activity and longer half-life radionuclides, but would not be required for waste routinely generated by hospitals.

Heat disinfection

Heat disinfection by maintaining a high temperature for a long period of time may be used to reduce the content of biological agents in certain types of clinical waste, so that material can be disposed of to landfill. This method would not be suitable for disposal of wastes containing pharmaceuticals included in the category of special waste and will therefore not be appropriate for most radioactive wastes from hospitals.

Alkaline hydrolysis

Waste containing tissue, pathogens, cytotoxic agents, and other toxic compounds would normally be disposed of by incineration. Alternative approaches such as alkaline hydrolysis may provide a more environmentally appropriate method for disposal of tissue and chemical waste and are suitable for waste containing radioactivity. The waste is mixed with water and alkali in a pressure-tight vessel, stirred continuously, and heated (110–170°C) for 6–18 h. The process breaks down the tissue and chemical molecules to produce a sterile solution which can be discharged to the drains [11].

Disposal to the supplier or specialized waste contractor

Most sealed sources will require to be disposed of either through the supplier or by a contractor with an appropriate authorization for disposal. The least expensive option is generally to have an arrangement for the supplier to collect a decayed source when delivering a new one. Higher-activity unsealed material, such as ^{192}Ir wire, may also be returned to the supplier in this way.

Hospitals which have their own ^{99}Mo/^{99m}Tc or ^{81}Rb/^{81m}Kr generators usually have an arrangement for regular delivery of new generators and return of old ones. A system will be agreed with the Environment Agency for a limited period of storage followed by collection by the supplier.

Choice of disposal route

Risk assessments are required under both health and safety and environmental legislation with regard to the management and choice of disposal route for radioactive waste. The factors which will need to be taken into account are:

- compliance with relevant legislation
- recommendations in established guidance
- methods available and relative costs
- facilities for storage
- risks from movement and transportation.

Most of the waste generated will require use of a contractor specializing in waste disposal with relevant authorizations. The organization disposing of the waste has a 'duty of care' with regard to the waste under the Environmental Protection Act (Box 5.2), under which there is an obligation to ensure that throughout the chain of production, transport, treatment, and disposal, all reasonable measures are taken to ensure that the waste is managed and disposed of properly.

9.3.6 Decay storage of radioactive waste

Since radioactivity decays naturally, storage for a limited period can reduce the risk associated with some radioactive wastes. Temporary storage of waste containing radionuclides with shorter half-lives (a few hours to a few weeks) allows the radionuclide activities to decay, thereby reducing the potential hazard and facilitating disposal. However, in order to utilize this, it may be necessary to transfer the waste to a storage area to minimize risks to staff. A waste storage facility (Box 9.2) and an appropriate system for management of the waste are needed. In addition there should be:

- experienced and trained personnel with responsibility for management of the waste
- labelling of waste containers with all relevant information
- secondary containment in the event of an accident such as leakage of liquid waste
- systems to ensure waste is kept for the appropriate time and then transferred for disposal
- detailed records of the radionuclide, activity, and history of all waste in the store
- regular contamination monitoring and recording.

The risks from storage of radioactive waste include operational exposure of personnel involved in maintenance and surveillance and a continuing risk of accidental releases. These, together with the cost of the store, must be weighed against the potential exposure and financial cost of disposal at an earlier stage. The

Box 9.2 Requirements for a radioactive waste store

An organization using a variety of open sources should have a separate store reserved for radioactive waste and associated containers and ancillary equipment, if a significant quantity of the radioactive waste is produced. Some requirements for this type of store are given.

- The store should have adequate resistance to fire and must not contain any explosive or flammable substances.
- Emergency equipment such as a fire extinguisher should be provided nearby.
- External stores should offer protection against the weather and against extreme temperature, flood, or mechanical damage.
- There should be adequate ventilation to prevent build-up of gases, vapour, or any accidentally dispersed radioactive material.
- Shielding should be provided to give adequate protection for persons using the store and reduce external dose rates to a level such that no external restrictions will be required.
- The store must be secure against theft or interference by outside persons.
- The store must be marked as containing radioactive substances and the radiation warning sign displayed.
- There should be adequate space and storage racks or shelves to allow convenient arrangement and segregation of sources and a suitable labelling system.
- A notice should give the name and telephone number of the person(s) responsible.
- Access to the store should be limited to authorized staff, who have been trained in precautions and procedures to be adopted.

licensing authority will only allow extended decay storage if the facilities and waste-management systems are adequate.

For smaller facilities it may be appropriate to use one radionuclide store for both waste and other sources, but the two must be well separated. The waste store may serve as a point to which waste is delivered from several departments, checked, monitored, and prepared for disposal. Contaminated glassware or other items may also be stored there. Storage of liquid waste should be minimized. Containers must be leak-proof and precautions taken against evaporation of the contents. Plans for disposal routes should be put in place before any radionuclide work is undertaken and disposals made as early as practicable after the material is declared to be waste. Biological material may be stored in a freezer but plans must be in place to deal with the material.

9.3.7 Record keeping for radioactive waste

One of the requirements for granting of an authorization to accumulate and dispose of radioactive waste is that an up-to-date record is kept of all the activity on site and all disposals made. This record should demonstrate that the user is complying with the terms of any authorization granted. This will include amounts of liquid waste discharged via designated sinks, as well as liquid waste from patients, and estimates of amounts of gaseous waste released. The amounts of liquid waste released from patients can be assumed to be either equal to those administered or a percentage of that value agreed with the Environment Agency. Values used in the UK are given in Table 9.2. Appropriate proportions can be determined by using radiopharmaceutical dosimetry data (Box 9.3).

For solid waste, records should include the activities of the various radionuclides being used and corrections to allow for decay before disposal. It is usually desirable to segregate waste into bags or containers according to radionuclide or at least separate groups of radionuclides with different half-lives. This will enable the decline in activity to be determined. Since waste contractors normally charge by the activity disposed of as well as the volume of waste, having a proper system for decay correction may have financial implications.

In a laboratory, where standard techniques are used, it should be possible to determine amounts of waste generated as a proportion of total usage. If each process can be defined so that known proportions of the total go as liquid, solid, and gaseous waste, then an estimate of the activity in the waste can be made by use of a computer program. Waste containing ^{14}C or ^{3}H, for which measurement of activity is difficult, must be dealt with in this way.

For waste containing a single radionuclide emitting γ-radiation, a practical technique should be established for measuring and performing an assessment of activity using available instrumentation, which might be a scintillation or Geiger contamination monitor (§4.4.2). This method should provide a good estimation of activity

Box 9.3 Calculation of proportions of administered radioactivity excreted by patients

A knowledge of proportions of radionuclide activities excreted is important for determining waste authorization limits required for administered radiopharmaceuticals. Values may be determined practically by collection and measurement. Theoretical values can be derived using data on radiopharmaceutical behaviour in the body contained in ICRP 53 [12]. The relevant quantities are:

- A_s/A_o equal to the ratio of the cumulative activity in the body (A_s) to the administered activity (A_o). The cumulative activity is the activity in the body integrated over all time and is in units of activity × time, e.g. MBq hours, so that A_s/A_o is measured in hours.
- The biological half-lives (T_{biol}) for radioactivity in various compartments, representing a fraction (a) of the total.
- The physical half-life $T_{1/2}$ of the radionuclide is required, from which the effective half-life of activity in the body (T_{eff}) is given by $1/T_{eff} = 1/T_{1/2} + 1/T_{biol}$. Quantities λ equal to $0.693/T$ will be used in the equations to describe the physical (λ_{phys}), biological (λ_{biol}), and overall effective (λ_{eff}) rates of decay.

If there was no excretion of radiopharmaceutical from the body, the activity A_o would decline as a simple exponential determined by the physical half-life, and integration over an infinite time would give a cumulative activity (A_n) of A_o/λ_{phys}.

An assessment of the proportion of administered activity that is excreted (p_1) can be obtained from the proportional decrease in the cumulative activity $(A_n - A_s)/A_n$. This can be determined from the equation:

$$p_1 = (A_n - A_s)/A_n = 1 - [\lambda_{phys} \times (A_s/A_o)].$$

For out-patients who spend limited times in hospital, a different approach is more appropriate. It can be assumed that the patient excretes activity on a limited number of discrete occasions at time t after administration and thereafter at intervals of t hours. This can be simulated by an equation of the form:

$$p_2 = \exp(-\lambda_{phys}t)\ [1 - \exp(-\lambda_{biol}t)]\ [1 + \exp(-\lambda_{eff}t) + \exp(-2\lambda_{eff}t) + \ldots].$$

Activity excreted by the patient at time t after administration is represented by the first term in the second bracket, that at time $2t$ is represented by the second, that at $3t$ by the third, and so on. For a patient attending for a scan, it may only be necessary to consider the first term with an appropriate value for t, such as 1 h. There may be several compartments (i) within the body where a radiopharmaceutical will accumulate, with a fraction a_i in each. The compartments may have different biological half-lives, so that different proportions p_{2i} of the radionuclide would be excreted from each. The overall proportion of activity excreted could then be obtained from the sum $\sum_i a_i\, p_{2i}$.

This method can be used to calculate excretion levels during the short visit to a nuclear medicine department or after a patient has returned to another hospital. Some values of p_2 for various radionuclides, calculated by assuming that out-patients remain in the hospital for up to 4 h, are given in Table 9.2 for comparison with percentages used for calculating liquid disposals. Values for ^{99m}Tc were derived using a typical weighted mix of examinations and assuming that patients remained in the administering hospital for 3–4 h and returned to a hospital or nursing home in which they are staying after 4 h.

but will generally only be used as a back-up. Some quantification for high-energy β-emitters such as ^{32}P is possible, but more difficult because of variations in bremsstrahlung yield. The method is particularly useful for nuclear medicine and radionuclide therapy, where the amount of activity present in the waste is variable, but will not be required in many laboratories, for which accurate assessments of activities can be made by other methods. The method should be set up and documented by the qualified expert. A check on the adequacy of the technique should be made using simulations with known activities of the relevant radionuclide. A similar system may be used for monitoring and assessing items contaminated by radioactivity, such as laboratory equipment, bed linen, or patients' belongings.

9.4 Radiological impact of waste disposal

9.4.1 Doses from waste disposal

Before an authorization can be obtained to dispose of radioactive waste from any facility, an assessment must be made of the impact on the environment. This is usually performed by evaluating doses that individuals outside the facility might receive from the disposals. These are then compared with the dose constraint for members of the public (0.3 mSv $year^{-1}$) and anything above this is regarded as intolerable. In addition, the principle of ALARP (as low as reasonably practicable) must be applied and in the UK a threshold of 0.02 mSv $year^{-1}$ may be employed, below which further optimisation is not considered necessary, provided that the operator is considered to be using BPM to limit discharges. This threshold is used in assessments of doses from hospital discharges.

A simplified methodology has been prepared by the National Radiological Protection Board (NRPB) [13] for use by hospitals and other small users of radioactive materials in making radiological assessments. This covers discharge of aqueous waste to sewers, discharge of radioactive gases and vapours, and incineration of radioactive waste. It models the initial dispersion and any subsequent accumulation, and evaluates the exposure of individuals. Simple equations have been developed that can be applied to different scenarios into which factors for specific radionuclides are inserted.

9.4.2 Critical groups

It is not usually practicable to assess doses to individual members of the public, so the approach adopted is to identify 'critical groups' within the population who would be expected to receive the highest doses. The critical group would normally consist of up to a few tens of individuals [14] but could be as small as one or two individuals. Hypothetical critical groups can be identified based on national survey data, although some information on local practices, based on general observation of habits and behaviour, will be required. Initially, it may be appropriate to assess more than one potential critical group. The group that receives the highest dose is then the true critical group for the purpose of the assessment and the mean dose to this group can be compared to the dose constraints and threshold dose.

The authorization limits sought should be used for the assessment. This will be a conservative assumption, since actual discharges are likely to be lower, but will provide a high level of confidence that the maximum dose constraint will not be exceeded. This assessment alone is acceptable where the assessed doses are below the threshold of optimisation (0.02 mSv $year^{-1}$). Further investigation and evaluation should be undertaken using more realistic environmental and critical group data if the doses are found to be above this level. Assessment of doses can only be carried out for specific radionuclides, so where there are limits for groups of radionuclides, it is necessary either to split the discharge between the radionuclides applied for or to use a representative one.

9.4.3 Aquatic discharges

The most significant discharges from hospitals are usually liquid discharges to the sewer system, primarily from patient excretion. The highest activity concentrations will usually occur close to the discharge point and the main critical group is often workers either involved in maintenance of the hospital sewer or working in the sewage plant. However, activities of other members of the public relating to the river downstream of the discharge point may need to be considered. The following data are required for the assessment:

- disposal rate of each radionuclide derived from the monthly limit (Bq $month^{-1}$) (A_{lim})
- flow rate of waste water from the site, equal to the water usage (m^3 day^{-1}) (V_{use})
- flow rate (dry weather) of waste through the sewage works (m^3 day^{-1}) (V_{works})
- details of disposal route from the hospital to the sewage works
- flow rate in the water course to which the sewage is discharged (m^3 day^{-1}) (V_{river})
- data on the river water usage downstream of the discharge point.

Simplified equations can be used to derive the effective doses and committed effective doses for potential critical groups [13]. Critical groups exposed and ranges of effective doses are described in Box 9.4. The equations presented here are rationalized versions of those used by NRPB [13] in terms of effective dose rather than effective dose equivalent. Selected data from this and various ICRP reports are reproduced in Tables 9.4–9.8 for use in calculations of doses to critical groups.

Sewage workers

Effective doses to sewage workers should be estimated for inhalation, inadvertent ingestion, and external radiation. The methodology is described and an example calculation given in Box 9.5. The committed effective doses ($E_{\mathrm{ing/inh}}$) from ingestion ($_{\mathrm{ing}}$) and inhalation ($_{inh}$) can be derived from equations with the form:

$$E_{\mathrm{ing/inh}} = C_{\mathrm{wt}}\, I_{\mathrm{ing/inh}}\, D_{\mathrm{ing/inh}}\, O \qquad (9.1)$$

where C_{wt} is the concentration of radioactivity (Bq kg^{-1}) derived from the values (A_{lim}/V) (see Box 9.5), $I_{\mathrm{ing/inh}}$ is the rate of intake via the particular route (inhalation or ingestion), $D_{ing/inh}$ is the committed effective dose per unit intake, and O is the occupancy in terms of the length of time for which an individual might be exposed during a year [13, 15, 16]. This differs from the occupancy used for shielding calculations, which is expressed in terms of the proportion of time for which persons might be exposed (Chapter 13). The rate of intake through

Box 9.4 Groups exposed from aqueous disposals of radioactive waste

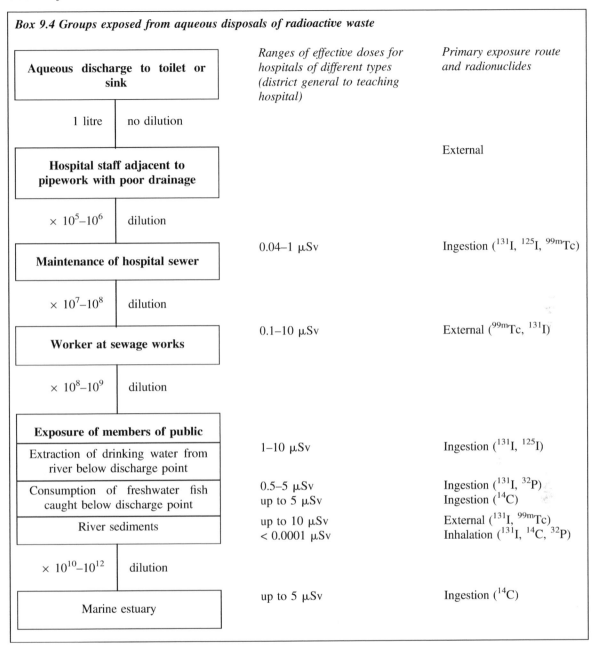

	Ranges of effective doses for hospitals of different types (district general to teaching hospital)	*Primary exposure route and radionuclides*
Aqueous discharge to toilet or sink		
1 litre — no dilution		
Hospital staff adjacent to pipework with poor drainage		External
$\times\ 10^5$–10^6 — dilution		
Maintenance of hospital sewer	0.04–1 μSv	Ingestion (^{131}I, ^{125}I, ^{99m}Tc)
$\times\ 10^7$–10^8 — dilution		
Worker at sewage works	0.1–10 μSv	External (^{99m}Tc, ^{131}I)
$\times\ 10^8$–10^9 — dilution		
Exposure of members of public		
Extraction of drinking water from river below discharge point	1–10 μSv	Ingestion (^{131}I, ^{125}I)
Consumption of freshwater fish caught below discharge point	0.5–5 μSv up to 5 μSv	Ingestion (^{131}I, ^{32}P) Ingestion (^{14}C)
River sediments	up to 10 μSv < 0.0001 μSv	External (^{131}I, ^{99m}Tc) Inhalation (^{131}I, ^{14}C, ^{32}P)
$\times\ 10^{10}$–10^{12} — dilution		
Marine estuary	up to 5 μSv	Ingestion (^{14}C)

inhalation is equal to the product of the resuspended sewage load (s_r) and the breathing rate (v).

$$I_{\text{inh}} = s_r\, v. \tag{9.2}$$

Typical values for quantities relating to human activities are given in Table 9.4 and values for $D_{\text{ing/inh}}$ are given in Table 9.5.

The equation used to calculate the effective dose from external radiation (E_{ext}) for a worker at a sewage plant is

$$E_{\text{ext}} = C_{\text{vol}}\, D_{\text{ext}}\, O \tag{9.3}$$

where C_{vol} is the concentration of radioactivity in Bq m^{-3} and D_{ext} is the effective dose rate from external γ-rays. D_{ext} for a semi-infinite slab of sewage contaminated at a level of 1 Bq m^{-3} is

$$D_{\text{ext/slab}} = 2.6 \times 10^{-13} \times E_{\text{output}} \tag{9.4}$$

where E_{output} for a radionuclide is the sum of the individual photon energies (MeV) multiplied by their probabilities of emission (Table 9.6) [17].

A worker maintaining a hospital sewer will be exposed to γ-rays from a pipe containing sewage and

Table 9.4 Recommended values of parameters for calculation of exposures from discharges

Liquid discharges—sewage workers	**Value**
Intake rate for inadvertent ingestion (I_{ing}, eq. 9.1)	5×10^{-5} kg h^{-1}
Resuspended sewage concentration sewage works (s_r, eq. 9.2)	10^{-7} kg m^{-3}
Resuspended sewage concentration sewer maintenance (s_r, eq. 9.2)	10^{-6} kg m^{-3}
Breathing rate (v, eq. 9.2)	1.2 m^3 h^{-1}
Occupancy at sewage works for inhalation (O, eq. 9.1)	2000 h $year^{-1}$
Occupancy at sewage works for ingestion and external exposure (O, eqs 9.1 and 9.3)	1000 h $year^{-1}$
Occupancy for sewer maintenance (all exposure pathways) (O, eqs 9.1 and 9.5)	200 h $year^{-1}$
Typical flow rate through sewer pipe (u_s, eq. 9.5)	0.5 m s^{-1}
Liquid discharges—general public	
Consumption of drinking water (M_{water}, eq. 9.7)	0.6 m^3 $year^{-1}$
Inadvertent ingestion of water (bathing) (M_{water}, eq. 9.7)	0.5×10^{-3} m^3 $year^{-1}$
Consumption of freshwater fish (M_{fish}, eq. 9.7)	20 kg $year^{-1}$
Riverbank occupancy (O, eq. 9.9)	500 h $year^{-1}$
Atmospheric disposals	
Occupancy for inhalation of gaseous releases (O, eq. 9.11)	8760 h $year^{-1}$
Inhalation rate (I_{atmos} O, eq. 9.11)	7300 m^3 $year^{-1}$
Dry deposition velocity (v_g, eq. 9.13)	10^{-3} m s^{-1}
Dry deposition velocity for inorganic form of iodine (v_g, eq. 9.13)	10^{-2} m s^{-1}
Dry deposition velocity for organic form of iodine (v_g, eq. 9.13)	10^{-5} m s^{-1}
Representative wet deposition rate for unit release of 1 Bq s^{-1} (x distance from release point in m) (r_w, eq. 9.13)	3.2×10^{-6} Bq m^{-2} s^{-1} (Bq s^{-1} m^{-1})$^{-1}$
Consumption of cereals ($M_{cereals}$, eq. 9.15)	100 kg $year^{-1}$
Consumption of green vegetables ($M_{vegetables}$, eq. 9.15)	80 kg $year^{-1}$
Consumption of root vegetables (M_{root}, eq. 9.15)	130 kg $year^{-1}$
Consumption of fruit (M_{friut}, eq. 9.15)	75 kg $year^{-1}$
Consumption of milk (M_{milk}, eq. 9.15)	240 kg $year^{-1}$

Data reproduced from McDonnell [13].

Table 9.5 Committed effective dose per radionuclide unit intake through ingestion and inhalation (Sv Bq^{-1}) (equations 9.1, 9.7, 9.11, and 9.15)

Radionuclide	Ingestion (D_{ing})	Inhalation (D_{inh})
^{3}H	1.8×10^{-11}	4.5×10^{-11}
^{14}C	5.8×10^{-10}	2.0×10^{-9}
^{14}C (as CO_2)	–	6.2×10^{-12}
^{32}P	2.4×10^{-9}	3.4×10^{-9}
^{35}S	7.7×10^{-10}	1.4×10^{-9}
^{99m}Tc	2.2×10^{-11}	1.9×10^{-11}
^{125}I	1.5×10^{-8}	5.1×10^{-9}
^{131}I	2.2×10^{-8}	7.4×10^{-9}
^{201}Tl	9.5×10^{-11}	4.4×10^{-11}

Note: Doses from ingestion and inhalation of ^{133}Xe are not significant compared to the external dose rate.
Data reproduced from McDonnell [13] and ICRP 72 [16].

an equation of the form

$$E_{ext} = C_L\, D_{ext}\, O \tag{9.5}$$

is appropriate here, where C_L relates to the concentration of activity along the length of the pipe. For a flow rate u_s, the concentration term C_L(Bq m^{-1}) can be derived from A_{lim}/u_s(Table 9.4) (see Box 9.5). D_{ext} for a line source is given by

$$D_{ext/line} = 3.6 \times 10^{-13} \times E_{output}. \tag{9.6}$$

The ranges of effective doses resulting from radioactive waste discharges that might be encountered in hospitals of varying size are given in Box 9.4. The most significant contributions usually arise from ^{131}I, because of its

Table 9.6 Values for radionuclide specific parameters for dose calculations

	^{14}C	^{32}P	^{99m}Tc	^{125}I	^{131}I	^{133}Xe	^{201}Tl
γ-ray energy output E_{output} (MeV Bq^{-1}) (eqs 9.4 and 9.6)	–	–	1.3×10^{-1}	4.2×10^{-2}	3.8×10^{-1}	4.6×10^{-2}	9.3×10^{-2}
Concentration factor for freshwater fish (k_{fish}) (Bq kg^{-1} [Bq $m^{-3}]^{-1}$) (eq. 9.8)	4.5	4.9	1.5×10^{-2}	2.0×10^{-2}	2.0×10^{-2}	–	9.8
Concentration factor for freshwater sediment (k_{sed}) (Bq kg^{-1} [Bq $m^{-3}]^{-1}$) (eq. 9.8)	2.0	1.4×10^{1}	2.0×10^{-1}	3.0×10^{-1}	3.0×10^{-1}	–	–
γ-ray dose rate from external exposure to semi-infinite cloud (D_{cloud}) (Sv h^{-1} [Bq $m^{-3}]^{-1}$) (eq. 9.12)	–	–	2.0×10^{-11}	6.7×10^{-12}	6.1×10^{-11}	7.4×10^{-12}	1.5×10^{-11}
β-ray dose rate from external exposure to infinite cloud (D_{cloud}) (Sv h^{-1} [Bq $m^{-3}]^{-1}$) (eq. 9.12)	–	3.3×10^{-10}	–	–	8.7×10^{-11}	6.2×10^{-11}	–

Data reproduced from McDonnell [13].

radiological and accumulation properties, and ^{99m}Tc because of the amounts used.

Members of the public

When the radionuclides are discharged to water bodies, they are dispersed through water movement and sedimentation processes. There may be groups exposed through abstraction of drinking water or fishing activity. A similar style of equation may be used to calculate committed effective doses ($E_{water/fish}$) to these groups from the annual consumption of drinking water (M_{water}) or fish (M_{fish}):

$$E_{water/fish} = C_{water/fish}\, M_{water/fish}\, D_{ing} \tag{9.7}$$

where C_{water} is the radionuclide concentration in filtered water, and C_{fish} is that in fish (see Box 9.5). A concentration factor (k_{fish}) is used to determine C_{fish} from C_{water} (Table 9.6).

$$C_{fish} = k_{fish}\, C_{water}. \tag{9.8}$$

This result can then be substituted into equation (9.7). Exposure is generally very low, but doses from ^{14}C disposal can be significant because of the relatively high concentration factor (Table 9.6). Another route which might be significant for liquid discharges is through external γ-ray exposure from river sediments (E_{ext}), given by

$$E_{ext} = C_{sed}\, D_{ext/slab}\, O \tag{9.9}$$

where C_{sed} is calculated using the concentration factor for sediment k_{sed} (Table 9.6) using an equation of the form of (9.8) and $D_{ext/slab}$ is the dose rate from a semi-infinite slab of material [equation (9.4)]. Radionuclides may also be concentrated in sewage sludge, which may be used for land treatment or disposed of by incineration.

9.4.4 Atmospheric releases

For releases to the atmosphere, a model is used to predict concentrations in the air at ground level under standard meteorological conditions. The information required is:

- the height of the release point
- the discharge rate (R) for each radionuclide (Bq s^{-1})
- the distance to the location of potential critical groups (If this is uncertain it may be appropriate to assume that the critical group is at the point of maximum ground level airborne concentration)
- information on food pathways through farm produce and cultivation of vegetables by local residents.

Atmospheric releases may occur from exhalation of radioactive gases used in diagnostic tests or from incineration of waste. The radionuclide concentration in the plume downwind from the release point (C_{plume}) (Bq m^{-3}) can be obtained from the equation

$$C_{plume} = R\, P \tag{9.10}$$

where R is the release rate in Bq s^{-1} and P is the radionuclide concentration in the plume per unit release [Bq m^{-3} (Bq $s^{-1})^{-1}$]. Values for P derived using the Gaussian plume diffusion model of atmospheric dispersion are plotted against distance in Figure 9.1 for different release heights, assuming a uniform release rate and average weather conditions [18]. Meteorological

Box 9.5 Environmental impact assessment for discharge of liquid waste containing ^{131}I

A hospital is applying to dispose of 10 GBq of ^{131}I to the sewer per month. An assessment of the resulting doses to critical groups is required.

Information on discharges, water flow rates and water usage (§9.4.3)

- disposal rate is 10 GBq per month
- flow rate of waste water from the site is 100 m^3 day^{-1}
- flow rate of waste through the sewage works is 20 000 m^3 day^{-1}
- the river has drinking water abstracted and is popular with anglers
- flow rate in the water course at the point of water abstraction is 1 000 000 m^3 day^{-1}.

Radionuclide concentrations

The concentration of ^{131}I at the hospital sewer $[C_{vol}] = 10 \times 10^9/(100 \times 30) = 3.3 \times 10^6$ Bq m^{-3}
$[C_{wt}] = 3.3 \times 10^3$ Bq kg^{-1}
The concentration of ^{131}I at the sewage works $[C_{vol}] = 10 \times 10^9/(20\,000 \times 30) = 1.7 \times 10^4$ Bq m^{-3}
$[C_{wt}] = 1.7 \times 10^1$ Bq kg^{-1}
The ^{131}I source strength in the sewage pipe $[C_L] = 10 \times 10^9/(30 \times 24 \times 60 \times 60 \times 0.5)$ Bq m^{-1}
$= 7.7 \times 10^3$ Bq m^{-1}
The concentration of ^{131}I in river water $[C_{water}] = 10 \times 10^9/(1\,000\,000 \times 30) = 3.3 \times 10^2$ Bq m^{-3}

Annual effective dose from maintenance of hospital sewer

Substituting in equations (9.1), (9.2), (9.5), and (9.6) from Tables 9.4 and 9.5, the annual effective doses from ingestion (E_{ing}), inhalation (E_{inh}), and external radiation (E_{ext}) are given by

$$E_{ing} = C_{wt}\, I_{ing}\, D_{ing}\, O = (3.3 \times 10^3) \times (5 \times 10^{-5}) \times (2.2 \times 10^{-8}) \times (200)\ \text{Sv} = 7.3 \times 10^{-1}\ \mu\text{Sv}$$
$$E_{inh} = C_{wt}\, I_{inh}\, D_{inh}\, O = (3.3 \times 10^3) \times (1.2 \times 10^{-6}) \times (7.4 \times 10^{-9}) \times (200)\ \text{Sv} = 5.9 \times 10^{-3}\ \mu\text{Sv}$$
$$E_{ext} = C_L\, D_{ext}\, O = (7.7 \times 10^3) \times (3.6 \times 10^{-13} \times 3.8 \times 10^{-1}) \times (200)\ \text{Sv} = 2.1 \times 10^{-3}\ \mu\text{Sv}$$

Thus the predicted annual effective doses from ^{131}I to a worker from maintenance of the hospital sewer is 0.7 μSv.

Annual effective dose to a worker in the sewage works

Substituting in equations (9.1)–(9.4) from Tables 9.4 and 9.5, the annual effective doses are given by

$$E_{ing} = C_{wt}\, I_{ing}\, D_{ing}\, O = (1.7 \times 10^1) \times (5 \times 10^{-5}) \times (2.2 \times 10^{-8}) \times (1000)\ \text{Sv} = 1.9 \times 10^{-2}\ \mu\text{Sv}$$
$$E_{inh} = C_{wt}\, I_{inh}\, D_{inh}\, O = (1.7 \times 10^1) \times (1.2 \times 10^{-7}) \times (7.4 \times 10^{-9}) \times (2000)\ \text{Sv} = 3.0 \times 10^{-5}\ \mu\text{Sv}$$
$$E_{ext} = C_{vol}\, D_{ext}\, O = (1.7 \times 10^4) \times (2.6 \times 10^{-13} \times 3.8 \times 10^{-1}) \times (1000)\ \text{Sv} = 1.7\ \mu\text{Sv}$$

Thus the predicted annual effective dose to a worker in the sewage works is 1.7 μSv.

Exposure of critical group among members of the public

A member of the public may be exposed through consumption of drinking water abstracted downstream of the discharge point (E_{water}) or from consumption of local fish (E_{fish}). The committed effective doses from these activities can be calculated from equations (9.7) and (9.8) using data from Tables 9.4–9.6.

$$E_{water} = C_{water}\, M_{water}\, D_{ing} = (3.3 \times 10^2) \times (0.6) \times (2.2 \times 10^{-8})\ \text{Sv} = 4.4\ \mu\text{Sv}$$
$$E_{fish} = C_{fish}\, M_{fish}\, D_{ing} = (2.0 \times 10^{-2} \times 3.3 \times 10^2) \times (20) \times (2.2 \times 10^{-8})\ \text{Sv} = 2.9\ \mu\text{Sv}$$

A member of the public exposed through both these routes could receive an annual dose of 7.3 μSv from ^{131}I. The total dose received by an individual would be the sum of contributions from all radionuclides discharged.

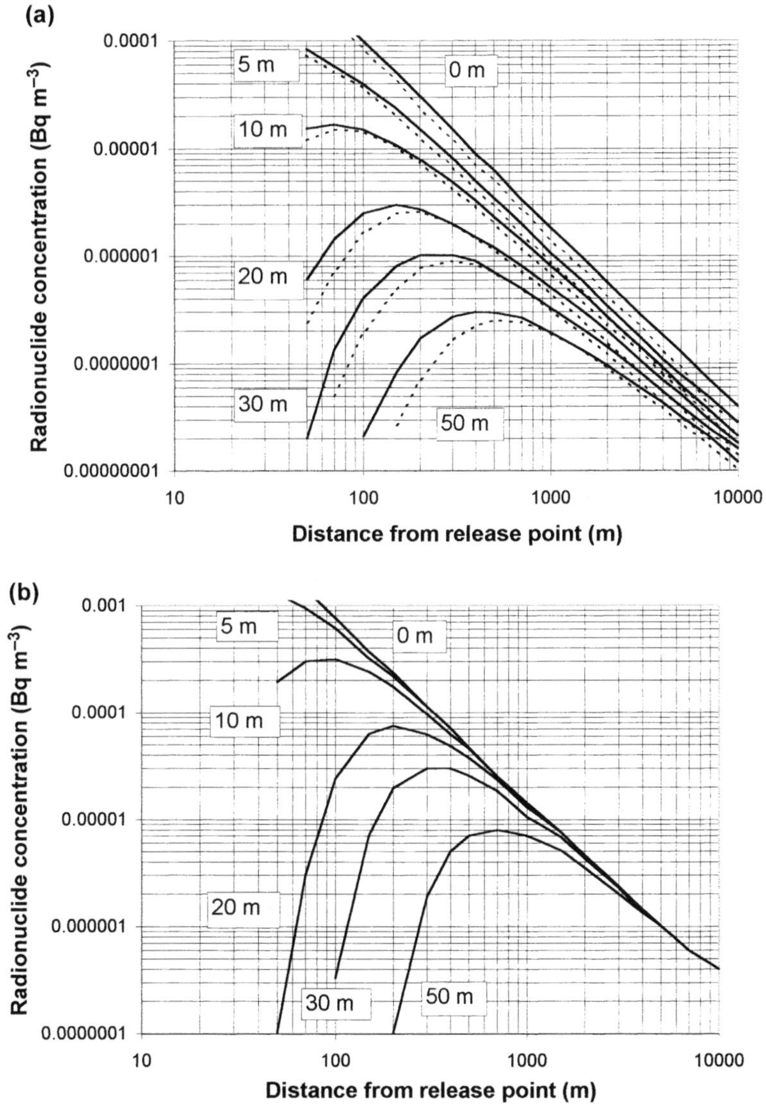

Figure 9.1 Variations in airborne radionuclide concentrations (Bq m^{-3}) per unit release of radioactivity (Bq s^{-1}) from stacks with a range of heights (0–50 m). These represent values of P [Bq m^{-3} (Bq $s^{-1})^{-1}$] for substitution into equation (9.10). Data are shown in (a) for Pasquill D 50% (bold line) and 70% (dashed line) stability (the boundaries of the typical range found in the UK) with a uniform distribution of wind direction and in (b) for Pasquill D with 60% stability downwind with a fixed wind direction over a 30° sector. *Note*: A fixed wind direction can give concentrations 5–50 times greater than a uniform distribution. Data are taken from NRPB reports M744 [13] and R91 [18].

conditions occurring most frequently in the UK fall into the Pasquill D classification. Plume concentrations are affected by the Pasquill stability category. Typical UK values range from 50% inland in south-eastern England, through 60% for inland areas in the remainder of England and Scotland to 70% in coastal regions [18]. The set of curves in Figure 9.1a assumes a uniform distribution of wind directions, which should give a sufficiently accurate result for most hospital assessments. Curves are shown in Figure 9.1b giving downwind values for P for a fixed wind direction. If the prevailing wind blows towards the critical area for exposure, an appropriate value for P would be a mean of the uniform and fixed wind direction values weighted according to the proportion of time the wind blew in the prevailing direction. For a release height of at least 10 m, a

Table 9.7 Factors relating radionuclide concentration to deposition rate (T) [Bq kg^{-1} (Bq m^{-2} s^{-1})$^{-1}$] (eq. 9.13) or air concentration (T^*) [Bq kg^{-1}(Bq m^{-3})$^{-1}$] (eq. 9.14)

	^{3}H [T^*]	^{14}C [T^*]	^{32}P [T]	^{35}S [T]	^{125}I [T]	^{131}I [T]
Cereals	1.3×10^{1}	2.4×10^{3}	1×10^{5}	3.7×10^{5}	3.1×10^{5}	4.2×10^{4}
Green vegetables	1.1×10^{2}	2.7×10^{2}	6.3×10^{4}	1.2×10^{5}	1.0×10^{5}	4.1×10^{5}
Root vegetables	1.0×10^{2}	5.3×10^{2}	3.0×10^{4}	1.2×10^{5}	8.9×10^{3}	1.1×10^{1}
Fruit	1.0×10^{2}	5.3×10^{2}	–	–	–	–
Milk	1.1×10^{2}	2.7×10^{2}	5.0×10^{5}	9.8×10^{5}	1.2×10^{5}	5.8×10^{4}

Data reproduced from McDonnell [13].

conservative concentration at most critical group distances is 10^{-5} Bq m^{-3} for a release rate of 1 Bq s^{-1}.

Plume exposure

Committed effective doses from inhalation (E_{inh}) can be derived from C_{plume} using the equation

$$E_{inh} = C_{plume}\, I_{atmos}\, D_{inh}\, O \qquad (9.11)$$

where I_{atmos} is the rate of intake through inhalation and O is the occupancy.

Effective doses from external exposure can be calculated from the equation

$$E_{ext} = C_{plume}\, D_{cloud}\, O \qquad (9.12)$$

using values for D_{cloud} giving exposure for a semi-infinite cloud for γ-rays or an infinite cloud for skin exposure from β-particles (Table 9.6) [13].

Food uptake

It may also be necessary to take account of uptake of activity in foods grown locally and transfer through the food chain. For most radionuclides, the concentration in produce is related to the rate of deposition through an equation of the form

$$C_{food} = D_{dep}\, T \qquad (9.13)$$

where D_{dep} is the deposition rate for each radionuclide (Bq m^{-2} s^{-1}) and T is a transfer factor (Table 9.7). The deposition rate during dry weather (D_{dry}) is the product of the air concentration C_{plume} and the deposition velocity v_g (Table 9.4). Deposition is enhanced in wet weather and the rate (D_{wet}) at distance d metres from a point of release can be approximated by r_w/d (Table 9.4). If it is assumed that it rains for 10% of the time, then $D_{dep} = D_{dry} + 0.1D_{wet}$. The reader is referred to the NRPB report [13] for a more detailed explanation.

^{14}C and ^{3}H are taken up directly from the air and uptake rates are related to the airborne concentrations through a concentration factor (T^*) (Table 9.7). This can lead to significant concentration levels.

$$C_{food} = C_{plume}\, T^*. \qquad (9.14)$$

The committed effective dose arising from ingestion of foodstuff (E_{ing}) is given by

$$E_{ing} = C_{food}\, M_{food}\, D_{ing} \qquad (9.15)$$

where M_{food} is the rate of intake of the particular food (Table 9.4) and D_{ing} is the committed effective dose per Bq from ingestion (Table 9.5).

If radioactive waste is accumulated in an external store, it may also be necessary to assess the potential exposure which could result from a fire in the store [13]. An example of a dose assessment for release of ^{14}C to the atmosphere is given in Box 9.6.

9.5 Transport of radioactive materials

The risks of accidents occurring or sources being lost are greater during transportation, so stricter controls need to be in place. Recommendations on requirements for transport of radioactive materials have been set out in documentation prepared by the IAEA [19], and these have been incorporated into national legislation [20, 21]. These include requirements for packaging, labelling, documentation, and precautions. In general, transport legislation only applies to radioactive materials with a specific activity greater than 70 kBq kg^{-1} [19, 20]. The containers used for transport are designed so as to minimize the risk of damage to the source, to contain any spillage of radioactive material, and to minimize the radiation exposure of any person handling or coming into contact with the container. Procedures must be in place to reduce the likelihood of anything going wrong and accompanying documentation should provide sufficient information to enable the safe transportation. Finally, each package should be adequately labelled, so that it can be readily identified and anyone who has to deal with it following an accident is made aware of the potential hazards. Most transport of materials from hospital sites is by road, so the majority of this section relates to road transport. Separate legislation covers transport by rail [22], air [23, 24], and sea [25], but requirements relating to package design and transport documentation are

Box 9.6 Environmental impact assessment for incineration of waste containing ^{14}C

A waste disposal contractor is applying to release 20 GBq of ^{14}C per month in the form of CO_2 from incineration. An assessment of the resulting doses to critical groups is required.

Information on discharges and distances to potential critical groups (§9.4.4)

- the height of the release point is 20 m
- the discharge rate is 20 GBq per month
- a potential critical group is located at 150 m, the distance at which the maximum ground level concentration occurs
- local residents grow their own vegetables in an allotment at a distance of 600 m from the release point.

Assuming that Pasquill D conditions with 60% stability apply, air concentrations in the plume at ground level can be derived from equation (9.10) with values for the factor P derived from Figure 9.1a.

At 150 m: $C_{\text{plume}} = RP = [(20 \times 10^9)/(30 \times 24 \times 60 \times 60)] \times (2.7 \times 10^{-6})\ \text{Bq m}^{-3} = 2 \times 10^{-2}\ \text{Bq m}^{-3}$
At 600 m: $C_{\text{plume}} = RP = [(20 \times 10^9)/(30 \times 24 \times 60 \times 60)] \times (1 \times 10^{-6})\ \text{Bq m}^{-3} = 7.7 \times 10^{-3}\ \text{Bq m}^{-3}$

Annual dose from inhalation

Substituting into equation (9.11) from Tables 9.4 and 9.5, the annual effective dose from inhalation (E_{inh}) by a person at 150 m is given by

$E_{\text{inh}} = C_{\text{plume}}\, D_{\text{inh}}\, (I_{\text{atmos}}\, O) = (2 \times 10^{-2}) \times (6.2 \times 10^{-12}) \times (7300)\ \text{Sv} = 9 \times 10^{-4}\ \mu\text{Sv}$

The external dose from ^{14}C is small and can be ignored, but this route should be considered for other radionuclides (Table 9.6).

Annual dose from consumption of vegetables grown 600 m away

The uptake of ^{14}C in produce is proportional to the air concentration (unlike most other radionuclides) and can be derived using equation (9.14) with the factor from Table 9.7

$C_{\text{vegetables}} = C_{\text{plume}}\, T^* = (7.7 \times 10^{-3}) \times (2.7 \times 10^2)\ \text{Bq kg}^{-1} = 2.1\ \text{Bq kg}^{-1}$

The annual committed effective dose from consumption of vegetables grown in the allotment ($E_{\text{vegetables}}$) can be obtained by substituting values from Tables 9.4 and 9.5 in equation (9.15)

$E_{\text{vegetables}} = C_{\text{vegetables}}\, M_{\text{vegetables}}\, D_{\text{ing}} = (2.1) \times (80) \times (5.8 \times 10^{-10})\ \text{Sv} = 0.1\ \mu\text{Sv}$

Note: P at 600 m downwind of the stack with a fixed wind direction is 30 times higher (Figure 9.1b). If the prevailing wind blew in the direction of the allotment for a third of the year, the annual dose from consumption of vegetables from the allotment would be 1 μSv.

similar. Patients who contain radioactive materials are not subject to the requirements of transport regulations but are subject to restriction under ionising radiation regulations (§16.8). Similarly, very low-level waste (Table 9.3) being transported to a refuse disposal site is exempt from the radioactive material transport regulations.

Where radioactive material is moved within a hospital site, the precautions taken must fulfil radiation safety requirements (Chapter 6). The material would normally be held in a container appropriate for the physical and chemical form of the source. The container should incorporate adequate shielding for the carrier, taking into account the distance that the material had to be moved, and be able to withstand minor accidents such as being dropped. Risk assessments relating to foreseeable incidents should be carried out and contingency plans put in place to ensure that appropriate action is initiated promptly and efficiently (§15.11.2). A report on incidents involving the transport of radioactive materials in the UK has been produced by the NRPB [26].

9.5.1 Packaging for radioactive materials

Specifications for packaging required for transport of radioactive materials have been set out by the IAEA [19]. The standard of package required relates to the amount of radioactive material. The package types, in order of increasing activity, are excepted, industrial, type A, and

Table 9.8 Activity limits for excepted packages [19, 21]

Physical state	Package limit
Solid	
special form	10^{-3} A_1
other form	10^{-3} A_2
Liquid	10^{-4} A_2
Gas	
tritium	2×10^{-2} A_2
special form	10^{-3} A_1
other forms	10^{-3} A_2

type B. Hospital users will generally only use excepted packages and type A ones. Industrial packaging relates to applications such as transport of large volumes of low specific activity (LSA) material, while type B packages are utilized by the nuclear industry to transport larger radiation sources and are designed to withstand more severe accidents.

The IAEA has prepared tables giving the maximum activities of different radionuclides which may be transported in a type A package. Two activities are given for each radionuclide, A_1 applies to 'special form' or sealed sources and A_2 to unsealed radionuclides, and values for some radionuclides used in hospitals are given in Table 9.1. If a package contains a mixture of radionuclides, the relevant limit on activity can be determined from a summation of the fractions $\{f(i)\}$ of activity $\{A_n(i)\}$ of each radionuclide (i) in the mixture using the equation

$$A_n = 1/[\textstyle\sum_i\{f(i)/A_n(i)\}]. \qquad (9.16)$$

Requirements for the design of packages include the following:

- the package can be easily and safely handled and transported
- the package can be properly secured during transport
- any lifting attachment should not fail and its removal should not impair the source containment
- the external surface can easily be decontaminated
- the outer layer should prevent collection and retention of water
- the package should be capable of withstanding mechanical impacts and vibration
- other dangerous properties of the contents should be taken into account.

Excepted packages

Excepted packages are used where the level of hazard is low. No indication that a package contains radioactive material is required on the outside of the package, since this may cause unnecessary alarm. However, the word 'Radioactive' must be written inside, so that anyone opening the package is warned of its radioactive contents. Only radioactive materials with activities less than those given in Table 9.8 may be transported in excepted packages. In addition, the dose rate on any external surface must be less than 5 μSv h^{-1} and the level of non-fixed contamination less than 0.4 Bq cm^{-2} for β/γ-emitters and 0.04 Bq cm^{-2} for most α-emitters. Excepted packages must retain their contents under conditions likely to be encountered in routine transport. The criteria for excepted packages containing an instrument or article incorporating a radioactive source are less stringent than for other materials and relevant limits are given in transport regulations [21]. Consignments of radioactive waste transported by road would normally come within the criteria for excepted packages, although careful packing of bins may sometimes be necessary to ensure compliance with the external dose-rate criteria.

Type A packages

The sources that hospitals need to transport should usually fall below the activity levels for type A packages (Table 9.1). The restriction on dose rate at any point on the external surface is 2 mSv h^{-1} and that on non-fixed contamination is 4 Bq cm^{-2} for β/γ-emitters and 0.4 Bq cm^{-2} for most α-emitters. Additional requirements for type A packages include:

- external dimensions should not be less than 10 cm
- a seal or other feature should be incorporated to show that the package has not been opened
- the design should take account of possible degradation from exposure to a wide range of temperatures and pressures
- there should be a securely fastened containment system which cannot be opened unintentionally.

For transport of liquid radioactive materials:

- the amount of liquid in the vessel and ullage should be chosen to take account of variations in temperature of contents, dynamic effects, and fluid dynamics
- the package should contain material able to absorb double the volume of liquid contents
- a secondary containment system should retain the liquid contents if the primary container leaks.

Type A packages must be able to retain their radioactive contents and maintain the integrity of their shielding (external dose rate should not increase by more than 20%) in an accident. A series of tests must be carried out to confirm that the design is adequate, for which detailed specifications are given in regulations [21]. These include:

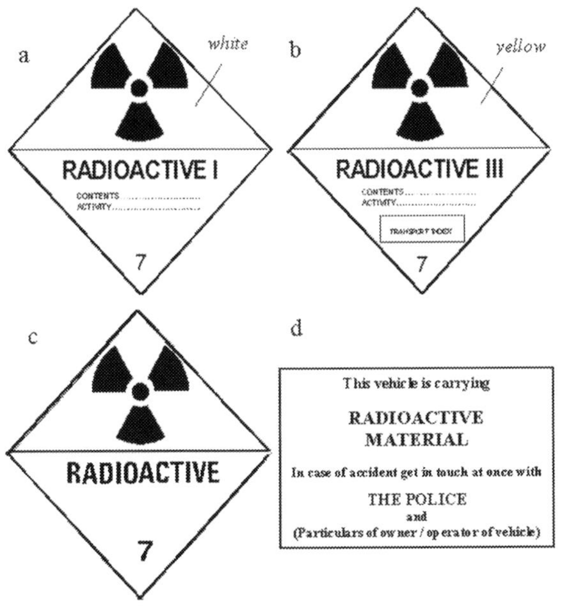

Figure 9.2 Labels used in transport of radioactive materials: (a) label for Category I package; (b) label for Category III package; (c) notice to be affixed to outside of vehicle transporting radioactive material; (d) notice for display inside driver's cab.

- water spray test (1 h)
- free drop test (up to 1.2 m)
- stacking test (compressive load for 24 h)
- penetration test (1 m drop onto weakest point).

Packaging for liquids requires additional strength, such that they will withstand a 9 m free drop and a 1.7 m drop penetration test.

It may be possible to reuse packaging in which radioactive material has been delivered from a reliable manufacturer. However, care must be taken to ensure that the packaging is undamaged and that all components, including polystyrene inserts and absorbent material, are retained or replaced. The packages must be inspected and tested periodically to ensure that their construction remains satisfactory.

9.5.2 Labelling and documentation

Labelling

The inner containers of any radioactive package such as, for nuclear medicine radiopharmaceuticals, the glass vial, the lead pot, and the sealed tin should all be labelled clearly with the word 'radioactive', the radiation trefoil, the radionuclide, its activity at a reference time, and the chemical form. This is important for avoiding misidentification of a vial at the point of delivery as well as providing information on the material during transport.

Table 9.9 Categories of radioactive packages [19, 21]

Transport index	Maximum surface dose rate (mSv h^{-1})	Category
0	0 – 0.005	I White
>0 – 1	>0.005 – 0.5	II Yellow
>1 – 10	>0.5 – 2	III Yellow
>10	>2 – 10	III Yellow (vehicle under exclusive use)

The outside of type A packages must be marked as 'Type A'. There is an internationally recognized system of labelling for radioactive packages (Figure 9.2a and b), with a classification I (white), II and III (yellow) relating to the external hazard. This is based on a measurement of the maximum radiation dose rate in air at 1 m from the external surface of the package (Table 9.9). The label for all type A packages must include the radionuclide and activity and categories II and III must also include a quantity known as the 'Transport Index', which is the dose rate at 1 m measured in μSv h^{-1} and divided by 10 (it was originally derived from the dose rate measured in mrem h^{-1}). The transport index should be rounded to the first decimal place and any values less than 0.05 taken as zero. The package must also have an identification mark and serial number.

Documentation

The person or organization consigning a package containing radioactive materials for transport to another hospital must ensure that the containment, packaging, and labelling are adequate and must complete a consignor's certificate to accompany the package (Box 9.7) [21]. They must also give the carrier a document setting out actions that need to be taken, including restrictions and emergency arrangements. The transport documents must be kept on the vehicle until the packages are delivered. Thereafter consignment certificates must be retained for a period of 2 years. Where radioactive materials are imported, additional forms relating to shipment of sources must be completed, which may be obtained from the Environment Agency.

9.5.3 Transport of packages

The majority of packages containing radioactivity are transported by road and this section deals primarily with the regulations covering this form of transportation. Separate regulations cover other modes of transport. There is not sufficient space to discuss these here and the reader is referred to relevant recommendations and legislation [22–25]. Basic requirements must be fulfilled, such as that packages must be securely stowed during transit. Packages of radioactive material must be

Box 9.7 Consignment certificates

The certificate for a type A package must include all the items listed below and those marked with an asterisk must be included in the certificate for an excepted package.

- Title of transport regulations
- Name, address, and telephone number of consignor (for contact in the event of an accident)*
- Name and address of consignee*
- Proper shipping name (see Table)*
- United Nations (UN) Class Number '7'
- Words 'RADIOACTIVE MATERIAL'
- UN number for material in package (see Table)*
- Name and symbol of each radionuclide
- Description of physical and chemical form
- Maximum activity of radioactive contents in Bq
- Category of package I—WHITE, II—YELLOW, or III—YELLOW
- Transport Index for categories II and III
- Identification mark for every competent authority approval certificate for material, package, etc.
- Declaration about accuracy of description of package contents, signed and dated by consignor.

UN number (IAEA 96) [19,21]	UN number (ADR 2001) [31]	Proper shipping name
		Radioactive material, except package
2910	2908	• Empty packaging
2975–2981	2909	• Articles manufactured from natural uranium, depleted uranium or natural thorium
2910	2910	• Limited quantity of material
2910	2911	• Instruments or articles
2912	2912, 3321 or 3322	Radioactive material, low specific activity (LSA I, II or III)
2913	2913	Surface contaminated objects (SCO I or II)
	2915	Radioactive material, type A package
2974	3332	Radioactive material, type A package, special form
2982		Radioactive material (not otherwise specified)

separated from any consignments of undeveloped photographic film to ensure that the dose to the film during transit is less than 0.1 mSv. Packages must be stowed so that the dose rate at any point on the external surface of the vehicle does not exceed 2 mSv h^{-1} and that at 2 m from the vehicle is less than 0.1 mSv h^{-1}.

The driver of any road vehicle has responsibility for the security of the vehicle and must ensure that no radioactive material is removed during transport. The driver should not leave the vehicle unattended in a place with public access while it has radioactive materials on board and must follow certain restrictions on parking in public places [21]. Anyone else travelling in a vehicle transporting radioactive material must have the permission of the carrier and travel in a personnel compartment separate from that in which the radioactive material is transported. Analogous requirements apply to transport by rail [22], where type A packages must be carried in the guard's van at least 1.5 m from passenger compartments and a restriction of 1.5 is placed on the transport index.

Certain requirements are relaxed for consignments containing smaller amounts of radioactivity where the following 'small load' conditions apply:

- transportation is in a car or small van
- less than 10 type A packages are transported
- the sum of the transport indices is less than 3.

A road vehicle transporting type A packages should display signs of the form shown in Figure 9.2c on the sides and rear and have a fire-proof notice fixed inside the vehicle cab of the form shown in Figure 9.2d. If the small-load conditions are met, then the vehicle need only display external signs (Figure 9.2c) measuring 150 mm × 150 mm. However, if the radioactive content or the vehicle is larger, three signs measuring 250 mm × 250 mm will be required.

Driver training

Any driver involved in the transport of radioactive materials other than solely excepted packages must have received appropriate training to ensure that they are aware of all necessary precautions that should be taken and are able to deal effectively with any incidents that may occur [27]. This training would have both theoretical and practical components and would include:

- the nature of the hazard posed by the radioactive material
- general requirements for carriage of dangerous goods
- preventative and safety measures
- precautions during loading and unloading
- what to do in the event of an accident
- environmental protection and control measures.

If the last two of the small-load conditions are met, the employer can provide the training and issue the certificate in the UK, but for transport of larger loads, a driver must have a national vocational training certificate. The driver should notify the police and the consignor of any loss or damage to a package during transport.

Quality assurance

Hospitals should have a documented organizational structure relating to the transport arrangements to enable the system to operate smoothly even when there are changes in staff. Transport regulations require quality assurance programmes to be in place for all aspects of transport, including packaging, documentation, use, maintenance, and in-transit storage, for which results should be documented. A qualified Dangerous Goods Safety Adviser [28] must be appointed to advise on general matters relating to transport of dangerous goods and carry out an annual audit of procedures if radioactive packages are transported regularly or the last two of the small-load conditions referred to above are exceeded.

9.5.4 Changes in transport legislation

Since the preparation of this text, a restructuring ADR has been published which is a European Agreement concerning the International Carriage of Dangerous Goods by Road [31]. This incorporates revised activity limites A_1 and A_2 for transport of radionuclides (Table 9.1) and revised United Nations numbers and proper shipping names for types of radioactive material (Box 9.7). The ADR also requires the appropriate UN number to be displayed on the outside of excepted packages. The new requirements are likely to be incorporated in revised UK legistation to come into force in 2003.

9.6 Medical administration of radioactive substances

Safeguards relating to the administration of radioactive materials to patients are required to provide protection for patients and for volunteers participating in medical research. Before any medical or dental practitioner may prescribe the administration of radioactive material to a patient for diagnosis or therapy, he/she must have received adequate training and have been granted a licence for the particular procedure. In therapy, the licence also applies to solid sources introduced into the body or body cavities or applied to the surface and the applicant must demonstrate extensive training, significant experience, and a high level of competence before a certificate would be granted. In the UK, the licence is in the form of a certificate issued under the Medical Administration of Radioactive Substances (MARS) Regulations [29]. The process of approval and certification is controlled by the Administration of Radioactive Substances Committee (ARSAC) which issues guidance on methodology, approved tests, and radiopharmaceutical activity levels [30].

9.6.1 Licensing of medical practitioners

Normally, licences or certificates to carry out procedures using radioactive materials will only be given to more senior clinicians, who wish to administer radioactive medicinal products on a regular basis. The licence is specific to one site and any procedure to be carried out must be applied for and listed on the certificate. Certificates for established procedures for diagnosis and treatment are granted for a period of 5 years, while those for research, where there is no direct benefit to the person to whom the activity is administered, are for 2 years. Details of the equipment and facilities must be given by the scientist responsible for the scientific support, normally the local Medical Physics Expert in nuclear medicine (or radiotherapy) and they and the scientist responsible for provision of the radioactive medicinal products must indicate that they are satisfied with the facilities and arrangements. The Radiation Protection Adviser (RPA) must sign to indicate that he/she is satisfied with the arrangements for radiation safety at the hospital. This would require inspection of the facilities and checking safety arrangements in detail for a new location, as well as assessing that limits on holdings in the hospital registration and disposal limits in the authorization are adequate for the tests applied for.

Occasionally, if for clinical reasons a certificate holder wishes to administer radiopharmaceuticals in different premises, he/she can do so with the agreement of the RPA, after ensuring that the conditions, staff, and facilities are adequate. However, if the alternative arrangement is to be a regular practice, approval must be obtained from ARSAC. There is also a mechanism for a certificate holder to obtain a particular patient request from ARSAC, where a procedure which is not included on the practitioner's certificate is required. However, in most hospitals the nuclear medicine clinicians will apply for a certificate to cover the full range of practices that they consider may be needed.

Ideally, two clinicians holding certificates for the same procedure at an establishment should be sufficient to provide a continuous service under all eventualities, including long-term absence of one certificate holder. Where there is a single certificate holder, administration of medicinal products can continue during periods when the certificate holder is temporarily absent, but in the case of a long absence, the employer must make alternative arrangements if administration of radioactive medicinal products is to continue.

9.6.2 Licences for research applications

ARSAC certificates must be obtained for all research projects which result in radiation exposure to subjects additional to that involved in their routine diagnostic or therapeutic management. This includes:

- all clinical trials
- administration of radioactive medicinal products where the subject is not expected to benefit from the test (i.e. non-therapeutic research and healthy volunteer trials)
- additional radiation exposure above that incurred in routine management of the patient.

However, research using a new or unestablished procedure intended to benefit a single patient would be considered under the category of diagnosis or treatment.

Every clinical research investigation involving the use of radioactive medicinal products should be checked and approved by the local research ethics committee and the procedures that should be followed are set out in Box 11.3.

9.7 References

1 International Atomic Energy Agency (1996). *International basic safety standards for protection against ionising radiation and for the safety of radiation sources.* Safety Series No. 115. IAEA, Vienna.

2 International Atomic Energy Agency (1995). *The principles of waste management.* Safety Series No. 111-F. IAEA, Vienna.

3 International Commission on Radiological Protection (1997). *Radiological protection policy for the disposal of radioactive waste.* ICRP Publication 77. Elsevier Science.

4 Radioactive Substances Act (1993). HMSO, London.

5 International Atomic Energy Agency (1988). *Principles for the exemption of radiation sources and practices from regulatory control.* IAEA Safety Guides No. 89. IAEA, Vienna.

6 The Radioactive Substances (Testing Instrument) Exemption Order (1985). SI No. 1049. HMSO, London.

7 The Radioactive Substances (Hospitals) Exemption Order (1990) (SI No. 2512) and Amendment (1995) (SI No. 2395). HMSO, London.

8 The Radioactive Substances (Substances of Low Activity) Exemption Order (1986). SI No. 1002. HMSO, London.

9 Ionising Radiations Regulations (1999). SI No. 3232. HSE, London.

10 Special Waste Regulations (as amended) (1996). SI No. 972. HMSO, London.

11 Kaye, G. I., Weber, P. B., Evans, A., and Venezia, R. A. (1998). Efficacy of alkaline hydrolysis as an alternative method for treatment and disposal of infectious animal waste. *Contemp. Top. Anim. Sci.*, **37**, 43–6.

12 International Commission on Radiological Protection (1987). *Radiation doses to patients from radiopharmaceuticals.* ICRP Publication 53. Pergamon, Oxford.

13 McDonnell, C. E. (1996) *Assessment of the radiological consequences of accumulation and disposal of radioactive wastes by small users of radioactive materials.* NRPB-M744. NRPB, Chilton.

14 International Commission on Radiological Protection (1985). *Principles of monitoring for the radiation protection of the population.* ICRP Publication 43. Pergamon, Oxford.

15 International Commission on Radiological Protection (1995). *Age dependent doses to members of the public from intake of radionuclides. Part 4. Inhalation dose coefficients.* ICRP Publication 71. Pergamon, Oxford.

16 International Commission on Radiological Protection (1996). *Age dependent doses to members of the public from intake of radionuclides. Part 5. Compilation of ingestion and inhalation dose coefficients.* ICRP Publication 72. Pergamon, Oxford.

17 International Commission on Radiological Protection (1983). *Radionuclide transformations: energy and intensity of emissions.* ICRP Publication 38. Pergamon, Oxford.

18 Clarke, R. H. (1979). *A model for short and medium range dispersion of radionuclides released to the atmosphere.* NRPB-R91. NRPB, Chilton.

19 International Atomic Energy Agency (1996). *Regulations for the safe transport of radioactive materials.* IAEA Safety Series No. 6 (1996 revision). IAEA, Vienna.

20 Radioactive Material (Road Transport) Act (1991). HMSO, London.

21 The Radioactive Materials (Road Transport) (Great Britain) Regulations (1996). SI No. 1350. HMSO, London.

22 Packaging, Labelling and Carriage of Radioactive Materials by Rail Regulations (1996). SI 2090. HMSO, London.

23 International Civil Aviation Organization (1998). *Instruction for the safe transport of dangerous goods by air.* ICAO.

24 International Air Transport Association (1997). *Dangerous goods regulations.* IATA.

25 International Maritime Organization (1994). *International maritime dangerous goods code.* IMO.

26 Hughes, J. S. and Shaw, K. B. (1996). *Accidents and incidents involving the transport of radioactive materials in the UK from 1958 to 1994 and their radiological consequences.* NRPB Report R282.

27 The Carriage of Goods by Road (Driver Training) Regulations (1996). SI No. 2094. HMSO, London.

28 The Transport of Dangerous Goods (Safety Advisers) Regulations (1999). SI No. 257. HMSO, London.

29 The Medicines (Administration of Radioactive Substances) Regulations (1978). SI No. 1006 and Amendment (1995). HMSO, London.

30 Administration of Radioactive Substances Advisory Committee (1998). *Notes for guidance on the clinical administration of radiopharmaceuticals and use of sealed radioactive sources.* Department of Health, London.

31 Economic Commision for Europe (2001). ADR European Agreement concerning the international carriage of dangerous goods by road. Volumes I & II. United Nations, New York.

Chapter 10

Intervention, incidents, and emergencies

A. R. Denman

10.1 Introduction

This chapter gives an overview of radiation sources outside healthcare and intervention, incidents, and emergencies with which a medical physicist might be involved. Natural sources contribute most of the dose received by the general public and are considered first. Radon, which gives the most significant dose, will be dealt with in more depth. Applications of artificial radioactive sources in industry are described, together with the potential for incidents which could lead to exposure of the public. Finally, the chapter considers emergency plans for dealing with radiation accidents, limiting exposure of the public, and treatment of radiation casualties. Medical physicists may be involved in providing assistance when an incident occurs. Situations where intervention may be appropriate, such as modifications to buildings to reduce radon levels, or recommendations relating to sheltering or evacuation of the public following a major release of radioactive material are considered. Here the dose saving from the intervention must be justified in social and economic terms.

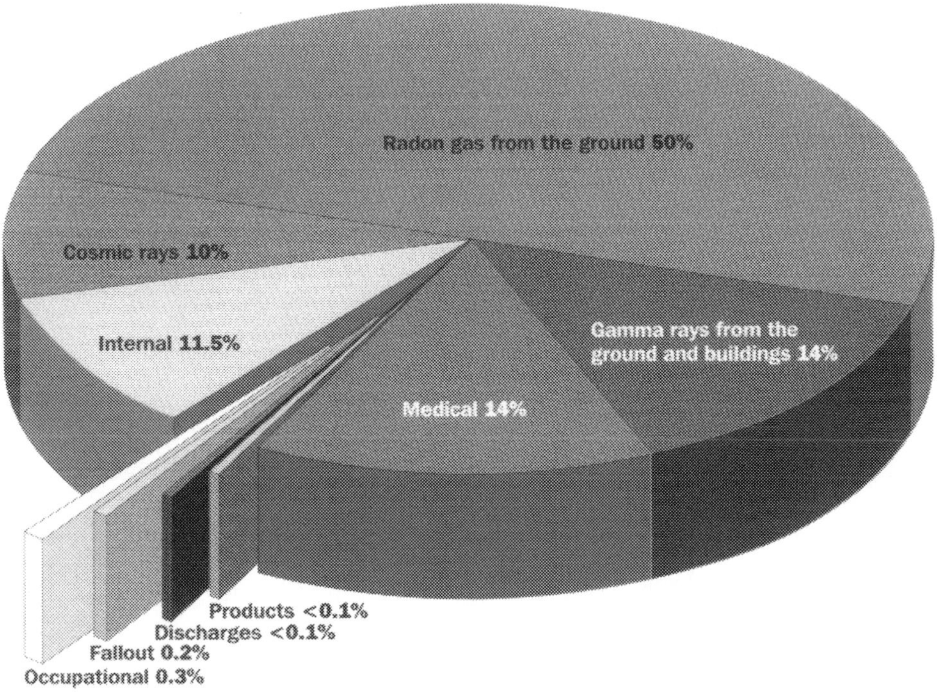

Figure 10.1 Contributions to the average radiation dose to the general public in the UK. Reproduced with permission from NRPB.

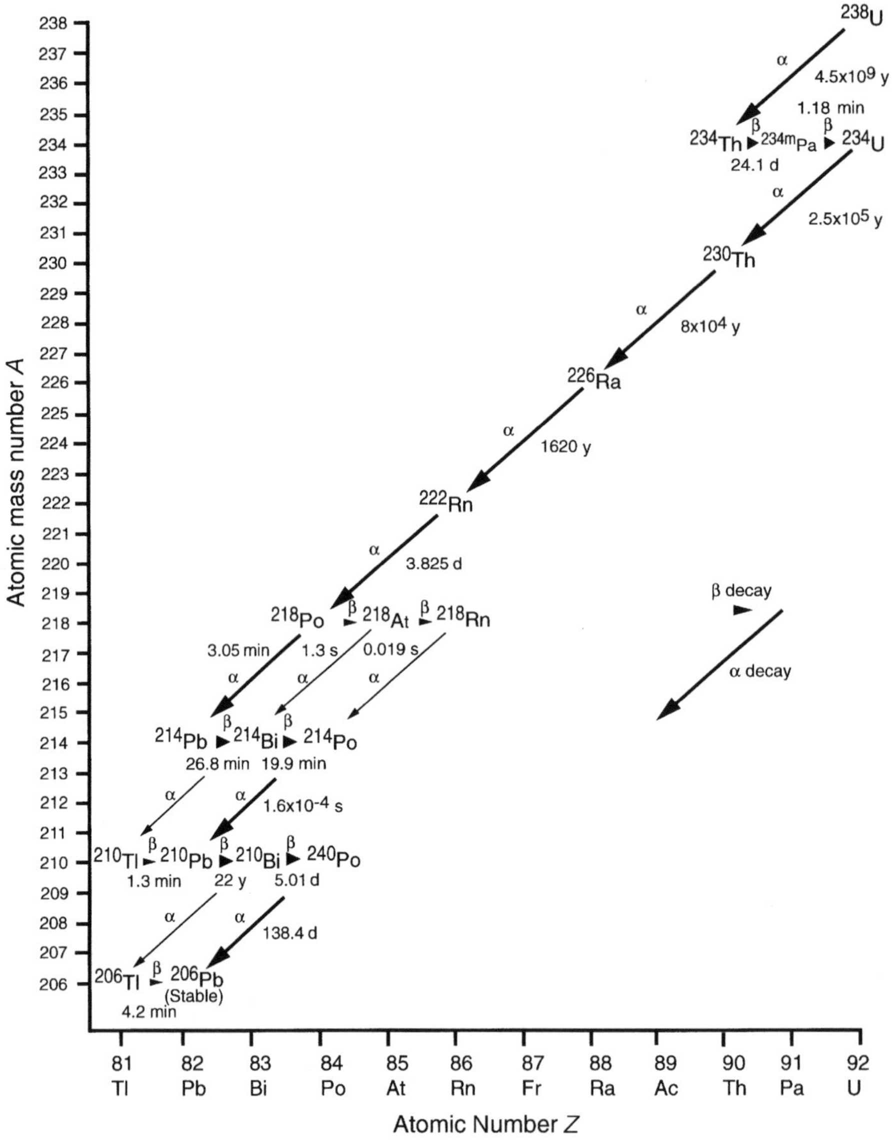

Figure 10.2 Uranium-238 decay series.

10.2 Natural background radiation

10.2.1 Terrestrial sources

Everyone receives a dose from background radiation, which is made up of doses primarily from natural sources (Figure 10.1). The dose amounts to 2.6 mSv per year on average in the UK [1]. Twelve per cent of the radiation dose is from man-made sources and the majority of this is from medical uses of radiation. Fifty per cent of the average background dose in the UK is from radon gas.

Natural radionuclides in rocks and soil were formed in supernovae before the earth was created. There are still significant quantities present, because certain radionuclides have long half-lives. For example ^{238}U has a half-life of 4.5×10^9 years, it decays by α-emission to ^{234}Th and then undergoes a further 13 disintegrations before eventually being transformed to the stable nuclide ^{206}Pb (Figure 10.2). When an atom undergoes a succession of radioactive disintegrations in this way, each generating another radioactive atom, the chain of disintegrations is called a *radioactive series*.

Box 10.1 Radioactive equilibrium

If a radionuclide with a long half-life has a daughter with a shorter half-life, then, after a certain time, the number of daughter atoms produced by decay of the parent will match the number of parent atoms decaying. Thus the number of daughter atoms present in the sample reaches a constant value, which is determined by the relative half-lives of parent and daughter and the initial activity of the parent. This state, known as radioactive equilibrium, occurs in the natural radioactive series and for many man-made radionuclides.

If $A \overset{\lambda_A}{\rightarrow} B \overset{\lambda_B}{\rightarrow} C$

When radioactive equilibrium is reached (from equation 2.4):

$$\frac{dN_A}{dt} = \frac{dN_B}{dt} \quad \text{or} \quad \lambda_A N_A = \lambda_B N_B$$

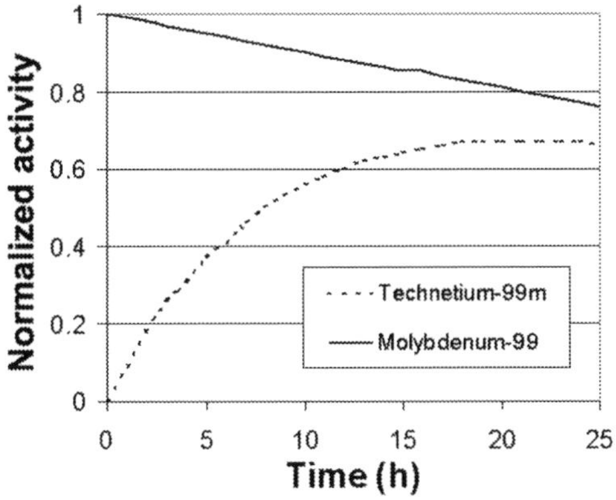

Figure B10.1 Radiation equilibrium. Example of growth of daughter radionuclide ^{99m}Tc (half-life 6 h) reaching radioactive equilibrium with parent ^{99}Mo.

The decay rates of parent and daughter are equal. The time to reach equilibrium is also a function of the relative half-lives of the two radionuclides. If the daughter half-life is greater than that of the parent, equilibrium will never be reached. ^{99m}Tc (half-life 6 h) comes into equilibrium with its parent radionuclide ^{99}Mo (half-life 2.5 days) within 2 days.

There are three naturally occurring series of radionuclides, called the uranium (^{238}U), thorium (^{232}Th), and actinium (^{235}U) series. The first member of each series has a half-life of the order of several thousands of millions of years, long enough for a significant proportion of the radionuclide present when the earth was formed to be still present. The final end-product from each series is a stable isotope of lead. The first long-lived member of each series is termed the *parent* and the radionuclides formed by the succession of disintegrations are called the *daughters* or *progeny* (see Box 10.1).

Several other radionuclides with lower atomic numbers are found in nature. ^{40}K, which has a half-life of 1.25×10^9 years, decays straight to a stable form (^{40}Ar). The isotopic abundance is 0.012% and the human body contains 0.03 g of ^{40}K, the highest activity of any radionuclide present. ^{14}C has a much shorter half-life of 5568 years, but the levels are constantly renewed by the nuclear transformation of ^{14}N induced by cosmic ray bombardment. This process maintains the level of ^{14}C in the atmosphere at roughly the same level. The carbon which forms living matter contains a similar proportion of ^{14}C, but when living matter dies, this gradually decays. The amount of ^{14}C can be used to date ancient artefacts.

10.2.2 Cosmic radiation

Atomic nuclei with energies up to 10^{20} eV from space are incident on the earth's outer atmosphere where they interact with air molecules to produce a mixture of particle and γ-radiation. At the earth's surface, the general public receive 0.24 mSv on average each year from cosmic radiation and 50% of this dose is from neutrons. Doses are much greater at high altitudes, so, for example, a flight from London to New York cruising at 35 000 feet would give a dose of 25–35 μSv. High-flying aircraft, such as Concorde, can be exposed to short bursts of radiation from solar flares, with an average dose rate of 10–15 μSv h^{-1}. Aircrew on long-haul routes receive 4–6 mSv annually and must be considered as radiation workers [1].

10.3 Radon

10.3.1 Introduction

The uranium decay series includes radon-222, which is a gas (Figure 10.2 and Box 10.2). If radon or its progeny decay while in the lungs, they will deliver a radiation dose from α- or β-particles. Radon progeny, rather than radon itself, deliver the greater dose to the respiratory tract. Radon gas in buildings delivers the largest component of the radiation dose to the population and raised levels in mines are linked to lung cancer in miners (Box 10.3).

Box 10.2 Radon

Radon is a colourless, odourless, and tasteless gas from Group 0 of the periodic table and has a density of 9.25 kg m^{-3}. The most abundant isotope is ^{222}Rn, which is part of the ^{238}U decay series (Figure 10.2), and is formed by the decay of ^{226}Ra. ^{222}Rn has a half-life of 3.8 days, and emits 5.5 MeV α-particles. The most significant of the progeny in health terms are ^{214}Po (half-life 1.6×10^{-4} s, 7.7 MeV α-particles) and ^{218}Po (half-life 3.05 min, 6 MeV α-particles).

Another isotope, sometimes called thoron (^{220}Rn), is found in the natural environment with a concentration about one-tenth of that from ^{222}Rn. It is part of the ^{232}Th decay series. It has a half-life of 54.5 s, and emits 6.8 MeVα-particles, decays to ^{216}Po (half-life 0.158 s, 6.7 MeV α-particles) and later ^{212}Po (half-life 3.7×10^{-7} s, 8.8 MeV α-particles).

10.3.2 Environmental influences

Radon is given off by soil where the underlying geology has high levels of the uranium decay series [2]. Radon is dissipated rapidly in outdoor air so that levels are on average around 4 Bq m^{-3}. However, it is concentrated in buildings so that in the UK, high radon levels would be expected above the granite in Cornwall, Devon, and Aberdeen. However, this is an oversimplification because the radon gas has to reach the surface layers of soil within a few half-lives to produce a significant concentration.

Radon gas rapidly reaches the surface through fissures, but is impeded by solid rock, which may include many granites and water-logged clay soils. Thus the phosphate nodules found at the base of the Northampton Sand Layer in the middle of England have only a moderate uranium content but there are significant radon levels at the surface because of the permeability of this soil, while radon levels around Aberdeen are low despite the far higher uranium content of the granite rock. Radon levels in Cornwall and Devon where the rock is fractured are the highest in the UK. The distribution of average indoor radon levels in parts of Europe is shown in Figure 10.3.

Box 10.3 Health risks from radon

Evidence shows that excessive levels of radon in mines cause lung cancer in miners. In 11 studies involving over 50 000 miners, 2299 lung cancer deaths were observed where 686 would be expected [4]. More recent studies have confirmed that the risk is related to the average radon level and the length of exposure, with a latency period of at least 15 years before lung cancers arise. Evidence also suggests that there is a multiplicative interaction between smoking and radon exposure [5, 6].

If lung cancer induction follows the linear no-threshold pattern there is a likelihood of a significant number of lung cancer cases among the general public even at moderate radon levels found in most houses. However, large numbers of cases are required to disentangle the effects of differing smoking habits. There have been a number of epidemiological studies of radon exposures in the home, some of which have not been able to demonstrate an increased risk of lung cancer. However, recently more detailed studies have demonstrated a risk in line with the miners' results [7, 8]. Between 15,000 and 22,000 lung cancer deaths each year in the USA may be radon-related [6].

A few researchers consider that the risk from radon in the home is either less than predicted by the linear no-threshold model or non-existent, due to a threshold. Cohen [9] has shown that in a number of counties in the USA, lung cancer incidence goes down as radon levels increase, although many researchers have criticized aspects of Cohen's work [10]. Bogen [11] suggests that Cohen's data are compatible with a two-stage cancer induction model.

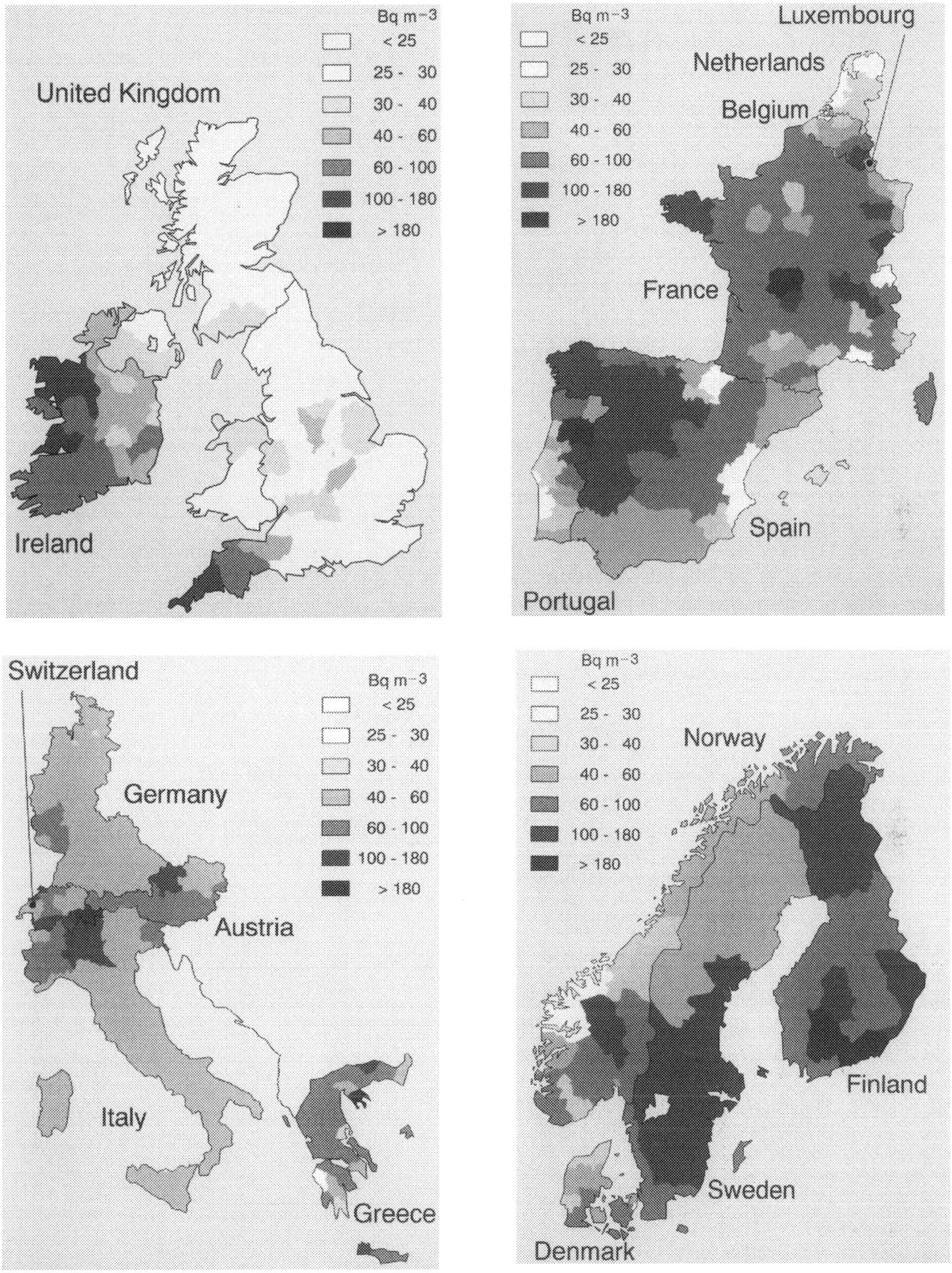

Figure 10.3 Average indoor radon levels in some European countries. Reproduced with permission from NRPB.

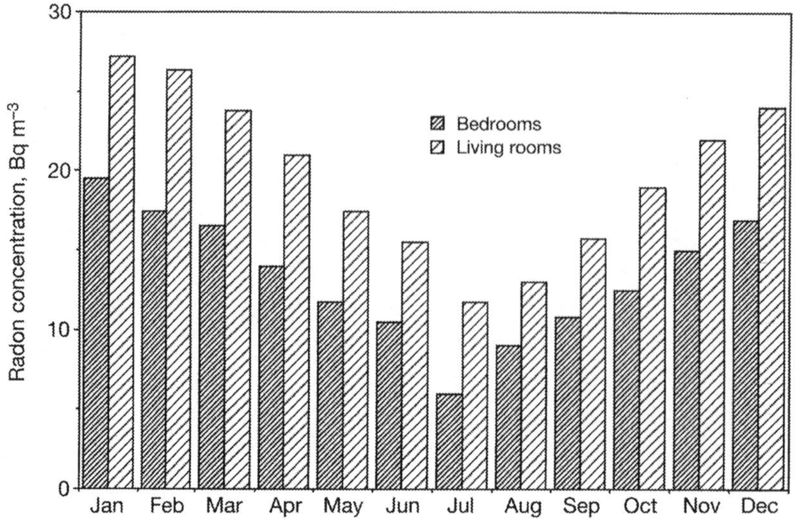

Figure 10.4 Seasonal variations in radon levels in houses. Reproduced with permission from *The Radon Manual* [15].

The average radon concentration in domestic homes in the UK is 20 Bq m^{-3}, although levels in individual houses can occasionally exceed 10 000 Bq m^{-3} [3]. Radon levels for a large number of houses in one area follow a log normal distribution. Pressure tends to be lower inside buildings and this draws radon from underlying soil. The pressure difference results from the higher indoor temperature which reduces indoor air density causing it to rise (*stack effect*). In addition, wind blows across chimneys, windows, and other gaps, and creates under-pressure (*Bernoulli effect*). Buildings may contain and concentrate the radon sufficiently to cause a health risk. Radon levels are much higher in winter, when windows are closed more often and there is a greater temperature difference between the inside and outside (Figure 10.4). Radon enters buildings in a number of ways. Concrete floors have cracks both around the edges and where pipes pass through. In homes with suspended timber floors the gaps between floorboards are the major route of entry (see Figure 10.5). Although the most widespread source of radon in buildings is from underlying soil, building materials with a high uranium decay series content may also contribute, particularly where rock has been used as a filler in wall construction.

Radon is soluble in water, especially at lower temperature, and can be transported for considerable distances dissolved in underground streams. The solubility drops as the temperature rises, and the air-to-water partition coefficient is low, so radon will readily leave water to enter air. Water from reservoirs will therefore be low in radon but water taken directly from wells can have substantial radon levels. This has implications for workers in the water and telephone industries.

10.3.3 Measurement techniques

The only way of identifying a building with raised radon levels is by measurement. There are a number of different ways of measuring radon and its progeny, all of which depend on the detection of α-particles (Box 10.4). Radon can be distinguished from the progeny either by energy discrimination or by filtration.

The simplest device is the etched track detector, which consists of a plastic sheet, usually CR-39 (polyallyl diglycol carbonate). An α-particle leaves a minute scratch when it is incident on the plastic, and this can be enhanced at the end of the exposure by immersion in caustic soda. The plastic is housed in a tight-fitting container with a gap between sections of less than 0.1 mm which permits only radon gas to enter. Detectors may be used to monitor an area or worn as personal dosemeters. The tracks can be viewed under a microscope and counted to give a measure of exposure. Counting is done automatically by pattern recognition computers. Detectors should be left in position for 3 months to obtain statistically valid readings at levels found in buildings. The detectors have a minimum detection limit of 10 kBq m^{-3} h and saturate at 2500 kBq m^{-3} h, which are equivalent to 4 and 1200 Bq m^{-3}, respectively, for a 3-month measurement.

A variety of other techniques are used for radon measurement over shorter periods. These include ionisation chamber systems, where the radon gas can enter the chamber, and semiconductor diodes and scintillation detectors which are used to count decay of progeny trapped in paper filters through which air from the room to be tested has been pumped.

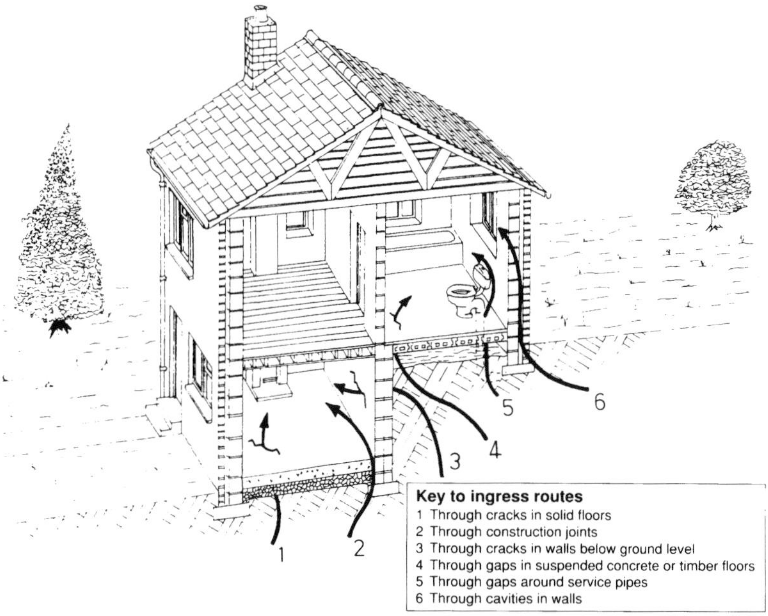

Figure 10.5 Where radon enters a home. Reproduced with permission from the Building Research Establishment.

Box 10.4 Radon measurement quantities

Radon gas and its progeny can be measured as activity concentration in air in Bq m^{-3} (1 pCi L^{-1} = 37 Bq m^{-3}). They emit α-particles with a range of energies and the concentration of radon decay products in air is known as the *potential α-energy concentration* (PAEC). The unit of PAEC is the *working level*, defined as any combination of short-lived decay products that results in the emission of 1.3×10^5 MeV in a litre of air or 2.08×10^{-5} J m^{-3} [12]. The time integral of PAEC gives a measure of exposure, with *1 working level month* being received from 1 working level experienced over 170 hours of a working month.

The degree of equilibrium that radon gas achieves with its airborne progeny in the measurement environment is variable. In an idealized model, where ^{222}Rn is in equilibrium with its progeny, the activity of radon is equal to that of each daughter product and the *equilibrium factor* (*F*), defined as the ratio of the activity of the radon progeny to that of radon gas, is equal to 1.0. However, in a real system, true equilibrium is never reached, as the radon progeny quickly become attached to aerosol particles, which then deposit on surfaces. Factors such as smoking affect the ratio of unattached to attached fractions, and the room volume to surface area ratio affects the equilibrium factor. In domestic properties and the overground workplace, the average value is around 0.5, with a range 0.4 to 0.6. However, in air-conditioned rooms such as hospital operating theatres the equilibrium factor is significantly reduced.

The *equilibrium equivalent radon concentration* is the activity of radon gas which, in equilibrium with its decay products, would give the same PAEC as the measured sample. This will be equal to the actual radon gas concentration multiplied by the equilibrium factor. Assuming an equilibrium factor of 0.5, a working level of 0.03 corresponds to an equilibrium equivalent radon concentration of 112 Bq m^{-3}, and an actual radon concentration of 225 Bq m^{-3}. Extreme care must be taken when using these units and applying them to intermittent occupancy, such as the occupation of offices by staff during the day-time when radon levels are usually at their lowest.

10.3.4 Radon action levels

In Europe employers are required to reduce radon levels in the workplace below an action level set at 400 Bq m^{-3} or restrict access by creating controlled areas. In the UK the levels are applied to concentrations averaged over the whole day, whereas in some European countries they are only applied to the working day. This has implications because radon levels in buildings vary during the day and are normally higher at night. Lower action levels are required in the home to account for this variation and greater occupancy. At present in the UK, the action level is 200 Bq m^{-3}, above which the householder is advised to take remedial measures.

The IAEA suggests the declaration of radon affected areas where 1% of houses are above the radon action level in homes. This has resulted in NRPB declaring a number of affected areas in the UK—including Devon, Cornwall, Somerset, Northamptonshire, Derbyshire, and parts of Scotland, Wales, and Northern Ireland.

In the UK, employers in radon affected areas are required to carry out radon surveys of the workplace (Box 10.5) to assess the risk under the Management of Health and Safety Regulations [13]. The radiation dose to health service workers in radon affected areas can be far higher than doses from working with diagnostic and therapeutic radiation. The use of a 400 Bq m^{-3} workplace action level ensures that 75% of staff receive less than 6 mSv per year [14]. Someone living in a house at the domestic action level of 200 Bq m^{-3} would receive an annual dose of about 10 mSv, with critical groups receiving up to 16 mSv. The UK has one of the lowest average radon levels in Europe (Figure 10.3). Average domestic radon levels, together with national action levels for other countries, are summarized in Table 10.1.

Table 10.1 Average domestic indoor radon levels and action levels in Europe

Country	Average radon level (Bq m^{-3})	Advisory action level (Bq m^{-3})
Austria[a]		400
Belgium[b]	48	400 (200)
Czechslovakia	70	400
Denmark[b]	68	400 (200)
Finland	90	400
Germany[b]		400 (200)
Ireland	68	200
Italy	55	None
Luxembourg		150
Netherlands	32	None
Norway[b]	90	400 (200)
Sweden[a]	100	200
UK	20	200
USA		148

[a]These countries have mandatory action levels: Austria 1000 Bq m^{-3} and Sweden 400 Bq m^{-3}.
[b]Belgium, Denmark, Germany, and Norway have two advisory levels: 400 Bq m^{-3} for existing houses and 200 Bq m^{-3} for new houses.

10.3.5 Intervention to reduce radon levels

Should raised radon levels be found, there are a number of methods which can be used to reduce them [15]. If the building has an underfloor cavity, ventilation of this space can be increased. Cracks in floors could be sealed, but in practice even the smallest residual crack will allow significant amounts of radon through. A simple fan in a ground-floor room with a reverse flow to blow air inwards to create a positive pressure is sometimes used. However, the most effective method is to create a sump under the floor, and fit a fan which draws radon to the external atmosphere (Figure 10.6; Table 10.2). In new homes, a heavy-duty rubber damp-proof membrane will prevent radon penetration. Since 1992 in the UK, it has been a requirement to fit a membrane in all new houses in affected areas [16].

Despite local publicity, in the UK only 30% of householders in affected areas have so far tested their homes, and only 10% of those finding raised levels have carried out remediation work. Remediation for schools in an affected area is the most cost-effective method of reducing risk. Similar programmes in the workplace are four times less effective [17]. The cost per life year gained for a domestic remediation programme in Northhamptonshire is projected to be £13 250 [18]. This compares with that for the Breast Screening Service using X-ray mammography of £6000 per life year gained.

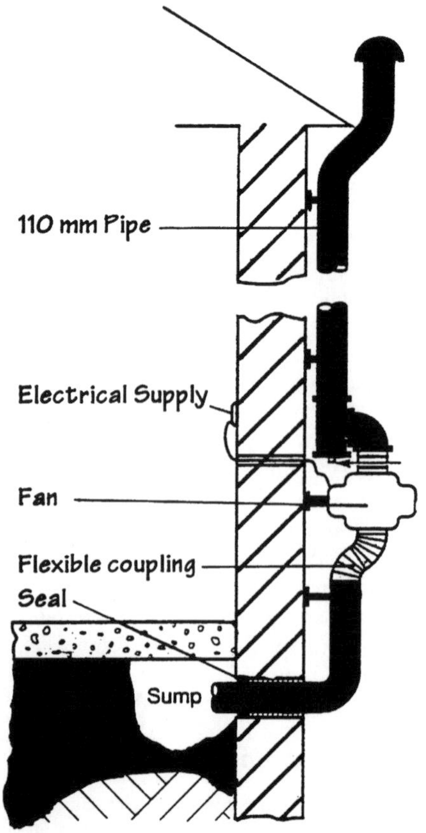

Figure 10.6 Typical domestic radon sump system. Reproduced with permission from Radon Centres Ltd.

Box 10.5 Planning a radon survey of the workplace

If a radon survey is required in a workplace, it must be sufficiently thorough to detect areas of raised radon levels. Radon concentrations above the action level may be restricted to a single small office, although if this is the case other rooms in the area are likely to have elevated concentrations. Radon gas levels are usually highest on the lowest floor, and so measurements should be made in the basement and ground-floor areas. Since the numbers of rooms to be surveyed may be large, an initial survey in which measurements are made in every other room is recommended. If any rooms with concentrations above half the action level are found, then all rooms in the area should be surveyed. Usually etched track detectors are placed for a 3-month period on cupboards or other surfaces about 1 metre from the floor away from windows and external doors. The detectors should be deployed during the winter months, as a hot spell in summer with all the windows open will reduce indoor radon levels considerably. It is prudent to measure radon levels in new buildings fitted with radon reduction precautions, once the building is heated and fully occupied. For assessment of domestic properties, the NRPB suggest that an average of levels measured in a main living room and a bedroom is calculated, weighted by occupancy (45% living room + 55% bedroom). The approved laboratory providing the detectors will normally apply a seasonal correction factor for domestic properties, to provide an estimate of the average annual radon level.

An alternative approach to the use of etched track detectors is to employ a direct reading radon meter taking 5-minute readings to identify rooms for further study. This requires a skilled operator and the measurement will depend on weather conditions and use of the room at the time. It is preferable to make the measurements at night or in the early morning, as radon levels are lower during the working day. Three-month measurements with the etched track detectors should then be made in suspect rooms, to determine whether the action level is exceeded.

Should a raised level be found, remedial action should be taken over the next few months. The urgency is related to the radon level found, and it is only appropriate to relocate staff immediately if levels over 5000 Bq m^{-3} are found. A specialist remediation firm can advise on the most appropriate action without the need for further extensive measurements.

If the employer is unable to reduce the radon level below the action level, staff safety must be ensured by operating a scheme of work which limits the time spent in the affected room. This may be appropriate for a basement used for long-term storage of files where access is low. In this instance dose assessments can be made knowing the time staff spend in the room, using the relation 1 mSv = 126 kBq m^{-3} h, which assumes an equilibrium factor of 0.5 which is generally applicable in the workplace. Personal etched track detectors could be considered, but storage of these detectors overnight in a low radon environment when not worn is critical.

A building should be tested when remediation work is complete. The definitive measurement is with a 3-month track etch detector, but it is useful to use a short exposure of 7 days, or use a direct-reading radon meter in sniff mode to give an early indication that remediation is likely to have been successful.

Table 10.2 Efficacy of radon remediation methods

Method	Reduction factor Geometric mean	Maximum	Number of samples
Positive ventilation	4.3	24	16
Additional natural ventilation	4.8	17	3
Underfloor void			
– with added natural ventilation	1.5	3.1	7
– with mechanical ventilation	1.1	2.5	3
Sealing only	2	2.6	4
Floor membrane		2.4	1
Sump	12	130	70
Sump with other methods	9.9	51	11

Initial radon level between 750 and 1500 Bq m^{-3}.
Source: NRPB.

10.4 Artificial sources and potential incidents

This section reviews general applications of radioactive sources outside specialist hospital departments and considers potential accidents that could place members of the public at risk.

10.4.1 Nuclear installations

These applications involve large quantities of radioactive material and must have emergency plans to deal with foreseeable accidents which could affect members of the public. These will be discussed in §10.6.2. Civil nuclear installations include nuclear power stations, plants preparing uranium fuel from ore, processing plants such as Sellafield, and research reactors. There are also Ministry of Defence bases for submarines powered by nuclear reactors.

10.4.2 Nuclear weapons

Detonators are stored separately from warheads to avoid the risk of explosion, so the main hazard in an accident involving nuclear weapons would be from release of plutonium particles in a fire. In addition to its radioactivity, plutonium is chemically toxic. It emits a low-energy γ-ray and requires thin-window monitors. When weapons are transported by road in the UK, a radiation safety team is included in the escort. The Ministry of Defence have comprehensive contingency arrangements and back-up plans if the escort is disabled. Contingency plans are designed to minimize risk of a conventional explosion with evacuation to 600 metres, radio silence within 50 metres and cooling the weapon with water spray. If a release of plutonium is suspected, then the escort commander could advise sheltering of the general public up to 5 kilometres downwind.

10.4.3 Gamma-irradiation systems

Gamma-irradiation plants contain arrays of ^{60}Co sources with a total activity of about 6×10^5 TBq. The high dose rates are employed to sterilize needles and syringes for hospital use. The plants are usually operated continuously with objects to be irradiated transported through the irradiation chamber on trucks with an automated drive (Figure 10.7). When not in use, the sources are lowered into a tank of water so that operators can enter the irradiation chamber in safety. Safety requirements include the use of trucks too small for human access, interlocked doors, and key entry. Seven exposure incidents with five fatalities occurred worldwide during the period 1975–94, caused by staff deliberately bypassing safety systems [19].

Blood product irradiators containing activities up to 60 TBq of ^{137}Cs are found in hospitals. The irradiation chamber is capable of holding a small number of blood bags which rotate in front of the exposed source. The shielding of the source is designed so that non-radiation workers can carry out their normal duties in the vicinity. Appropriate safety checks and contingency plans for a blood irradiator are given in Box 10.6.

10.4.4 Industrial radiography

Industrial radiography is the use of portable γ-ray sources such as ^{60}Co, ^{192}Ir (up to 740 GBq), or ^{170}Tm (20 GBq) to produce an image on film. The technique is applied to assessment of welds in metal objects and checking the uniformity of concrete. The source is housed in a shielded container and connected to a wire so that it can be manually exposed using a winding handle. Several incidents have occurred where sources have jammed in the open position, including occasions when a source has been left on site in the open position for several days.

Box 10.6 Radiation protection requirements for blood irradiators

Safety checks

A radiation safety survey will be carried out at least once a year to ensure that no deficiencies arise in the radiation shielding and that no radioactive material is detectable at the irradiation chamber. This latter check gives an indirect assurance that no radioactive material is leaking from the source.

Contingency plans

The training schedule for operators must include instructions for the action to be taken in the event of power failure or equipment breakdown. If the equipment cannot be returned to normal operation, it must be switched off at the mains supply and contact made with the service organization. It should be noted that the radioactive source remains in its fixed position at all times and that no radiation hazard arises from machine breakdown.

The worst credible incident would be a fire in the vicinity of the equipment. A severe fire could lead to some loss of shielding or leakage of radioactive material, but it is unlikely that a severe radiological hazard would arise. Nevertheless, the area, once evacuated, should not be re-entered until a radiological safety check has been carried out.

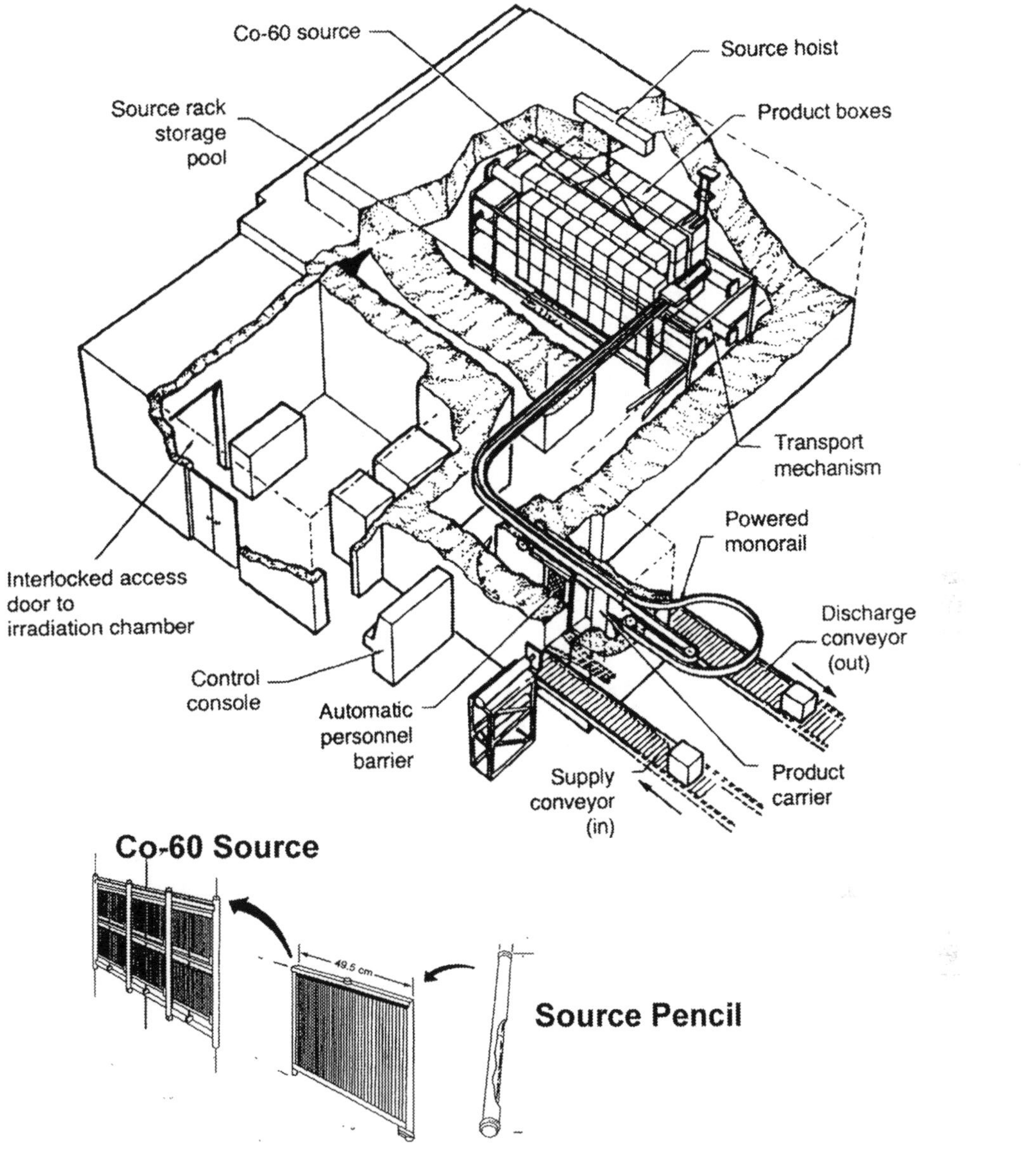

Figure 10.7 Industrial irradiation plant layout; cobalt source array in an industrial irradiator shown as inset. Reproduced with permission from MDS Nordion.

Portable X-ray units are used by security firms for radiography of suspicious packages and by veterinary surgeons. Fixed devices are used for examination of luggage at airports.

10.4.5 Small users of radioactivity

Many different types of radioactive source are used in industry, the majority of which are small sealed sources (Table 10.3). Incidents can result from loss or damage to sources. Members of the public have received significant localized radiation doses from keeping stray sealed sources in their pockets. Hospitals are the major users of unsealed radionuclides but they are also used in universities, research laboratories of pharmaceutical companies, gas supply companies, and factories producing tritium light sources.

Table 10.3 Common uses of radioactive sources in industry

Use	Radionuclide	Activity	Form	Industries
Thickness gauges	^{90}Sr	4 GBq	SS	Cigarettes, paper, plastic, mag tape
	^{85}Kr	55 GBq	SS	Paper, board, plastic, mag tape
	^{204}Tl	3.7 GBq	SS	Paper and board
	^{241}Am	10 GBq	SS	Metal strip
	$^{226}Ra/Be$	2 MBq	SS	Road coatings
	$^{241}Am/Be$	2 MBq	SS	Road coatings
Level gauges	^{137}Cs	10 GBq	SS	Sugar, flour, oil, petrol, food
	^{60}Co	1 GBq	SS	Sugar, flour, oil, petrol, food
	^{90}Sr	555 MBq	SS	Package
	^{241}Am	4 GBq	SS	Bottling
Moisture	$^{241}Am/Be$	2 GBq	SS	Steel industry
Strata density	^{137}Cs	74 GBq	SS	Gas and oil
	^{60}Co	4 GBq	SS	Well logging
Gas detection	Tritium (^{3}H)	40 GBq	SS	Oil and gas
	^{63}Ni	40 MBq	SS	Oil and gas, valve and CRT manufacture
Dust emission	^{14}C	4 GBq	SS	Coal, cement, etc.
	^{147}Pm	1 MBq	SS	Coal, cement, etc.
Industrial Radiography	^{192}Ir	740 GBq	Wire	Pipe welds
	^{170}Tm	20 GBq	SS	Pipe welds
Smoke detector	^{241}Am	37 MBq	Metal disc	Any
Gas flow studies	^{82}Br	1.5 GBq	Bromine gas	Gas supply company
	^{85}Kr	80 MBq	Gas	Gas supply company
Medical supplies	^{125}I	7.4 MBq	Stock solution	Radioisotope supplier
Luminous exit signs	Tritium (^{3}H)	1110 TBq	Tritiated water	Sign manufacturer

10.4.6 Radioactivity in scrap metal

A relatively common cause of radiation emergencies is the presence of radioactivity in scrap metal. Major scrapyards monitor incoming loads for radioactivity. About 50 reports are recorded each year in the UK, of which 50% are due to naturally occurring radioactive materials and 25% to small industrial sealed sources. Most sealed sources can survive the majority of manipulations in a scrapyard, apart from the smelting process, which will lead to widespread contamination. Several incidents in different parts of the world have involved removal of large sources from radiotherapy equipment when medical facilities have been closed down and have had major radiological consequences (Box 10.7).

10.4.7 Historical uses

Residues from historical applications of radioactivity can still give rise to incidents. There were many factories where radium was refined or used for the radium paint industry. Larger factories have been identified and decontaminated but smaller concerns, often in single houses, are still found. Several hundred nuclear-powered cardiac pacemakers, which contained 110 GBq ^{238}Pu, were fitted to patients in the UK during the 1970s. The casing was designed to withstand high temperatures, such as in cremation. Such patients should be identified so that the power pack can be removed at post-mortem, and disposed of safely to an authorized agency. Other historical items such as radon emanators are handed in to the police from time to time and need to be safely disposed of.

10.4.8 Transport

Transport of radioactive materials is covered by legislation (§9.5) based on IAEA guidance. Transport accidents are foreseeable events so that packages must be designed to withstand subsequent damage by impact and fire. In addition, vehicles and packages must be clearly labelled. Sources transported range from small quantities of radionuclides for hospital use to spent nuclear fuel. Transport of spent nuclear fuel in the UK comes under the Nuclear Industry Road Emergency Response Plan (NIREP).

Box 10.7 The Goiânia incident, Brazil 1987

The incident started when people entered premises formerly used as a private radiotherapy clinic that had been partially demolished. The premises contained a teletherapy unit that had been abandoned without notification of the licensing authority. The source capsule contained 51 TBq ^{137}Cs in the form of caesium chloride powder and this was ruptured as the machine was dismantled. The powder gave off a blue light and caused great fascination. Small parts of the source were given to friends and family, resulting in external irradiation, personal contamination, and ingestion. Contaminated scrap metal was sold on and further dispersed. It was only when those involved developed acute radiation injuries and part of the source was taken to the local hospital that a medical physicist discovered that the object was highly radioactive [20].

This started a major evacuation and decontamination programme involving 500 staff monitoring 120 000 people, using the local football stadium as a decontamination unit. A total of 249 people were found to be contaminated, with 21 requiring treatment for acute radiation syndrome. Four people died and one had an amputation of the forearm. Large areas of the city had to be decontaminated, including the removal of top soil.

10.4.9 Nuclear-powered satellites

Nuclear power is used in some orbital satellites and in satellites for deep space missions. There are two types of power systems. In the first, the heat associated with decay is extracted. The activity used depends on the power required, with 7800 TBq of ^{238}Pu used for the Voyager mission to Jupiter, while orbiting satellites employ about 100 TBq. The second type uses ^{235}U in a small nuclear reactor to provide higher power and produces standard fission products.

Problems arise when satellite orbits decay prematurely. The satellite may not burn out completely in the atmosphere and a large fragment could reach the ground. The decaying orbit would be detected several days before it entered the earth's atmosphere but the point of impact can only be estimated to within a crash window 2000 miles (3000 km) long and 200 miles (300 km) wide. COSMOS 954 crashed on 23 January 1978 in an unoccupied part of Canada, but despite a major search effort, only 1% of the radioactivity had been recovered by 2000, and it is likely that the remainder is in small fragments spread over a wide area.

10.5 Dealing with radiation incidents

10.5.1 Hospital radiation incidents

Hospitals use radiation in many forms and incidents will occur from time to time. There are important lessons to be learned from incidents, as they show how procedures can fail. A system must be in place whereby incidents involving ionising or non-ionising radiation are reported to the Radiation Protection Service. A form should be completed by the local person responsible for radiation safety. The type of questions that should be asked include:

- What happened?
- When did it occur?
- Where did it happen?
- Who was involved?
- Was anyone exposed or injured?
- Was any radioactive contamination produced?
- If YES, what monitoring and decontamination was carried out?
- Who was notified?
- What action was taken?
- Is any further action required?

Every incident will require an investigation by local or area radiation protection personnel, depending on its type, nature, and severity, and all action taken should be documented. The radiation protection adviser (RPA) will be required to give advice on steps that should be taken to deal with the incident and on changes in procedures which should be made. Lessons learned from minor mistakes can help to prevent more major ones. An assessment of any radiation dose received and the risk to the health of any individual as a result of the incident should also be made. More significant incidents must be reported to the appropriate regulatory authority. A system operated in the west of Scotland for many years has recorded 12–15 radiation incidents per year per million population served. The number will depend on the threshold criteria used to signify that an incident has occurred. While patient overdoses are of concern at diagnostic levels, it must be remembered that a patient underdose in radiotherapy is as significant for the patient because of the increased risk of local recurrence, and so must be reported and investigated [21].

10.5.2 Incidents in the community

When police in the UK are called to an incident and discover that radioactivity or radiation is involved, they

Box 10.8 Planning for incidents in the community

- Ensure that appropriate mechanisms are in place so that a physicist with radiation protection experience can be contacted by the police at any time to provide advice. A list of telephone numbers may be held by the hospital switchboard or included in the plan.
- Ensure up-to-date communication links are maintained with the emergency services.
- Devise a radiation incident plan which dovetails into the hospital major accident plan. This should include arrangements for dealing with radiation casualties (§10.6.3) and setting up radiation monitoring units (§10.7.2).
- Identify technicians from nuclear medicine and other departments who have experience with radioactive materials, so that in the event of a major contamination incident, all available monitors and staff can be utilized, and a shift system established if necessary.
- Draw together a kit of useful equipment, including protective clothing, gloves, wellington boots and a safety helmet, a torch, notebook, waterproof pens, calculator, resealable plastic bags of various sizes, PVC tape, filter papers for taking wipes, tongs for handling sources, a lead pot for containing a source, and a camera for recording the incident.
- Ensure physics staff know where contamination monitors and personal dosemeters can be obtained.
- Find out what unsealed and sealed sources are used locally and confirm that contamination monitors will detect them.
- Visit sites with off-site action plans and be familiar with their plans and capabilities.

can obtain advice through the National Arrangements for Incidents involving Radioactivity (NAIR) (Box 10.8). This scheme is designed to provide assistance to the police for incidents involving radioactivity where the operator responsible for the source cannot immediately be contacted and where no emergency plan exists, or where an emergency plan fails. It is invoked when members of the general public are at risk, so that a spill of radioactive material within a factory would be the responsibility of the employer, but if the factory caught fire and the fire brigade were concerned about their own exposure, or the spill spread to nearby houses, then NAIR would be invoked.

The NAIR scheme has two stages, the first is a response by local medical physics departments who, because of their wide distribution, may be able to reach the scene of an accident rapidly and provide immediate advice (Box 10.9). Staff from such departments are only required to respond within their own resources. They would confirm whether a hazard existed and advise the police on appropriate action. Stage II is provided by health physics teams at nuclear power stations or research facilities who have the experience, training, and equipment to deal with major spills. The NRPB coordinate the scheme, and can provide expert advice or equipment should this be required. In a major incident the medical physicist may simply advise the police to set up an exclusion zone and request that Stage II should be called out.

The most common types of occurrences where NAIR is invoked are ones where small sources have found their way into the public domain, empty source containers

Box 10.9 Practical responses to radiation incidents

When a physicist is first called for advice following an incident, he/she needs to find out what is involved and then to give preliminary advice over the telephone. The type of information required is:

- Is it known what the radionuclide and its activity are?
- Is the radionuclide shielded and does the shielding appear to be intact?
- Is there any obvious sign of spillage and contamination?
- Are there any casualties and could they be contaminated?

If it is clear that an incident has occurred, immediate advice may be needed on:

- whether barriers need to be erected at the accident site to restrict access
- whether further precautions are required to restrict spread of contamination
- whether the incident requires specialist help, such as Stage II of NAIR.

Table 10.4 The international nuclear event scale

Level	Type	Extent	Examples
7	Major accident	Major release of radioactivity. Widespread health and environment effects	Chernobyl, USSR, 1986
6	Serious accident	Significant release of radioactivity. Full implementation of local countermeasures	
5	Accidents with off-site risks	Limited release of radioactivity. Partial implementation of local countermeasures	Windscale, UK, 1957 Three Mile Island, USA, 1979
4	Accidents without significant off-site risks	Minor release of radioactivity in the order of prescribed limits. Local protective measures unlikely except for some food monitoring and control. Significant plant damage, Fatal exposure of a worker	Saint-Laurent, France, 1980 Tokaimura, 1999
3	Serious incident	Very small release of radioactivity, a fraction of the prescribed limits. Local protective measures unlikely. Possible acute health effects to a worker	Vandellos, Spain, 1989 Sosndy Bar, 1992 Tomsk 7, FSU, 1993
2	Incident	Incident with potential safety consequences on site. Insignificant release of radioactivity off site	
1	Anomaly	Variation from permitted procedures	
0	Below scale	No safety significance	

have been found, or false alarms. Incidents have involved damaged sources, vehicle accidents, and dumping of material of low specific activity. One incident of the latter type resulted from dumping of one tonne of depleted uranium tailings in a field with extensive public access [22]. A specialist contractor dealt with removal of the uranium and, following an appeal by the public health department, contamination monitoring was carried out on 134 people in their own homes.

In the acute phase of a more serious incident, medical physicists may need to consider the implication of any decontamination process in providing advice to the police. This may include whether aqueous washings can go directly to local water courses at the accident scene. Solid waste similarly needs to be made safe and secure, and possibly shielded, although final disposal can usually be delayed until the acute phase is over. Consultation with the organization responsible for authorization of waste disposal will be required.

The emergency services may need advice about where contaminated casualties should be taken. The physicist may need to alert the accident and emergency department at the hospital and arrange for physics staff to assist in decontamination. The fire brigade have portable chemical decontamination facilities, and it may be appropriate for these to be used at the scene to deal with a serious incident.

In an incident the police or hospital will use their press officer to brief the media and others should only say what has been agreed with the press officer. However, current wisdom is that the press should be briefed as soon as possible to avoid the accusation that 'the authorities are hiding something'. At the request of the police, the physicist, as the local radiation expert, may be called upon to give an opinion before the incident is fully evaluated. It is important that the risks from the incident are put in simple terms, perhaps compared to the dose from a few weeks additional exposure to natural radiation or to the dose from routine patient X-rays (§11.6).

10.6 Major nuclear radiation emergencies

Accidents involving radioactivity are graded on an international scale (Table 10.4). The accident at Chernobyl has been the most significant to date [23]. It was level 7 with a major release of radioactivity and widespread health and environmental effects (Box 10.10). The criticality accident at Tokaimura, Japan, in September 1999 was classified as level 4.

10.6.1 Risks of a major accident

Major users of radioactivity should carry out assessments of the risks from foreseeable accidents. Requirements for the provision of information to the public about plans to

Box 10.10 The Chernobyl incident

The Chernobyl incident happened on 25 April 1986, when operators running the Number 4 reactor in the Chernobyl complex near Kiev, Russia, overrode safety systems. The nuclear reaction went out of control, blowing the roof off the reactor building and releasing 3 700 000 TBq of mixed radioactivity into the atmosphere. Use of helicopters to drop sand, lead, boron, and carbon into the open reactor restricted the release to 3.5% of the total activity in the core. The residue was entombed in a sarcophagus. A total of 134 of the emergency personnel suffered acute radiation sickness, from which 28 died.

The primary radionuclides released were ^{137}Cs and ^{131}I and the latter was responsible for the major health consequence—a large increase in childhood thyroid cancer in the three nearest Russian states. A contributory factor was the slow and variable distribution of iodine tablets following the incident (Box 10.13).

A total of 24 700 local people were evacuated and relocated. However, an extension to a further 130 000 people in 1990–91 was politically motivated and of dubious radiological value. Enforced and unsympathetic relocation had a major effect on stress levels, and one of the major lessons of Chernobyl is that psychological damage from the handling of an incident can be the most significant health detriment.

The radiological consequences extended well beyond USSR, and by 2000 there were still 10 farms in Wales where lambs contained ^{137}Cs above the action level of 1000 Bq kg $^{-1}$.

deal with radiation accidents with off-site implications are determined in the UK by the Radiation (Emergency Preparedness and Public Information) Regulations 2001. These regulations contain a schedule of radionuclide limits above which risk assessment and hazard evaluation must be performed. If an accident could result in doses of 5 mSv over the following year to members of the public, off-site emergency plans must be prepared by the operator and the local authority. This will include responsibilities for the local public health department and the local hospital, and liaison with the emergency services. Civil nuclear installations and gamma-irradiation plants must have plans under these regulations and these must be exercised regularly, including exercises in which off-site releases are simulated [24].

The radionuclide limits in these regulations are such that hospital radiopharmacies using short-lived β- and γ-ray-emitting unsealed sources are unlikely to require assessment. Large ^{137}Cs sources in blood irradiators (§10.4.3) or radiotherapy departments or ^{241}Am sources which emit α-particles may in some cases require risk assessments, but are unlikely to require emergency plans as the radioactive material is sealed in such a manner that it is not readily dispersible.

10.6.2 Plans for major radiation incidents

In the UK, plans for conventional major emergencies have been established, with cooperation between the fire, police, and ambulance services, hospitals and local councils, and these are tested through regular exercises. In a major incident a system of strategic, tactical, and operational controls will be adopted by all emergency services, with strategic involving the chiefs in a control centre off-site, tactical being the on-site commanders, and operational being the section heads with specific responsibility, such as fire brigade radiation safety officers. In England these three controls are designated gold, silver, and bronze, and officers wear suitably coloured tabards for identification. Should such an incident involve radioactive contamination, medical physicists would have to work within these patterns, and may need to provide a presence at the strategic control centre, as well as on site.

Medical physics departments are required to respond to radiation emergencies and specialist hospitals with an accident and emergency department and medical physics support must be identified to accept radiation casualties [25] (Box 10.8). The area around a nuclear plant which may be affected by an incident is known as the detailed emergency planning zone. Hospitals within this zone are required to have an emergency plan for responding to an incident at the nuclear plant. Other hospitals should have radiation incident plans as part of their general response to major incidents.

In a radiation accident it may be necessary for emergency service personnel or workers to enter a high-dose-rate area to reduce the risk to others. These personnel might only attend one significant radiological accident in a lifetime and in such cases a single-event effective dose limit is adopted, which must be defined in the employer's emergency plan and agreed with HSE.

10.6.3 Treatment of radiation casualties

As a result of a radiation incident there may be casualties who have received a significant radiation dose or been contaminated with radioactivity or both. Moreover, the casualties may have other injuries. If it is suspected that a casualty may be contaminated, they should be taken to an area set aside for decontamination (§10.6.4) in the specialist hospital identified in the emergency plan. Life-threatening injuries must take precedence over deconta-

Box 10.11 Preparation for monitoring and decontamination

- Suitable non-slip, disposable floor covering should be laid along the route through which contaminated casualties will enter.
- An adequate supply of swabs and cleaning materials must be available.
- Large polythene bags should be available for contaminated garments and waste.
- Small polythene bags for swab samples taken from the nose and contaminated skin should be provided.
- Appropriate signs to indicate location, entry, exit, and prohibiting unauthorized entry should be provided.
- Staff identified for treating the patient must put on appropriate protective clothing (boots or overshoes, gloves, gowns, caps, and face masks). These items must be used only in the area(s) designated for decontamination or treatment of a contaminated patient.
- Physics staff will need to obtain appropriate contamination monitors.
- Barriers may need to be erected to prevent access between clean and contaminated areas.
- Movements into and out of the area must be restricted, with care taken when removing soiled overshoes, etc.
- Forms should be provided for recording details of casualties and the activity and distribution of contamination found. Diagrams with parts of the body likely to be heavily contaminated expanded (Figure 10.8) may be useful for this.

mination, but care must be taken to prevent the spread of contamination to the emergency services or hospital staff. Ambulances should take patients with life-threatening injuries to the nearest accident and emergency department, even if it is not approved to take contaminated casualties, so that the patient is treated rapidly. All hospitals with accident and emergency departments must have basic plans for dealing with suspected contamination situations, including means of contacting medical physics support. The medical physicist will then need to catch up with the ambulance and patient to ensure both are subsequently monitored and decontaminated. A casualty suspected of being contaminated may be wrapped in a plastic sheet or blanket before transfer to the ambulance to contain the spread of contamination as much as possible.

Casualties will be assessed rapidly on arrival at the accident and emergency department (triage) and those critically injured will be treated immediately, with precautions to minimize spread of contamination. Others with minor injuries will be decontaminated before being admitted for treatment.

10.6.4 Decontamination

The aims of decontamination are to remove the radioactive material from the contaminated individual before it gives rise to a significant dose, while containing the contamination and minimizing its spread to staff or surroundings [26]. Once the accident and emergency department learns that contaminated casualties are on their way, the department should prepare the area designated for decontamination in the hospital plan (Box 10.11).

Other points to be considered include:

- It may be necessary to turn off air conditioning if air is circulated to other parts of the hospital and a significant quantity of particulate contamination is likely to be present. Contingency plans should include a procedure for disabling the air conditioning.
- Items such as X-ray cassettes which may need to be brought into the room should be covered, and the cover removed and the cassettes monitored before they leave the area.

Once injuries have been stabilized, decontamination can begin (Box 10.12).

- Individuals who will undertake the decontamination should be identified.
- Scribes should be designated to record the extent of contamination and progress of decontamination for each casualty (Figure 10.8) so that a retrospective estimate of radiation dose can be made.
- All non-essential personnel should be excluded from the area.
- Patients should be monitored to ascertain the extent and distribution of contamination.
- Nose blows and nose and mouth swabs should be taken where contamination is found and placed in labelled polythene bags for assessment of probability of internal contamination.
- Contaminated clothing should be removed (by cutting if necessary) and placed in polythene bags.
- Decontamination should be carried out under the direction of a clinician or physicist using procedures

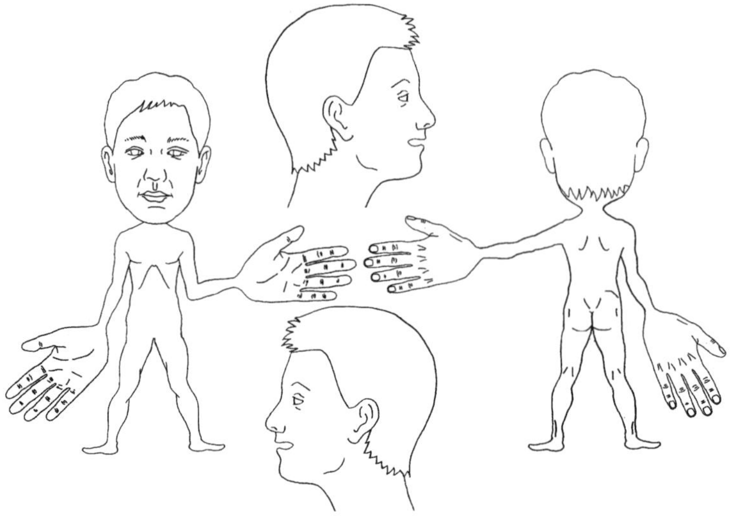

Figure 10.8 Diagrams suitable for recording the distribution of contamination found during monitoring of patients

similar to those described in §15.10. In cases of modest contamination, it should be acceptable to dispose of the radioactivity to the drains. With unknown radionuclides, or higher activity, it may be necessary to keep all washings and store them for future disposal.

- When decontamination is complete, ambulances and their crews and persons assisting in decontamination must be monitored and decontaminated, before they can return to normal duties.

10.6.5 Internal contamination

Radionuclides may be taken into the body by ingestion or inhalation, or through breaks in the skin. An assessment of the likelihood of intake through different routes may be derived from mouth, nose, and wound swabs and measurements of uptake. The chemical form of the contamination, the radionuclides involved, and the amounts are important in determining treatment. Some radio-elements and critical organs are listed in Table 10.5. Methods for reducing absorption and speeding up excretion are described in §15.10.2 and §15.10.3. Intake of stable iodine may reduce uptake of iodine radioisotopes (Box 10.13). If the chemical form is insoluble in the gastrointestinal tract, only a small amount will be absorbed which will not usually justify action, but chelating agents may be used for soluble metallic radionuclides, such as Prussian Blue for caesium contamination. If the intake results from inhalation of gaseous or particulate material, factors such as particle size, solubility, and respiration rate will affect the dose. Almost 50% of clearance from the lung is through the pharynx and this may give rise to secondary digestive absorption. Serious contamination of a wound should be treated as soon as possible. If the radionuclide is in a soluble form, it should, if possible, be made insoluble at the wound site to prevent diffusion into

Box 10.12 Design of a decontamination unit

A similar decontamination unit can be used for both radioactive and chemical decontamination. It should be in an area that can be readily partitioned off from the rest of the accident and emergency or other department and should preferably have a separate entrance and exit. All rooms should have sealed floors which can be readily decontaminated and a dedicated decontamination room, with sealed walls and a drain, is an advantage. Additional showers for staff and patients are appropriate, but do not usually provide the best approach for initial decontamination of a casualty.

Some units are fitted with holding tanks for aqueous waste (§15.4.2), into which the decontamination room drains. However, the amount of radioactivity involved in most incidents is unlikely to be sufficiently large to make such tanks essential, unless the authorization to dispose of aqueous waste is insufficient for certain foreseeable accidents. It may be necessary to discuss these matters with the agency with responsibility for disposal of radioactive material to the environment.

Table 10.5 Critical organs for some radio-elements

Lung	Bone	Thyroid	Gastrointestinal tract	Whole body
Inhaled insolubles	Phosphorus			
	Calcium	Iodine	Cobalt	Carbon
	Strontium	Astatine	Ruthenium	Sodium
	Radium		Silver	Zinc
	Plutonium (soluble)		Rare earths	Caesium
			Ingested insolubles	

the body. If the contamination is insoluble, the injury should be treated with a local therapeutic agent, before surgery is considered. For contamination by solid particles, surgical excision is the sole option and an assessment should be made as soon as possible.

10.6.6 Irradiated casualties

Deterministic effects of ionising radiation are described in §3.3. Casualties suspected of receiving a whole-body dose over 1 Sv should be transferred to a specialist hospital, where they can be nursed in germ-free conditions, given blood transfusions, assessed for bone marrow transplant, and provided with psychological support [28]. Temporary hospitalization may be considered in burns units or transplant units until transfer to a specialist radiation unit can be organized. It is important for subsequent treatment to evaluate the dose received by such casualties. Chromosome aberration analysis, which is conducted by national laboratories (NRPB in the UK), will detect whole-body radiation exposures above 300 mSv (§3.2.5). A drawback is that the test takes over a week to give a result. In addition, its accuracy depends on a knowledge of the patient's previous radiation history and the best estimate may eventually come from a reconstruction of the circumstances of the irradiation if this is possible.

A radiation exposure may be highly localized and information on the source and circumstances of the accident is important for assessing this. The skin is particularly vulnerable from exposure to β-particle contaminant or low-energy X- or γ-rays. Effects will not usually be apparent for many hours following exposure. The medical treatment of casualties with localized radiation damage has advanced rapidly in recent years. It is now possible to excise a necrosing area and apply a graft with artificial skin, as in a specialist burns unit, where once only amputation of the limb would be successful. This treatment requires rapid assessment of the patient, including a dose reconstruction of the radiation dose distribution, using Monte Carlo code or treatment planning computers to judge whether underlying structures, such as the bone, had received sublethal doses [29]. This treatment is only available in one or two specialist hospitals in the world.

10.7 Release of radioactivity

10.7.1 Protection of the public in the short term

If radioactivity is released into the atmosphere by a fire or major explosion, there is a potential for radioactive contamination to be spread over a wide area. The deposition of radioactivity depends on the size of radioactive particles, their nature, the wind speed, and the likelihood of rain washing out particles from the atmosphere and enhancing deposition. Intervention may be necessary in the form of advice given to the public to minimize their exposure. This may be a simple recommendation to stay indoors, but in the case of a large incident could involve evacuation. In the UK, two-stage levels for sheltering, evacuation, and provision of

Box 10.13 Iodine tablets

The distribution of iodine tablets would be undertaken following a major release of radioactive iodine in order to block uptake by the thyroid. Practices vary in different countries, but in the UK authorization for distribution would be given by the local director of public health. Stocks may be held by the nuclear reactor operator or other local centres, and may be predistributed to remote householders. The aim is for tablets to be distributed within a few hours of an incident. If taken 3 hours after an ^{131}I release, a thyroid dose reduction of 60–70% has been estimated. Recent findings [27] show that in the absence of stable iodine distribution, significantly more cancers occur where the normal diet is deficient in iodine. The protective effect of iodine tablets may be lower for incidents in developed parts of Europe and the USA where dietary iodine intake is above average.

Table 10.6 UK emergency reference levels (ERLs) for early countermeasures

Countermeasure	Body organ	Lower ERL (mSv)	Upper ERL (mSv)
Sheltering	Whole body	3	30
	Thyroid, Lung, Skin	30	300
Evacuation	Whole body	30	300
	Thyroid, Lung, Skin	300	3000
Stable iodine	Thyroid	30	300

stable iodine tablets (Box 10.13) have been established (Table 10.6). Action should be taken above the lower level if the risk in doing so is small. Action is justified in almost all circumstances at the upper level. Advice to the public will be issued by the medical director of the local health authority or consultants in public health medicine. They will act on advice provided by expert personnel at an off-site centre set up to coordinate emergency actions. These personnel will include a government technical adviser (normally from NRPB), health physicists, medical physicists, police, and other experts such as meteorologists.

Computer models have been developed to assist in projecting the content of plumes of radioactivity and they can estimate the extent and direction of any fallout. In the UK, data should be available from the NRPB and similar information is provided in other countries; for example, by the French ASTRAL program. This information can be utilized in making decisions about appropriate action to minimize the dose to the public.

10.7.2 Public (validation) monitoring

If a significant amount of radioactive material has been released into the atmosphere, it may be appropriate to establish one or more temporary radiation screening units in local schools or sports centres. Such a site may also serve as a reception centre for evacuees. This would allow individuals who might be contaminated to be assessed and decontaminated if necessary, and provide reassurance for others. The centre would require a segregated waiting area, a room in which the monitoring was carried out, a room with hot and cold running water for decontamination, and a reporting area with a telephone and ideally a fax and computer link (Figure 10.9). There should be a separate exit and toilet facilities for persons who have been decontaminated. It is important to establish a route through the unit which minimizes the risk of transfer of contamination between individuals. This should be thought out beforehand and plans prepared showing positions at which barriers must be set up to restrict access. Two areas for monitoring may be advisable, the first to identify persons with higher levels of contamination who require immediate decontamination and the second to carry out low-level monitoring after decontamination, before the person is discharged. Contaminated outer clothing and shoes may have to be removed and stored, with replacements supplied by the local council or voluntary services. Responsibility for operation of the unit would normally lie with the most senior medical physicist present.

Typical staffing would be one clerk for the waiting area, two physics staff to carry out monitoring, two nurses to assist with patient changing and decontamination, and one clerk to assist the physicist in charge in the reporting area. Material that would be required for setting up the unit is outlined in Box 10.11.

Monitoring should be in accordance with an agreed protocol, outlining the instruments to be used, the sequence of areas to be monitored, and techniques to be used. The protocol should contain criteria for action, for example:

1. Net count rate zero: Person sent away
2. Net count rate 0–10 cps: Person sent away to wash and change
3. Net count rate 10–100 cps: Person instructed to wash and change at screening unit and return for further monitoring.

Box 10.14 Environmental dose monitoring

Civil nuclear power station operators are required to monitor for potential off-site radioactive releases by siting automatic gamma dose monitors around the site perimeter. In addition, there will be extensive monitors within the plant, which will include real-time monitoring of radioactivity in air. In the UK, the Department of the Environment has also established 91 sites around the country with automatic gamma dose monitors, known as the Radioactive Incident Monitoring Network (RIMNET). The sites feed regular readings to a control centre, to give early warning of any radioactive release, specifically from overseas accidents, and its spread.

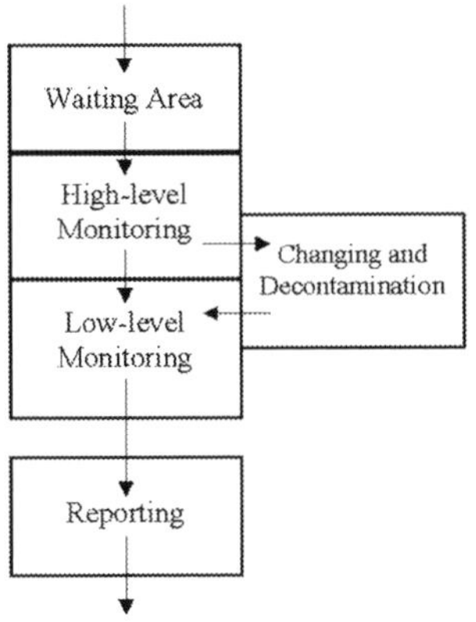

Figure 10.9 Possible layout of unit suitable for monitoring of the public.

4. Net count rate > 100 cps: As for (3). If contamination on exposed skin, person requested to attend unit for measurement of uptake at a later date.
5. Net count rate > 1000 cps: As for (3) and arrangements made for transfer to unit for measurement of uptake.

The criteria should be determined locally for the instruments available. Those quoted here are for a Mini Instruments monitor with a 44B probe.

Forms showing the distribution of contamination from monitoring (Figure 10.8) should be passed to the next staff member dealing with the person. Procedures for removal of contamination are described in §15.10. If contamination is still present on low-level monitoring, it may be necessary for the person to return for further decontamination. The location and final count rate for any remaining contamination should be recorded. It will be necessary to carry out a clean-up, decontamination, and final monitoring before staff leave the unit.

10.7.3 Long-term measures

Release of radioactivity can have continuing consequences in the environment which become the concern of government environmental and agricultural agencies, and may result in long-term restrictions on foodstuffs and milk. Derived levels and limits are used to provide guidance during emergency situations. Individual radionuclide limits for concentration in air, for amounts which could be ingested annually, and for maximum concentrations in foodstuffs, such as milk, vegetables, and meat, and drinking water are given in Table 10.7 [25, 30]. Monitoring of the environment and of foodstuffs would be conducted by government agencies, and advice given on the need for restrictions on consumption.

10.8 References

1 Hughes, J. S. (1999). *Ionising radiation exposure of the UK population: 1999 review.* NRPB Report R311. NRPB, Chilton.
2 Gates, A. E. and Gunderson, L. C. S. (eds) (1992). *Geological controls on radon.* The Geological Society of America, Boulder.
3 Bradley, E. J., Lomas, P. R., Green, B. M. R., and Smithard, J. (1997). *Radon in dwellings in England: 1997 review.* NRPB Report R293.
4 National Radiological Protection Board (1993). Estimate of late radiation risks to the UK population. *Doc. NRPB*, **4** (4), 15–157.
5 Phillips, P. S. and Denman, A. R. (1997). Radon: a human carcinogen. *Sci. Prog.*, **80** (4), 317–36.
6 Committee on Health Risks of Exposure to Radon (BEIR VI) (1999). *Health effects of exposure to radon.* National Academy Press, USA.
7 Lubin, J. H. and Boice, J. D. (1997). Lung cancer risk from residential radon: meta-analysis of eight epidemiological studies. *J. Natl. Cancer Inst.*, **89** (1), 49–57.
8 Darby, S., Whitley, E., Silcocks, P., Thakrar, B., Green, M., Lomas, P., *et al.* (1998). Risk of lung cancer associated with residential radon exposure in south west England: a case control study. *Br. J. Cancer*, **78** (3), 394–408.
9 Cohen, B. (1995). Test of the linear no-threshold theory of radiation carcinogenesis for inhaled radon decay products. *Health Phys.*, **68** (2), 157–74.

Table 10.7 Drinking water limits

Radionuclide	Action level (Bq l^{-1})	Derived limits (Bq l^{-1})
Strontium (notably Sr-90)	125	–
Strontium-89	–	200
Strontium-90	–	50
Iodine-131	500	20
Plutonium and trans-plutonium elements	20	7
Caesium-137	–	100
Ruthenium-106	–	80

10 Health Physics (1998). Forums with contributions from Lubin *et al.* and Smith *et al.*, and responses from Cohen. *Health Phys.*, **75** (1), 4–33.

11 Bogen, K. T. (1998). Mechanistic model predicts a U-shaped relation of radon exposure to lung cancer risk reflected in combined occupational and US residential data. *Hum. Exp. Toxicol.*, **17**, 701–4.

12 International Agency for Research on Cancer (1988). *Man-made mineral fibres and radon.* Monographs on the evaluation of carcinogenic risks to humans. Vol. 43. WHO, Geneva.

13 Health and Safety Executive (1992). *The Management of Health and Safety Regulations.* SI 2051. HMSO, London.

14 Denman, A. R., Barker, S. P., Parkinson, S., Marley, F., and Phillips, P. S. (1999). Do the UK workplace radon action levels reflect the radiation dose received by the occupants? *J. Radiol. Prot.*, **19** (1), 37–43.

15 Phillips, P. S. (ed.) (1995). *The radon manual* (2nd edn). The Radon Council.

16 Building Research Establishment (1999). *Radon: guidance on protective measures for new dwellings.* BRE Report BR 211. BRE, Watford.

17 Denman, A. R. and Phillips, P. S. (1998). The cost effectiveness of radon mitigation in schools in Northamptonshire. *J. Radiol. Prot.*, **18** (3), 203–8.

18 Kennedy, C., Gray, A., Denman, A. R., and Phillips, P. S. (1999). A cost analysis of a residential radon remediation programme in the United Kingdom. *Br. J. Cancer*, **18** (7), 1243–7.

19 International Atomic Energy Agency (1996). *Lessons learned from accidents in industrial irradiation facilities.* IAEA, Vienna.

20 International Atomic Energy Agency (1988). *The radiological accident at Goiâ nia.* STI/PUB/815. IAEA, Vienna.

21 British Institute of Radiology (1996). *Radiation incidents: papers from the meetings on radiation incidents in hospital, 5 December, 1994, and uncertainties, errors and accidents in radiotherapy, 24 April 1995* (ed. K. Faulkner and R. M. Harrison). BIR, London.

22 Denman, A. R., Morgan, P., and Tomlinson, S. (1998). *The response to depleted uranium turnings dumped in Northamptonshire.* Meeting Proceedings of the International Radiological Post-Emergency Response Issues Conference, Washington, DC, USA, 9–11 September 1998. US Environment Protection Agency, EPA 402-S-98-001, pp. 43–7.

23 Haywood, J. K. (ed.) (1986). *Chernobyl: response of medical physics departments in the United Kingdom.* IPSM Report 50. IPSM, London.

24 International Atomic Energy Agency (1986). *Emergency planning and preparedness for nuclear facilities.*

25 NHS Executive (1998). *Planning for major accidents: the NHS guidance.* ID 98C 173/235.

26 National Council on Radiation Protection and Measurements (1979). *Management of persons accidentally contaminated with radionuclides.* NCRP Report 65. NCRB, Washington, DC.

27 Parshkov, E. M., Tsyb, A. F., Sokolov, V. A., and Chebotareva, I. V. (1998). *A model explaining thyroid cancer induction from Chernobyl radioactivity.* Meeting Proceedings of the International Radiological Post-Emergency Response Issues Conference, Washington, DC, USA, 9–11 September 1998. US Environment Protection Agency, EPA 402-S-98-001, pp. 195–8.

28 International Committee for Radiation Protection (1978). Report 28: The principles and general procedures for handling emergency and accidental exposures to workers. *Ann. ICRP*, **2** (Part 1).

29 Bottollier-Depois, J. F., Gaillard-Lecanu, E., Roux, A., Chau, Q., Trompier, F., Voisin, P., *et al.* (2000). New approach for dose reconstruction: application to one case of localised irradiation with radiological burns. *Health Phys.*, **79**, 251–6.

30 International Committee for Radiation Protection (1979–82). Report 30: Limits of intake of radionuclides by workers. Parts 1–3 each with supplements, and index. *Ann. ICRP*, **2** (Parts 3–4), **8**.

Part III

Ionising radiations in medicine and research

Part III is concerned with radiation protection relating to the applications of ionising radiations in hospitals. Chapter 11 considers the risks arising from diagnostic medical exposures and aspects to be taken into account in justification and optimisation of medical exposures. The other chapters deal with areas of application; namely diagnostic radiology (Chapters 12–14), radionuclide applications (Chapters 15 and 16), and radiotherapy (Chapters 17 and 18). Chapter 12 covers specification, testing, and use of X-ray equipment with emphasis on achieving a balance between patient dose and image quality, while Chapter 13 deals with the radiology facility, specification of shielding, and the protection of staff, and Chapter 14 covers patient dosimetry for all types of X-ray equipment. Chapter 15 contains information on radionuclide facilities and general precautions required for handling unsealed radionuclides and Chapter 16 covers dosimetry relating to the nuclear medicine patient and others involved with their care. Radiotherapy is divided into two parts: external beam therapy (Chapter 17) and therapy ward treatments (Chapter 18).

Symbols

absorbed dose	D (Gy)
air kerma incident on barrier/film	K_b/K_f (Gy)
air kerma rate at boundary due to primary beam	$\dot{K}^{pr}$
air kerma rate at boundar due to secondary radiation	$\dot{K}^{sc}$
angle of incidence / reflection	ϕ/Θ
area (cross-section of maze)	A (m^2)
area of field at phantom/patient	A_f (cm^2)
attenuation factor	η
barrier thickness in TVLs or HVLs	n_{TVL}, n_{HVL}
body surface area	B (m^2)
concentration of radioactivity	c (Bq volume^{-1})
cumulative activity in source organ	A_h (Bq h)
decay constant	λ (time^{-1})
distances from source to points of exposure	d (m)
duty cycle	C
effective dose	E (Sv)
effective energy	E_{eff} (eV)
effective half-life of activity in body	T_{eff} (days, h)
effective half-life of activity in source organ	$t_{1/2}$ (days, h)
effective ingest volume for breastfeeding	K (volume)
energy of β-particle	E_β(eV)
energy of γ-ray	E_γ(eV)
equivalent dose to tissue T (ICRP)	H_T (Sv)
equivalent activity of radionuclide to ^{131}I	A_{eq} (Bq)
factor equal to ratio $(\mu_{en}/\rho)_{medium}:(\mu_{en}/\rho)_{air}$	F
film speed	S (mGy^{-1})
fraction of administered activity passing through source organ	F_s
fraction of energy emitted in source organ	ϕ
fraction of time beam irradiates barrier	f_o
half-life (radioactive decay)	$T_{\frac{1}{2}}$ (s,d,h)
height of child	h (cm)

ingested activity from resumption of breastfeeding	I (Bq)
instantaneous dose rate (acceptable)	D'_{inst} (Gy h^{-1})
instantaneous dose rate at isocentre	D'_o (Gy min^{-1})
instantaneous dose rates	D' (Gy min^{-1})
instantaneous dose rate (unattenuated)	D'_B (Gy h^{-1})
length of CTDI chamber	L (mm)
mass	m (kg)
mass energy absorption coefficient	μ_{en}/ρ (kg^{-1} m^2)
number	n, N
radiation reflection coefficients	α (m^{-2})
radioactivity administered	A_o (Bq)
radioactivity initially in source organ	A_s (Bq)
residence time	τ (h)
scatter coefficient for 400 cm^2 field	α_{pat}
scatter fraction (for DAP)	S mGy (Gy cm^2)$^{-1}$
scatter kerma	K_s (Gy)
slice dose profile (CT)	$D(z)$ (Gy)
slice thickness (CT) (nominal)	T (mm)
S-value, mean dose to target organ per unit activity	$S(r_k < r_h)$
time	t (s)
tissue weighting factor	w_T, $w_{remainder}$
thickness of shielding material	x (mm)
time for breastfeeding to be interrupted	P (h)
transmission (material density ρ)	B, B_ρ
weight of child	w (kg)
workload	W_L (Gy $week^{-1}$)
X-ray tube current	A, mA (A)

Chapter 11
Risk control in medical exposures

C. J. Martin, D. G. Sutton, P. J. Mountford, and A. P. Hufton

11.1 Benefit versus risk

All medical exposures involve a balance between benefit and risk for the patient. Diseases of many types can be detected by X-ray or nuclear medicine examinations and their progress monitored, enabling appropriate treatment to be given at the correct stage. The patient benefits through successful treatment of disease, which may both prolong life and improve its quality. The benefit must be balanced against the radiation risk associated with the exposure. Failure to carry out an examination that is indicated can place a patient at significantly greater risk than that from radiation exposure. On the other hand, a procedure is of no value if it will not influence the management of the patient in any way and such an exposure will contribute an unnecessary risk.

11.2 Doses from medical exposures

Medical exposures contribute the largest component of the radiation dose to the population from artificial sources [1]. In the UK, 95% of the population dose for medical exposures comes from diagnostic examinations. The magnitude of the effective dose to the population from medical exposures depends on the frequency with which individual examinations are performed and the dose for each examination (Figure 11.1). There are

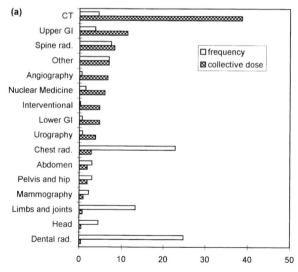

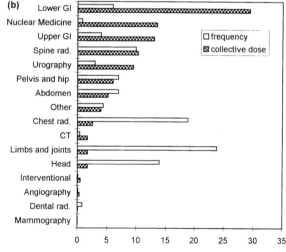

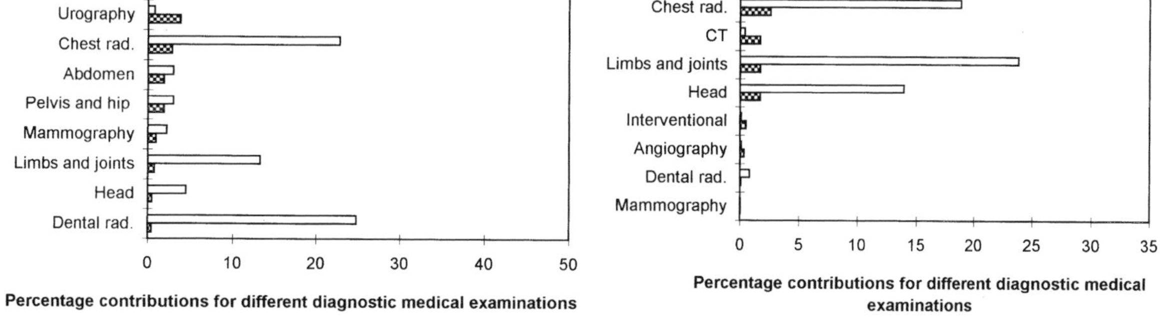

Figure 11.1 Relative frequencies and collective doses for groups of diagnostic medical radiation examinations, expressed as percentages of the total, during the period 1991–96 taken from UNSCEAR [2]. The data are for countries within healthcare levels as defined by UNSCEAR: (a) level I (more than 1 medical practitioner per 1000 population); (b) levels III and IV (less than 0.3 medical practitioner per 1000 population).

significant differences in the frequency and pattern of examinations in different countries. The United Nations Scientific Committee on the Effects of Radiation (UNSCEAR) define healthcare levels for global evaluation of practices. In countries within level I, where there is more than one medical practitioner per 1000 persons, there are on average 920 medical and 310 dental X-ray examinations per million population each year, while in countries in levels III and IV, where there is less than one doctor per 3000 persons, there are less than 20 medical and 0.2 dental radiation examinations per 1000 population each year. Average doses from medical exposures are estimated to be 0.4–0.5 mSv per year to each individual in Denmark, Finland, and the UK, 0.6–0.8 mSv per year in Australia, the Netherlands, Romania, Sweden, and the United States, 0.8–1.0 mSv per year in Australia and Russia, 1.1 mSv per year in Canada, and 2.0 mSv per year in Germany [2], while countries with less developed radiology provision have annual doses from medical exposures of less than 0.1 mSv per year, e.g. 0.09 mSv in China, 0.04 mSv in Malaysia, and 0.02 mSv in India [3]. The type of examination which contributes most to the collective dose in the developed world is computed tomography (CT) (Figure 11.1), which increased steadily during the 1990s. Angiography and interventional radiology also make substantially greater contributions to the collective dose in these countries. Within each country there are large variations in individual doses and certain persons will receive substantially higher doses than others. The number of examinations performed tends to increase with patient age; data collated by the National Radiological Protection Board (NRPB) during a survey of UK radiographic examinations showed the number of examinations peaking between ages 60 and 74 years [1] (see Figure 11.2).

Exposure to ionising radiation carries with it an increased risk of malignant disease (§3.4) and a risk of hereditary disease in descendants of the exposed person (§3.5). There is also the possibility of inducing deterministic effects (§3.3). However, the overall benefits from the diagnostic use of ionising radiation in medicine greatly exceed the small risks to the individual from the radiation exposure. The health of the population would decline if ionising radiation techniques were not available to diagnose disease and detect trauma. Nevertheless, there is no excuse for complacency and it is a basic premise of radiation protection practice that any exposure should be justified by weighing the potential harm against the perceived benefit. Furthermore, it is requisite that procedures should be adopted to ensure that techniques are optimised so that doses to individual patients are as low as compatible with the medical requirements of each examination.

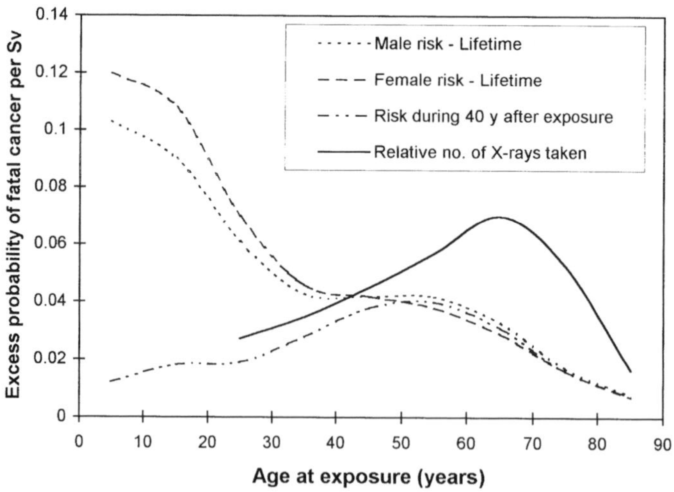

Figure 11.2 The mean lifetime excess probability of fatal cancer for males and females after an exposure giving a 1 mSv effective dose as a function of age at exposure from NRPB data [6]. In addition, the excess risk (mean for both sexes) during the 40 years following a 1 mSv exposure is shown. Data on the relative number of diagnostic radiology examinations as a function of age are also given on an arbitrary scale. These were derived from a patient dose survey based on data supplied to NRPB for national collation, where patient age was specified [1]. These data give an indication of the age distribution of patients examined, but the trend is likely to be biased towards that for the small selection of examinations included in the survey and is not necessarily representative of general UK practice.

Table 11.1 Probability coefficients for use in risk estimation from effective doses (Sv^{-1})

Effect	Whole population	Working population
Fatal cancer (worldwide) [5]	5.0×10^{-2}	4.0×10^{-2}
Fatal cancer (UK) [6]	5.9×10^{-2}	5.0×10^{-2}
Non-fatal cancer [5]	1.0×10^{-2}	0.8×10^{-2}
Severe hereditary effects [5]	1.3×10^{-2}	0.8×10^{-2}

Multiply cancer coefficients by 2 for paediatric patients and divide by 5 for patients over 60 years [8].

11.3 Risks from medical exposures

11.3.1 Stochastic risk and effective dose

The concept of effective dose was developed by ICRP [5] as the basis of risk estimation for occupational exposure, and was later adopted as a quantity which could be used to compare the risks to patients from different diagnostic examinations. It represents the uniform whole-body dose which would result in the same radiation risk as the non-uniform absorbed dose. Effective dose is relatively difficult to assess since it requires absorbed doses to a variety of organs to be estimated, and then weighted and summed according to the ICRP scheme outlined in Chapter 3. It is also impossible to measure directly, and has to be approximated in occupational exposure metrology with the operational dose quantities described in Box 4.1 and §8.1. Nevertheless, in concept it is directly related to stochastic radiation risk and provides an easy to understand link between radiation dose and the probability of harm associated with that dose. As such, it would appear to be an appropriate quantity to use when comparing relative risks from different diagnostic procedures, provided that its conceptual basis and genesis in the field of occupational exposure is kept in mind. In particular, it should be appreciated that effective dose is not a tool which can be used to determine with any degree of certainty the probability of harm to a specific individual resulting from a medical exposure. Examples of the methodology used to calculate effective dose are given in Boxes 11.1 and 16.1.

The harm experienced by an exposed group of persons and their descendants as a result of medical exposure, combined with an estimate of the severity of that harm, is termed the detriment. In its adoption of effective dose as a measure of harm, the ICRP used an aggregate representation of detriment which takes into account five factors. These are the probability of inducing a fatal cancer, the probability of inducing a non-fatal cancer, the probability of inducing hereditary effects, the severity of the last two effects compared to a fatal cancer, and the relative length of life lost for fatal cancers and hereditary effects. Detriment is dependent on the age at exposure, so the risk factors depend on the population group exposed. The probability coefficient (risk) for the overall (aggregated) detriment for the whole population is 7.3×10^{-2} Sv^{-1} and for the working population it is 5.6×10^{-2} Sv^{-1} [5]. Within the aggregated detriment there is a component which represents the excess risk of contracting a fatal cancer. The excess risks of fatal cancer vary with sex and age at the time of exposure and this is shown in Figure 11.2. However, more specific factors should be treated with caution because of the large uncertainty associated with their derivation.

11.3.2 Estimating stochastic risk

For the purpose of evaluating risks, the probabilities of stochastic radiation effects are assumed to be proportional to the effective dose with no dose threshold. Coefficients which may be used to estimate risks of inducing cancer or severe hereditary effects in adult patients are given in Table 11.1 [5]. The overall probability coefficients for radiation-induced cancer in the UK [6] are somewhat higher than the world average used by ICRP [5], reflecting the higher baseline cancer rates in the UK. The National Council on Radiation Protection and Measurements (NCRP) have published similar data for the US population, and also for Japan, Puerto Rico, the UK, and China [9]. Probability coefficients have also been derived relating to induction of fatal cancer for doses received by individual organs (Table 3.6), which may be used where exposure is predominantly of a single organ. Risks from fetal irradiation are discussed in Box 11.2.

One method for estimating the risk of inducing a fatal cancer is to determine the effective dose and multiply it by the fatal cancer risk probability coefficient (for example, 5.9×10^{-2} Sv^{-1} for the UK population, Table 11.1). However, this is an approximation, since effective dose includes weighted contributions from non-fatal cancers and hereditary effects. Table 11.2 illustrates the difference between this approximate method and the more precise one, whereby the product of the individual organ doses and organ-specific fatal cancer probability coefficients (Table 3.6) are summed to give the overall fatal cancer risk. Use of the approximate method is recommended as it is relatively easy to apply, and gives an order of magnitude indication of the fatal cancer risk, which is sufficient for

Box 11.1 Calculation of effective dose

The effective dose (E) is derived from the sum of the equivalent doses to individual organs (H_T) multiplied by their tissue weighting factors (w_T):

$$E = \sum_T w_T H_T$$

Twelve organs are given specific weighting factors (see table) and a further group of organs are included in the remainder and doses must be determined for all of these. For X-ray exposures, computer simulations using Monte Carlo techniques have been used to derive coefficients linking measurements of entrance surface dose or dose–area product to individual organ doses for different exposure parameters (§14.2.4), while for nuclear medicine procedures, similar data can be derived from the MIRD scheme (§16.2).

In ICRP 60, which introduced the concept of effective dose, 10 organs, namely the adrenals, brain, upper large intestine, small intestine, kidney, muscle, pancreas, spleen, thymus, and uterus, were included in the remainder. ICRP 80 [7] redefined the calculation method by including both lower and upper large intestine equivalent doses in the colon equivalent dose. The tissue weighting factor for the colon is applied to the mass average of the equivalent dose to the walls of the upper and lower large intestine (ULI, LLI) so that the colon dose is given by $D_{colon} = 0.57D_{ULI} + 0.43D_{LLI}$. As a result, there are now only nine remainder organs. It should be noted that some software used to calculate effective dose does not incorporate this modification.

Two examples are given here to illustrate the method used to calculate effective dose for radiological examinations and an example for nuclear medicine is given in Box 16.1. Example 1 is for an abdomen anterior posterior (AP) radiographic exposure made using an X-ray unit with 3 mm of aluminium filtration. The entrance surface dose is 4 mGy and the doses to individual organs have been obtained using NRPB report 262 [4]. The weighted sums of the doses to individual organs are summed to give the effective dose. ICRP recommend that the remainder organ dose should usually be taken as the mass weighted average of the doses to the nine organs included in the remainder. In this case, the bladder and stomach, which have their own weighting factors, received a higher dose than any of the remainder organs. However, if one of the remainder organs receives a higher dose, then a different method is used for the calculation. Example 2 shows a similar calculation for a right lateral lumbar spine radiograph taken with the same X-ray unit. The spleen, which is a remainder organ, receives a higher dose than any of the organs with their own weighting factors and it is given a weighting factor of 0.025 while the mean dose for the other eight remainder organs is given a weighting factor of 0.025. Because different criteria are used for calculating effective dose, depending on whether one of the main radiosensitive organs or one of the remainder organs has the highest dose, the effective dose should strictly be evaluated from the weighted sum of the doses to each organ for the whole of an examination or series of exposures given at one time.

On occasions, the method of calculation may produce somewhat artificial jumps in effective dose for particular radiological projections when tube potential is adjusted, because the organ receiving the highest dose changes. This occurs as a more superficial organ may receive the higher dose at a lower tube potential. For example, in

most circumstances. However, differences in risks derived from the two methods are often of the order of 50% and expression of results in a form which suggests a greater degree of precision is not justified and should be avoided. Typical doses for a selection of diagnostic medical examinations and lifetime risks calculated using the above approximate approach are given in Table 11.3.

The lifetime risk of radiation-induced cancer increases steadily with decreasing age below 40 years, but the risk in the 40 years following exposure is in fact greatest for those irradiated between 40 and 60 years of age, because they are entering the period of life when they are more likely to develop cancer (Figure 11.2, Table 3.7) [6]. The use of age-dependent probability coefficients is not recommended, but the application of simple correction factors, which involve multiplying the derived risk by 2 for paediatric patients or dividing by 5 for geriatric patients, is appropriate [8].

11.3.3 Risk from deterministic effects

In recent years the advent and increasing use of complex lengthy interventional X-ray procedures has meant that entrance surface doses can be sufficiently high to cause deterministic effects, such as skin erythema or temporary hair loss [12–14]. Procedures which have been associated with deterministic effects include RF cardiac catheter ablation, transjugular intrahepatic portosystemic stents, renal angioplasty, and coronary angioplasty [15]. In nuclear medicine, deterministic effects such as pruritus,

Box 11.1 *(Continued)*

paediatric AP chest radiographs, the thymus may receive a higher dose than the breast when higher kVs are used, but the breast, being more superficial, receives a higher dose at low kVs.

Calculations of effective dose depend critically on the proportions of the most radiosensitive organs exposed. Thus there may be significant differences in effective doses determined using Monte Carlo factors depending on the positions chosen for the X-ray field boundaries. This is particularly significant where a boundary falls within the abdominal area, which includes a number of radiosensitive organs, or where a boundary lies just above or below the thyroid. Care and judgement should therefore be used when carrying out such calculations. It is also important that the results of such calculations are not used in too prescriptive a manner, given the artificial nature of the quantity calculated.

Examples of effective dose calculations for two single radiographs

Organ or tissue	Example 1: Abdomen AP[a]			Example 2: R Lat Lumbar spine[b]		
	H_T (mSv)	w_T	$H_T w_T$ (mSv)	H_T (mSv)	w_T	$H_T w_T$ (mSv)
Gonads*	0.425	0.20	0.085	0.211	0.20	0.0422
Colon	0.995	0.12	0.1194	0.361	0.12	0.0433
Lung	0.023	0.12	0.0028	0.038	0.12	0.0046
Red bone marrow	0.111	0.12	0.0133	0.197	0.12	0.0236
Stomach	1.208	0.12	0.1450	0.474	0.12	0.0569
Bladder	1.62	0.05	0.0810	0.057	0.05	0.0028
Breast	0.01	0.05	0.0005	0.0054	0.05	0.0003
Liver	0.656	0.05	0.0328	0.042	0.05	0.0021
Oesophagus	0.032	0.05	0.0016	0.056	0.05	0.0028
Thyroid	0.00	0.05	0.0000	0.00	0.05	0.0000
Bone surface	0.161	0.01	0.0016	0.237	0.01	0.0024
Skin	0.266	0.01	0.0027	0.337	0.01	0.0034
Nine remainder organs: mean dose**	0.327	0.05	0.0164			
Remainder organ with highest dose				2.72	0.025	0.068
Eight remainder organs excluding organ with highest dose: mean dose				0.258	0.025	0.0065
Effective dose (E)			0.5			0.26

[a]Entrance surface dose = 4 mGy; tube potential = 70 kVp.
[b]Entrance surface dose = 10 mGy; tube potential = 80 kVp.
*Mean of ovary and testes. If the sex is known then either testes or ovary should be used.
**Masses of the remainder organs (ICRP 23) are: adrenals (14 g), brain (1400 g), small intestine (640 g), kidney (310 g), muscle (28 000 g), pancreas (100 g), spleen (180 g), thymus (20 g), and uterus (80 g).

Box 11.2 Fetal irradiation

The greatest risk from radiation exposure during pregnancy is the early induction of cancer in the offspring. The excess risk of fatal cancer up to age 15 years from exposure *in utero* is taken as 3×10^{-2} Sv^{-1} (1 in 30 000 per mSv) and the risk for all cancers during this period is double this (§3.6), while the possible risk of heritable disease is about 2.4×10^{-2} Sv^{-1} (1 in 40 000 per mSv) [6]. The incidence of cancer in later life, following irradiation *in utero*, is likely to be comparable to that for exposure of children (Table 11.1). Typical fetal doses from a selection of examinations are given in Table 11.3. In the first 3 weeks post-conception when pregnancy may not yet have been confirmed, it is considered that although the risk of cancer cannot be assumed to be zero, it should be much lower than during later stages. The most likely effect of exposure at this early stage is failure of the pregnancy to develop further. Possible deterministic effects to the fetus from 3 weeks onwards include gross malformations and fetal death [5, 6], but the threshold doses for these are well in excess of fetal doses from diagnostic investigations. For gestational ages between 8 and 15 weeks, there is a possible no-threshold response for the induction of severe mental retardation, with a predicted intelligence quotient (IQ) loss of 0.03 IQ points mSv^{-1} (§3.6.1). These predicted IQ losses would not be detectable on an individual basis for the fetal doses associated with diagnostic procedures.

Table 11.2 Comparison of methods for estimating fatal cancer risk

Examination	Probability of inducing a fatal cancer per 100 mGy entrance surface dose		
	Method A	Method B	Method A/Method B
Lateral skull	63.9×10^{-6}	45.6×10^{-6}	1.40
PA Chest	683×10^{-6}	520×10^{-6}	1.31
AP Abdomen	817×10^{-6}	675×10^{-6}	1.21
AP Pelvis	470×10^{-6}	805×10^{-6}	0.58

Calculations performed using NRPB-SR262 [10] and XDOSE [11] with typical kVs and filtrations.
Method A (accurate method): fatal cancer risk = individual organ dose × organ risk factor.
Method B (approximate method): fatal cancer risk = effective dose × overall fatal cancer risk (5×10^{-2} per Sv).
ICRP risk factors for the general population used.

Table 11.3 Effective doses and lifetime risks of cancer for an adult, a 5-year-old child, and exposures *in utero* from some common diagnostic medical examinations in the UK

Examination	Mean effective dose (mSv)	Risk of fatal cancer	Mean fetal dose (mGy)	Risk of cancer to age 15 for *in utero* exposure
Natural incidence		1 in 4.5		1 in 1300
Radiography (adult)				
Skull (PA)	0.03	1 in 700 000	< 0.01	< 1 in 3 million
Chest (PA)	0.02	1 in 1 million	< 0.01	< 1 in 3 million
Abdomen (AP)	0.7	1 in 30 000	1.4	1 in 24 000
Lumbar spine (AP and Lat)	1.0	1 in 20 000	1.7	1 in 20 000
Pelvis (AP)	0.7	1 in 30 000	1.1	1 in 30 000
Fluoroscopy/radiography (adult)				
Barium swallow	1.5	1 in 13 000		
Barium meal	3	1 in 7000	1.1	1 in 30 000
Barium enema	7	1 in 3000	6.8	1 in 5000
IVU	2.5	1 in 8000	1.7	1 in 20 000
X-ray CT (adult)				
Head	2	1 in 10 000	< 0.005	< 1 in 3 million
Chest	8	1 in 2500	0.06	1 in 500 000
Abdomen	10	1 in 2000	8.0	1 in 4000
Pelvis	10	1 in 2000	25	1 in 1300
Radiography (5-year-old child)				
Chest (PA)	0.01	1 in 1 million		
Abdomen (AP)	0.12	1 in 80 000		
Pelvis (AP)	0.08	1 in 120 000		
Nuclear medicine (adult)				
^{99m}Tc bone scan (phosphate)	3	1 in 7000	3.3	1 in 10 000
^{99m}Tc lung perfusion (MAA)	1	1 in 20 000	0.2	1 in 160 000
^{99m}Tc lung ventilation (aerosol)	0.4	1 in 50 000	0.3	1 in 110 000
^{99m}Tc dynamic cardiac scan (RBC)	7	1 in 3000	3.4	1 in 10 000
^{201}Tl myocardial perfusion	18	1 in 1000	3.7	1 in 9000
^{99m}Tc kidney MAG3	0.7	1 in 20 000	0.7	1 in 20 000

Data taken from various sources including references [1, 22, 23] and surveys performed by the authors, as representing typical doses.

Box 11.3 Research

The general principles stated in the context of biomedical research on human subjects by the World Medical Assembly (the Helsinki declaration) form the ethical basis for decisions on research and related aspects. In the UK, all research must be approved by a Local Research Ethics Committee, whether or not it has been submitted to a Multi-centre Research Ethics Committee. Proposals to ethics committees for research involving radiation usually require the effective dose to be stated. However, in some instances it may be more appropriate to give the dose to a single organ, if irradiation is largely limited to that organ. When a research project is of direct diagnostic or therapeutic relevance to the individual patient, the ethical problems involved tend to be simple ones. When, however, a project is intended to extend medical and scientific knowledge without specific benefit to the individual concerned, the problem becomes more complex.

No one should be subject to medical or other investigation without giving free and informed consent. This means that the risks and likely benefits of the research should be explained in advance. The most suitable approach is to include an explanation of the risk in the information leaflet supplied to subjects. The subject has the right to accept the risk voluntarily and has an equal right to refuse to accept. It is therefore difficult to carry out research on children or those of diminished mental capacity since they may well not be able to give appropriate consent. Pregnant women should not be asked to take part in research projects involving irradiation of the fetus unless the pregnancy itself is central to the research and then only if other techniques involving less risk cannot be used. It is usually prudent to consider the possibility that a woman may be pregnant but not know it. The protocol involved in the investigation should recognize this possibility. Within the European Community dose constraints must be set for volunteers participating in research projects to whom there is no direct medical benefit. For other participants in research, target doses must be set when planning the project.

ICRP have produced a scheme to aid in the assessment of research projects. The risk categories are given below. In the ICRP scheme, the lowest risk is of the order of one in a million and is in the region where people are usually content to dismiss the risk as trivial. ICRP conclude that 'the level of benefit needed as the basis for approval of investigations with risks or doses in Category I will be minor and would include those investigations expected only to increase knowledge.'

ICRP categories of risk and corresponding levels of benefit (from ICRP 62 [17])

Level of risk	Risk category	Corresponding effective dose range (adults) (mSv)	Level of societal benefit
Trivial	Category I ($\sim 10^{-6}$ or less)	< 0.1	Minor
Minor to intermediate	Category II		Intermediate to moderate
	IIa ($\sim 10^{-5}$)	0.1–1	
	IIb ($\sim 10^{-4}$)	1–10	
Moderate	Category III ($\sim 10^{-3}$ or more)	> 10[a]	Substantial

[a]To be kept below deterministic thresholds except for therapeutic experiments.

The highest risk category includes risks of the order of 1 in a 1000 or greater. The category covers exposures of 10 mSv or more—greater than the current annual dose limit for unclassified radiation workers. ICRP consider that to justify investigations involving doses or risks in Category III, the benefit would have to be substantial and usually directly related to the saving of life or the prevention or mitigation of serious disease. In circumstances in which the potential benefit is directly to the participant, an investigation in this category may be appropriate.

Between these two there is a category in which the risks, although neither trivial nor unacceptable, cannot readily be either accepted or used as the basis for refusal. ICRP make a distinction between (a) Category IIb similar in magnitude to those doses typically received by (some) workers each year, for which a moderate benefit is needed, and (b) Category IIa, a minor level of risk from doses similar in magnitude to those which might be received by members of the public from controlled sources, for which an intermediate benefit is nonetheless required. As further guidance, to justify risks in Category IIa the benefit will probably be related to increases in knowledge leading to health benefit. For risks in Category IIb the benefit will be more directly aimed at the cure or prevention of disease.

Box 11.4 Pregnant and breastfeeding patients

Advice about radiation exposure of women of childbearing age has varied with time. In the 1950s and early 1960s exposure of patients known to be pregnant was avoided where possible. Reservations about irradiation of the fetus during the early phases of pregnancy led to the widespread adoption of a 10-day rule in the mid-1960s. This involved restriction of exposures to the abdomen of women of childbearing age to the 10 days following the last menstrual period. In the 1980s ICRP concluded that radiosensitivity was minimal during the early weeks after fertilization and a revised 28-day rule approach was recommended. In the 1990s, evidence of possible radiobiological damage from irradiation during the first few weeks of pregnancy led to use of a version of the 10-day rule for higher dose examinations. Changes in recommendations with time have led to confusion about which practice should be adopted.

Current advice is that there is no risk from diagnostic medical exposures during the first 10 days of the menstrual cycle, and no special limitations need apply during the remainder of the cycle for most radiation examinations. A woman should be treated as though she was pregnant if her period is overdue or clearly missed. The National Radiological Protection Board (NRPB) considers that exposures of 'tens of mGy' approximately double the natural risk of childhood cancer in the unborn child [6] from an age of about 3 weeks onwards. NRPB recommends that procedures resulting in such fetal doses should be avoided even in early pregnancy unless there is an overriding clinical need, and that one way of eliminating this risk is by restricting these procedures to the first 10 days of the menstrual cycle. Examples of procedures which may result in such doses are pelvic and abdomen CT examinations and barium enemas.

It should be remembered that if an essential examination is rearranged because of this recommendation, and if the patient subsequently proves to be pregnant, the fetal risk will increase following the first missed period. High-dose procedures for a pregnant patient should only be rescheduled if they are not essential to the patient management and can be safely postponed until after delivery of the child [22].

In the case of nuclear medicine examinations it is also important that steps should be taken to ensure that the patient is not breastfeeding since some activity will appear in the milk (§16.5).

The following procedures may be adopted to reduce the likelihood of giving a medical exposure to a female patient without realizing that she is pregnant or breastfeeding.

- The request form should ask whether the patient may be pregnant and, for a nuclear medicine examination, breastfeeding. The date of the last menstrual period should also be requested on the card.
- Signs should be displayed prominently in waiting areas asking patients to inform staff if they are pregnant (or breastfeeding). These signs may need to be written in more than one language, and may include an appropriate pictorial representation of the question in case of reading difficulties.
- Female patients of childbearing age (12–55 years) should be questioned directly and discretely just before the X-ray examination or administration of radiopharmaceutical.

erythema, and ulceration are observed occasionally when all or part of a radiopharmaceutical injection has been extravasated (a misadministration) (§16.4.2).

The induction of deterministic effects is the aim of radiotherapeutic exposures. The prescribed dose should be delivered to the treatment volume and optimisation performed to minimize the dose to the surrounding healthy tissue and organs. There is considerable risk to the patient should the exposure be too large or, indeed, smaller than prescribed. This topic is central to radiotherapy physics and is well covered in more specialized texts [16] .

11.4 Justification of exposures

Justification of medical exposures is primarily the responsibility of the medical profession. As pointed out in §6.2 the process involves decisions at two levels, the generic and the individual. At the generic level, one is concerned with practices. These are defined in broad terms relating to their objectives which include the following.

Examinations or treatments directly associated with illness or injury

The expected clinical benefit associated with each type of procedure should have been demonstrated to be sufficient to offset the radiation detriment. The benefit of practices using ionising radiation for treatment or diagnosis can be assessed by considering how the practice will influence the subsequent patient management. In the case of diagnosis consideration should be given to whether other types of examination which do not involve ionising radiations such as ultrasound, magnetic resonance imaging (MRI), or endoscopy can be used to provide the necessary information. In the case of treatment, complex clinical factors must be taken into account.

Box 11.4 *(continued)*

- For high-dose procedures where the average fetal dose would be some tens of mGy, it is recommended that the examination is undertaken in the first 10 days following the last menstrual period, when the patient is unlikely to be pregnant (see above).
- A pregnancy test may be carried out as a matter of routine for high-dose procedures.

If the patient is, or is likely to be, pregnant or breastfeeding, then the justification for the examination should be reviewed. The justification process should acknowledge that a radiation exposure of benefit to the mother may or may not be of indirect benefit to the fetus or infant. ARSAC recommends that a radionuclide procedure resulting in an absorbed dose to the fetus of more than 1.0 mGy requires particular justification [23]. Any procedure should be justified and optimised by considering the following questions:

- Is the requested procedure essential?
- Is there an alternative procedure not involving a radiation exposure?
- Can the procedure be delayed until after childbirth or until the mother has given up breastfeeding?
- Is there an alternative procedure which would give a lower dose to the fetus or infant?
- What is the possibility of further medical exposures which will result in a dose to the fetus? If the mother is to have any further radiation procedures, then the total effective dose to the fetus from these must be considered. Similar methods should be applied to consideration of the implications for a potential nuclear medicine patient who is breastfeeding (§16.5).

If it is decided to proceed with an examination, then special attention needs to be given to ways of minimizing the dose, consistent with the clinical requirements. For example, in diagnostic radiology:

- a posterior anterior (PA) projection might be used for an abdominal radiograph of a pregnant patient
- lower dose options may be employed for computed radiography, CT, or fluoroscopy, where practicable (§12.3)
- particular attention should be paid to beam collimation
- additional shielding may be employed.

In the case of a nuclear medicine patient, less than the usual administered activity might be used provided that a diagnostic result can be assured or an alternative technique employed (e.g. Box 11.5). Recommendations for reducing the dose to a breastfed infant are given in §16.5.4.

Periodic health checks or mass screening of asymptomatic patients and employees

Mass screening must be justified by weighing the total benefit against the total detriment of the radiation exposure, including health detriment and economic cost of the programme.

Examinations for medico-legal or insurance purposes

Critical assessment of the need for exposures for medico-legal or insurance purposes is particularly important because of the lack of direct medical benefit to the individual. However, benefits to society as a whole can be considered in the justification process.

Examinations or treatments forming part of a medical research programme

There is considerable guidance on research involving medical exposures [17–20] and the subject is considered in Box 11.3.

The second level of justification is in respect of individual patients for whom there must be a net benefit. This will be the responsibility of a trained healthcare professional who may or may not be medically qualified. This person is often called a practitioner and is usually a radiologist or an oncologist, but in some cases may come from another group, e.g. a cardiologist or a radiographer. The clinician who refers the patient must supply the appropriate relevant clinical information such as the patient's personal details, symptoms, medical history, current treatment, and details of any previous radiological investigations. Guideline referral criteria have been published [21]. Appropriate referral procedures should enable the practitioner who is responsible for justification to assess the relevance of the investigation and how the diagnosis or treatment will affect subsequent management of the patient. A diagnostic procedure is not justified if it cannot be carried out, and, in particular, a report issued within a timescale to affect the clinical management of the patient. Part of the justification process is to consider whether there are alternative methods which either do not give a radiation dose to the patient or give a lower radiation dose. Of particular concern is the female patient who is or might be pregnant, and for nuclear medicine, the female patient who is breastfeeding (Box 11.4).

11.5 Optimisation

11.5.1 Optimisation of technique

For optimisation to be successful, appropriate decisions must be made about what is reasonably achievable. Adoption of systematic procedures and standardization of criteria for making judgements will assist in the optimal use of resources. Appropriate procedures must be in place and adequate resources allocated to ensure that delays in conveying information from examinations are minimized. If a report reaches the referring clinician too late to affect clinical management, then the patient has had an unnecessary radiation exposure. The optimisation process includes design, selection, and maintenance of equipment (§12.5) as well as adoption of procedures commensurate with obtaining the necessary diagnostic information using the lowest radiation dose that can be reasonably achieved (§12.3). The quality of clinical images must be maintained at a level which is sufficient for the intended purpose [24].

The wide variation in doses for diagnostic radiology procedures reported in surveys shows that there is significant scope for optimisation. For example, improvements in sensitivity of film/screen combinations and image intensifiers and refinement of techniques resulted in a 30–40% reduction in effective doses for most common radiographic and fluoroscopic examinations in the UK over the period 1984 to 1995 [1]. Particular care is required in optimisation of techniques for procedures where skin doses may be high enough to induce deterministic effects [14, 25].

Another important aspect of optimisation is protection of other organs near to the examination site. In diagnostic radiology, specialized shielding is used for radiosensitive organs such as the gonads, and protocols which minimize the exposure of the eyes are used for examinations such as head CT to reduce the risk of deterministic effects in the eye lens. In addition, projections may be chosen in which radiosensitive organs are further from the surface on which the X-ray beam is incident, such as posterior anterior chest (to protect the breasts) and left lateral lumbar spine (to protect the sigmoid colon). Care must be taken to ensure that such strategies do not compromise the diagnostic quality of the image. In nuclear medicine, doses to the thyroid are reduced by use of thyroid-blocking agents when a radio-iodine labelled compound is employed for investigation of another part of the body. Doses to the bladder and surrounding organs are minimized by encouraging patients to drink after a procedure is completed and to empty their bladder as frequently as possible.

11.5.2 Diagnostic reference levels

It is not appropriate to apply dose limits to medical exposures since there is by definition a direct benefit to the patient. Instead, quantitative guidance on levels of dose for different examinations are available in terms of reference dose levels. These are clinical audit tools and can function as local investigation levels and provide a practical device for use in dose optimisation by helping to identify poor practice.

In diagnostic radiology, reference levels are set on the basis of observed practice from surveys of measured dose levels for patients of average size in hospitals, preferably at national but conceivably at regional or local levels. An internal investigation might be triggered if the mean dose for a radiographic procedure in a department exceeds the reference level. For complex examinations involving both fluoroscopy and radiography, the reference level might be used as an investigation level for individual practitioners or as a warning indicator during an examination to highlight to the practitioner that the dose level is significant. If reference levels are exceeded frequently, steps should be taken to improve practice by changing technique or equipment or even by re-evaluation of the reference dose if it is shown to have been set at too low a level.

In nuclear medicine diagnostic reference levels are established in terms of administered activity. Guidance notes produced in the UK by the Administration of Radioactive Substances Advisory Committee (ARSAC) recommend maximum activities for established diagnostic procedures using specific radiopharmaceuticals [23]. Since the majority of hospitals use the levels recommended or lower, there is less interdepartment variation in dose than in diagnostic radiology. ARSAC certificate holders have the discretion to vary the administered activity for individual patients through special justification where there are sound clinical reasons.

Dose reduction must be combined with assessment of image quality [26]. Doses must not be reduced to the level where the quality of images is inadequate for the intended purpose, but the level of image quality should be adapted to the clinical problem. A concept of achievable doses has been proposed [27], based on mean doses from departments meeting image quality criteria.

These represent realistic dose levels that should be readily achievable using good practice, rather than those that are achievable with full optimisation.

11.5.3 The paediatric patient

The risk coefficient for fatal cancer associated with radiation exposure of children under 15 years is more than double that for adult patients (Figure 11.2). Therefore, the balance between radiation risk and benefit to the patient is of greater significance, and special facilities should be available for carrying out paediatric procedures. In radiology, specialized techniques and exposure factor options on equipment are used for paediatric examinations. However, because patients are generally smaller, the radiation intensity and the radiation dose are lower for radiographic and fluoroscopic procedures, and the associated risks are less than in adult examinations (Table 11.3). Nevertheless, optimisation is important, because certain individuals may have large numbers of X-ray examinations in the early part of life. Doses for CT examinations on paediatric patients may not be lower than for adults and particular attention should be paid to optimisation in this case.

In nuclear medicine lower activities may be administered (§16.6). There may sometimes be a competing factor that the time required for the child to keep still needs to be kept to a minimum and this may require the administered activity to be increased. This must be considered in optimisation of the technique. If necessary, a sedative can be administered, and for very young infants, withholding their feed until just before the scan may be sufficient for them to fall asleep.

11.5.4 Avoidance of repeat investigations

In optimising the strategy for each patient, failure to obtain a diagnostic outcome after the patient has received a radiation dose must be avoided. Factors that need to be taken into account include the following.

- When a diagnostic outcome requires more than one type of investigation, then they must be carried out in a sequence which ensures that an earlier study does not interfere with the outcome of a later one.
- All the images recorded from a procedure should be checked before the patient leaves the department, and preferably before getting off the imaging couch.
- A programme should be in place in diagnostic radiology departments, in which reasons for rejected films are analysed and action is taken to remedy any poor practices identified.
- Where possible, previous radiographs should be obtained since this may avoid repeating an examination.
- For nuclear medicine investigations staff should ensure that instructions for stopping medication, food, or drink which may interfere with the investigation are issued to the patient before the procedure, and that they are understood by the patient. Where practicable, a copy of the report should be kept in the department.

11.5.5 Incidents

It is important to have an agreed policy for dealing with incidents relating to patient exposure, such as an accidental overexposure. This should include the reporting chain and the level of responsibility at each stage of that chain (§10.5.1). All staff must be familiar with the procedures to follow in the event of an incident, particularly the need to record all actions taken and all necessary data, and the need to notify immediately the clinician responsible for the patient and/or the head of department. Unless there are overwhelming reasons to the contrary, it is advisable for the clinician to inform the patient as soon as possible in order to maintain their confidence. A decision has to be taken as to whether the incident is notifiable to external statutory agencies (see §10.5.1). A preliminary investigation should be carried out at the earliest opportunity. Attention should be directed at whether procedures should be revised, particularly the use of additional checking, whether staff need to be retrained, or whether equipment should be modified or even replaced.

11.6 Explanation of risk

Explanation of risk may need to be given in a variety of circumstances such as:

- where a patient is concerned about the risk from an exposure he/she needs to undergo
- where a patient who is pregnant needs to have an examination involving a fetal exposure
- where a patient who is breastfeeding needs to undergo a nuclear medicine procedure
- following an unintended patient exposure or an overexposure
- when ionising radiation is used in a research project.

It is important to explain risks to the patient, members of the patient's family, and even the referring clinician in a form which can be readily understood. People are concerned with the risk for an individual and want to know the chance that they might become ill. A large body of epidemiological data exists on the risk from radiation exposure on which an assessment can be based (Chapter 3). An evaluation may be carried out in terms of relative or absolute risk. The problem with both of these methods is that the general public's perception of risk is usually very poor.

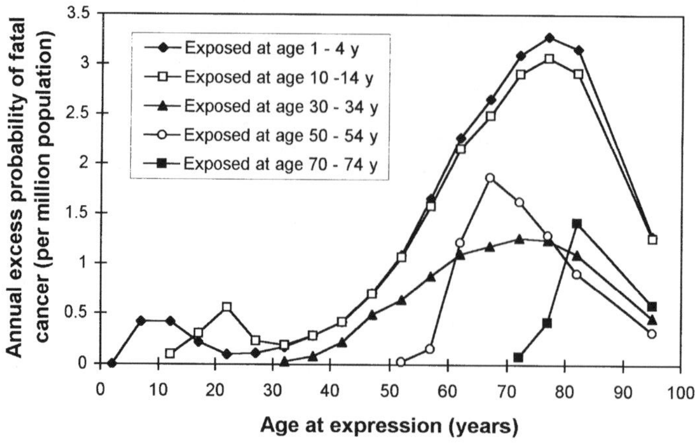

Figure 11.3 Predicted probabilities of radiation-induced fatal cancer as a function of age, following a single exposure giving an effective dose of 1 mSv to a female for five different ages taken from NRPB report 261 [28]. There are two components to the risk portrayed in these results. The probabilities of leukaemia and bone cancer start to increase about 2 years after exposure, reaching a peak after about 8 years, while the increased risk of solid tumours, following a latent period of 10 years or more, is related to the natural incidence in the population (§3.4.1).

11.6.1 Relative and absolute risk

There are a variety of ways in which an indication of risk can be conveyed. A simple explanation can be given by comparing the effective dose from the medical procedure with that from another, more familiar, source of radiation exposure. This could involve comparison with the dose from exposure to natural background radiation for an appropriate length of time (2.3 mSv $year^{-1}$ or 0.05 mSv $week^{-1}$ in the UK) (§10.2) or that from a number of X-rays of the chest or lumbar spine (Table 11.3). Alternatively, a comparison can be made with doses received from other activities. For example, an additional dose of 0.1 mSv will be incurred by a resident of the UK for every week spent in Cornwall or for a return transatlantic flight. This technique provides a comparison with another activity from which the risk is usually perceived as being low or acceptable, but does not give a direct indication of risk.

The risk of potential harm associated with radiation exposure can be evaluated in absolute terms using the probability coefficients in Table 11.1. Average effective doses and lifetime risks for a variety of diagnostic examinations are given in Table 11.3. These risks of cancer occur over a lifetime and are derived using the multiplicative risk model (§3.4) in which the additional risk is related to the natural incidence of cancer in the population. According to this model, the risks associated with most cancers vary with age in relation to the natural incidence. In Figure 11.3, a series of curves are shown which portray how the mean probability of death from radiation-induced cancer varies with age following single radiation exposures [28]. Each curve represents an exposure received at a different age. Exposures received below the age of 20 years have a higher lifetime risk associated with them, although the period when death resulting from the radiation exposure is most likely to occur will be when the individual reaches an age of 60–90 years. Lifetime risks are usually quoted for radiation exposures, because of the variation in risk with age.

The lifetime probability coefficients (Table 11.1) allow the risk to be defined in terms of effects on populations with statements about the incidence of disease. However, the numbers can give a false impression of precision and there is no indication that they may be highly uncertain or hotly disputed. Small risks, such as 1 in 10 000 or a probability of 0.0001 are difficult to conceptualize. A study comparing public perception of the number of individuals who died each year with the actual number, for a wide range of activities and occurrences, showed that individuals placed all events within a narrower probability range of 10^3 compared with the actual one of over 10^6 (Figure 11.4) [29]. Thus, if the aim is to give a rough idea of orders of magnitude, familiar comparators such as 'about one person in a small town' for 1 in 10 000 may be

Table 11.4 Community risk scale

Risk	Comparable population
1 in 10	Family
1 in 100	Street
1 in 1000	Village
1 in 10 000	Small town
1 in 100 000	Large town
1 in 1 million	City
1 in 10 million	Small country
1 in 100 million	Large country

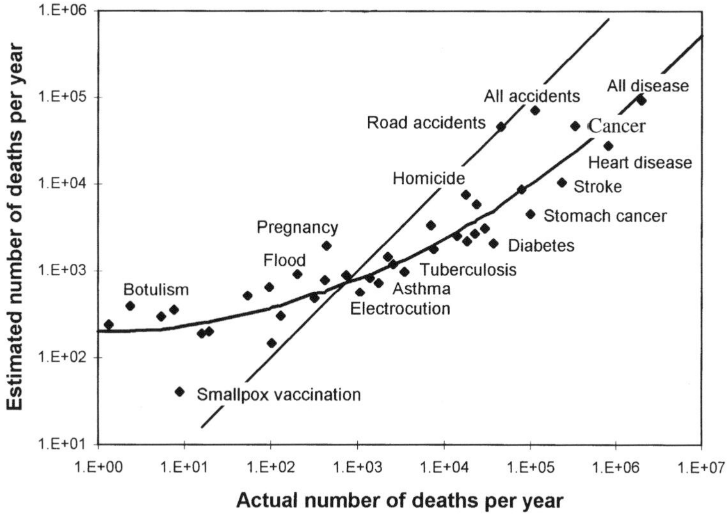

Figure 11.4 Plot of the perception of the number of deaths in a year from various causes in the United States (population 2.3E+08), derived from the averaged responses given by a sample from the population, against the actual number of deaths [29]. If the estimated number equalled the actual one, the data would lie on the straight line rather than follow the curve. The estimates were within a range of 10^3, whereas the actual range covered was over 10^6. Data were taken from the results of Fischhoff *et al.* [29].

preferable. These and other risk factors have been developed into a community risk scale (Table 11.4), which may be useful to set probabilities in context [30].

Another popular way of communicating risk is to compare risks from different sources, such as smoking 10 cigarettes per day or driving a car. Such comparisons are thought of as calibrating public perceptions of risk against real mortality statistics. They may be useful in providing a sense of perspective and some risks associated with other activities are given in Table 11.5. However, the brain tends to manipulate these risks in ways that can ignore this logic. Risk comparisons have a poor reputation as practical aids to communication [30, 31], since they omit the effects of the 'fright factors' associated with radiation (§1.3) and do not take account of the values of the audience. One problem is that there is generally a significant overestimate of the likelihood of death due to unusual or dramatic causes, such as floods or plane crashes. These events have a high profile in the press and are easily brought to mind and so are perceived to be more frequent. On the other hand, there is an underestimation of common killers such as heart disease and cancer (Figure 11.4). A problem where comparisons are made with risks from leisure activities is that there is a greater willingness to accept voluntary risks, which may reflect the value placed on personal autonomy. Risks taken by mountaineers and racing drivers may have a positive attraction. Thus responses to risk are intimately bound up with wider values.

Probabilities can also be given in relative terms (the chance has doubled) rather than absolute terms (the chance was 2% and is now 4%) and this may have a significant effect on the perceived message. For example, if 1 million people are exposed to two fatal risks, news that risk A has doubled may sound more alarming than news that risk B has increased by 10%. But if the baseline probabilities of death from A and B are 1 in 10^6 and 1 in 10^4 respectively, doubling risk A produces one extra fatality, while the apparently smaller increase in risk B will kill 10 more people. This type of relative risk explanation is sometimes used in discussion of the risk of childhood cancer following fetal exposure, but is not applied to the overall risk of malignancy because of the high natural incidence.

11.6.2 Communication of risk

When communicating an idea of the risk to a patient or guardian, it is important to adopt an open approach. A candid account of the situation should be given, making all the information available and answering all the questions raised. This type of approach is more likely to elicit the trust of the patient. An explanation of the benefit from the exposure and the potential risk if it is not carried out must be given. Care should be taken that the message is compatible with the action taken. An important element of the consultation is being ready to listen. This enables the concerns of the individual to be addressed and avoids taking too narrow a view of the issues. Some patients may be absorbed by the risks inherent in their disease while others may be more

Table 11.5 Lifetime risks of death from radiation exposure and other causes (unless otherwise stated, the risks relate to an individual aged 40 and activities undertaken within the remainder of their life)

Term for risk	Range of risks	Example causes	Risk estimate
Negligible	Less than 1:1 million	Hand or foot X-ray	< 1:10 million
		Chest X-ray	1:1 million
		Drinking 30 cans of diet soda (saccharin)	1:1 million
Minimal	Between 1:1 million and 1:100 000	Skull (PA) X-ray	1:700 000
		Killed by lightning	1:300 000
		100 hours of rail travel	1:200 000
Very low	Between 1:100 000 and 1:10 000	Anaesthesia (risk from single administration)	1:50 000
		Flood	1:30 000
		Commercial aviation from 1000 miles jet travel per year	1:30 000
		Eating one peanut butter sandwich per week	1:30 000
		Lumbar spine X-ray	1:20 000
Low	Between 1:10 000 and 1:1000	Barium meal	1:7000
		Work in service industry	1:6000
		Electrocution	1:4000
		Murder	1:3000
		Work in manufacturing industry	1:2500
		Abdomen CT scan	1:2000
		Accident at work	1:2000
Moderate	Between 1:1000 and 1:100	Cycling for 300 miles per year for next 30 years (accident)	1:1000
		Additional risk of fatal cancer from work with ionising radiation 1 mSv per year from 40 to 65 years	1:800
		Work in construction	1:800
		Accident on the road	1:500
		Accident at home	1:400
		Suicide	1:200
		Living in large city (air pollution)	1:160
High	Greater than 1:100	Chronic liver disease	1:90
		Pneumonia and influenza	1:30
		Additional risk of fatal cancer in Japanese survivors of atomic bombs over first 40 years per Sv	1:20
		Smoking 10 cigarettes per day	1:5
		All cancers	1:4
		Heart disease	1:3

Data were derived for the UK population [30, 32] but were supplemented with some data derived from the US population on specific risks. Where lifetime risks were not available, annual risks were multiplied by 35, assuming that on average a 40-year-old individual will live to age 75 years.

concerned about the side-effects of treatment. In most cases, the explanation would be given by the referring clinician, since the risks will depend on the patient's clinical condition and circumstances. Descriptive terms that have been developed to describe risks of different magnitude [33] and might be used in explanations to patients are included in Table 11.5.

11.6.3 Advice to a pregnant patient

Before appropriate advice can be given to a pregnant patient, an estimate must be made of the fetal dose, and the stage of the pregnancy must be established. The corresponding risks of deterministic and stochastic effects can then be estimated and the mother advised of these risks. A comparison can be made with the natural incidence of babies born with congenital malformations, which is estimated to be 1–3 in 100, and the cumulative risk for fatal childhood cancer up to the age of 15 years, which is 1 in 1300 [6]. Fetal doses of tens of mGy more than double the natural cancer risk in the unborn child. The patient must also be advised of the risks associated with not carrying out the procedure. Even the highest fetal doses from diagnostic procedures are unlikely to justify the risks associated with invasive fetal diagnostic procedures (such as amniocentesis) or to justify termination of pregnancy [6]. In nuclear medicine, advice should also be given to the patient on any further steps which she can take to reduce the fetal dose. An example of the formulation of advice on risks and dose reduction for a nuclear medicine patient is given in Box 11.5.

11.6.4 Advice on avoidance of conception

There may be a need to avoid conception for a period of time after a medical exposure, because of irradiation of a parent's germ cells or, in nuclear medicine, the potential for irradiation of the embryo by a longer half-life radionuclide retained in the mother or appearing in the father's ejaculate and sperm. Precautions for diagnostic examinations are required only for nuclear medicine procedures where a radionuclide with a half-life greater than 7 days has been administered to a female patient. However, restrictions may be required in therapeutic procedures and these are discussed in §16.4.3.

Box 11.5 An example of the formulation of advice to a pregnant patient

A ventilation–perfusion lung scan is requested for a female patient who is 10 weeks pregnant for a suspected pulmonary embolism. [This is probably the most frequently requested nuclear medicine procedure for a pregnant woman.]

The routine practice at this particular hospital is to inhale about 30 MBq ^{99m}Tc–DTPA (aerosol) for the ventilation scan, followed by an intravenous administration of 100 MBq ^{99m}Tc–MAA for the perfusion scan.

What is the appropriate advice?

Dose estimate

At 10 weeks, it can be considered that the fetal absorbed dose is the same as the uterine absorbed dose. Using data in ICRP 53 and 80 [7, 34]:

Total fetal absorbed dose = 0.18 (ventilation scan) + 0.24 (perfusion scan) mGy = 0.42 mGy

Deterministic effects

The predicted IQ loss in the fetus = 0.03 IQ points mGy^{-1} × 0.42 mGy = 0.01 IQ points
(not detectable on an individual basis)

Stochastic effects

The risk of heritable disease = (2.4×10^{-5} mGy^{-1}) × (0.42 mGy) = 1 in 100 000
The risk of fatal cancer = (3.0×10^{-5} mGy^{-1}) × (0.42 mGy) = 1 in 80 000
[These risks can be reduced to about 1 in 170 000 and 1 in 140 000 respectively by the use of ^{81m}Kr gas for the ventilation scan, and can be reduced even further if it is diagnostically acceptable to use a lower activity of ^{99m}Tc-MAA.]

Comparison

The risk of a baby being born with a congenital malformation was about 1 in 56 in England and Wales during 1989, and the natural cumulative risk of fatal childhood cancer is about 1 in 1300 in England and Wales.

What is the risk of not carrying out the investigation?

This example represents a potentially fatal condition, and therefore the risks associated with not carrying out the investigation can be given as the number of deaths from pulmonary embolism during pregnancy (16 in the UK during the period 1985–87).

Dose reduction

The ^{99m}Tc-DTPA will be absorbed through the lung and excreted by the kidneys. Free ^{99m}Tc-pertechnetate will dissociate from the ^{99m}Tc-MAA and will also be excreted by the kidneys. Therefore, to reduce the contribution of the bladder activity to the fetal dose, the patient should be encouraged to drink plenty of fluid and to empty her bladder as often as possible in order to hasten excretion.

11.7 References

1 Hart, D., Hillier, M. C., Wall, B. F., Shrimpton, P. C., and Bungay, D. (1996). *Doses to patients from medical X-ray examinations in the UK–1995 review*. NRPB Report R289. NRPB, Chilton.

2 United Nations Scientific Committee on the Effects of Atomic Radiation (2000). *Sources and effects of ionising radiation. Vol. I Sources, Vol. II Effects*. United Nations, New York.

3 Ng, K.-H., Abdullah, B. J. J., and Sivalingam, S. (1999). Medical radiation exposures for diagnostic radiology in Malaysia. *Health Phys.*, **77**, 33–6.

4 Hart, D., Jones, D. G., and Wall, B. F. (1994). *Estimation of effective dose in diagnostic radiology from entrance surface dose and dose–area product measurements*. NRPB-R262. NRPB, Chilton.

5 International Commission on Radiological Protection (1991). 1990 Recommendations of the International Commission on Radiological Protection. ICRP Publication 60. *Ann. ICRP*, **21** (1–3).

6 National Radiological Protection Board (1993). Board statement on diagnostic medical exposures to ionising radiation during pregnancy and estimates of late radiation risks to the UK population. *Doc. NRPB*, **4** (4).

7 International Commission on Radiological Protection (1999). Radiation dose to patients from radiopharmaceuticals. Addendum to ICRP 53. ICRP Publication 80. *Ann. ICRP*, **28** (3).

8 National Radiological Protection Board (1993). Occupational, public and medical exposure. *Doc. NRPB*, **4** (2).

9 National Council on Radiation Protection and Measurements (1993). *Risk estimates for radiation protection*. NCRP Report 115. NCRP, Bethesda.

10 Hart, D., Jones, D. G., and Wall, B. F. (1994). *Normalised organ doses for medical X-ray examinations calculated using Monte Carlo techniques*. NRPB-SR262. NRPB, Chilton.

11 Le Heron, J. C. (1994). *XDOSE: Program utilizing NRPB data to calculate organ doses and effective doses*. Available from J. C. Le Heron, National Radiation Laboratory, Ministry of Health, Christchurch, New Zealand.

12 Huda, W. and Peters, K. R. (1994). Radiation induced temporary epilation after a neuroradiologically guided embolization procedure. *Radiology*, **193**, 642–4.

13 Wagner, L. K., Eifel, P. J., and Geise, R. A. (1994). Potential biological effects following high X-ray dose interventional procedures. *J. Vasc. Interv. Radiol.*, **5**, 71–84.

14 Norbash, A. M., Busick, D., and Marks, M. P. (1996). Techniques for reducing interventional neuroradiologic skin dose: tube position, rotation and supplemental beam filtration. *Am. J. Neuroradiol.*, **17**, 41–9.

15 Shope, T. B. (1996). Radiation-induced skin injuries from fluoroscopy. *Radiographics*, **16** (5), 1195–9.

16 Williams, J. R. and Thwaites, D. (2000). *Radiotherapy physics in practice* (2nd edn). Oxford University Press.

17 International Commission on Radiological Protection (1991). 1990 radiological protection in biomedical research. ICRP Publication 62. *Ann. ICRP*, **22** (3).

18 European Commission (1998). *Radiation protection 99. Guidance on exposures in medical and biomedical research*. European Communities, Luxembourg.

19 European Commission (1997). Council Directive 97/43/Euratom of 30 June 1997 on health protection of individuals against the dangers of ionising radiation in relation to medical exposure, and repealing Directive 84/466/Euratom. *Off. J. Eur. Communities*, No. L180/22. European Commission, Luxembourg.

20 Department of Health (2000). *The Ionising Radiation (Medical Exposure) Regulations 2000*.

21 Royal College of Radiologists (1998). *Making the best use of a department of clinical radiology – guidelines for doctors* (4th edn). RCR, London.

22 Sharp, C., Shrimpton, J. A., and Bury, R. F. (1998). *Diagnostic medical exposures. Advice on exposure to ionising radiation during pregnancy*. NRPB, Chilton.

23 Administration of Radioactive Substances Advisory Committee (1998). *Notes for guidance on the clinical administration of radiopharmaceuticals and use of sealed radioactive sources*. Department of Health, London.

24 Martin, C. J., Sutton, D. G., and Sharp, P. F. (1999). Balancing patient dose and image quality. *Appl. Radiat. Isot.*, **50**, 1–19.

25 Food and Drug Administration (1994). *Avoidance of serious X-ray induced skin injuries to patients during fluoroscopically guided procedures*. Public Health Advisory: September 30, 1994, FDA, Washington, DC.

26 Martin, C. J., Sharp, P. F., and Sutton, D. G. (1999). Measurement of image quality in diagnostic radiology. *Appl. Radiat. Isot.*, **50**, 21–38.

27 National Radiological Protection Board (1999). Guidelines on patient dose to promote the optimisation of protection for diagnostic medical exposures. *Doc. NRPB*, **10** (1).

28 Stokell, P. J., Robb, J. D., Crick, M. J., and Muirhead, C. R. (1993). *SPIDER-1: Software for evaluating the detriment associated with radiation exposure*. NRPB Report R261. NRPB, Chilton.

29 Fischhoff, B., Lichtenstein, S., Slovic, P., Derby, S. L., and Keeney, R. L. (1981). *Acceptable risk*. Cambridge University Press.

30 Department of Health (1998). *Communicating about risks to public health: pointers to good practice*. DoH, London.

31 Osei, E. K., Amoh, G. E. A., and Schandorf, C. (1997). Risk ranking by perception. *Health Phys.*, **72**, 195–203.

32 National Radiological Protection Board (1998). *Living with radiation* (5th edn). NRPB, Chilton.

33 Harrison, J. R. (1996). *Health of the nation*. Radiation Protection Bulletin No. 184, pp. 10–13. NRPB, Chilton.

34 International Commission on Radiological Protection (1994). Radiation dose to patients from radiopharmaceuticals (including Addendum 1). ICRP Publication 53 (2nd edn). *Ann. ICRP*, **18** (1–4).

Chapter 12
Diagnostic radiology: equipment

J. R. Williams

12.1 Introduction

When selecting X-ray equipment, the purchaser bases their choice on a number of factors including cost, ergonomics, technology level, compatibility, image quality, patient dose, and user safety including radiation protection.

In general, user safety is not a significant issue in equipment selection provided that compliance with relevant national and international standards is specified. It is important, however, to ensure that the equipment is capable of restricting the radiation exposure to patients as far as reasonably practicable consistent with the clinical purpose. In the context of diagnostic radiology, this is a requirement for the dose to the patient to be no greater than is required to produce images which are adequate for the clinical purpose.

Optimisation of patient dose and image quality is a compromise because, generally, a reduction in dose leads to poorer image quality. This chapter is concerned with the selection and testing of equipment in respect of these two parameters. It also considers those aspects of design which influence the radiation protection of staff using the equipment.

In the UK requirements for radiation protection are laid down in the Ionising Radiations Regulations 1999 [1] and the Ionising Radiation (Medical Exposure) Regulations 2000 [IR(ME)R] [2]. Although reference will be made to this legislation and associated guidance in this chapter, the principle of keeping doses as low as reasonably achievable (ALARA) [3], which underpins these regulations and influences radiation protection in practice, applies equally to legislation in other countries.

12.2 Patient dose and image quality

12.2.1 Dose assessment

The underlying purpose of reducing dose is to reduce risk. In general, the principal concern is the risk of stochastic effects, in particular cancer induction. However, other risks may need to be considered. High radiation doses above a threshold level will result in deterministic effects. This is particularly relevant for lengthy interventional procedures which have the potential for causing injury to the patient's skin (§11.3.3).

The risk of stochastic effects is proportional to the effective dose. However, effective dose cannot be used for dose optimisation because it cannot be measured directly. The purpose of dose assessment is to determine whether the dose has been kept as low as reasonably practicable (ALARP). Simple, measurable parameters are sufficient for this. In practice, three dosimetry quantities may be used in diagnostic radiology. These are summarized below.

Entrance surface dose

Entrance surface dose (ESD) is the parameter most commonly used in radiography. It has the advantage that it can be measured fairly easily (usually with thermoluminescence detectors, TLDs) or it can be calculated from the radiographic factors (kVp and mAs) coupled with measurements of equipment output. The ESD rate is a useful parameter to characterize the dose efficiency of a fluoroscopy system. Fluoroscopy sets are almost always operated under automatic exposure control (AEC). This varies kVp and mA so as to maintain a constant output light intensity from the image intensifier with changes in radiological thickness. The ESD rate for standard phantom thicknesses provides information on the relative dose efficiency of the X-ray set. ESD is also an important quantity for the assessment of the likelihood of deterministic effects on the skin. This is particularly important for equipment used for interventional procedures for which ESD may be in the region of 1 Gy or more, i.e. approaching the threshold dose for skin erythema (see §3.3.4).

Dose–area product

Dose–area product (DAP) is the most easily measured parameter provided that a DAP meter is fitted to the equipment. It can be used both for radiography and fluoroscopy. An additional advantage compared with ESD is that DAP is more directly related to effective dose because it includes the beam area and it can be assessed for examinations with multiple projections.

ESD and DAP may both be converted to effective dose using Monte Carlo derived factors. These have been published for a range of kVp values and filtration by NRPB [4].

Computed tomography dose index

For CT scanners the most commonly used dosimetry parameter is the computed tomography dose index (CTDI). It is defined as:

$$CDTI = 1/T \int D(z).dz$$

in which *T* is the nominal slice width (in mm) and *D*(*z*) is the absorbed dose at position *z* measured parallel to the scanner's axis of rotation. There are variants on this basic definition depending on the geometry of measurement (in-air or in-phantom), the material in which the absorbed dose is stated, and the limits of integration.

CTDI is normally measured with a pencil ionisation chamber calibrated in terms of air kerma. The chamber measures the integrated dose profile over its length which is normally 100 mm. The reading is multiplied by the chamber calibration factor and the ratio of chamber length to nominal slice thickness to give $CTDI_{100}$, the subscript denoting integration length.

For any region of the body, effective dose is approximately proportional to dose–length product (DLP). DLP is calculated as the product of the normalized, weighted CTDI ($CTDI_w$) for the relevant body section phantom and the operator-selected parameters, i. e. slice thickness (*T*), number of scanned slices (*N*), and mAs per slice.

$$DLP = CTDI_w \times T \times N \times mAs$$

The operator-selected parameters, together with the reconstruction algorithm, also influence image quality. $CTDI_w$ is derived from measurements of $CTDI_{100}$ in a standard, cylindrical perspex phantom. The measurements are made at the centre of the phantom and at four points around the periphery at depths of 1 cm. The results are normalized to mAs and weighted as one-third of the central dose plus two-thirds of the average peripheral dose.

Full details of dosimetry methods are given in Chapter 14 and further information can be found in [5]. In this chapter these parameters will be discussed in relation to the selection and testing of equipment.

12.2.2 Image quality assessment

The assessment of image quality is notoriously difficult. The arbiter of quality is the radiologist who requires an image which is sufficient to provide an accurate diagnosis within the limitations imposed by the diagnostic technique. The judgement of image quality by the radiologist is by definition subjective. However, there may be defined criteria which can be used for this purpose. For example, the European Commission have produced guidelines on quality criteria for diagnostic radiographic images for both adults and children [6, 7]. These give image criteria for particular examinations which include aspects concerned with technique and patient positioning and with the visibility of normal anatomic structures.

For assessing the performance of equipment, such criteria are not useful and much effort has been dedicated to the design and production of image quality phantoms which have the advantage of structural consistency but which may lack clinical significance. In general, phantoms are designed to measure threshold spatial and contrast resolution. For spatial resolution a line pair test device may be used with groups of metal strips with varying width and spacing. The limiting resolution corresponds to the maximum number of line pairs per millimetre which can be resolved by the observer. In practice, spatial resolution is assessed with optimal conditions (minimum kVp) using a magnifier if necessary, for example for film/screen radiography where resolution in the range 6–10 lp mm^{-1} may be observed. Threshold contrast test phantoms use larger details with varying thickness set into the phantom in a regular array. These phantoms are used at a set kVp which should be checked prior to use and the observer scores the number of details which they are able to distinguish. Use of phantoms with varying detail size and contrasts enables the observer to construct a contrast-detail diagram. A set of phantoms for testing image intensifier performance has been described by Hay *et al.* [8].

Phantom scoring relies on a trained observer making a subjective assessment of the image. Alternatively, there are measurable parameters such as modulation transfer function or detective quantum efficiency which may be used to describe image quality [9, 10].

12.2.3 Interaction between patient dose and image quality

The most critical factor influencing dose is the sensitivity of the imaging device. Generally a reduction in dose brought about by an increase in sensitivity will increase noise due to quantum mottle. Noise limits the detection of low contrast detail. As an example, increasing the gain on the TV system of an image intensifier means that a less bright image can be viewed on the output screen of the intensifier resulting in a lower input dose rate and a consequent increase in quantum mottle.

Sensitivity and noise

The relationship between noise and detector sensitivity is, however, not always as simple as this. For example, the manufacturer may use a thicker layer of phosphor in an intensifying screen. The effect is to increase the detection efficiency of the screen allowing a reduction in dose to produce the same optical density on the film. In this situation, the number of X-ray photons detected by the faster film/screen system to produce an image will be similar to the number detected using the thin phosphor screen to produce an image of the same density. Thus the noise, which is a function of the number of photons detected, remains essentially unaltered. However, image quality is made worse because of the effect of screen thickness on sharpness. Similarly, changing from ionisation chamber to solid state or ceramic detectors in CT scanners allows a reduction in dose without any increase in quantum noise because the solid-state detectors have a greater detection efficiency. In this example there is no change in any other factor which would affect image quality.

Radiation quality

A second important influence on dose is the radiation quality. It is unfortunate that the word 'quality' is used in several different contexts in radiology. It is used in terms such as image quality to characterize the diagnostic potential of the image. It is used in the field of quality assurance to describe the process of image production. Here we use the term beam quality to express the penetrating ability of the X-ray beam. This is a complex situation because it is difficult to express penetrating ability as a single, measurable number. In theory it can only be fully described by the photon spectrum but such information is impossible to use.

For analogue imaging devices (film/screen systems, image intensifiers) the X-ray fluence at the detector is critical in terms of the image display. Increasing the penetration of the X-ray beam by, for example, increasing kVp, requires a reduction in the photon fluence reaching the patient, i.e. there is a reduction in ESD. However, this is at a cost in terms of the intrinsic contrast in the image because contrast is mainly provided by the photoelectric interaction process and increasing tube potential reduces its significance (§2.4.2). Choice of tube potential is generally under the control of the operator or may be determined by automatic selections preprogrammed into the generator in accordance with the user's requirements. There are very limited circumstances in which kVp selection is completely taken out of the control of the operator and is determined by the selection of equipment. The main instance where this happens is in the automatic exposure control for fluoroscopy where the relationship between kVp and mA is a function programmed into the system by the manufacturer. However, even then there may be a choice of programmes designed for different clinical situations. Other major factors influencing dose and radiation quality which are determined by the equipment specification are waveform and filtration (see §2.5.1). However, these have a secondary influence compared to kVp selection and their effects may to a certain extent be mimicked by changes in kVp. The use of copper filters is considered in more detail in §12.3.2.

Anti-scatter grids are designed to improve image quality by minimization of scatter but they also increase dose. Grids are considered in §12.3.7.

12.3 Factors influencing patient dose and image quality

12.3.1 Tube potential

Beam quality is mainly determined by tube potential (kVp). It is then further influenced by kV waveform, filtration, and by anode target angle. Figure 12.1 is an example of the relationship between ESD and kVp for radiographic exposures taken on a lumbar spine dosimetry phantom. The phantom, made of perspex and aluminium, was designed to provide the same relative attenuation as a patient over a range of kVps [11]. It can be seen that at potentials less than about 80 kVp, the dependence of ESD on kVp is very strong. This is due to the strong keV dependence of the interaction

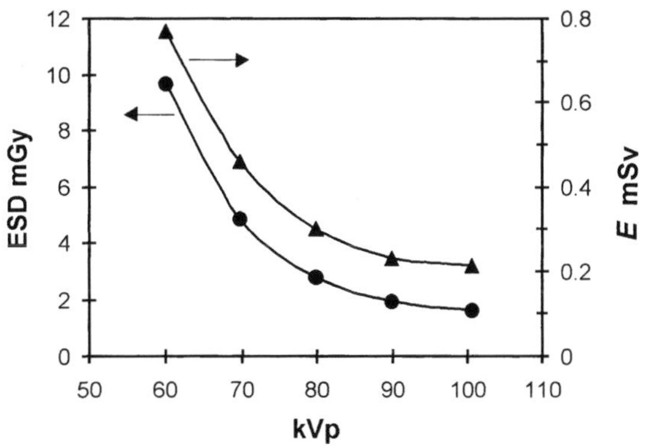

Figure 12.1 The variation of dose with tube potential measured on a lumbar spine dosimetry phantom [11]. (•) represents the measured values of entrance surface dose (ESD) and (▲) represents the calculated values of effective dose (*E*) using the data presented by Hart *et al.* [4].

probability for the photoelectric effect when compared to the relatively weak dependence for the Compton effect. The crossover, in terms of the relative importance of the two effects, occurs in the energy range 15 to 40 keV for soft tissue and bone (§2.4). This illustrates the dilemma caused by the trade-off between dose and image quality. The maximum tissue contrast will be demonstrated in the image in the energy range where the photoelectric effect has a significant influence on attenuation. However, it is in this energy range where the highest doses are required.

The European Guidelines on Quality Criteria for Diagnostic Radiographic Images [6] recommend that the tube potential for lumbar spine radiography should be in the range of 75 to 90 kVp. It can be seen in Figure 12.1 that this corresponds to the energy region in which the slope of the ESD vs. kVp curve begins to flatten out. For this phantom, ESD varies by a factor of 2.0 between these two settings. However, the relationship between ESD and kVp is an overstatement of the relative risk. The ratio between ESD and the dose to tissues below the surface reduces towards unity with increasing kVp. This means that the effective dose, which is calculated from the doses to organs and tissues at depth in the body, shows less variation with kVp. Figure 12.1 includes the variation of effective dose (*E*) with kVp. *E* was calculated from ESD using the conversion factors given by Hart *et al.* [4] for the AP view of the lumbar spine. The ratio of effective doses between 75 and 90 kVp is 1.6.

12.3.2 Filtration

In radiography, the selection of tube potential is an operational procedure and is not related to equipment specification. When purchasing radiographic equipment, the principal factors influencing radiation quality are waveform and filtration. With modern, high- or medium-frequency generators, it is only filtration which may have a significant influence and this is generally only related to the option of using copper filtration in addition to aluminium. The effect of additional filtration is to increase average keV. For example, it can be shown using the software of Sutton and Reilly [12] that the average energy of the X-ray spectrum generated at 70 kVp is increased from 40.5 to 47.0 keV with the addition of 0.2 mm of copper to a 3 mm aluminium filter (Figure 12.2a). Without the addition of copper, an increase in potential to 88 kVp would achieve the same average photon energy. Similarly in Figure 12.2b an increase in average energy from 50.2 to 58.1 keV is shown when 0.2 mm Cu is added to a 100 kVp X-ray beam.

The effects of copper filtration and kVp on ESD have been demonstrated using a 22 cm water phantom [13]. In that report it is also noted that the addition of the copper filter has a significant adverse effect on image quality as assessed using test objects, although this was not noted in the clinical context of cardiac catheterization. EUR 16261 [7] gives recommendations for the use of copper filters in paediatrics although part of the rationale is that it permits the use of higher average energy to reduce dose which cannot always be achieved in practice by raising kVp because of equipment limitations imposed by the very low exposure times.

12.3.3 Film–screen systems

The sensitivity of a film–screen system is specified in terms of speed. Speed is inversely proportional to the air kerma to produce a density of 1 above base plus fog. The problem with speed as a parameter is that there are available very many film and screen combinations with different performance characteristics. Assessment of speed on the same film–screen system will produce a variety of results depending on measurement parameters (e.g. kVp) and processing chemistry and conditions. There is no commonly applied standard methodology and the manufacturers themselves use different assessment methods. The speed class system provides a method for comparing film–screen systems. This classifies systems on a logarithmic scale with 100 as the benchmark figure based on calcium tungstate screens. The log of successive speed class number is incremented by 0.1 leading to speed classes (after rounding) in the sequence 100, 125, 160, 200, 250, 320, 400, etc.

Increase in speed results in an increase in noise due to quantum mottle. Although film–screen combinations in speed class 800 or higher are available, the deterioration in image quality leads to a general recommendation that 400 speed film is used for radiography [14]. In specifying a system it is essential that the intensifying screens, films, and processing chemistry are chosen in accordance with manufacturer's recommendations.

In conventional radiography, contrast is determined by the film's characteristic curve (Figure 12.3). This shows the base plus fog, i.e. the optical density of the unexposed film and the film latitude which is the range of exposures which provide adequate contrast when the film is viewed on a light box. The film gamma (or slope of straight line part of the curve) determines the contrast. Although high contrast is desirable there are disadvantages:

- There is a narrow latitude which increases the likelihood of over- or underexposure and therefore the number of retakes.
- The narrow latitude means that information is missed in a high contrast subject.

The best example of this is chest radiography in which the radiologist is looking for information in both the lung and the mediastinum. For this reason low-contrast or

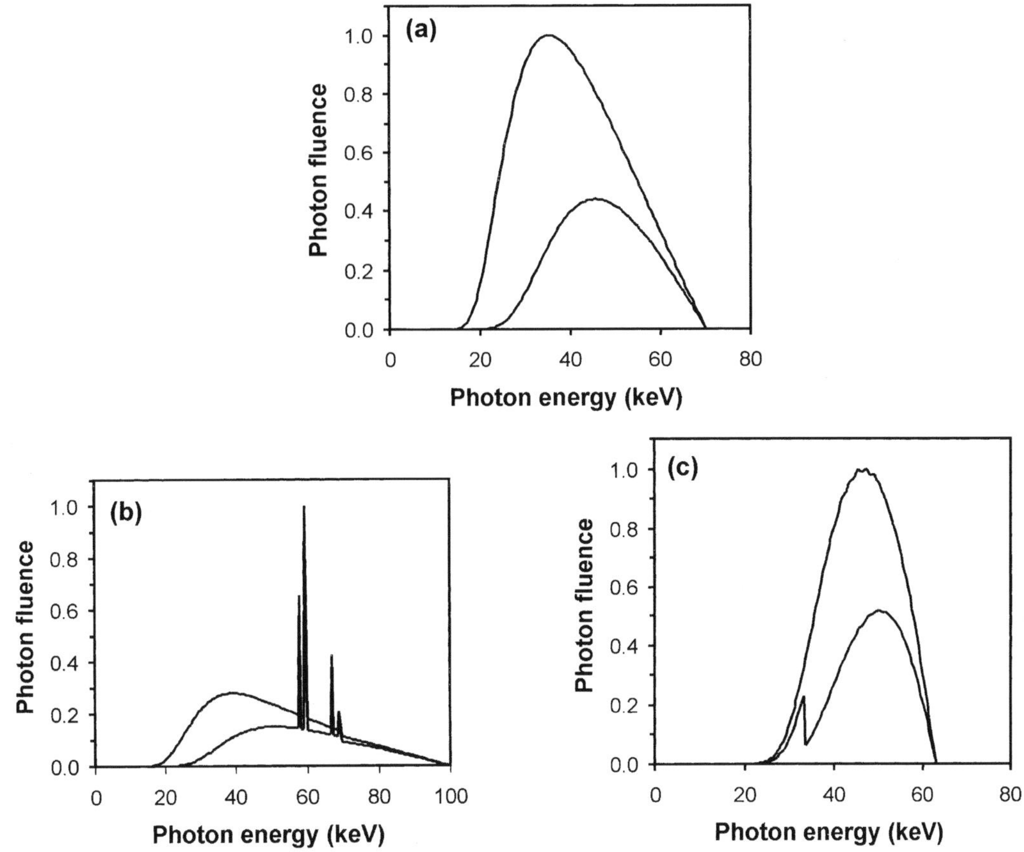

Figure 12.2 X-ray spectra calculated using the software of Sutton and Reilly [12] for generating potentials of (a) 70 kVp and (b) 100 kVp with a 3 mm aluminium filter with and without an additional 0.2 mm copper filtration, and (c) 63 kVp with a 3 mm aluminium filter after transmission through a 150-mm-thick block of soft tissue showing the effect of the addition of 0.1 mm of iodine.

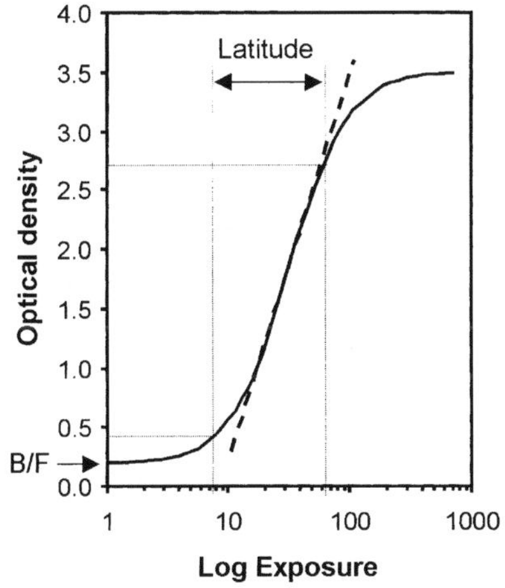

Figure 12.3 The characteristic curve for a film–screen system. The dashed line shows the maximum slope of the curve which represents the film gamma. B/F is the base plus fog.

latitude films are commonly used for chest radiography. Where such films are used they are generally in combination with the same specification of screen which is used for general radiography. A more complete discussion about the characteristic curve may be found in [15].

Increasing the sensitivity of a film–screen combination can be at the cost of reduced spatial resolution because the increase in sensitivity is achieved by increasing the phosphor thickness. This may be detrimental for those investigations where finer detail is being investigated such as in the examination of extremities. It is therefore common practice for such examinations to use so-called 'detail' screens which have thin phosphor layers and significantly reduced speeds. Typically the speed class of a detail cassette is in the region of 100 to 150. The resultant increase in dose are acceptable for such examinations because they are low in any case.

12.3.4 Digital radiography systems

There is an increasing trend towards digital systems for all medical imaging modalities. For radiography the two main systems for digital image capture are computed radiography (CR), using photostimulable phosphor plates, and direct digital radiography (DR), which gives almost instantaneous images. DR systems are of several types. Some use phosphors backed by silicon photodiode arrays or CCDs. An alternative system has direct X-ray detection using selenium photoconductive plates. The full potential of DR technology is yet to be realized and this chapter is only concerned with CR systems.

CR has the potential for lower doses than film–screen radiography because of the linear dose–response curve and wide dynamic range (about 10 000:1). The captured image can be windowed retrospectively with optimisation of the characteristic curve for the particular clinical situation. The dose cannot be lowered indefinitely because of quantum limits. However, quantum noise is less at the same dose level because of the greater pixel size.

It should be possible to set up the CR system to match 400 speed class film and commissioning tests should establish this. The problem with digital systems is that the user is not immediately aware whether or not the dose for an individual patient has been adequately controlled. It is therefore essential that lifetime testing programmes are established to ensure that the performance is maintained. Such tests are considered in §6.3.

12.3.5 Image intensifier systems

With an image intensifier, the dose to the patient is determined by:

- image intensifier input air kerma rate
- preprogrammed variation of kVp and mA with radiological thickness
- the use of additional features such as pulsed fluoroscopy.

For continuous fluoroscopy most manufacturers specify an input air kerma rate in the range 0.2–0.4 μGy s^{-1} for the largest field of view of the image intensifier. This is an important parameter to measure when a set is commissioned and as part of a performance testing programme. It is a parameter which should be checked by service engineers at scheduled service visits. Testing methods are described in §12.6.4. It is important to recognize that the automatic brightness control of an image intensifier is driven by the energy imparted to the caesium iodide input screen and that the relationship between this and input air kerma is strongly influenced by photon energy. Therefore, input air kerma rate varies with kVp and with filtration by the patient or by the attenuators used in the test programme.

The kVp/mA programmes available depend on application. The purpose is to maintain a fixed image intensifier signal by altering the two parameters with varying radiological thickness. There are two standard types of curve. The most common is the so-called 'anti-isowatt' curve in which both kVp and mA are progressively increased with radiological thickness (see Figure 12.4a). The alternative, which is favoured by one manufacturer, is a curve with which the mA is increased at a fixed kVp until a preset maximum mA is reached at which stage the kVp is increased with associated reduction in mA maintaining effectively the same wattage (Figure 12.4b). The starting kVp (i.e. minimum value) for this type of system can be selected by the operator with a default value which needs to be set by an engineer on the advice of the user.

Other programmes may be available for specialist purposes. Figure 12.4c (similar to Figure 12.4b) is a curve which would be used for iodine contrast studies in which a potential of 63 kVp is maintained for a wide range of radiological thicknesses. The choice of this energy is to give maximum attenuation by iodine which has a K-edge at 33 keV which is approximately the peak energy of the 63 kVp bremsstrahlung spectrum. In practice, the peak energy of the spectrum is much greater after filtration by the patient and the K-edge of iodine is at the lower end of the transmitted bremsstrahlung spectrum. This is illustrated in Figure 12.2c which shows the significant attenuation produced by 0.1 mm of iodine in a 150 mm thickness of soft tissue. A fourth example control programme is a paediatric low-dose curve which uses high kVp (Figure 12.4d).

12.3.6 CT scanners

In selecting a CT scanner, important data to consider are the manufacturer's specification of CTDI. This information is generally based on the FDA definition of CTDI which differs from the value required for DLP calculation (§12.2.1). $CTDI_{FDA}$ is defined as the absorbed dose to PMMA (perspex) integrated over 14 times the nominal slice width. The standard CTDI ionisation chamber is calibrated in terms of air kerma and measures the integrated dose profile over the length of the chamber which is normally 100 mm ($CTDI_{100}$). It is possible to convert from $CTDI_{FDA}$ to $CTDI_{100}$ by dividing by the appropriate ratios in Table 14.5 which were derived from data given on the ImPACT website (http://www.impactscan.org/). Alternatively, measured CTDI data may be available on the ImPACT website. The intending purchaser is then able to calculate $CTDI_w$ and DLP for the standard examination protocols specified by the manufacturer. It is also useful to ascertain the examination protocols used on scanners which may be clinically assessed by radiologists/radio-

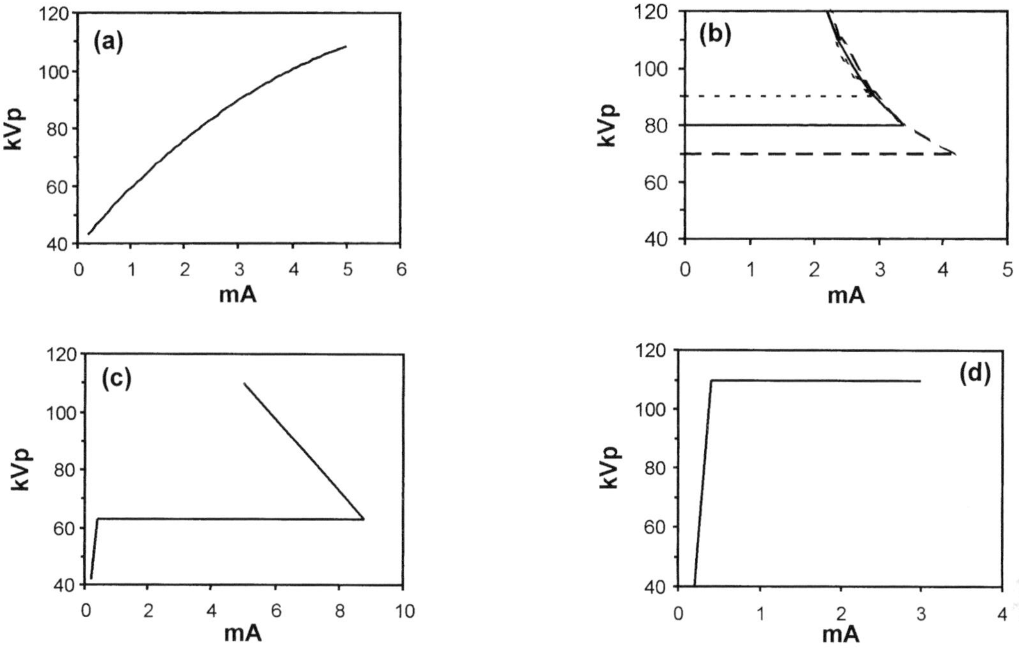

Figure 12.4 Dose control curves for fluoroscopy systems: (a) standard anti-isowatt curve in which kVp and mA are progressively increased with the radiological thickness; (b) curve with user-selected starting kVp, the three curves shown are for starting values of 70, 80, and 90 kVp; (c) iodine contrast curve with kVp held at 63 kVp up to maximum continuous power rating of X-ray tube; (d) low-dose paediatric curve.

graphers. This will allow a comparison to be made of doses between scanners for the image quality which is seen by the assessment team.

The principal hardware feature influencing dose is detector type. Solid-state and ceramic detectors have a greater detection efficiency than xenon ionisation chamber detectors and give a potential dose saving in the region of 25%. In the past they were less commonly used because ionisation detectors had greater stability and detector response could be more easily matched. In addition, there were response time problems with solid-state detectors due to afterglow. These disadvantages have largely been overcome and manufacturers are increasingly offering solid-state detection systems and these are obligatory on rotate-fixed (fourth generation) scanners and with multi-slice CT.

12.3.7 Ancillary devices

Any item placed between the patient and the detector increases dose. Dose saving can be achieved with low attenuation table-tops and NRPB [14] recommended the use of carbon fibre. However, Sutton and Cranley [16] demonstrated that the potential for dose saving in adult radiography is small (generally less than about 6%) because of beam hardening following transmission through the patient. In general, it is recommended that table-tops should have less than 1 mm Al equivalence. Any further reduction in attenuating properties would not be cost efficient.

Grids are used to remove scatter radiation and improve image quality. When purchasing equipment the specification of the grid is a key factor influencing dose. Both dose and contrast improvement increase with increasing grid ratio [17]. Generally, grid ratios between 8:1 and 12:1 are selected for routine radiography and image intensifier systems. It is also important to select grids with low attenuation covers and interspace material and carbon fibre is generally the material of choice [18]. Dance *et al.* [19] have described the benefits of using carbon fibre cassette covers. These are in terms not only of dose but also of image quality due to the lower scatter production.

12.4 Factors influencing staff dose

Staff radiation protection is generally assured by operating equipment while staff remain outside the X-ray room. Radiation doses are restricted by the use of shielding in the walls, doors, and floors of the room and the provision of fixed radiation protection screens. The design of shielding for diagnostic X-ray rooms is described in Chapter 13. In these situations the safety of staff is assured by ensuring that equipment can only be operated from behind the protective screen and by the use of strict operating protocols (local rules).

There are certain circumstances in which there are no protective screens (e.g. for ward radiography) and/or there is a requirement for staff to be in the controlled area during the procedure. Ward radiography and dental radiography are generally associated with relatively low levels of potential exposure to staff. Protection is assured by ensuring that the primary beam is not directed towards any person who is not behind a protective barrier, by relying on inverse square law to reduce scatter, and, where appropriate, requiring staff close to the controlled area to wear a lead apron. Other than compliance with leakage standards, equipment design has a small influence on staff dose.

In diagnostic radiology the most significant exposure to staff is during fluoroscopy. The three potential sources of exposure (primary, leakage, and scatter) will be considered separately.

12.4.1 Primary radiation

It is a requirement that fluoroscopy equipment is designed to provide the equivalent of 2 mm of lead shielding in the image intensifier casing and in the film cassette carriage which may be incorporated into the system [20]. A member of staff standing behind the image intensifier during fluoroscopy or for a radiographic exposure will therefore be adequately protected.

It is possible for the operator to put their fingers in the primary beam. On the entry side dose rates may be 50 mGy min^{-1} or greater. It is essential that the operator is aware of this and the absolute imperative of never putting their fingers in the direct beam. Fortunately, this is very unlikely to happen in the normal undercouch tube configuration. It is more likely for the fingers to be in the transmitted primary for which the doses are much lower although still to be avoided. To reduce the possibility of significant finger dose the operator should be advised always to watch the image with the beam on so that they will be able to see their fingers if they are in the beam. In addition, the equipment should be designed so that the X-ray beam is always limited to the field of view on the TV monitor. To achieve this, there should be automatic collimation to adjust beam size with focus intensifier distance (FID) variation and with magnification. In addition, there should be circular collimation so that the corners of a rectangular field are not outside the circular field of view. These are standard features on modern equipment.

It is important that the collimation is adjusted so that the beam size is no greater than the field of view. This should be tested as part of the critical examination and of the ongoing performance testing programme (see §12.6).

12.4.2 Leakage radiation

It is a requirement that X-ray tubes should be designed so that the leakage air kerma at a distance of 1 m from the focus cannot exceed 1 mGy h^{-1} [20]. The tube will have been designed to this standard at its maximum design kVp so that under normal operating conditions leakage is much lower. In general, the exposure to leakage radiation is very small compared to the exposure from scatter [21] and it can therefore be ignored. Testing for leakage is considered in §12.6.1.

12.4.3 Scatter

The amount of scatter at any position in the room is approximately proportional to DAP [22] and is a function of kVp and scattering angle. It represents the principal source of radiation dose to staff. The main feature of the fluoroscopy system which influences staff dose is the orientation of the tube and image intensifier. With an undercouch system (i.e. with the X-ray tube beneath the patient) the dose to staff standing beside the patient may be reduced by a factor of 10 or more in comparison with overcouch geometry [23, 24]. There are three main reasons for this:

- The intensity of scatter from a human trunk increases with angle of scatter, defined as the angle between the direction of the primary beam and the direction of scatter (Chapter 7). For example, at 120° the scatter intensity is nearly three times greater than at 60°. Therefore, with overcouch geometry, the operator standing beside the patient has the upper part of their body exposed to the greater levels of scatter and the upper part of the body contains most of the organs and tissues having a high weighting factor in the calculation of effective dose. There is also maximum irradiation of the unprotected eyes.
- With undercouch geometry the image intensifier should be positioned as close as possible to the patient and its structure provides local shielding, particularly for scatter directed towards the operator's eyes.
- With undercouch systems designed for barium contrast studies, the table structure provides additional shielding from large-angle scatter below the table and an additional shield can be readily suspended from the image intensifier carriage. This is a requirement of IPEM [20]. The shield is generally made from lead rubber with minimum dimensions 45 × 45 cm^2 and 0.5 mm lead equivalence.

Because of the radiation protection implications, it is a general recommendation that overcouch systems are not used with staff in the X-ray room. Some radiologists prefer to carry out barium contrast studies remotely using an overcouch system with table and exposure controls behind the protective screen. Provided that there is no requirement for other staff to be in the room, there should be no radiation protection concerns for this type of examination. There is the advantage that the lateral decubitus films required as part of a barium enema examination and which need 43 × 35 cm^2 films can be taken on the same table with the same tube. However, the equipment is restricted in its use and it should not be used for interventional types of examination such as ERCPs and line insertions which require staff to remain close to the patient during fluoroscopy.

Angiography and interventional radiology are potentially associated with high doses to both staff and patients. The potential exposure of staff to scatter radiation is directly related to patient dose (DAP) as shown by Williams [25]. Reduction in staff exposure can be achieved by using standard radiation procedures as discussed in Chapter 7. The C-arm system should be designed to operate with the tube under the patient and, for oblique views, the tube should be angled away from the operator. Additional shielding should be added, including a flexible lead shield attached to the table to reduce dose to the lower part of the body and a ceiling-mounted screen. The screen should incorporate a lead glass or acrylic window which can be supplied with an additional flexible apron. The mounting of this screen can be difficult due to potential interference with the free movement of other ceiling-mounted equipment such as the TV monitors and theatre lights. When designing an angiography room, it is recommended that the equipment manufacturer install the ceiling-mounted screen. This helps to avoid collision between the screen and the equipment particularly if an experienced radiographer is involved in the discussions.

12.5 Specification of equipment

12.5.1 General considerations

At the initial stage of the procurement process it is necessary to prepare a technical specification based on user requirements. The specification should state what the equipment is to be used for, where it is to be installed, the major system components, any accessories to be part of the purchase, maintenance and repair arrangements, and key performance parameters. As far as possible an 'output' specification should be used. This describes the user requirements and not the means by which these requirements are achieved. For example, it may be a requirement to have a low attenuation table-top but it would be wrong to require the table-top to be made of carbon fibre.

In writing a technical specification, it is necessary to make clear what is a requirement and what is a desirable option. It is important to pay particular attention to the language which is used. A helpful approach is to clarify this at the beginning. One way to classify the individual requirements is the following.

- **Essential** features which the equipment must have. In writing a specification it is necessary to ensure that the classification of a feature as essential will not exclude the choice of equipment which may be fit for the clinical purpose.
- **Important** features are those elements which the user considers should be included but which may not be available on every model. For example, specification of pulsed fluoroscopy as an essential requirement automatically excludes equipment which does not comply but which may have alternative features to reduce patient dose.
- **Desirable** features may be optional extras which are priced separately. They might also include the 'bells and whistles' offered by particular manufacturers.

This section is concerned with equipment specification and radiation protection. Many of the required features for radiation protection are established in standards (e.g. published by the IEC) and in guidance [20]. If the intending purchaser writes into the specification that the equipment must comply with these standards and requires the intending purchaser to confirm compliance, then it should not be necessary to list every feature such as tube leakage, filtration, tube markings, interlocks, etc.

12.5.2 Technical specification and patient dose

It is necessary to specify that the equipment is designed so as to be capable of reducing the dose to the patient as far as reasonably practicable [1]. Patient dose is strongly influenced by the mode of use, for example kVp selection in radiography, mA selection in CT, screening time in fluoroscopy. However, these factors may be influenced by image quality. It is important to consider the design features which will impact on the dose to the patient.

Radiographic equipment

In radiography the principal influences on dose are the imaging device and kVp selection. The following equipment-related features may be included in the specification.

- High-frequency generator, although it is now standard for all equipment to produce almost constant potential.
- It may be the choice to specify additional copper filtration. This may be user-selectable and purchasers should be aware that if the radiographer is able to

change the filter manually, then there is a risk of the wrong filter being used, leading to repeat radiographs.

- Low-attenuation table-top (< 1 mm Al at 100 kVp) and grid cover and interspaces.
- Table-top to cassette tray spacing, ideally this should be less than 80 mm.

It is recommended that DAP meters for radiographic sets should be able to read down to 1 mGy cm^2. This is important if the meter is to be used for low-dose examinations or in paediatrics.

The overall dose efficiency of radiographic systems has been assessed by Williams and Catling [26] who showed that dose could be related to the measurable factors concerned with beam quality, transmission of a heavily filtered beam through the table-top and grid, and geometric factors.

CR systems

When specifying a CR system, the purchaser is likely to be concerned with issues such as throughput, user interface, post-processing, interconnectivity, and cost. It is important to ask the manufacturer the equivalent speed class of the system to provide adequate image quality. This should be 400 or faster. The manufacturer should state the dose to the cassette for normal operation and include the irradiation conditions, particularly phantom geometry and kVp. Generally the dose should not be greater than 3 μGy.

Fluoroscopy equipment

Some essential features are:

- circular collimation
- automatic collimation to field of view with focus–intensifier distance and with magnification
- last image hold
- provision of local shielding
- interlock to prevent screening when the image intensifier is parked.

To assess the dosimetric aspects, data measured in accordance with the protocol published by Martin *et al.* [27] may be requested. However, supplier's may not have this information and responses need to be considered carefully. It is suggested that as a minimum the following information should be requested:

- input air kerma rate to the image intensifier for all fluoroscopy modes with details of measurement conditions
- input air kerma to the image intensifier for image acquisition
- details of kVp/mA curves for all programmes
- details of dose-saving features, e.g. pulsed fluoroscopy
- ESD rate for a standard phantom (20 cm water).

CT equipment

Essential features might include solid-state or ceramic detectors, all slice widths to be achieved using pre-patient collimation. Information required from the manufacturer relating to patient doses would include focus–detector distance, CTDI data for standard head and body phantoms, and examination protocols for standard examinations.

12.6 Equipment testing

A critical examination is required for equipment to be used for the production of ionising radiations (Regulation 31(2) [1]). The critical examination must be carried out in consultation with a radiation protection adviser (RPA) who may be employed by the installer/manufacturer/supplier of the equipment or be the hospital's own RPA. However, the responsibility for the examination rests with the installer. It is common practice for the hospital's RPA to oversee the critical examination because he/she will be involved with commissioning and acceptance tests of the equipment. These various tests overlap and it is more efficient for the same person to take responsibility for the whole procedure. In addition, for the equipment supplier it may not be cost effective to appoint their own RPA. It is important to establish with the installer at the stage that the supply contract is signed who the RPA will be for the critical examination. The RPA should obtain a list of tests from the supplier which they consider should be included.

The critical examination is concerned with the radiological safety of the equipment but it may be associated with tests of electrical and mechanical safety. The RPA or medical physicist may be asked to supervise this testing on behalf of the hospital.

Acceptance testing is concerned with ensuring that the equipment installed meets the contractual agreement, i.e. that what has been ordered is that which is supplied and that the performance matches the technical specification. Acceptance testing may be a simple paper exercise involving the recording of serial numbers, observation of the operation of the equipment, and inspection of the engineer's test sheets to ensure that the manufacturer's test protocols have been followed and the results are within their tolerances.

Commissioning tests are the responsibility of the purchaser and are generally carried out by the medical physicist. The tests serve two purposes: to establish

Table 12.1 Features to be checked in a critical examination (adapted from IPEM 79 [28])

Warning signs, etc.	Room warning lights
	Control panel indicators
	Tube selection
Exposure switches	Position
	Operation
	Protection against accidental exposure
Fluoroscopy alarm/termination	Audible warning
	Exposure termination
Emergency off-switches	Position and operation
Image intensifier collimation	Centring
	Maximum size
	Automatic adjustment
Safety interlocks	
Documentation and labelling	
Leakage radiation	
Radiological performance	Filtration
	AEC termination
	kVp, timer, mA linearity, output, etc.—all part of commissioning tests

baseline measurements for the lifetime performance testing of the equipment; and to establish optimum settings to ensure that the overall aim of keeping doses ALARP consistent with adequate image quality. These tests may need the involvement of the equipment engineer and/or the application specialist who is responsible for user training.

12.6.1 Critical examination

Guidance on the critical examination of safety features in X-ray installations can be found in IPEM 79 [28]. The installer is required to consult with the RPA on the nature and extent of the examination and on the results [1]. The RPA does not need to be present but he/she should inspect the results before the equipment is put into use. In practice, the RPA will normally choose to carry out the critical examination in person but can delegate the inspection task to a member of his/her staff and this may be appropriate for simpler items of equipment. UK regulations [1] allow the RPA to inspect the installation engineer's test records and to agree that the nature of the tests and the results are sufficient.

The critical examination is required for 'installed' equipment. IPEM 79 suggests that this does not include equipment which is fully assembled prior to delivery and which only needs to be plugged into a mains socket to be ready for use on the customer's premises. Such equipment would include mobile equipment as well as image intensifier systems. It may be noted, however, that there is conflicting guidance given elsewhere. NRPB [29] states that dental X-ray equipment, which is not installed in the terms described by IPEM 79 [30], requires a critical examination. It is therefore prudent for the RPA to test all such equipment in the manner suggested here.

Table 12.1 lists those items which might be included in any critical examination of X-ray equipment. It has been adapted from IPEM 79 [28]. This chapter is concerned with equipment so that references to the examination of shielding in the room structure or protective screens are not included. Methods of assessing room shielding can be found in [31]. Specific requirements and associated test procedures will be considered here. This list is not intended to be exhaustive and should be used in association with the specific recommendations of the equipment manufacturer, recommendations given in guidance [28], and the judgement of the RPA.

Warning devices

Indication is required to show that the equipment is switched on in readiness to make an exposure and to show when X-rays are being emitted. Such visual indication should be given at the control panel and at the entrance to the room in the case of fixed equipment. The X-rays-on light outside the room should be activated in the 'prep' stage, whereas the light on the control panel should only be illuminated when exposure is initiated. This is an indicator for the radiographer not only that the exposure has terminated but also that an exposure has taken place. It is essential that the minimum illumination time is such that this indication can be seen so that the light should be tested for the shortest available exposure time.

The position of the lights outside the room will have been specified by the RPA at the planning stage. It is recommended that if there is more than one X-ray tube in the room, then the X-rays-on light should be checked for each tube.

It is necessary to check that there is an audible warning after 5 minutes of screening and that the exposure will terminate after 10 minutes of continuous fluoroscopy [20]. Not all equipment complies precisely with this standard. Previous UK guidance required termination after an integrated screening time of 10 minutes with an audible warning given at least 30 seconds prior to termination. On such equipment resetting the audible warning also reset the cumulative timer. This was not an international standard and non-compliance could be noted for equipment from manufacturers with limited experience of the UK market. It is advisable to test with the assumption that continuous screening is required and not reset audible warning in case the equipment complies with the older standard. It is advisable to inform the engineer of the test as they will otherwise eagerly demonstrate how to reset the timer to get rid of a very ear-piercing sounds.

Exposure switch

For radiographic exposures check that the exposure terminates if the switch is released in mid-exposure. This can be done by using a long exposure time and either observing the exposure warning light or measuring output. Check each switch to ensure that a second exposure does not occur when the switch continues to be pressed for several seconds following termination. Switches behind the protective screen should be positioned so that the operator is able to observe the patient in any imaging location in the room and to observe any room door, and it should not be on a cable such that the operator can make an exposure while standing outside the protected area. For mobile equipment the cable should be at least 2 m long to allow the operator to stand outside the controlled area. Check that screening will not occur if a footswitch is overturned.

Image intensifier collimation

The following requirements should be tested:

- the beam is centred on the image intensifier
- the collimation is such that the fluoroscopy beam is no larger than the field of view
- the collimation on fluoroscopy equipment is such that the beam cannot extend past the edges of the image intensifier shield when the tube is used for radiographic exposures
- the collimation adjusts automatically for magnified fields of view and when the focus to intensifier distance (FID) is altered.

Centring can be tested by closing the beam down to about 5 cm diameter and checking that the image is in the centre of the monitor display. A useful method of testing beam size is to have a stand which can be placed on the patient table so that test objects can be positioned close to the cover of the image intensifier mount. Use an appropriate test object such as M1 from the Leeds test object set, and assess the beam size seen on the viewing monitor. Then place a film in the same position as the test object and screen for no more than 1 s. Measure the beam size on the film and compare it with the size on the TV screen. Acceptance criteria may depend on the application but it is suggested that the ratio of X-ray beam to image diameters should be no greater than 1.05 for any equipment. For equipment used for interventional procedures, where there is a greater risk of operators putting their fingers in the beam, the edges of the beam should be coincident with the edge of the image on the screen. This measurement should be made for all fields of view.

If the collimation is centred correctly and the beam size is no more than 5% greater than the maximum field of view, then the beam will be confined to the area of the image intensifier field of view during fluoroscopy. For sets used for conventional spot film imaging, i.e. using film–screen radiography with the cassette in front of the image intensifier, the collimation should be tested for the largest film size to ensure that the beam is restricted to the area of the cassette.

To check that collimation adjusts with FID is best done by viewing the beam edges directly using a fluoroscopic screen positioned on the table-top. Generally the light emitted from the screen can only be viewed with the room lights dimmed and may require relatively high factors. To screen at high kVp/mA requires an attenuator to be placed between the fluorescent screen and the intensifier face. It is useful to have a 0.5 mm lead plate (lead stuck on perspex or section of lead apron) for this. It can be placed on top of the stand used for the test objects.

Interlocks

The equipment will have a number of safety interlocks which should be tested. Certain of these are installed to prevent damage to the equipment itself, for example collision interlocks on rise and fall tables, and interlocks to inhibit table tilt in a fluoroscopy room unless the ceiling-mounted X-ray tube is parked in an appropriate position. They may be to protect the patient, for example proximity detectors to prevent C-arm collision with the patient in an angiography suite. And they may be designed for radiation safety such as the interlock to prevent exposures from an undercouch X-ray tube when the image intensifier is moved to the parked position. The RPA should ascertain from the engineer what interlocks are installed and should test them appropriately.

Emergency switch-off

Switches should be positioned in the room to remove the power from the equipment in the case of an emergency.

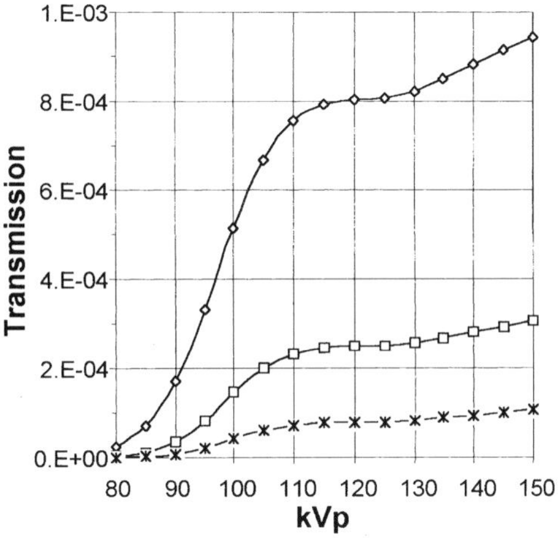

Figure 12.5 X-ray transmission for varying kVp: (◇) 2 mm lead; (□) 2.5 mm lead; (*) 3 mm lead.

Generally there are one or two such switches in the room with a further switch behind the control panel. The function of at least one of these should be tested.

Documentation and labelling

Check that full documentation is provided, including instruction manuals and records of the installers own tests. Check that controls are satisfactorily labelled.

Leakage radiation

The manufacturer will provide leakage technique factors. These correspond to the maximum design kVp for the tube and the maximum continuous tube current which can be sustained at that potential. At these settings, leakage at 1 m should not exceed 1 mGy h^{-1}. Measurements should be carried out with the collimators closed and it is recommended that they are made at a shorter distance (50 cm). If a significant dose is measured, an inverse square law correction can be applied to determine the value at 1 m. Measurement on four sides and at the top of the tube is probably sufficient provided that no significant leakage is noted. Ideally the measurements should be at the maximum kVp and about 10 mAs. The measurements can be scaled up to the leakage technique mA-hours. It may not be possible or desirable to test the equipment at the maximum tube potential and a setting between 10 and 25 kVp below the maximum may be used instead. For tubes with a maximum of 120 kVp or greater, the leakage is decreased by no more than about 25% for a reduction of 10 kVp below the maximum (see Figure 12.5). When testing at a lower kVp than the maximum, it is recommended that further investigation is carried out if the measured values are greater than 30% of the specified maximum.

Radiological factors

The critical examination should include testing of kVps, filtration, timer and mA settings, and operation of the AEC system. Such tests will also form part of commissioning and these are considered in §12.6.4.

12.6.2 Electrical and mechanical safety

Although this is not included in radiation protection, the RPA/medical physicist may be involved in testing for electrical and mechanical safety to ensure that relevant safety requirements are met [32]. Testing by the representative of the customer may involve inspection and witnessing the installer's own tests of earth bonding.

CE marking is a guarantee of design and manufacturing standards which are concerned with issues of safety. However, there are aspects of installation which may compromise safety. It is recommended that equipment is moved over its full range to ensure that end-stops function correctly, that the movements are smooth, that brakes operate correctly, and that power failure will not cause any hazardous movement when brakes are released. Movements to be tested include the horizontal movement of a ceiling-suspended gantry, tube height and rotation, table height and tilt, table-top movement, vertical bucky height, movement of explorator on fluoroscopy systems, C-arm rotation, and CT gantry tilt.

The tester should also be aware of manual handling issues as these are of significant concern to operators in imaging departments. Movements should not require excessive force and installations may be compromised by, for example, difficulty in covering the full range of the ceiling suspension or rotation of the X-ray tube due to inappropriate cable runs. Some of these ergonomic problems may be a feature of the equipment design, e. g. the positioning of switches and controls. Such problems should have been addressed at the stage of equipment selection. However, if the problems appear to have been affected by the way in which the equipment was installed, then the hospital's manual handling adviser may be consulted.

12.6.3 Acceptance test

The acceptance test is carried out by a representative of the purchaser to determine that the equipment supplied is what was ordered and that it meets the specification specified in the purchase contract. This test could be carried out by the medical physics expert [2].

To be able to carry out the test, it is necessary to have a copy of the purchase contract which will list the model names of each element of the system, accessories, etc. The tester needs to check that each of these has been supplied and make a note of serial numbers. He/she should have a copy of the technical specification drawn up by the customer and should use this as a basis of ensuring that the equipment supplied complies with this specification. The engineer or manufacturer's representative can be asked to demonstrate compliance with any particular item. This may be by observation of the engineer's own tests or inspection of his/her records. It is unlikely that there will be sufficient time to test all aspects of performance against the specification. It is a matter of judgement of the tester to cover an appropriate range of features. It is important that there is a demonstration of the operation of software, for example different reconstruction algorithms on CT scanners or subtraction on an angiography system.

12.6.4 Commissioning tests

The purpose of commissioning tests is:

- to provide a baseline for the lifetime performance testing programme
- to provide evidence of performance at the time of purchase in order to be able to demonstrate deteriorating performance
- to inform users of dosimetric options.

It is not the intention to provide comprehensive guidance on performance testing programmes. Recommendations have been made in IPEM 79 [30] and tests described in many publications [33, 34]. Some specific tests of performance which are directly related to patient dose are covered here.

Fluoroscopy dose control

Measurement of the input air kerma rate to the intensifier is an essential quality control test. The assessment method is in principle straightforward but in practice there are certain problems which may be encountered. A parallel-plate (flat) ionisation chamber should be used which is capable of measurement at the low-dose rates encountered. To achieve this level of sensitivity the chamber has to have a volume of at least 150 cm^3 and this is associated with a diameter of about 10 cm. The chamber should be positioned as close as possible to the image intensifier face with the grid removed. The measurement should be made with an attenuator in the beam and most protocols use a copper filter between 1 and 3 mm in thickness. The input air kerma rate can then be measured for each field of view. In making this measurement the following practical difficulties will be encountered.

- It is not always possible or desirable to position the chamber directly on the cover over the image intensifier face. For example, there may be a reluctance to insert the chamber into the cassette slot of the intensifier carriage on an undercouch screening system due to concerns over the potential damage to the chamber or the imaging system. In such cases positioning the chamber over the lower cover of the system and applying the inverse square law may be satisfactory.
- It may not be possible to remove the grid particularly with C-arm systems. It is recommended that in these circumstances either a grid factor is established for the system at the time of commissioning or a standard factor (1.5 is typical) is applied for all measurements.
- The measurement protocol used by the physicist is likely to be different from that used by the X-ray engineer. This can lead to significant differences in the measured values of input air kerma rate. Differences may include type and position of detector (one manufacturer uses a solid-state detector positioned on the periphery of the image intensifier field of view for these measurement) and the thickness of attenuator.

It is suggested that in-house test protocols adapt a consistent technique to be used for all types of equipment and for all manufacturers. This satisfies the need to establish reliable constancy tests. At the time of the commissioning test, the physicist should compare results with those of the engineer to reconcile any differences. This initial measurement can be used when interpreting the results of the routine programme with values reported by the engineer.

The operation of the automatic exposure control system should also be tested through measurement of skin dose rates for a standard phantom. A measurement protocol has been given by Martin *et al.* [27]. A particular problem is phantom size which should be 20 cm thick and large enough to cover the full field of view which may be as great as 40 cm in diameter for some angiography systems. It may be convenient to use water-filled phantoms with the required cross-section. Alternatively the use of smaller phantoms (20 to 25 cm cross-section) made up of slabs of perspex can be satisfactory for constancy tests with the beam coned down to the edges of the phantom. The measurements should be made under consistent geometry (i.e. focus–intensifier and focus–surface distances) for each exposure control programme and field of view. Tolerance limits of about $\pm 30\%$ from baseline should be set.

Maximum entrance surface dose rate should be tested by adding a lead sheet (1 mm) to the phantom. The dose rate must not exceed 100 mGy min^{-1} for any field of view [20] and should not be greater than 50 mGy min^{-1} for the largest field.

Automatic exposure control (radiography)

The performance of AEC systems is critical for both image quality and dose control. The test procedure involves taking films of a homogeneous test phantom

Table 12.2 Test programme for radiographic automatic exposure control system

Parameter	Conditions	Tolerance
Baseline density	3 chambers	OD = 1.1–1.5[a]
Reproducibility	3 exposures	OD variation < 0.05
Relative chamber sensitivity		Left/right chambers OD variation < 0.05 Central chamber OD < 0.20 from L/R[b]
kVp variation	60–100 kVp	OD $\pm$ 0.15
Thickness variation	$\pm$4 to 6 cm	OD $\pm$ 0.15
Density steps	$\pm$1, $\pm$2, $\pm$3	OD change 0.07 to 0.15 per step

[a]Baseline density is likely to be determined by a local clinical decision on the optimum density for a specific examination.
[b]AEC systems are generally designed to take paler films on the central chamber.

and measuring the resultant optical density at the centre of the film. Testing the AEC is particularly important if used in conjunction with CR because the user has no direct indication even if there is a significant fault.

In principle, the tests are straightforward and a protocol is given by IPEM [32]. However, there are significant practical problems. It is important that the phantom is tissue equivalent in order to reproduce the performance that would be seen in clinical practice and ideally it should not be less than about 15 cm thick. To provide adequate coverage of the chambers, the phantom should be at least 25 × 25 cm^2. Such a phantom, if made of perspex, weighs more than 10 kg. Even if this is made up of thinner slabs of material, it represents a significant manual handling problem for the tester, who may be required to transport it between hospitals. In addition, comprehensive testing requires many films to be taken (up to 20 or 30), this is time-consuming since ideally the same cassette should be used for each exposure, and there is an associated cost.

One solution for the phantom transport is to use a bucket of water. However, this cannot be used with a vertical Bucky system. The optimum solution is to equip each hospital with its own test phantom to a standard specification. This can be used for regular performance checks by radiographers using a limited protocol as well as a more comprehensive programme by the physicist annually.

To limit the number of films for film-based radiography, it is recommended that a jig of the kind described by Hunt and Plain [35] is used. This comprises a 1 mm thick lead disc (diameter equal to 20 cm) out of which a 12° to 20° sector is cut. This can be fixed on top of a 24 × 30 cm^2 cassette using a perspex plate with a circular cut-out. Provided that the perspex plate is no more than 2 mm thick, the cassette with the plate and disc attached will fit into the Bucky tray [36]. The perspex plate is marked with 18 to 30 disc positions (depending on sector angle) and it should incorporate lead numbers to indicate the disc position on the processed film. After each exposure the disc is turned through the appropriate angle permitting multiple exposures to be taken on a single film.

A test protocol is given in Table 12.2. It is recommended, however, that before carrying out this programme, a single exposure is tested and the film processed to ensure that the overall operation and set-up is correct. If they were not correct, then the first series of exposures would have been wasted. This is particularly advisable for a new set which may have not been calibrated adequately by the installation engineer.

CR systems

Recommendations on the testing of CR systems are not generally available. When commissioning a system it is important to ensure that the AEC system is set up to match 400 speed film. To test this it is recommended that a 20 cm thick water phantom or equivalent is used. Direct measurement of dose in the cassette tray should be made at potentials between about 70 and 100 kVp. The air kerma should be no greater than 3 μGy. Repeat measurements will be the basis of future performance tests. It is also important to establish a regular performance test which can be done by radiographers to ensure that there is no drift in the AEC and this may be based on post-exposure mAs.

Most CR systems record and display an indicator which is related to the quantity of radiation reaching the imaging plate. The consistency of display of this parameter can be tested by the radiographers using a suitable copper filter for a uniform irradiation of a cassette at 80 kVp and a set mAs chosen to give approximately 3 μGy to the imaging plate. The plate should be read with an appropriate test protocol and the exposure indicator recorded. Periodic audit of the exposure indicator for selected common examinations will then demonstrate whether patient exposures are being maintained at an acceptable level. Audit is facilitated on the CR workstation provided that the exposure index is stored with the clinical information.

It is difficult for the radiographers to establish optimum exposure protocols for those examinations carried out without an AEC system. As a starting point they can base their protocols on existing experience with

400 speed class film–screen systems but they will also need to take the advice of the company's application specialist.

Annual tests of image quality may be made using contrast-detail test objects of the type used for digital subtraction fluoroscopy and a line pair test tool with maximum 5 lp mm^{-1}.

The role of patient dose audit is particularly crucial with digital imaging systems and to assist this all equipment using CR should be fitted with DAP meters.

Film-based radiography

Purchase of new intensifying screens and processors is likely to become increasingly uncommon as CR and direct digital radiography become the systems of choice. However, where film–screen systems continue to be used it is important to recognize that the speed may differ from the manufacturer's specification, particularly if the processing system is not optimised, and may deteriorate with time. Speed should be measured when new screens or processors are purchased and as part of an annual performance testing programme. A practical method of measurement is described in Box 12.1. This assumes a definition of speed as the inverse of air kerma in mGy required to produce a density of 1 above base plus fog. A sensitometry film should be taken at the same time to measure the speed index and detect the influence of any change in processing conditions. For this test the same cassette should be used each year. The results of such tests can be compared with the nominal speed class but some caution should be exercised because of the influence of the measurement method on the results obtained with different film–screen combinations.

CTDI assessment

When accepting a CT scanner, the tester should check that the manufacturer's specification of CTDI for the set is met. $CTDI_{100}$ is measured using a pencil ionisation chamber in standard CTDI head and body perspex phantoms. The methods are described in Chapter 14. These data can be converted to $CTDI_{FDA}$ using the conversion factors in Table 14.5 and the values can be compared with the manufacturer's specification.

At the time of commissioning it is recommended that in-air measurements of CTDI at the isocentre are also made. For in-air measurements, $CTDI_{100}$ should not vary with slice width and any variation is most probably due to inaccurate collimation. Measurement at all slice widths

Box 12.1 *Assessment of film speed*

Equipment: Ionisation chamber suitable for measurement of dose = 1 μGy
Foam block 5–10 cm thick
Lead (2 mm) mask with four pairs of holes each approximately 1 cm diameter
2 mm lead sheet to cover mask

- Set the focus to table distance to 100 cm,
- Centre the X-ray beam over the centre of the chamber which should be on the table-top.
- With a 1 mm copper filter taped to the light beam diaphragm, make a series of exposures at 80 kVp to determine the mAs setting required to deliver a dose of approximately 1 μGy (mAs_1). If the set is not able to deliver a sufficiently low dose, the focus to chamber distance can be increased but this may necessitate placing the cassette on the floor.
- Place a 24 × 30 cm^2 cassette on the table-top with the short edge parallel to the anode–cathode axis
- Position the ionisation chamber on the foam pad on one side of the cassette so that the edge of the chamber is adjacent to the beam centre.
- Position the mask on the opposite side of the cassette equidistant from the beam centre as the centre of the chamber.
- Expose at mAs_1 and record the dose. Repeat the exposure with the first pair of holes covered by the lead sheet. Make two further exposures at 2 × mAs_1 with the second and third pair of holes covered respectively, recording the dose each time.
- Process the film and measure the average optical density under each pair of holes. Use the surrounding area to measure base plus fog.
- Plot optical density against the log of the dose and from the graph interpolate the dose (D_0 μGy) required to deliver a density of 1 + base plus fog. Correct the interpolated value by the inverse square law from the position of the chamber to the film.
- Calculate film speed as $S = 1000/D_0$.

is therefore recommended. It is common experience that CTDI for the smallest slice thickness is high by up to 30% due to the difficulty of accurate collimation at widths less than about 2 mm. On some CT models post-patient collimation is used for these narrow slices and the reading may be double that for other settings. Annual performance checks could repeat the in-phantom measurements. However, it should be sufficient to measure in-air CTDI at all slice widths as a constancy test. When an X-ray tube is replaced, a fuller set of measurements using the phantom should be done.

12.7 References

1 Department of the Environment, Transport and Regions (1999). *Ionising Radiations Regulations 1999.* SI No. 3232. HMSO, London.
2 Department of Health (2000). *Ionising Radiation (Medical Exposure) Regulations 2000.* SI No. 1059. HMSO, London.
3 International Commission on Radiological Protection (1991). 1990 Recommendations of the International Commission on Radiological Protection. ICRP Publication 60. *Ann. ICRP*, **21** (1–3).
4 Hart, D., Jones, D. G., and Wall, B. F. (1994). *Estimation of effective dose in diagnostic radiology from entrance–surface dose and dose–area product measurements.* NRPB-R279. NRPB, Chilton.
5 Medical Devices Agency (1998). *Type testing of CT scanners: methods and methodology for assessing imaging performance and dosimetry.* MDA/98/25. MDA, London.
6 European Commission (1996). *European guidelines on quality criteria for diagnostic radiographic images.* EUR 16260 EN. EC, Luxembourg.
7 European Commission (1996). *European guidelines on quality criteria for diagnostic radiographic images in paediatrics.* EUR 16261 EN. EC, Luxembourg.
8 Hay, G. A., Clarke, O. F., Coleman, N. J., and Cowen, A. R. (1985). A set of X-ray test objects for quality control in television fluoroscopy. *Br. J. Radiol.*, **58**, 335–44.
9 International Commission on Radiation Units and Measurement (1996). *Medical imaging–the assessment of image quality.* ICRU Report 54. ICRU, Bethesda.
10 Martin, C. J., Sharp, P. F., and Sutton, D. G. (1999). Measurement of image quality in diagnostic radiology. *Appl. Radiat. Isot.*, **50**, 21–38.
11 Conway, B. J., Duff, J. E., Fewell, T. R., Jennings, R. J., Rothenberg, L. N., and Fleischman, R. C. (1990). A patient-equivalent attenuation phantom for estimating patient exposures from automatic exposure controlled X-ray examinations of the abdomen and lumbo-sacral spine. *Med. Phys.*, **17**, 448–53.
12 Sutton, D. and Reilly, A. J. (1997). *Spectrum processor.* IPEM Report 78 (CD-ROM). Institute of Physics and Engineering in Medicine, York.
13 Nicholson, R., Tuffee, F., and Uthappa, M. C. (2000). Skin sparing in interventional radiology: the effect of copper filtration. *Br. J. Radiol.*, **73**, 36–42.
14 National Radiological Protection Board (1990). Patient dose reduction in diagnostic radiology. *Doc. NRPB*, **1** (3).
15 Haus, A. G. and Jaskulski, S. M. (1997). *The basics of film processing in medical imaging.* Medical Physics Publishing, Madison.
16 Sutton, D. and Cranley, K. (1996). The potential for dose reduction in diagnostic radiology using low attenuation materials in table tops. *Br. J. Radiol.*, **69**, 249–55.
17 Sandborg, M., Dance, D. R., Alm Carlsson, G., and Persliden, J. (1993). Monte Carlo study of grid performance in diagnostic radiology: factors which affect the selection of tube potential and grid ratio. *Br. J. Radiol.*, **66**, 1164–76.
18 Sandborg, M., Dance, D. R., Alm Carlsson, G., and Persliden, J. (1993). Selection of anti-scatter grids for different imaging tasks: the advantage of low atomic number cover and interspace materials. *Br. J. Radiol.*, **66**, 1151–63.
19 Dance, D. R., Lester, S. A., Alm Carlsson, G., Sandborg, M., and Persliden, J. (1997). The use of carbon fibre materials in radiographic cassettes: estimation of the dose and contrast advantages. *Br. J. Radiol.*, **70**, 383–90.
20 Institute of Physics and Engineering in Medicine (2002). Medical and dental guidance notes: a good practice guide to implement ionising radiation protection legislation in the clinical environment. (IPEM, York)
21 Simpkin, D. J. and Dixon, R. L. (1998). Secondary shielding barriers for diagnostic X-ray facilities: scatter and leakage revisited. *Health Phys.*, **74**, 350–65.
22 Williams, J. R. (1996). Scatter dose estimation based on dose–area product and the specification of radiation barriers. *Br. J. Radiol.*, **69**, 1032–7.
23 Faulkner, K. and Moores, B. M. (1982). An assessment of the radiation dose received by staff using fluoroscopic equipment. *Br. J. Radiol.*, **55**, 272–6.
24 Law, J., Inglis, J. A., and Tolley, D. A. (1989). Radiation dose to urological surgeons during X-ray fluoroscopy for percutaneous stone extraction. *Br. J. Radiol.*, **62**, 185–7.
25 Williams, J. R. (1997). The interdependence of staff and patient doses in interventional radiology. *Br. J. Radiol.*, **70**, 498–503.
26 Williams, J. R. and Catling, M. K. (1998). An investigation of X-ray equipment factors influencing patient dose in radiography. *Br. J. Radiol.*, **71**, 1192–8.
27 Martin, C. J., Sutton, D. G., Workman, A., Shaw, A. J., and Temperton, D. (1998). Protocol for measurement of patient entrance dose rates for fluoroscopic X-ray equipment. *Br. J. Radiol.*, **71**, 1283–7.
28 Institute of Physics and Engineering in Medicine (1998). *The critical examination of X-ray generating equipment in diagnostic radiology: guidance on the interpretation of the Ionising Radiations Regulations 1985, Regulation 32(2)a.* IPEM Report 79. IPEM, York.
29 National Radiological Protection Board (1994). Guidelines on radiological standards for primary dental care. *Doc. NRPB*, **5** (3).
30 Institute of Physics and Engineering in Medicine (1997). *Recommended standards for the routine performance testing of diagnostic X-ray imaging systems.* IPEM, York.
31 Sutton, D. G. and Williams, J. R. (ed.) (2000). *Radiation shielding for diagnostic X-rays: report of a joint BIR/IPEM working party.* BIR, London.
32 Department of Health NHS Procurement Directorate (1989). *Technical requirements for the supply and installation of equipment for diagnostic imaging and radiotherapy.* Document TRS 89. DoH, London.

33 Institute of Physics and Engineering in Medicine (1996). *X-ray intensifying screens, films, processors and automatic exposure control systems.* IPEM Report 32, Part IV (2nd edn). IPEM, York.
34 British Institute of Diagnostic Radiology (1988). *Assurance of quality in the diagnostic X-ray department.* BIR, London.
35 Hunt, A. J. and Plain, S. G. (1993). A simple solution to the problems of testing automatic exposure control in diagnostic radiology. *Br. J. Radiol.*, **66**, 360–2.
36 Ison, J. E., Bridge, L. R., and Hennessey, R. M. (1999). Testing automatic exposure control devices used in diagnostic radiology. *Br. J. Radiol.*, **72**, 319.

Chapter 13
Diagnostic radiology: facility

G. Hart, D. G. Sutton, and C. J. Martin

13.1 Introduction

Adequate restriction of exposure to radiation for staff and members of the public can be achieved by seeking suitable compromises between the three basic elements of shielding, distance, and time. Procedural controls are sufficient to ensure that the time of exposure is minimized. Both procedural and design controls are required to ensure that the distance and shielding elements are used appropriately. The major objective of this chapter is to discuss the design controls which can be put into place to ensure that radiation doses to staff and members of the public can be maintained at levels which conform to the 'as low as reasonably practicable' (ALARP) principle. The factors that must be considered in designing the radiation protection for an X-ray room are discussed in §13.2. The methodology is described in §13.3 and practical examples of room design and shielding calculations are given in §13.4. Elements of personnel radiation protection are discussed in §13.5.

13.2 X-ray room design

13.2.1 Rationale

X-ray rooms must be designed to provide flexible and efficient working areas for different types of imaging procedure. In radiation protection terms, they must be capable of containing the radiation produced by the X-ray tube to within a set of criteria and limits determined by relevant legislation (see §13.3.1).

The radiation arises from three main sources—the primary beam, leakage, and scatter. Leakage and scatter are referred to as secondary radiation.

- The primary beam will usually be directed from the X-ray tube towards a patient and image receptor, and ideally all the beam should always fall within the bounds of that image receptor.
- Leakage radiation from the X-ray tube may be either in specific directions or relatively isotropic, although usually at a low level (maximum of <1 mGy h^{-1}, typically <0.2 mGy h^{-1}). It is more penetrating than the primary beam, since its softer, low-energy components are attenuated by the tube housing.
- Scattered radiation will occur whenever the X-ray beam meets any solid object, including the patient, the imaging table or bucky, and the image receptor itself. It has a strong angular dependence and may or may not be more penetrating than the primary radiation, depending on the angle of scatter (§2.5.2).

13.2.2 Workload assessment

In judging the radiation protection requirements of any X-ray facility, consideration must be given to the expected workload within the room.

The key factors to be considered are:

- technique factors for the range of studies to be performed in the room, such as average and maximum kVp, together with average and maximum dose–area product (DAP), entrance skin dose (ESD) or mAs values
- projected patient throughput.

The design must encompass as much flexibility as possible to allow for future changes of use, variations in technique, or increases in room workload. Designing too close to the borderline of the design criteria will limit this future flexibility.

13.2.3 Equipment location and orientation

The placement of radiological equipment within a room can have a profound impact on the radiation protection requirements. Factors which must be considered include:

- asymmetrical positioning of the equipment which may mean that one or two walls receive more scattered radiation than the others

- preferred directions for firing of the X-ray beam, such as towards a chest stand, which may mean that one particular wall receives more primary or scattered radiation than others, or the floor or ceiling carries a greater radiation weighting.

The location of the X-ray room within the whole building is also important. It is not uncommon for X-ray facilities to border rooms or areas that have a relatively high occupancy. The shielding to these areas must be designed so that accumulated radiation exposures to individuals within these rooms are kept to an acceptable level.

13.2.4 Protective barriers

Walls

Careful consideration should be given to the materials used for the construction of the walls. A wide range of materials is available, from stud partition walls with plasterboard through to brick and concrete blocks of varying densities and textures. Lead incorporated into plywood or plasterboard may be added to increase the protection. In addition, finishing methods such as the use of 'barium plaster' may be used to enhance the radiation attenuation properties.

Windows

In an X-ray room that has been purpose-designed and built, windows are generally positioned more than 2 m above floor level. At this height, it is usually possible to ignore any scattered radiation that may be transmitted through the window which can therefore be made from normal glass.

If an existing room is to be converted to X-ray use, however, it may contain normally-glazed windows at lower levels. An assessment will then have to be made as to whether anyone external to the window might receive significant radiation exposures from the projected use of the room. If this is possible, the lower portion of the window below a height of 2 m will need added protection. This can be achieved either by the use of lead glass (expensive, but preserves the light transmission) or by boarding the area concerned with a wood or plastic panel incorporating lead sheet of an appropriate thickness.

Floors and ceilings

The construction methods employed will need careful consideration to ensure that they provide both contiguous and sufficient protection to keep radiation doses in rooms above and below the X-ray room less than the required design criterion. The use of concrete slabs with a density of the order of 2350 kg m^{-3} and with a thickness of about 150 mm will generally provide sufficient protection against high-dose interventional procedures or even high-kVp modalities such as computed tomography (CT). However, lightweight concrete is increasingly being used and this will provide less protection. In addition, floors and ceilings are often poured onto metal bases with ridged cross-sections. These give a trapezoidal variation in concrete thickness that at its minimum may be only 80 mm. It is these minimum thicknesses that need to be considered in calculating the X-ray transmission.

Table 13.1 Standard lead sheet thicknesses

BS code	Lead thickness (mm)
3	1.32
4	1.80
5	2.24
6	2.65

Doors

Doors into X-ray rooms, which usually are custom-made by specialist suppliers, incorporate sheet lead into the door construction. Sheet lead is subject to a British Standard and the use of standard thicknesses (Table 13.1) will tend to be more cost-effective. However, lead sheet is also available from manufacturers in 0.5 mm increments. Shielding based on multiples of 0.5 mm lead may therefore turn out to be as cost-effective as using the standard thicknesses.

It is important during the room construction process that unleaded gaps are not left between the door and the frame. Stops and architraves will therefore need to be leaded to ensure protection is contiguous. For double or sliding doors there need to be lead rebates to ensure no gaps remain.

Protective screens

Protective screens are an important part of radiographic, fluoroscopic, and CT rooms. They should provide an area behind which dose rates are sufficiently low that members of staff would need no additional protective equipment. Screens should be at least 2 m high and usually consist of a solid base panel of lead-lined laminate material and an upper section of lead glass with a lead equivalence of 1.5, 2.0, or 2.5 mm, typically 40–50% of the total screen height. Screens may contain a mixture of flat and angled panels as required, but need to be large enough to provide sufficient shielding for all those who may need to be behind them (typically 2–4 people). The screen must also allow clear visibility to all entrances into the room, so that the operator can maintain effective control of the set in the event of unauthorized entry during an exposure.

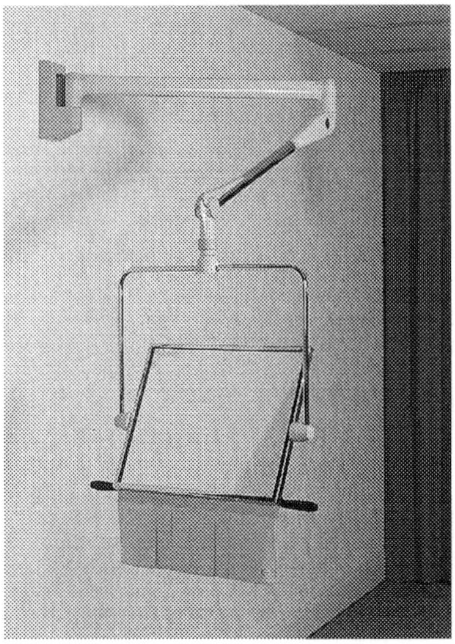

Figure 13.1 Overhead suspension shielding to reduce upper body exposure in high-dose fluoroscopic procedures. (Courtesy of Kenex Ltd.)

Consideration may be given in some circumstances to the use of lead acrylic material instead of lead glass. At diagnostic X-ray energies it has a relatively low lead equivalence (0.5 mm for a 12 mm thickness of acrylic) but this may be sufficient for some applications.

In certain circumstances, such as in the resuscitation room in an accident and emergency department, working practices may dictate the need for different protective systems. In such rooms equipment may be very mobile and move between treatment bays—some hospitals have installed ceiling-suspended tubes on long tracks for this purpose. The use of fixed protective screens may well not be appropriate because of the need to achieve flexible but rapid access all around the patient. In these circumstances the use of a protective curtain or mobile protective screens may provide the most appropriate solution, although it should be noted that these typically provide only 0.5 mm lead-equivalent protection. Mobile screens are sometimes also used to provide radiation protection in operating theatres.

Overhead suspended shields like the example in Figure 13.1 are increasingly being used in angiographic and interventional procedures to reduce radiation doses to the head and upper body of staff who may need to remain close to the patient during the procedure. These may be wall-, ceiling-, or equipment-mounted for flexibility of use, and typically use lead glass with 1.0 mm or 1.5 mm lead-equivalent protection. The optional use of a lead curtain underneath the shield may be useful in some situations.

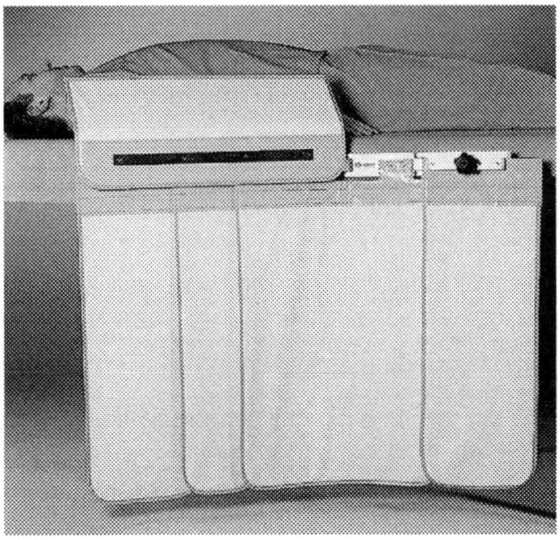

Figure 13.2 Table-mounted shielding for undercouch C-arm fluoroscopic systems to reduce lower body exposure. (Courtesy of Kenex Ltd.)

Table-mounted shields such as those shown in Figure 13.2 are particularly useful in areas such as fluoroscopy, where undercouch C-arm intensifier systems are used (§12.4.3). The legs of interventional radiologists or others working close to the X-ray beam from an undercouch X-ray unit may receive significant doses from scattered radiation. These may be substantially reduced by the use of lead drapes hung from the table or a short mobile screen. The protection afforded is typically equivalent to 0.5 mm lead. A rule of thumb that can be applied to determine whether doses are likely to be significant is that a DAP of 10 Gy cm^2 will give a radiation dose of 1 mGy to the legs of a radiologist working near to the X-ray field, if leg shielding is not used.

13.2.5 Warning signs

All entrances to rooms containing X-ray equipment should carry a warning sign designed to alert all concerned to the presence of ionising radiation within the area. Such signs should incorporate the radiation trefoil symbol and indicate that the hazard refers to X-rays. The signs should be in a prominent location, preferably at eye level, where they cannot be easily ignored.

For all types of X-ray sets with the exception of specimen cabinets and dental units, the preference is for illuminated warning signs. Such signs are usually connected in parallel with the electrical power supply to the X-ray unit and are two-stage signs:

- The first stage should illuminate whenever the mains power is connected to the X-ray set. In the UK it usually displays the trefoil and words such as 'Radiation Controlled Area' or an equivalent message, and is coloured yellow on a black background, or black on a yellow background, to give an approximate coincidence with the standard 'yellow = warning' in safety signs.

- The second stage should illuminate whenever the X-ray set is preparing to operate or is in operation. This typically bears the message 'X-Rays On, Do Not Enter' or an equivalent, usually displayed in red on a black background or black on a red background. Red is used here again to give a parallel with the 'red = danger' in safety signing.

Illuminated warning signs ideally contain multiple bulbs to guard against lamp failure but need regular checks to ensure they remain functional. It is good practice to display an adhesive warning sign in the middle of the door panel in addition to the illuminated sign.

13.2.6 Access and egress

The design of the X-ray room must incorporate easy access for the patient, and consideration must be given as to whether patients will be ambulant, in a wheelchair, on a trolley, or in a hospital bed. If imaging is to take place on an imaging table, consideration must also be given to whether the room design permits good access to the patient, both for the routine procedures that are to take place and in an emergency.

The room design must take into account arrangements for emergency egress from the room, both for patients and for any staff within the room. The position of the control panel must be carefully considered so that in the event of an emergency, such as fire or a potentially violent patient, staff are not trapped because of poor design. One simple option is for the point of entry for staff to be sited within the control cubicle.

13.3 Room shielding

13.3.1 Criteria for the shielding assessment

It is a requirement under most regulatory systems that X-ray rooms are shielded to ensure that all those who may come into contact with ionising radiation as a result of the use of the room receive radiation doses consistent with ALARP. In practice, there are two distinct groups of people that must be considered and the design methodology must satisfy the radiation protection requirements for both groups:

- members of the public or employees not directly concerned with the work of the room
- employees who will be using the particular room in question.

When considering the radiation protection requirements of the first group, it is clear that the annual radiation dose of any non-radiation employee should not exceed that of any other member of the public (1 mSv). To design an X-ray room to this radiation level, however, is not likely to represent an ALARP solution. The concept of dose constraints (§6.7) should be applied, such that a member of the public will not receive any more than 30% of their maximum permissible dose from any one source–that is, no more than 0.3 mSv per annum. This would place an upper bound on the radiation dose in any design calculation.

The application of the dose constraint must be made using realistic assumptions regarding the occupancy of areas which are relevant in terms of the shielding problem. The occupancy factor for an area should not be considered as being an indication of the time during which it is occupied by a group of people (such as patients in a waiting room). Instead, it is the fraction of time spent by the single person who is there the longest. Consequently, the occupancy factor is best defined as being the fraction of an 8-hour day, 2000-hour year, or other relevant period (whichever is most appropriate) for which a particular area may be occupied by a single individual. Occupancy factors should, wherever possible, be based on realistic data obtained from the installation site. In this context it is important to consider the fact that the use to which an adjacent space is put may change over the lifetime of the X-ray installation. It is also important to consider all of the surrounding rooms, not just those immediately adjacent to the area being shielded. Indicative values of occupancy factor are given in Table 13.2.

It should be noted that the product of the design constraint and the reciprocal of the occupancy factor should not exceed any dose limit used to define a controlled area. For example, if areas are designated as being controlled when the potential dose exceeds 6 mSv then consequent to the design criterion of 0.3 mSv per annum must be the adoption of 5% as the lowest occupancy factor. Furthermore, if controlled area classification has to be based on dose rate due to low usage of the room, then it may not be appropriate to consider occupancy.

The second group of people to be considered are the employees who will have to work within the X-ray room. Wherever possible, the room design should incorporate features that minimize their radiation doses. One example is the siting of the control panel behind a protective barrier (§13.2.4), so that those who operate the set are in a low-radiation area.

Another factor which must be taken into account is avoidance of fogging of film stored adjacent to an X-ray room. A design limit of 0.3 mSv should be sufficient for a film store. However, film in a cassette is much more sensitive and significant fogging can occur at exposures

Table 13.2 Occupancy factors provided for general guidance[a]

Location	Possible occupancy factor (%)
Adjacent X-ray room, reception areas, film reading area, X-ray control room	100
Offices, shops, living quarters, children's indoor play areas, occupied space in nearby buildings, staff rooms	100
Patient examination and treatment rooms	50
Corridors, wards, patient rooms	20
Toilets or bathrooms, outdoor areas with seating	10
Storage rooms, patient changing rooms, stairways, unattended car parks, unattended waiting rooms	5

[a]Assessment of occupancy in the local situation should be made whenever possible.

as low as 0.4 μGy. Thus for a barrier behind which a loaded cassette may be stored and remain unused for a day, a design criteria of 100 μGy per year should be used.

13.3.2 Calculation of radiation doses from workload

Protection must be provided against primary and secondary (scatter and leakage) radiations. The doses from each are closely linked to the amount of radiation to which patients are exposed. In the method recommended, assessments for primary radiation are based on patient ESD and those for scatter derived from patient DAP data. The methodology used follows that of the BIR/IPEM report on *Radiation shielding for diagnostic X-rays* [1], which discusses the whole topic of diagnostic X-ray shielding in some depth. Alternative methodologies based on workload in mAs may be used, where patient dose data are not available [2, 3].

Dose

Dose limits and associated constraints are expressed in terms of effective dose. However, although some radiation protection instruments are calibrated in terms of the ICRU operational quantity ambient dose equivalent (Chapter 4), most X-ray output and transmission data are measured in terms of air kerma or air kerma ratios using ionisation chambers. It is therefore not practical or realistic to use effective dose (or its associated operational quantities) when calculating shielding requirements. All calculations described here and the underlying theory are based on air kerma measurements. An approximate equivalence is made between effective dose (mSv) and air kerma (mGy). This is a conservative assumption since air kerma represents a significant overestimate of effective dose [4].

Primary barrier

In the majority of radiology procedures, the primary beam is entirely intercepted by an attenuator and so is not incident directly on a wall or other barrier. For example, in fluoroscopy, the beam should always fall within the boundary of the image intensifier, which provides an adequate primary barrier [2], except for the special case of radiotherapy simulators, where this assumption cannot be made. A similar assumption can be made for CT scanners. The same is not the case for plain film radiography where two situations can arise: (a) all of the X-ray beam is attenuated by the patient and cassette and (b) some of the beam is not intercepted by the patient, cassette, etc., and unattenuated radiation is incident on the primary barrier. The methods for addressing the transmission properties of the two types of primary radiation differ and are described in §13.3.3.

Primary radiation which has passed through a patient

In radiography the beam will in most cases be entirely intercepted by the patient's body and the cassette so the kerma incident on the film (K_f) can be used for assessments. A conservative assumption is that $K_f = 10$ μGy for film/screen combinations with speed indices >400, while $K_f = 20$ μGy for a film/screen system with a 200 speed index. The inverse square law can be applied to allow for the different distances from the X-ray tube focus of the wall (FWD) and the film (FFD) to calculate the dose at the barrier. The primary radiation kerma incident on the barrier (K_b) over a given period can be determined from the number of films (n) taken in that orientation:

$$K_b = n \times K_f \times (\mathrm{FFD}/\mathrm{FWD})^2. \qquad (13.1)$$

Unattenuated primary radiation

In certain situations, such as chest and skull radiography, the body and/or cassette may not intercept the entire beam. In this case the primary air kerma (K_b) at the barrier can be calculated from the sum of ESDs (§14.1.1) for the appropriate number (n_i) of each type of radiograph (i). An inverse square law correction using the focus to skin distance (FSD) can again be applied to determine the kerma at the barrier:

$$K_b = \sum_i (n_i \times \mathrm{ESD}_i) \times (\mathrm{FSD}/\mathrm{FWD})^2. \quad (13.2)$$

This method is an explicitly conservative approach since it equates ESD and air kerma, neglecting the backscatter component of approximately 30%.

Secondary barrier

Secondary radiation is present in all shielding problems and comprises components arising from scattered and leakage radiation which should both be taken into account. The method for dealing with the transmission of secondary radiation is described in §13.3.3.

Scatter contribution

The scatter kerma (K_s) is closely related to the DAP (§14.1.1) and can be determined from the equation [5]:

$$K_s = S \times \mathrm{DAP} \quad (13.3)$$

where S is the scatter fraction. The use of DAP to derive the scatter component implicitly integrates over all technique factors, so that no assumptions need to be made concerning field size. The amount of scatter varies with angle (§2.5.2) and the maximum scatter incident on a wall will be at approximately 120° to the direction of the incident beam when the inverse square law is taken into account. In the general case the maximum value of the scatter factor at 1 metre can be calculated using the equation:

$$S = (0.031\ \mathrm{kVp} + 2.5)\ \mu\mathrm{Gy}(\mathrm{Gy\ cm}^2)^{-1}. \quad (13.4)$$

This equation is applicable in most situations, but for examinations where all exposures are similar such as intra-oral dental radiographs or mammography, assumptions may be made that the same amount of scatter/primary is produced for all exposures to simplify the calculation.

Leakage contribution

Leakage is usually defined at the maximum operating potential of an X-ray tube/generator combination and is specified at the maximum continuous tube current possible at that potential (the leakage technique factors). Normally the scattered radiation component exceeds that from leakage radiation by at least an order of magnitude at kVps above 100 kVp [6]. At kVps below 100 kVp, the ratio of scatter to leakage radiation gradually increases to more than 10^8. However, because leakage radiation generally passes through at least 2 mm of lead, it will be considerably harder than radiation in the primary beam.

The majority of radiological examinations are performed at less than 100 kV and, consequently, it is safe to assume that the amount of leakage radiation will be substantially less than that of scattered radiation and can be neglected. At 100 kV and above, this is not necessarily the case and allowance should be made for leakage by using secondary radiation parameters in the transmission equation (§13.3.3).

Table 13.3 Example values of DAP and ESD for various examinations

Examination	DAP (Gy cm^2)	ESD (mGy)
Chest (PA)	0.15	0.17
Chest (lateral)	0.5	0.8
Skull (AP/PA)	0.8	2.8
Skull (lateral)	0.5	1.5
Pelvis (AP)	3.3	4.7
Abdomen (AP)	3.8	5.8
Lumbar spine (AP)	3.2	6.4
Lumbar spine (lateral)	3.4	15.0
ERCP	11	–
Barium swallow	10	–
Barium meal	13	–
IVU	16	–
Barium enema	27	–
Coronary angiography	40	–
Cerebral angiography	53	–
PTCA	55	–
Femoral angiography	60	–
Cerebral embolization	110	–
Abdominal angiography	120	–
TIPS	260	–

ERCP, endoscopic retrograde cholangiopancreatogram; IVU, intravenous urogram; PTCA, percutaneous transluminal coronary angiography; TIPS, transjugular intrahepatic portosystemic shunt.

Workload data

The most appropriate source of information for estimating workload is local dose audit. If this information is not available, then published data can be used. Alternatively, ESD or DAP can be calculated using either output data obtained from the equipment to be used in the room or calculation from theoretical spectral data [7]. Examples of DAP and ESD values for a range of examinations are given in Table 13.3. The table uses UK data and as such may not be applicable elsewhere. Provided that the dose information is known, then the only other requirement of the method is a knowledge of the number of patients (§7.4.3).

13.3.3 Attenuation properties of materials

A number of authors have addressed the issues surrounding the attenuation of primary and secondary radiation from diagnostic X-ray equipment by various shielding materials [6, 8–11]. From a combination of empirical measurement and theoretical modelling, they

Table 13.4 Transmission parameters for lead and concrete

	kVp	α	β	γ	Limiting HVL (mm)
Primary beam					
Lead	30	38.80	178	0.347	0.018
	50	8.801	27.28	0.296	0.079
	70	5.369	23.49	0.588	0.13
	90	3.067	18.83	0.773	0.23
	100	2.500	15.28	0.756	0.28
	125	2.219	7.923	0.539	0.31
Concrete	30	0.3173	1.698	0.359	2.2
	50	0.0903	0.1712	0.232	7.7
	70	0.0509	0.1696	0.385	14
	90	0.0423	0.1137	0.469	16
	100	0.0393	0.0857	0.427	18
	125	0.0352	0.0711	0.697	20
Secondary radiation					
Lead	100	2.507	15.33	0.912	0.28
	125	2.233	7.89	0.730	0.31
	150	1.791	5.48	0.568	0.39
Concrete	100	0.0395	0.084	0.519	18
	125	0.0351	0.066	0.783	20
	150	0.0324	0.078	1.566	21

have provided realistic data on which to base shielding calculations.

The method is based around an empirical equation describing the broad-beam transmission of X-rays through a material, given three parameters:

$$B = [(1 + \beta/\alpha).\exp(\alpha\gamma x) - \beta/\alpha]^{-1/\gamma} \quad (13.5)$$

where B is transmission, x is the thickness of material, and α,β,γ are constants for any given material. Values for these constants have been determined over a range of kVs used in general radiography for the key X-ray shielding materials, including lead, concrete, glass, wood, and gypsum and barium plaster [1]. Parameters for primary transmission through lead and concrete are shown in Table 13.4.

These parameters can be used to generate curves showing the transmission of primary X-radiation through lead of varying thickness, as shown in Figure 13.3. They can be incorporated into a spreadsheet to enable explicit calculations using equation (13.5) and its inverse (§7.4.3).

Since the transmission depends on the degree of hardening of the X-ray beam incident on the barrier, the approach that should be adopted will depend on the source of radiation.

- *Unattenuated primary.* The primary beam coefficients given in Table 13.4 can be applied directly. Allowance can be made for attenuation by a cassette, which is equivalent to about 0.15 mm of lead, or a grid and cassette (0.2 mm of lead) [1].
- Primary which has passed through a patient. When the X-ray beam has passed through larger thicknesses of material, it is hardened. The relationship between transmission and thickness tends towards a simple exponential one (Figure 13.3), which can be defined in terms of the limiting half-value layer (HVL), equal to $\ln 2/\alpha$. Where protection is being assessed for primary radiation hardened by transmission through the patient, the limiting HVL (Table 13.4) should be used to calculate the thickness of shielding.
- In the case of table radiography, the cassette and table assembly can be considered to provide attenuation equivalent to 0.8 mm of lead (75 mm concrete) [9], while for cross-table radiography the cassette can be taken to have a transmission of 0.5 [1], which conservatively is equivalent to 0.15 mm of lead.
- *Secondary radiation.* The coefficients in Table 13.4 for the primary beam can be applied for secondary radiation energies below 100 kVp, but for higher

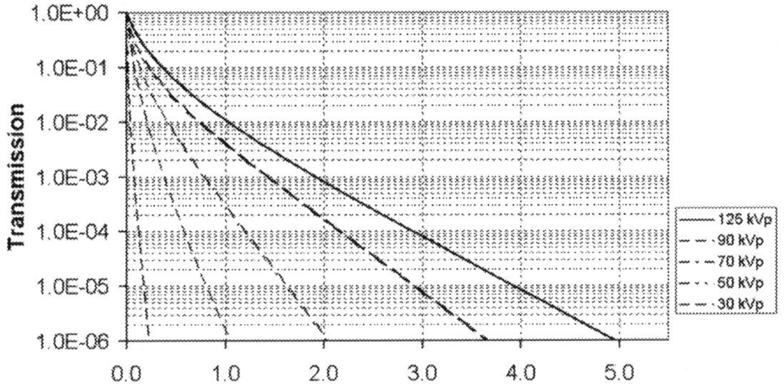

Figure 13.3 Transmission of primary radiation through lead.

Table 13.5 Approximate lead equivalences for thistle X-ray plaster

Plaster thickness (mm)	X-ray tube potential (kVp) 50	75	100	125	150
15	0.77	1.96	1.87	1.16	0.83
20	1.03	2.62	2.50	1.55	1.10
25	1.29	3.27	3.12	1.94	1.38

energies separate coefficients should be used to take account of the harder beam for the leakage component. These coefficients, which are also given in Table 13.4, should be used when calculating transmission for shielding in CT installations.

Coefficients given in Table 13.4 are for transmission through concrete of density 2350 kg m^{-3}. However, there is not one substance called 'concrete'. In fact, concrete comes in various densities, from the US standard concrete at 2350 kg m^{-3}, through UK standard concrete at 2200 kg m^{-3} to lightweight concrete at 1840 kg m^{-3}. Other forms of aerated concrete with even smaller densities are increasingly being used as building materials and are unlikely to provide sufficient protective shielding for most diagnostic X-ray rooms. An approximate assessment of transmission (B_ρ) for concrete of density ρ kg m^{-3} can be obtained by scaling according to density:

$$B_\rho = B_{2350}(2350/\rho). \qquad (13.6)$$

Barytes (or thistle X-ray) plaster may be used as an undercoat plaster where added radiation protection is required. Table 13.5 gives approximate lead equivalences at various kVps for differing plaster thicknesses.

If the acceptable barrier transmission has been determined from a knowledge of the quantities of incident radiation (§13.3.2), data in §13.3.3 can then be used to calculate the thickness of a particular shielding material required in any given situation.

13.3.4 Assessment of shielding

The aims of the practical assessment of shielding are (a) to detect any places where there are gaps in the shielding provided and (b) to check that the protection is of the level specified. After the installation is complete, the integrity of the shielding can be investigated using a radionuclide source or an X-ray generator. However, it is advisable to visit the site during the construction period to ensure that problems do not occur.

Use of a radiation source and detector allows the integrity of all parts of the shielding in a completed installation to be checked. The most suitable, although not necessarily the most available, source is a sealed source of ^{241}Am which has a γ-ray energy of 60 keV which is within the energy range used in general radiography. A vial of ^{99m}Tc may be used as an alternative if the ^{241}Am source is not available. The ^{241}Am source can be calibrated in a defined geometry using differing thicknesses of lead and the results used to infer the lead equivalence of any installed protection. The same is not strictly true in the case of ^{99m}Tc since the K-edge of lead (88 keV) occurs significantly below the main γ-ray at 141 keV. Circumspection must be applied if shielding is assessed using ^{99m}Tc unless the shielding material is lead or a calibration exists for the material used [1].

It is also possible to use an X-ray set to assess shielding integrity. In theory this is the best solution since the energy spectrum is correct. However, there are many practical problems associated with this approach. These include availability of a set to perform the assessment and the difficulties associated with positioning measuring equipment, given the short duration of the exposures.

13.4 Protection assessments for specific installations

This section comprises examples of shielding calculations to illustrate use of the methodology described. No account has been taken of occupancy in any of the examples given, but realistic assumptions about occupancy may enable shielding to be reduced [1].

13.4.1 Radiography

General radiography

An example is given in Box 13.1 to demonstrate application of the principles described in §13.2 to the primary beam and scatter in table radiography. An occupancy of 1.0 has been assumed but values for transmission could be reduced proportionately for lower occupancies.

Dental radiography

Although dental radiography produces relatively low radiation doses, room shielding must be considered since dental X-ray rooms are often small and rarely purpose-built. This means that the X-ray set may be close to one or more walls. A simple assumption that the dose from primary and scattered radiation at 1 m from the patient is 1 μGy can be made, because of the similarity between all intra-oral exposures. An example calculation is given in Box 13.2.

- 20 mm of plasterboard transmits approximately 25% of a 70 kVp X-ray beam. Partition walls with 10 mm plasterboard on both sides will provide sufficient protection in most circumstances.

Box 13.1 Example for table radiography (primary and scatter)

Parameter	Example values
Applied voltage	90 kVp (DAP weighted average)
Example workload (table radiography)	500 films per week
Primary air kerma at film (K_f)	15 μGy (300 speed index)
Distance to person on floor below	4.5 m
Annual primary kerma [eq. 13.1]	20 mGy [$(500 \times 52 \times 15)/(4.5)^2$ μGy]
Transmission to achieve 0.3 mGy	0.015 [0.3/20]
Protection recommended for primary beam provided by table and floor	**96 mm concrete [6 HVLs]** (*Note*: table provides 75 mm concrete equivalence)
Total workload (DAP)	600 Gy cm^2 per week
Scatter factor (at 1 m) [eq. 13.4]	5.3 μGy (Gy cm^2)$^{-1}$ [(0.031x 90 + 2.5) μGy (Gy cm^2)$^{-1}$]
Distance from patient to nearest wall	2 m
Annual scatter kerma at wall [eq. 13.3]	41 mGy [$(600 \times 52 \times 5.3)/4^2$ μGy]
Transmission to achieve 0.3 mGy	0.007 [0.3/41]
Protection recommended for scatter	**0.9 mm of lead or 65 mm of concrete [eq. 13.5]**

Box 13.2 Example for dental radiography

Parameter	Example values
Applied voltage	70 kVp
Primary/scatter kerma	1 μGy per film
Example workload	1000 films per annum
Distance to nearest wall from patient/X-ray tube	1.5 m
Annual primary/scatter kerma	440 μGy [1000/1.5^2]
Transmission to achieve 300 μGy	0.65 [300/440]
Protection recommended	**10 mm plasterboard [eq. 13.5] [1]**

- Walls greater than 2 m from the patient would not need to be shielded for a workload of 1000 films per annum.
- Brick or blockwork walls should provide sufficient protection in most circumstances.
- For panoramic dental radiography, the entire beam is intercepted by the patient. The scatter dose from a unit operating at 70 kVp may be assumed to be 0.65 μGy per examination. However, these units are usually mounted close to a wall, so that the scatter kerma at the wall is between 1 and 2 μGy per examination.

Mammography

Mammography only produces relatively low radiation doses and dose rates, with the additional advantage from a radiation protection perspective of low-energy X-rays. Room shielding must still be considered since mammography rooms are often quite small. However, the primary beam is intercepted by the image receptor, so only scattered radiation need be considered.

Standard values may be assumed for the maximum scatter kerma (K_s) at 1 m of 7.6 μGy for the back wall (in front of the patient) and 1.3 μGy for the side wall. A simple approach of the type adopted for dental radiography (Box 13.2) can then be used. A few points concerning appropriate shielding materials are worth noting.

- Given the low ratio of air kerma to effective dose at mammographic energies, these calculations are likely to be pessimistic. Normal building materials should therefore suffice under most circumstances.
- At mammographic energies, materials such as plasterboard and glass can provide a protection solution as demonstrated in Table 13.6.
- The wall behind the patient will receive almost no radiation. Thus, if the room is small, protection of the door can be avoided by positioning the equipment so that the patient faces away from the entrance.

13.4.2 Fluoroscopy

A requirement of fluoroscopic equipment design, other than radiotherapy simulators, is that the primary beam is absorbed entirely by the image receptor. Thus only

Table 13.6 Transmissions for mammographic X-rays (30 kVp) of different thicknesses of light construction materials

Transmission	Gypsum plaster board (mm)	Plate glass (mm)	Wood (mm)
0.1	4	2	50
0.01	10	5	110
0.001	22	10	

scattered radiation needs to be considered for radiation protection purposes.

General fluoroscopy

Most fluoroscopic X-ray systems use an undercouch X-ray tube with the image intensifier gantry mounted above the table. The gantry usually possesses some lead curtains to reduce scattered radiation in lateral directions from the patient. Some systems use an overcouch tube with the intensifier underneath the patient and imaging table. This latter arrangement frequently gives rise to higher scattered dose rates within the room which will need to be considered for room shielding purposes. An example calculation is given in Box 13.3.

C-arm/interventional fluoroscopic equipment

There is a wide range of equipment, of varying degrees of complexity, using a tube and intensifier at opposing ends of a C-arm. The systems are used in several clinical situations, including mobile units in operating theatres and endoscopy rooms to dedicated vascular angiographic and interventional suites. In normal practice, the tube is used in an undercouch position, although some techniques will require beams angled more horizontally. The method for calculating shielding requirements is the same as that for standard fluoroscopy equipment. The workloads can, however, differ markedly [1].

- There are large differences in DAP values for such procedures, depending on their complexity and the techniques used.
- For more complex interventional procedures, the maximum annual scattered doses at the nearest wall surfaces may reach 140 mGy. Assuming 100% occupancy, the radiation protection requirement for the wall would be in the region of 1.0–1.5 mm of lead-equivalent material.
- In the case of orthopaedic theatres, X-ray guided endoscopy and cardiac pacemaker insertions, sizes of rooms and workloads suggest a maximum annual scatter dose of 2 mGy at wall surfaces. Given relatively low occupancy factors for adjacent rooms, even standard plasterboard walls are likely to provide sufficient attenuation to ensure the design criteria are met.

13.4.3 Computed tomography (CT)

The whole of the primary beam in CT will be absorbed by the radiation detectors and equipment gantry. Thus, the only radiation to be considered in CT room design is that scattered by the patient and imaging table. CT produces a well-defined pattern of scattered radiation, which is dependent on exposure parameters, beam collimation, and filtration, and most importantly the design of the scanner gantry. Figure 13.4 gives one example of plotted isodose contours from a CT scanner. The pattern, shown here in two dimensions, is similar in the third dimension. Greater protection may be necessary in directions of higher dose rate.

Some specific points to be considered are listed below and an example calculation is given in Box 13.4.

- The location and orientation of the scanner within the room are important.
- The high kVps and more heavily filtered X-rays used in CT mean that the scattered radiation produced is of

Box 13.3 Example exposure data for fluoroscopy

Parameter	Example values
Applied potential	100 kVp
Dose–area product	Barium meals 15 Gy cm^2 Barium enemas 30 Gy cm^2
Scatter factor (at 1 m) [eq. 13.4]	5.6 μGy (Gy $cm^2)^{-1}$ [(0.031 kVp + 2.5) μGy (Gy $cm^2)^{-1}$]
Example workload	20 cases/week (Barium meals) 30 cases/week (Barium enemas)
Distance to nearest wall from patient/X-ray tube	3 m
Annual scatter kerma [eq. 13.3]	37 mGy [{([20 × 15] + [30 × 30]) × 52 × 5.6}/3^2] mGy
Transmission to achieve 0.3 mGy	0.008 [0.3/37]
Protection recommended	**1.0 mm lead [eq. 13.5]**

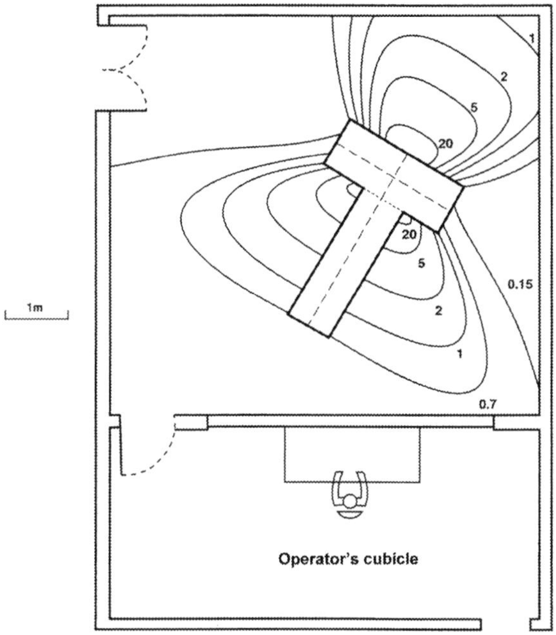

Figure 13.4 Isodose curves for scattered radiation from a CT scanner.

a higher average energy than in other radiological techniques. This tends to increase the shielding requirements.

- Scattered dose rates are generally proportional to the slice thickness and mAs. Differing case-mixes of head and body examinations will therefore result in different scattered dose profiles and totals. Narrower slice thicknesses may use detector collimation without additional source collimation so that the relationship to slice thickness may not always be followed. CTDI values will provide guidance on this (§14.8.1).
- Scatter plots will differ for head and body sections, but the relationship depends on the scanner. Conservative assumptions are that when only data for a head scan are available, the scatter dose per mAs should be multiplied by two to obtain a value for the body, while when only data for a body scan are available, the same value per mAs should be applied to head scans.
- New multi-slice scanners enable examinations to be performed more quickly and are likely to lead to increased workloads. Consideration may need to be given to the issue of instantaneous dose rates.
- Shielding of the roof and/or floor is likely to be required.
- It is likely that the entry into the room from the control cubicle will need a shielded door. Otherwise, scattered dose rates from adjacent walls may well be significant within the control room.
- The higher levels of scattered radiation will usually require shielding of walls and control cubicle to extend to the full height of the room to avoid radiation being scattered from the ceiling slab into adjacent areas. About 1% of the radiation incident on a concrete roof slab or wall may be scattered into an adjacent area.

13.4.4 Temporary and mobile facilities

The above requirements for shielding X-ray rooms are based on the equipment being sited in permanent buildings. They will need to be modified when dealing with X-ray units in mobile trailers or in temporary structures such as portacabins.

For mobile units the design, weight, and space limitations of the trailer will almost certainly place restrictions on the amount of shielding that will be provided with the unit. As such, much of the limitation

Box 13.4 Example exposure data for a CT scanner

Parameter	Example values
Applied voltage	140 kVp (filtration typically 6–7 mm Al)
Example workload	120 body exam/week (based on 22 × 10 mm slices at 250 mAs/slice) and 70 head exam/week (12 × 10 mm slices at 350 mAs/slice)
Distance from centre of scanner	2.5 m
Scatter kerma in position for assessment	1.5 μGy per 250 mAs, 10 mm body slices (from scatter diagram)
Annual scatter kerma	298 mGy [(120 × 22) + (70 × 12 × 350/250)] × 52 × 1.5 μGy]
Transmission to achieve 300 μGy	0.001 [0.3/298]
Protection recommended	**2 mm lead or 190 mm concrete [eq. 13.5]**

on radiation dose may need to be achieved by careful siting of the trailer. If the trailer is not parked adjacent to buildings or directly underneath areas with significant overhang, distance can almost certainly be used to achieve the necessary reduction in radiation dose rate, in conjunction with the shielding provided by the walls of the nearest buildings.

It is unlikely that temporary structures will have sufficient shielding to provide the necessary dose reduction, so distance will again be used to achieve this. Mobile protective screens may have to be used for certain directions and to provide protection for the operators.

Where distance is used, consideration will have to be given to the use of fencing to delineate boundaries at which radiation dose rates will be at an acceptable level.

13.5 Personnel radiation protection

13.5.1 Strategies for dose reduction

In general, staff should never be exposed to the primary X-ray beam, but in many situations scattered dose rates will be significant and steps must be taken to reduce this exposure. As discussed in §7.3, there are three basic personnel dose-reduction strategies—time, distance, and shielding. With regards to equipment factors, the following should be noted.

Time

Individuals controlling the length of exposures (e.g. during a fluoroscopic procedure) must be aware that they are controlling this most basic aspect of radiation exposure and seek to minimize it, as this will reduce exposures to both the patient and staff in the radiation field. Optimisation of equipment factors such as pulsed fluoroscopy also form part of the dose-reduction strategy.

Distance

When an individual is close to the radiation source (e.g. close by the imaging table during interventional procedures), even small increases in distance can produce significant dose reductions. Examples include keeping the hands away from the imaging or theatre table and taking a pace back from the patient whenever practicable. Clearly there are instances where the needs of the patient mean that staff must be close at hand but this should be kept under constant review by those concerned and especially by the operator of the X-ray set.

Shielding

Protection is provided by fixed protective barriers (§13.2.4) and personal protective equipment (§13.5.2). Personal protective equipment uses stated lead equivalences of 0.25, 0.35, and 0.5 mm. With a normal diagnostic X-ray beam, even a 0.25 mm lead equivalence will attenuate about 97% of the radiation at 70 kVp. As the kVp climbs, the protective value of the shielding equipment starts to fall, and at 105 kVp the attenuation will only be of the order of 90%. Thus a greater lead equivalence is required to maintain a similar level of protection at higher kVps.

13.5.2 Personal protective equipment

Personal protective equipment is needed whenever staff or others have to remain in radiation fields because they cannot stand behind fixed or mobile protective screens. One basic example in radiography is a parent or member of staff supporting a child undergoing X-ray examination. In fluoroscopy, angiography, or interventional radiology there may be a number of staff performing many different functions at varying distances within the radiation field. In such situations assessment of the potential for radiation exposure, and hence the degree of personal protective equipment required, should be carried out by a qualified radiation protection physicist.

Lead aprons

A lead apron is a basic requirement for all those who need some mobility while working in significant radiation fields. Lead aprons come in a variety of designs, which can be subdivided into front-only, front and half-back, double-sided, or wrap-around styles. The style chosen will depend to some extent on the working practices used, but designs that do not provide complete protection for the torso must be used with some caution to prevent exposure of unprotected areas. Even double-sided aprons can sometimes allow significant exposures to lateral aspects of the body if not designed or used correctly.

Weight reduction in lead aprons is an important issue. Depending on size and lead equivalence, a lead apron may weigh anywhere from 5 kg to more than 10 kg. The weight is often taken entirely on the shoulders, which has consequences for members of staff who may have to wear them for any length of time. Lumbar spine supports or belts are often used to take some of the weight on the hips. Other materials are also used to achieve some degree of weight reduction, such as barium and tungsten to replace some of the lead, although the effect on the attenuation properties at higher energies must be considered.

Lead aprons must be stored carefully because if they are folded repeatedly they will be likely to develop cracks that will seriously reduce their effectiveness as protective equipment. Either flat storage or vertical hanging from specialist hangers is recommended.

Thyroid shields

Most lead aprons are designed specifically to protect the torso and have a relatively free neckline to aid easy movement of the head. They do, however, leave the thyroid gland exposed to any radiation that may be present.

In circumstances where scattered radiation fields may be large and/or where staff must remain close to the radiation source, thyroid shields may provide a valuable source of protection. Typically made of the same material as lead aprons and with a velcro fastener around the back of the neck, they usually provide 0.5 mm lead-equivalent protection. They will restrict head and neck movement to some degree and give some loading to the lower cervical spine.

Lead gloves

Lead gloves are designed to protect the hands, wrists, and lower arms of any member of staff (typically a radiologist) who must get close to the primary beam or perhaps even be within the beam, for example to palpate an area under fluoroscopic exposure. Modern lead gloves typically provide 0.5 or 1.0 mm lead-equivalent protection and have increased flexibility than older designs, but will nevertheless restrict movement significantly.

Some designs of lead gloves are thinner and provide a greater degree of flexibility and sensitivity at the expense of some degree of protection. These designs use multilayer materials that provide attenuation levels between 20% and 60%, depending on the kVp used and the glove thickness.

Lead glasses

Lead glasses are designed to reduce radiation exposure to the eye in situations where staff must remain close to the radiation source. Styles vary widely, depending on the lead equivalence of the lead glass used (range 0.25–1.0 mm lead equivalence), whether there is side shielding, whether they are plain or prescription lenses, and whether they are designed to fit over existing spectacles. As a consequence, the weight varies considerably but is typically in the range 75–200 g.

Gonad shields

Gonad shields are designed specifically to protect patients undergoing X-ray examinations around the pelvis that would otherwise irradiate the gonads. They are available in various sizes and with 0.5 mm or, more typically, 1.0 mm lead equivalence. They need careful placement to absorb the primary beam.

13.6 References

1 Sutton, D. G. and Williams, J. R. (2000). *Radiation shielding for diagnostic X-rays*. Working Party Report. British Institute of Radiology.

2 National Council on Radiation Protection and Measurements (1976). *Structural design and evaluation for medical use of X-rays and gamma-rays of energies up to 10 MeV.* NCRP Report 49. NCRP, Bethesda.

3 Dixon, R. L. and Simpkin, D. J. (1998). Primary shielding barriers for diagnostic X-ray facilities: a new model. *Health Phys.*, **74**, 181–9.

4 International Commission on Radiological Protection (1997). Conversion coefficients for use in radiological protection against external radiation. ICRP Publication 74. *Ann. ICRP*, **27** (2).

5 Williams, J. R. (1996). Scatter dose estimation based on dose–area product and the specification of radiation barriers. *Br. J. Radiol.*, **69**, 1032–7.

6 Simpkin, D. J. and Dixon, R. L. (1998). Secondary radiation shielding barriers for diagnostic X-ray facilities: scatter and leakage revisited. *Health Phys.*, **74**, 350–65.

7 Sutton, D. G. and Reilly, A. J. (1997). *Spectrum processor.* IPEM Report 78 (CD-ROM). Institute of Physics and Engineering in Medicine, York.

8 Archer, B. R. (1994). Attenuation properties of diagnostic X-ray shielding materials. *Med. Phys.*, **21**, 9.

9 Dixon, R. L. (1994). On the primary barrier in diagnostic X-ray shielding. *Med. Phys.*, **21**, 1785–93.

10 Petrantonaki, M., Kappas, C., Efstathopoulos, E. P., Theodorakos, Y., and Panayiotakis, G. (1999). Calculating shielding requirements in diagnostic X-ray departments. *Br. J. Radiol.*, **72**, 179–85.

11 Simpkin, D. J. (1995). Transmission data for shielding diagnostic X-ray facilities. *Health Phys.*, **68**, 704–9.

Chapter 14

Diagnostic radiology: patient dosimetry

A. P. Hufton

14.1 Introduction

Protection of the patient in diagnostic radiology is of key importance in minimizing risks, both to individual patients and to the population at large. For example, in the UK, diagnostic radiology contributes over 96% to the average annual effective dose from artificial sources. The main purpose of this chapter is to discuss the principal reasons for assessing patient dose, and to give some practical methods for its determination.

There are many reasons why it may be necessary to make an assessment of patient dose. These include the need to ensure compliance with national legislation and guidance, to compare different techniques, to evaluate the effectiveness of dose reduction methods, to satisfy the requirements of research proposals and ethics committees, and to assess individual organ or effective doses in order to evaluate risk. In the majority of routine cases dose figures will be adequate, and it will be unnecessary to estimate the absolute risk of inducing a fatal cancer, for example. However, particularly where detailed risk–benefit or justification calculations are required, estimates of radiation detriment are essential. High-dose examinations, or screening programmes of largely asymptomatic individuals, are cases in point.

Consideration of the objectives is important because it determines the appropriate dose quantity to be measured and the techniques to be used. This chapter outlines the most useful dose quantities and their applications and develops the various ways of estimating these quantities. Specific details of how these techniques may be applied in different areas of diagnostic radiology are given in later sections.

14.2 Dose quantities

For an assessment of risk to the patient, organ equivalent doses and effective dose are the quantities of choice. However, it is rarely possible to measure any biologically relevant dose directly. Absorbed dose to the skin is an exception, and may be important in lengthy interventional procedures. It may also be possible to estimate the dose to a superficial organ from a direct measurement (e. g. the testes and eyes), although usually some allowance will need to be made for attenuation of overlying tissue. However, ultimately it is the detriment to the patient which is important, and selection of the appropriate dose quantity must reflect this. The two measurable quantities which have proved to be most useful for evaluating patient dose are entrance surface dose and dose–area product.

14.2.1 Entrance surface dose (ESD)

The absorbed dose at the point where the X-ray beam enters the patient can usually be measured directly, or easily estimated. Decisions will need to be made about whether to include backscatter (Box 14.1), and what medium to use for absorbed dose. This is particularly important when comparisons are made with published data, since different authors may have quoted doses to air, skin, water, or ICRU soft tissue (§2.7.4). In this chapter, ESD is defined as the absorbed dose to air at the surface of the patient, including backscatter. Unfortunately, ESD is not, in most cases, a good indicator of risk, although if used with care it can be of value for quality control purposes or comparative measurements. Importantly, it is often a useful starting point for estimating organ doses and effective dose.

14.2.2 Dose–area product (DAP)

As the name implies, dose–area product is the product of absorbed dose to air and X-ray field area. The dose is averaged over the X-ray field, in a plane perpendicular to the beam axis, and the beam area is specified in this same plane. Dose is measured without backscatter, and due to the inverse square law DAP is independent of distance from the X-ray tube. The units are Gy cm^2, or

Box 14.1 Backscatter factor (BSF), percentage depth dose (PDD), and tissue–air ratio (TAR)

Dose measurements made on the surface of a patient (or phantom) not only record the primary radiation incident on the patient but also measure the additional radiation scattered back from the patient. Therefore, output or dose measurements made free in air need to be increased by a factor, known as the *backscatter factor* (BSF), in order to obtain the entrance dose at the surface of the patient. The *backscatter fraction* is simply one minus the backscatter factor. Extensive data have been published in the literature: Hart *et al.* [1, 2] give backscatter fractions calculated by Monte Carlo methods for realistic clinical conditions, and Harrison [3] tabulates data measured in a water phantom.

The *percentage depth dose* (PDD) is the dose at a given depth, usually in a uniform phantom, as a percentage of the dose at the surface. It is a function of beam quality, focus to skin distance (FSD), and field size at the surface. Depth doses measured in water have been published by Harrison [4], who also cites a method of converting PDD measured at a given FSD to PDD at a different FSD.

The *tissue–air ratio* (TAR) is the ratio of the dose at a specified depth in a phantom to the dose in air at the same point but in the absence of the phantom. It is independent of FSD, provided field size is specified at the depth of interest. TARs can be measured directly or derived simply from corresponding PDD and BSF data [5].

submultiples thereof. DAP is more closely related to overall risk than ESD. It has found most use in assessing dose and risk in complex examinations, where the position of the X-ray beam, relative to the patient, may change during the course of the examination. It can be converted into energy imparted to the patient (in mJ) or, more conveniently, directly into effective dose by the use of suitable published data.

14.2.3 Energy imparted

Energy imparted is the total energy, in joules, absorbed by the patient. It can be estimated from the measured DAP, if the beam quality and fraction of energy scattered and transmitted out of the patient are known.

$$\text{Energy Imparted} = \text{DAP} \times \text{IF}/(\mu_{en}/\rho)\ \text{joules}$$

where DAP is in Gy m^2, IF is the fraction of incident radiation imparted to the patient, and μ_{en}/ρ is the mean mass energy absorption coefficient for air, for the X-ray spectrum in use. If the primary beam is fully intercepted by the patient, the imparted fraction is independent, to within 2–3% of the part of the body being examined. Typical values are included in Table 14.1 along with other useful data. However, the fraction of the beam which misses the patient must also be taken into account. For many examinations this is insignificant, but for skull X-rays 30–35% of the beam will not be intercepted by the patient's head.

It is not now commonly used because extensive data exist to convert DAP to effective dose. However, it may be useful to give an approximate idea of effective dose in those circumstances where the examination details do not match any of the published data. This can be done simply by dividing the energy imparted by the total mass of the body or trunk.

14.2.4 Organ dose

The absorbed dose to individual organs is clearly biologically relevant, but can rarely be measured directly (§3.2.2). However, it can be estimated, either from published data relating organ dose to ESD (normalized organ doses) or from measured or published depth dose data. An estimate of individual organ dose may be particularly relevant if a single organ receives a high dose, has a high sensitivity to radiation damage, or receives most of the dose in an examination, such as the breast in mammography.

14.2.5 Effective dose

Effective dose embodies, in a single figure, a measure of the radiation detriment. It can be calculated from a knowledge of the doses to individual organs and tissue weighting factors (Table 3.8) or from published conversion factors relating ESD and DAP to effective dose. Example effective dose calculations for diagnostic radiology and nuclear medicine are given in Boxes 11.1 and 16.1. The evaluation of risks is the natural conclusion of a radiation dose assessment and this is discussed in §11.6. Since detriment includes hereditary damage (§3.5), and weighted allowances for non-fatal cancers and years of life lost (§3.4), effective dose should not strictly be used to estimate the probability of fatal cancer induction. However, as discussed in §11.3.2, the estimate obtained is sufficiently close to the actual result to allow its use for conveying risk in most circumstances.

14.3 Requirements for patient dose estimation

This section gives examples of circumstances which require patient doses to be estimated.

Table 14.1 Some typical data for diagnostic X-ray beams

	Typical values for 3 mm total filtration at the following tube potentials					
	60 kVp	70 kVp	80 kVp	90 kVp	100 kVp	120 kVp
Output (μGy/mAs at 1 m)	46	61	78	96	115	155
Half-value layer (mm Al)	2.3	2.7	3.2	3.6	4.1	5.0
Backscatter factor[a]						
Field sizes:						
10 cm × 10 cm	1.27	1.29	1.30	1.33	1.37	1.42
15 cm × 15 cm	1.30	1.32	1.34	1.37	1.40	1.45
20 cm × 20 cm	1.31	1.33	1.35	1.38	1.41	1.46
30 cm × 30 cm	1.33	1.35	1.37	1.40	1.43	1.48
Imparted fraction	0.77	0.74	0.70	0.67	0.65	0.61
Energy imparted to adult trunk per dose–area product (mJ/Gy cm^2)	7.30	8.56	9.59	10.6	11.4	12.8
Percentage depth dose						
Depth[b] (mm)						
0	100	100	100	100	100	100
20	76	77	78	79	81	83
50	37	40	42	43	45	49
100	11	13	14	15	17	20
150	3.2	4	4.5	5.1	5.7	7.5
200	0.96	1.2	1.4	1.8	2.3	3.3

[a]Adapted from Harrison [3].
[b]Depth in a 25 cm × 25 cm water phantom, 70 cm FSD.

14.3.1 Legislation and guidance

The requirement to keep doses 'as low as reasonably practicable' (ALARP) applies as much to patients as to staff. As an aid to restricting doses from medical exposures, the International Commission on Radiological Protection (ICRP) introduced the idea of diagnostic reference levels (DRLs) in diagnostic radiology [6] (§11.5.2, Box 14.2). Legislation in Europe requires member states to promote the establishment of DRLs (Article 4), assess and evaluate patient dose as part of the optimisation process (Article 3), include patient dose measurements as part of a quality assurance programme (Article 8), and ensure that the distribution of individual dose estimates is determined for the population [7–9]. In the UK there is also a legal requirement to carry out a detailed investigation and assessment of dose if a patient receives a dose much greater than intended, either as a result of equipment malfunction [8] or as a result of operator error [9] (Box 14.3).

14.3.2 Dose comparisons and optimisation

Comparisons of patient dose may be necessary as part of an evaluation of different techniques, or in order to assess the effectiveness of dose reduction strategies. In some instances, all that may be required is a relative, qualitative assessment of dose: for example, which of two techniques gives the higher dose. At the other extreme a quantitative evaluation of the change in radiation detriment may be needed. A professional judgement needs to be made as to what dose quantity to use. In the simplest cases, where, for example, the only change is in the mAs delivered, it will be possible to use an estimate of the ESD for comparative purposes. DAP is likely to give a more realistic comparison of risks, since it takes into account changes in field size. However, if the kV or filtration changes, the energy imparted will be a better indicator of risk, but even this does not allow for the irradiation of different organs and tissues. Only an assessment of effective dose can allow for all these factors, and in order to be confident about any conclusions it may often be simpler to use this as the dose quantity for comparative purposes.

14.3.3 Research

Proposals to ethics committees for research involving radiation usually require the effective dose to be stated.

Box 14.2 Diagnostic reference levels (DRLs)

The purpose of DRLs is to help to identify potentially poor radiation protection practice. Thus they function in a similar way to investigation levels and give a quantitative guide to optimizing patient doses. An internal investigation should be carried out if the average dose for a particular type of examination exceeds the relevant DRL. The investigation should either identify ways of improving practice to reduce doses or clinically justify the use of such higher doses.

DRLs must relate to the average dose to a representative sample of typical patients. They should not be applied to individual patients, since it is acknowledged that some patients will receive higher doses than others due to their size or the difficulty of the investigation.

There is, as yet, no accepted way of setting DRLs. Those originally derived for some common examinations were based on the third quartile of the dose distributions from national surveys. The establishment of local DRLs, set lower than the national figures, is encouraged. Such a procedure would drive doses ever downwards, and there is a danger that at some stage image quality would be compromised. There is therefore a move towards the establishment of 'achievable doses', which would represent levels of dose that should be accomplished with reasonable practice, without necessarily implying optimum performance.

Box 14.3 Exposures much greater than intended

An exposure is considered to be much greater than intended if the ratio of the suspected exposure to the intended exposure exceeds the appropriate value given below [10]. These factors are to be applied to the whole examination.

Barium enemas, barium meals, IVUs, angiography, and other such procedures involving fluoroscopy (including digital radiology) and computed tomography	3
Lumbar spine, abdomen, pelvis, mammography, and all all other examinations not otherwise listed	10
Extremities, skull, chest, dental examinations, and other simple examinations such as elbow, knee, and shoulder	20

The above factors are broadly based on an additional cancer incidence of 0.1%, i.e. this is the risk due to the unintended, excess part of the exposure. Although developed for unintended exposures due to equipment faults, the intention is that these ratios should be used for the time being for other causes of unintended exposures, such as operator error.

However, in some instances it may be more appropriate to give the dose to a single organ, if irradiation is largely limited to that organ. Further details on research exposures can be found in Box 11.3.

14.4 Dosimetry techniques using patients and phantoms

There are many ways of estimating patient doses, and the method chosen will depend on several factors; principally, the dose quantity required, the resources and equipment available, and the type of X-ray examination. Doses can be obtained by measurement or calculation, or more usually by a combination of both.

When dose estimations are derived from measurements, these may be made on real patients or on phantoms designed to simulate a patient in some relevant realistic way. Estimations from patients have the advantage that variations in dose due to variations in the size of individual patients, or in differences in technique between different operators, can be quantified. This knowledge may be particularly useful when trying to optimise doses. Patient measurements also give some confidence that the doses reflect what patients are really receiving. Alternatively, phantoms offer the advantage of fixed shape, size, and composition, making it easier to compare doses when given sets of parameters are varied. Nevertheless, if possible, doses should always be assessed finally on patients. A large number of patients may be required to demonstrate statistically significant dose differences, which may well be much smaller than the spread in doses due to patient size.

For dosimetric purposes, phantoms should ideally match tissue in terms of atomic composition. However, in general this is very difficult to achieve, so instead an attempt is made to simulate the interaction properties of tissues in terms of mass attenuation coefficients. Table 14.2 lists some materials suitable for use in the diagnostic energy range. All of these can be acquired commercially or are otherwise easily obtainable. Their interaction properties and those of the ICRU selected body tissues are given in ICRU Report 44 [11]. Because of differences in density, the thickness of phantom material may not be the same as the tissue thickness required to give the same total attenuation, even if the mass attenuation coefficients are very similar. As can be seen from Table 14.2, very good tissue substitutes for a variety of applications can be obtained by appropriate epoxy resin mixtures. These are commonly available in square sheets of different sizes and thicknesses, but can be cut to different shapes if desired. For many applications less expensive alternatives, such as plastic or perspex containers filled with water, can be used. While these may not be very realistic in terms of mimicking the shape and heterogeneity of a real patient, they are useful for measuring simple depth dose curves or for estimating ESDs, particularly when exposure factors are set automatically.

For more complex or realistic measurements, anthropomorphic phantoms are available. These consist of a human skeleton or plastic substitute embedded in soft tissue equivalent material, with reasonably realistic air and lung cavities. Different body sections, such as skull or pelvis, can be obtained separately if the high cost mitigates against purchase of a whole body. Solid phantoms can look quite realistic when radiographed, but the sectioned type, with cavities for dosimeters, are likely to be more useful for extensive dosimetric measurements (Figure 14.1). ICRU Report 48 [12] gives the specifications for a number of these types of phantoms, both adult and child sized, and including the well-known 'Rando' type of anthropomorphic phantom. The latter was originally intended for use in radiotherapy but has been used extensively for diagnostic applications. However, the rubber material of these phantoms is less attenuating than water, the effective attenuation being up to 9% less than water at low kilovoltages. Possible differences in attenuation properties should therefore be borne in mind when choosing any phantom. Other anthropomorphic phantoms have been developed for special applications, such as mammography (§14.9.1).

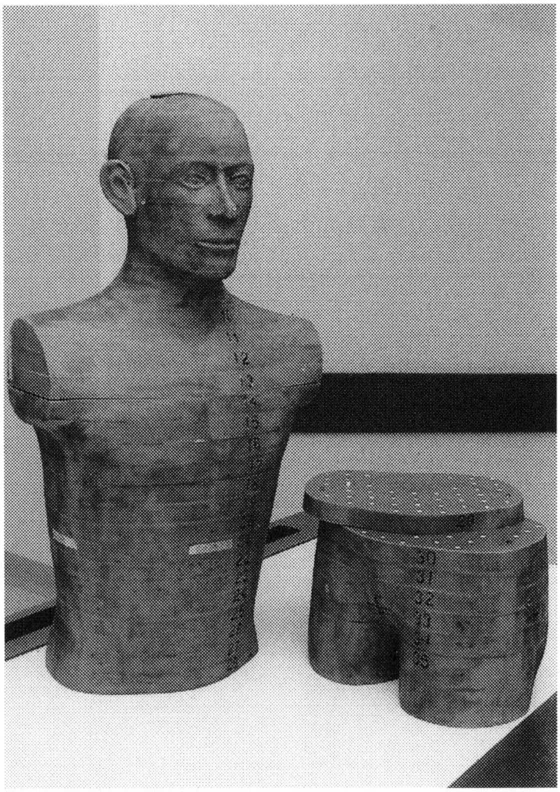

Figure 14.1 The 'Rando' phantom, showing the 25 mm thick transverse sections each containing a grid of plugs which can be replaced with TLDs for dosimetry measurements.

14.5 Radiation measurements

The reader is referred to Chapter 4 for a detailed discussion of radiation measurement techniques. This section is confined to practical considerations relating to patient dose measurements in diagnostic radiology.

When choosing a suitable radiation detector for dose measurements a number of factors need to be considered. The main ones are the required accuracy and precision, the sensitivity, and the energy response. Other important practical points include the robustness of the detector, whether, if measurements are being made on patients, the detector will be visible on the image, directional dependence of the detector, linearity, and dose-rate dependence. Such data are usually given in the manufacturer's technical information.

The calibration of dosemeters should be traceable to national standards, and should ideally be carried out under similar conditions to those in which field measurements will be undertaken. Spectra defined for radiation protection instruments are generally unsuitable, and those defined in IEC 61267 are more relevant [13]. Calibration laboratories may also be able to offer additional combinations of kV, waveform, and filtration to suit particular needs. Often the dose rates used for calibration are lower than those encountered in radiographic exposures, although this is less of a problem now that suitable facilities exist for diagnostic in-beam

Table 14.2 A selection of tissue substitutes suitable for diagnostic radiology

Tissue substitute	Density (kg m^{-3})	n_0, number of electrons per m^3	Comments
General radiography			
Muscle (ρ = 1050 kg m^{-3}, n_0 = 3480 × 10^{26})			
Polymethylmethacrylate	1170	3800 × 10^{26}	PMMA, also known as acrylic, plexiglass, perspex, and lucite
Water	1000	3340 × 10^{26}	
WT1	1020	3310 × 10^{26}	Same as MS20
Alderson	1000	3270 × 10^{26}	Rubber material used in Rando anthropomorphic phantoms
Temex	1010	3310 × 10^{26}	Rubber material used in some anthropomorphic phantoms
Paraffin wax	930	3210 × 10^{26}	
Polystyrene	1050	3400 × 10^{26}	
Cortical bone (ρ = 1920 kg m^{-3}, n_0 = 5950 × 10^{26})			
Aluminium	2700	7840 × 10^{26}	
Polytetrafluoroethylene	2100	6070 × 10^{26}	PTFE
SB5	1870	5770 × 10^{26}	
Adipose (fat) (ρ = 950 kg m^{-3}, n_0 = 3180 × 10^{26})			
AP6	920	2990 × 10^{26}	
Polythene	920	3160 × 10^{26}	
Paraffin wax	930	3210 × 10^{26}	
Nylon-6	1130	3730 × 10^{26}	
Lung (*inflated*: ρ = 260 kg m^{-3}, n_0 = 86 × 10^{26}; *deflated*: ρ = 1050 kg m^{-3}, n_0 = 3480 × 10^{26})			
LN10	310	1000 × 10^{26}	Alderson lung
Mammography			
Average breast (ρ = 1020 kg m^{-3}, n_0 = 3390 × 10^{26})			
BR12	970	3170 × 10^{26}	BR12 is more representative of the average breast in older women, i.e. 50% fat + 50% glandular tissue by weight. For such breasts the mass attenuation coefficient differs from that of BR12 by no more than 2%
Adipose (fat) (ρ = 950 kg m^{-3}, n_0 = 3180 × 10^{26})			
AP6	920	2990 × 10^{26}	Mass attenuation coefficient within 3–10% of that for adipose tissue
Fibroglandular (ρ = 1050 kg m^{-3}, n_0 = 3480 × 10^{26})			
WT1	1020	3310 × 10^{26}	Same as MS20. Mass attenuation coefficient differs from fibroglandular tissue by < 3%

ICRU Report 44 [11].

Notes: Most materials have a mass attenuation coefficient which differs by less than 3% from that for the tissue concerned, over the range 50–150 keV. The exceptions are acrylic, paraffin wax (as a muscle substitute), polystyrene, aluminium, PTFE, LN10, and AP6 which all fall within the range 3–10% at the lower energies.

calibrations. A local reference standard, which may be a secondary or tertiary standard, will be used to calibrate field instruments and other dosemeters, such as thermoluminescence dosemeters (TLDs).

The required accuracy and precision of a dose measurement will, to some extent, depend on the purpose of the measurement. In view of the large uncertainties in risk factors and organ positions, and the errors introduced by patient sizes differing from standard phantom sizes, it seems unlikely that an absolute accuracy of greater than ±30% would be required (at the 99% confidence level). However, for most other purposes, such as providing meaningful comparisons between different units or for comparing different techniques, ±10% would be preferable, although it is recognized that this can be difficult to achieve.

The most commonly used detectors for radiation dose measurements are ionisation chamber instruments and TLDs, but solid-state detectors and film may be suitable for some applications.

14.5.1 Ionisation chambers

Ionisation chambers have long been the instrument of choice for making measurements in the direct beam of diagnostic X-ray equipment, largely because of their flat energy response over the diagnostic energy range. This property is important because the energy spectrum of the radiation incident on a detector is generally quite broad and ill defined, particularly if scattered radiation is present. The report of the AAPM Task Group No. 6 [14] contains much useful information on the required performance characteristics of ionisation chamber instruments.

Ionisation chambers are ideal for measuring equipment output (air kerma in μGy mAs^{-1} at a specified distance) for use in subsequent dose calculations. Measurements on the surface, or at a depth in a suitable phantom, can also be made, in which case the usually uniform directional dependence is an advantage because the backscattered radiation is correctly measured. Although not impossible, measurements on the surface of patients have the disadvantages that the cable connection to the electrometer may prove cumbersome, and the chamber and cable may obscure important detail on the image.

Special thin-window chambers are available for low-energy measurements, such as in mammography, and pencil-type chambers have been designed for certain measurements in computerized tomography (CT). The DAP meter is an ionisation chamber instrument specially designed to measure the product of absorbed dose to air, and X-ray field area (Box 14.4). Normally, in order to measure absorbed dose or air kerma, the chamber size is relatively small, and the X-ray beam size must be larger than the chamber. However, this is not the case for a DAP meter, where instead the chamber must be larger than the maximum X-ray beam size.

14.5.2 Thermoluminescence dosimetry

TLDs are used mainly for measuring ESD, with backscatter, in radiographic examinations and CT. Their small size, relative transparency to radiation at diagnostic beam qualities, and self-contained nature mean that they do not significantly interfere with the examination and are not usually visible on radiographs. For the same reasons, they are the dosemeter of choice for measuring dose distributions within anthropomorphic phantoms. Also, by using several carefully positioned TLDs it is possible to investigate the pattern of doses on the surface of a patient arising from a radiation field which varies in a relatively unpredictable way, such as in fluoroscopy.

The most common TL material in use is lithium fluoride (LiF), doped with magnesium and titanium (known as TLD-100). It is reasonably tissue equivalent, its sensitivity being about 35% higher at 30 keV and below, compared with that at 100 keV and above. TLDs are usually calibrated against an ionisation chamber instrument, which in turn has a calibration traceable to national standards. It is easy to perform the calibration annually at a range of diagnostic energies (60 to 120 kV) using one of the methods described in Box 4.7. An average energy correction for diagnostic X-ray energies may be adequate for most purposes, since the sensitivity does not vary significantly over a broad spectral energy range (see Table 2.1). A single dose level of about 10 mGy would be suitable. It may then be convenient to relate the calibration to one obtained from a more simple check device, such as a ^{90}Sr irradiator, so that regular more frequent checks on sensitivity can be undertaken easily. The minimum dose that can be measured reliably (i.e. distinguished from zero with 95% confidence) is about 50 μGy (see Box 4.7). This is not as low as a typical ionisation chamber instrument, and may well be unacceptable in low-dose situations such as chest radiography, paediatric radiology, or when measuring doses attenuated by significant amounts of tissue. However, it is possible, by careful analysis of the glow curve, to improve the sensitivity significantly [15]. Although available in a number of different forms, probably the most convenient for routine patient dosimetry are the extruded chips, approximately 3 mm square. Like other TLD materials, the response of LiF is linear over the range of doses likely to be encountered in diagnostic radiology.

14.5.3 Solid-state dosemeters

In recent years, dosemeters incorporating solid-state detectors, based on silicon diodes, have become widely available but are in general more suited to equipment quality control than patient dosimetry. Although having good sensitivity, their energy dependence is not as good as ionisation chamber instruments, particularly at low X-ray energies. Nevertheless, with care they could prove useful in some circumstances. They are generally robust, compact, and do not require corrections for temperature or pressure. The small size of the detector may be of

Box 14.4 Calibration of DAP meters

A DAP meter gives a measurement proportional to the product of the air kerma averaged over the X-ray beam and the beam area. This is independent of the distance from the X-ray tube focus, as the decline in air kerma is compensated by the increase in beam size. Thus a DAP meter can be calibrated from measurements of the air kerma and the beam area made at the same distance from the focus. The precise position is not critical, but it is recommended that the beam is directed vertically downwards for a ceiling-mounted or overcouch tube with a focus to detector distance of 0.5–1 m and a beam size at the detector of 200–800 cm^2. For undercouch tubes a position a few centimetres above the couch is recommended for the measurement.

An ionisation chamber is usually employed and should be placed in the centre of the X-ray field. The air kerma and the DAP should then be measured for the same exposures with a tube potential near the centre of the range used clinically, with an mAs within the range appropriate for the equipment, but large enough to give a DAP reading with three digits if possible. The field size may be increased to raise the DAP. This measurement should be repeated several times to improve accuracy and minimize the chance of errors. The beam area should be recorded with a film cassette placed at the same height as the midpoint of the measuring chamber, using a low exposure. The product of the air kerma measurement and the beam area measured from the film should equal the DAP. The calibration of the meter may be adjusted to correct any discrepancy in the result. If the field size has not been changed, this can be checked by direct comparison of the DAP and ionisation chamber measurements. A calibration factor should be applied to results if adjustment of the meter is not possible.

Important points to be taken into account are the following.

- Ideally the ionisation chamber should be supported free in air as backscatter will increase the air kerma measurement. A purpose-built jig which can support the chamber or cassette is an advantage. Alternatively, the chamber may be placed on a slab of light, rigid material, such as polystyrene, or, if the chamber is placed on a couch and exposed from above, a sheet of lead may be placed behind the chamber to reduce scattered radiation.
- The calibration may vary by $\pm 20\%$ with tube potential, so it is important to select a value of clinical relevance.
- The air kerma will decline towards the edge of the field, because of the heel effect. Use of too large a field may give a slightly higher calibration factor, but use of too small a field may give too low a DAP reading to achieve the required accuracy.
- The calibration of DAP meters fitted to overcouch and undercouch tubes will be significantly different because of the position of the treatment couch, so it is important to ensure that the chamber is plugged into the correct input in the meter.
- With C-arm units the calibration factor will depend on whether the exposure is through the couch, and for thicker couches supported at one end, will vary with oblique views. Adjustment factors may be required to take account of such differences if DAP data are to be used to derive effective dose.
- Allowance must be made for any filter material introduced between the DAP chamber and the patient.

considerable advantage in measuring small X-ray beams, such as in dental panoramic radiography. However, they are not radiotransparent, nor are they sensitive to backscattered radiation. MOSFET devices have also been produced for patient dose measurements, initially in radiotherapy. Their use for measuring ESDs in diagnostic radiology has been investigated, but at the present stage of development they do not appear to offer any advantages over existing methods.

Dosemeters consisting of a small scintillation detector connected to an optical readout unit by a fibre optic have been introduced specifically to monitor skin dose in fluoroscopic procedures. The detector correctly includes backscattered radiation but, although small in size, is visible on the image.

14.5.4 Film

Film is rarely used for patient dosimetry for a variety of reasons. Accuracy may be difficult to ensure because of processing variations and very poor energy sensitivity. With non-screen film the response per gray is a maximum at about 40 keV, falling rapidly at lower and higher energies. Also, its response is non-linear, and due to the shape of the characteristic curve, film has a relatively limited dynamic range. Sensitivity is much poorer than, for example, ionisation chamber detectors. Nevertheless, in spite of all these drawbacks, envelope-wrapped film may be useful for mapping highly non-uniform dose distributions, such as those arising in the head from dental panoral radiography. This information may then be used as an aid to positioning TLDs to obtain more accurate dose results.

14.6 Dose calculation

14.6.1 Calculating dose from technique factors

It is a simple matter to calculate the entrance air kerma without backscatter (incident air kerma) at the point where the central ray enters the patient. The information required is the kV, mAs, and focus–patient distance.

$$\text{IAK} = [\text{output} \times \text{mAs}]/\text{FSD}^2 \text{ mGy}$$

where IAK is the incident air kerma, output is the air kerma per mAs at 1 m (in mGy mAs^{-1}) at the kV used, mAs is the product of X-ray tube current and exposure time, and FSD is the distance from the focus to the surface of the patient, in metres.

Output can be measured using an ionisation chamber or other instrument with suitable properties. Errors can occur if the output is not measured under exactly the same conditions as the clinical exposures. For example, significant differences may exist between broad and fine focus and between different mA stations. In addition, in the case of retrospective calculations the FSD is unlikely to be known, and the individual kV and mAs may also not have been recorded. (Whether or not the resultant error is significant will depend on the purpose of the dose estimations and will require some professional judgement.) For retrospective calculations, in the absence of direct measurements, quality control output data may be usable. Where output data at the kV used (kV_{Pat}) are not available, an adjustment can be made based on the proportionality to the square of the kV.

$$\text{IAK} = [\text{output}_{\text{kVo}} \times \text{mAs} \times (\text{kV}_{\text{Pat}}/\text{kV}_{\text{o}})^2]/\text{FSD}^2 \text{ mGy}.$$

As a last resort published output data can be utilized.

Clearly, the difference between a direct measurement of ESD, using TLD for example, and this method is the inclusion of backscatter in the former. Care needs to be taken when comparing data from different sources in establishing whether backscatter has been included, and in what medium dose has been calculated (e.g. water, air, ICRU muscle, etc.). The backscatter factor depends on beam quality and examination conditions, such as beam size and part of body being irradiated. For thick body parts the backscatter factor will be in the region of 1.35 ± 10% (Table 14.1).

14.6.2 Monte Carlo methods for estimating organ and effective doses

Monte Carlo techniques have been used extensively in diagnostic radiology to investigate patient doses and image quality. In summary, the method involves the computer simulation of the transport of X-ray photons through the patient, selecting photons at random from the relevant spectral distribution, and using cross-section data for the various interaction processes. Several million photons may need to be tracked in order to give acceptable statistical accuracy in the calculated quantities, such as absorbed dose in a particular organ. The patient is represented by a mathematical phantom, in which the various body parts, tissues, and organs are modelled by simple mathematical shapes of appropriate composition (Figure 14.2). Phantoms derived from cross-sectional data provided by CT or magnetic resonance (MR) images have also been developed [12]. Space does not permit a detailed discussion of the method: the interested reader is recommended to consult reviews or other texts [16, 17]. Monte Carlo techniques are generally used where analytical methods are unavailable or impractical. They have the advantage that results can be generated relatively easily for a wide variety of scenarios. Such results may be almost impossible to obtain by direct measurement or at best would be exceedingly time-consuming to collect.

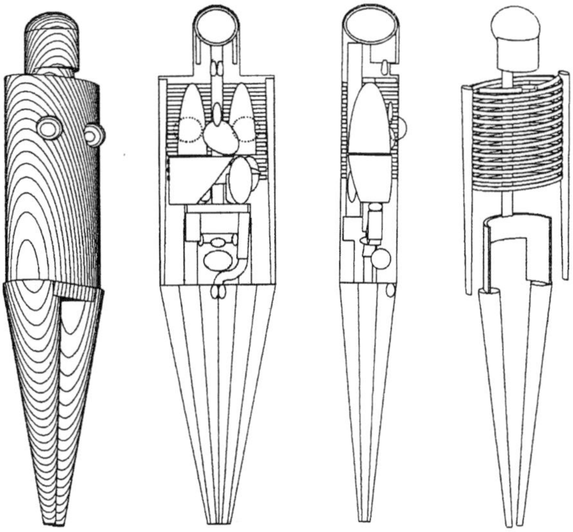

Figure 14.2 External, internal, and skeletal views of the hermaphrodite mathematical phantom used by Jones and Wall [18]. (Reproduced courtesy of NRPB.).

For the purposes of this chapter, the most useful form of the results generated by Monte Carlo programs is in terms of normalized organ doses, that is, organ dose per unit ESD or incident air kerma. There are a number of published compilations of normalized doses for common radiological procedures, which can be used in most circumstances.

The most extensive data, in terms of numbers of projections and organs included, are those which have been produced by the UK National Radiological Protection Board (NRPB). They used an adult hermaphrodite phantom, based on the MIRD-5 phantom [18]. Factors for estimating effective dose from ESD and DAP are given in NRPB-R262 [1] for 68 common X-ray projections and 40 X-ray spectra. Complementary software also gives normalized doses to all the ICRP and remainder organs [19]. In addition, the NRPB have produced similar information for children of ages 0, 1, 5, 10, and 15 years [2], and for adult CT examinations [20] (§14.8). The specifications for the mathematical phantoms mentioned above, along with a number of others, have been summarized in ICRU Report 48 [12]. A number of authors have published factors to convert entrance air kerma (or similar) to mean glandular dose for mammographic examinations and these are discussed in §14.9.1.

A problem which may be encountered when using published Monte Carlo data is the absence of data for the examination, projection, or field size under consideration. Nevertheless, it may still be possible to find an adequate match for most purposes, although it should be noted that there can be substantial differences for organ and effective doses between AP and PA projections, and between left and right laterals.

Errors will also be incurred due to differences between patient and phantom dimensions, and the positions and sizes of organs. Such errors are difficult to quantify, especially if a small organ is near to the edge of the primary beam, in which case small changes in beam or organ position can significantly affect the dose. The magnitude and sources of uncertainties in different circumstances have been discussed in [18].

14.7 Dosimetry in radiography and fluoroscopy

The following sections give some indications of how the techniques described above can be applied in common situations to estimate effective dose and relevant organ doses. The Monte Carlo methods for estimating organ doses take into account the different compositions of different organs. This is usually straightforward, except for bone, where calculation of bone marrow dose has to take into account the elevated dose due to photoelectrons generated in the surrounding high atomic number bone (Box 14.5).

14.7.1 Radiography

Patient dose estimations for radiographic exposures are usually relatively straightforward. For effective dose and organ doses the most convenient method would be to use the Monte Carlo generated data described in §14.6.2. Key requirements as input for the calculation are details of the examination and projection, the X-ray tube voltage (kVp), tube filtration, and the incident exposure, either in terms of ESD or DAP. Sometimes information on mAs may be unavailable if automatic exposure control (AEC) is used, although most new X-ray equipment now gives post-exposure readout of mAs. An alternative would be to use typical values employed in the department, taken from the exposure charts and possibly modified if the patient is known to be particularly large or small.

For simple radiographic examinations DRLs have been defined primarily in terms of ESD, with backscatter. However, much new X-ray equipment is provided with DAP meters, and by estimating the field size at the patient it is possible to convert from one quantity to the other. It is also possible to obtain DAP meters which use ultrasound to measure the distance to the patient, hence enabling entrance air kerma as well as DAP to be obtained. In the UK, publication of the *National protocol for patient dose measurements in diagnostic radiology* [22] was instrumental in initiating routine measurements of patient dose for comparison with DRLs. Typical patient doses and the current UK national DRLs for a range of examinations are given in Table 14.3.

When a patient receives a dose which may be 'much greater than intended' (Box 14.3), arising from an

Box 14.5 Bone dosimetry

The sensitive parts of trabecular bone, as far as cancer induction is concerned, are the bone surfaces and bone marrow. Because of the complex structure of trabecular bone, the calculation or measurement of dose to these tissues is extremely difficult. The dose to both the endosteal tissues and the marrow is enhanced as a result of photoelectrons produced by photoelectric interactions in the high atomic number bone. The dose enhancement depends on the distance of the sensitive tissues from the bone and is therefore higher for the endosteal tissues, which lie within 10 μm of the bone surfaces, whereas the marrow cavities vary from 50 μm to 2000 μm in size. Another factor to consider is the shielding effect of bone, which reduces the dose to tissues beyond (as well as to the soft tissues within the bone itself). In fact, for the dose to bone marrow, the shielding effect may outweigh the enhancement effect. Spiers [21] discusses bone and bone marrow dosimetry at much greater length, and gives tables of dose enhancement factors for different bones, at different ages, and for a range of X-ray energies. On average, the marrow dose enhancement is about 10% in the diagnostic energy range, whereas the enhancement to endosteal tissues is over 100%, except at the highest X-ray energies.

Table 14.3 Typical patient doses and provisional diagnostic reference levels for radiographic procedures

Examination		Entrance surface dose (mGy)	Dose–area product (Gy cm^2)	Effective dose (mSv)	Diagnostic reference level[a] (mGy)
Limbs and joints (except hip)				<0.01	
Chest	PA	0.16	0.08	0.02	0.2
	Lat	0.37	0.24	0.04	0.7
Skull	AP/PA	3.0	0.75	0.03	4
	Lat	1.5	0.37	0.01	2
Cervical spine				0.08	
Hip				0.3	
Thoracic spine	AP	4.7	1.7	0.4	5
	Lat	13.0	2.6	0.3	16
Pelvis	AP	4.4	4.0	0.7	5
Abdomen	AP	5.6	5.6	0.7	7
Lumbar spine	AP	6.1	2.6	0.7	7
	Lat	16.0	2.7	0.3	20
	LSJ	29.0	2.9	0.3	35
IVU (kidneys and bladder)			13.4	2.5	25[b]

[a]Entrance surface dose.
[b]Dose–area product (Gy cm^2).

equipment fault or human error, it is necessary to obtain an estimate of the patient dose. Initially, the requirement is to establish by what factor the actual dose exceeded the intended dose. It may be possible to make an adequate estimate by comparing mAs values, or DAP readings, for example. Assuming the exposure needs to be repeated to obtain a diagnostic film, the intended dose is best based on the factors used for the repeat film or from previous films taken on the same patient. A relatively common equipment fault is the failure of the AEC to correctly terminate the exposure. The operator may realize that something is wrong and release the handswitch, or the exposure may be terminated by the back-up timer. In either case the actual mAs given will probably be known. If it is not available a crude estimate of exposure time may be all that is possible. Alternatively, if the film is not completely black the increased dose may be estimated from the film density. If this initial investigation shows that the dose was ‘much greater than intended’, then a detailed estimate of effective dose is required, using the methods already described.

14.7.2 Fluoroscopy and fluorography

It is generally more difficult to estimate the dose to patients from image intensifier based examinations, mainly because the field size and projection tend to vary throughout the examination. In addition, exposure factors also vary and are less likely to be known: screening time and number of films, or digital images, may be the only parameters recorded. However, for prospective measurements, such as one-off dose surveys or special projects, it may be feasible to record complete information. The total examination can be divided into a number of discrete projections, and organ doses estimated for each projection, using the methods described in §14.7.1. Since most fluoroscopic equipment is fitted with DAP meters, doses will most conveniently be based on DAP meter readings for each projection. Strictly speaking, calculation of effective dose should then be based on the total doses to each organ over the complete examination, and should not be derived by summing the separate effective doses for each projection. This is because of the possibility of one of the remainder organs receiving the highest dose. If calculations are being performed using purpose-written software, such as that provided as an adjunct to the NRPB compilations [19], then this approach is straightforward. If, however, such software is not being used, it is often easier to sum the effective dose for each projection and make an estimate of the error involved. Care may be needed if the projections and field sizes used do not coincide with those available in the literature. However, several publications do give normalized organ doses appropriate to fluoroscopic procedures [1, 23, 24].

For retrospective dose estimations it may be necessary, and easiest, to determine the doses by simulating the examination using a phantom. If phantom measurements are undertaken care needs to be taken to reproduce clinical conditions as closely as possible, since exposure parameters are usually automatically controlled and can be quite critical on the techniques used.

DRLs for examinations involving fluoroscopy can be specified in terms of DAP, and UK national DRLs that have been set for barium enemas and barium meals are given in Table 14.4. Studies of more complex diagnostic and interventional procedures have taken place, and

Table 14.4 Typical patient doses and provisional diagnostic reference levels for fluoroscopy procedures

Examination	Dose–area product (Gy cm^2)	Effective dose (mSv)	Diagnostic reference level[a] (Gy cm^2)
Barium swallow	9.8	1.5	
Barium meal	13.0	3	17
Barium follow	12.0	3	
Barium enema	25.8	7	35

[a]Dose–area product.

should provide useful information in this developing area. At present, local dose surveys should be undertaken both for local guidance and to contribute to the setting of national levels. Since most dosimetry in fluoroscopic procedures is based on DAP readings, it is important that DAP meters fitted to equipment are calibrated regularly (Box 14.4). Some manufacturers display DAP readings based on calculation rather than direct measurement, and calibration is particularly important in these cases to allow for changes in X-ray output. Corrections may also need to be made for any special or additional tube filtration such as copper which may be introduced into the beam during an examination with the aim of reducing patient ESD.

With some lengthy interventional procedures it is possible to deliver skin doses high enough to cause deterministic effects, ranging from mild transient erythema to secondary ulceration (§11.3.3). Skin doses of up to 20 Gy have been reported. Normally, patient skin dose rates will be in the range 20–50 mGy min^{-1}, but could exceed 100 mGy min^{-1} under certain conditions: in fact UK legislation requires the dose rate at the surface of the skin not to exceed 100 mGy min^{-1}. Measurements should be undertaken to see if there is likely to be a problem, and where areas of the skin could receive more than about 1 Gy, such areas, along with dosimetric information, should be recorded for individual patients. Skin dose measurements on patients suffer from the difficulties already mentioned for fluoroscopy, particularly not knowing beforehand which area of skin will receive the highest dose. The options include placing one or more TLDs at appropriate positions on the patients or using one of the commercial instruments designed for this purpose (§14.5). Measurements of incident radiation derived from DAP readings could be used. They do not take into account the variation of beam position on the skin but would at least indicate the maximum possible skin dose.

14.8 Computed tomography

It is well recognized that CT delivers some of the highest doses to patients, compared with other radiological techniques. In the UK, although CT accounted for only about 4% of all procedures, its contribution to the collective effective dose due to diagnostic radiology was approximately 40% in 1998 and may now be greater. Estimation and control of doses in CT is therefore particularly important.

14.8.1 Computed tomography dose index (CTDI)

Because of differences between conventional radiography and CT, in particular in the shape of the X-ray beam and geometry of irradiation, it is not possible to use the same practical methods for assessing patient dose. ESD, with backscatter, can be measured with TLDs placed at appropriate locations on the patient's skin surface or on a suitable phantom. Various quantities, such as multiple scan average dose (MSAD) and multi-slice surface dose (MSSD), have been introduced to describe the average surface dose, over a slice width, from a series of contiguous slices. However, it is not easy to convert such a measurement to organ doses or effective dose, and it is not currently being proposed as a suitable quantity for DRLs in CT. Instead, it is usual to base CT dosimetry on measurements of the CTDI, a quantity which is a measure of the total dose from a single slice, and which is effectively a combination of tube output and slice width collimation. It is defined in general terms as:

$$\mathrm{CTDI} = 1/nT \int_{z_1}^{z_2} D(z)\,\mathrm{d}z$$

where z_1 and z_2 are the limits of integration, $D(z)$ is the single-slice dose profile, T is the nominal slice thickness in cm, and n is the number of slices irradiated simultaneously (for multi-slice CT).

CTDI is usually measured with a pencil ionisation chamber. The chamber is positioned parallel to the scanner axis at the centre of the field and a measurement taken for a single slice. The measurement performs the necessary integration, with limits determined by the length of the chamber. The length commonly used is 100 mm, and a number of suitable chambers are available commercially.

In terms of the chamber reading the CTDI is therefore given by

$$\mathrm{CTDI} = D \times F \times L/T \qquad \mathrm{mGy}$$

where D is the chamber reading in mGy, F is a factor to convert the chamber dose quantity to dose in the medium required, and L and T are the length of the ion chamber and the nominal slice thickness, respectively. F is unity in air and for other media is given by the ratio of the mass energy transfer coefficients in air and the appropriate medium: $(\mu_{en}/\rho)_{medium}/(\mu_{en}/\rho)_{air}$ (§2.7.4). The quantity is therefore energy dependent and it is

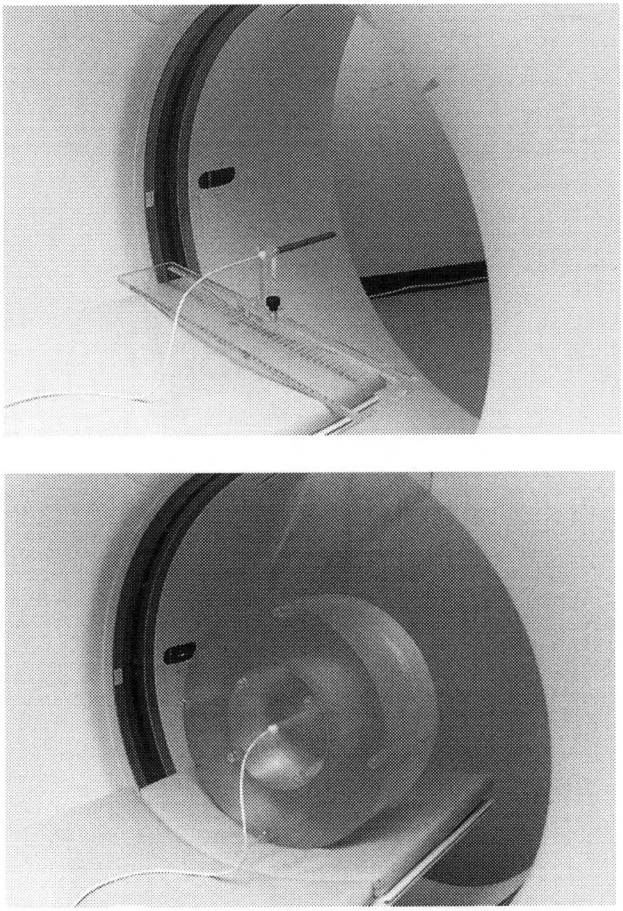

Figure 14.3 The set-up for measuring CTDI: (a) the 100 mm pencil ionisation chamber is positioned on-axis to measure CDTI free in air; (b) the chamber is inserted in a perspex phantom for a measurement in perspex. The phantom is 320 mm in diameter to simulate the body but the outer annulus can be removed to leave the central 160 mm diameter phantom to simulate the head. Four plugged cavities exist around the periphery of each phantom for additional measurements required to calculate $CTDI_w$.

customary to assign CT scanners an average energy of 70 keV (in a phantom) to aid in its determination. Apart from air, the most common medium used in CT dosimetry is perspex which has an approximate *F* value of 0.887. The ion chamber calibration should be undertaken at realistic beam qualities representative of CT practice.

CTDI can be measured free in air or in a suitable phantom, and either on the axis of rotation of the scanner or near the periphery of the phantom, depending on the purpose of the measurements (Figure 14.3). If performed in a phantom, it is equivalent to the average dose across the central scan width from several surrounding contiguous scans.

Phantoms suitable for dosimetry measurements are usually constructed from polymethylmethacrylate (acrylic or perspex), with a number of removable plugs for the insertion of TLDs or ionisation chambers. Standard diameters are 160 mm to simulate the head, and 320 mm for the body. The design has been recommended by the IEC and is described in more detail by Edyvean [25].

A CTDI value measured as described above depends on the usual factors, such as mAs, kV, and scanner geometry. It does not depend strongly on slice width, except that the smallest nominal slice width on a scanner may be determined by post-patient collimation, resulting in a higher CTDI compared with larger slice widths. Often it is useful to normalize the CTDI by dividing by the mAs. However, care needs to be taken if patient examination protocols employ overscan, since it is common for the scanner to give the nominal scan time for a 360° rotation, rather than the actual time. Thus, the dose may be underestimated if the CTDI is calculated from the normalized CTDI multiplied by the indicated mAs, since the true mAs may be slightly greater.

14.8.2 Estimation of organ doses and effective dose

The most convenient way of estimating organ doses and effective dose is to make use of published data relating organ doses to measurements of CTDI per mAs in air. Such data have been calculated using Monte Carlo methods [20], and are available as computer data files, providing a very convenient way of estimating effective dose [26]. It should be noted that the CTDI required for the data, although measured in air, is quoted as an absorbed dose to ICRU muscle. Therefore, a correction factor of 1.07 will need to be applied if measurements have been made in terms of absorbed dose to air, or air kerma, as is usually the case. The normalized organ doses are scanner specific, and so a potential problem arises if doses are required for patients examined on a scanner introduced after the work of Jones and Shrimpton [20]. However, it may be possible to find a matched older scanner to estimate effective dose, based on a knowledge of the different scanner models, filtration, kV, and geometry [27].

It should be noted that to comply with regulatory requirements in the United States, CT manufacturers provide data on CTDI in their technical literature. However, the definition of CTDI used by the Federal Drug Administration (FDA) differs in some significant aspects from that used above. The main difference is in the integration limits, which are $\pm 7T$, where T is the slice thickness, rather than the ± 50 mm normally used for practical patient dose measurements. The two quantities will only agree for a slice thickness of 7 mm. CTDI_{FDA} is determined in standard 16 cm and 32 cm diameter perspex phantoms, and is quoted as absorbed dose to perspex. In order to compare measurements of CTDI_{100} made using a 100 mm pencil chamber with respect to air with values of CTDI_{FDA} derived according to the FDA definition in perspex, correction factors given in Table 14.5 can be used. These factors allow measurements at acceptance to be compared with values quoted in the manufacturers' literature and can be used in dose evaluation.

Table 14.5 Ratio of $\text{CTDI}_{\text{FDA(perspex)}}$ to $\text{CTDI}_{100\text{(air)}}$

Slice thickness (mm)	Head phantom			Body phantom		
	C	P	S	C	P	S
10	0.98	0.93	0.92	1.03	0.93	0.92
5	0.77	0.82	0.84	0.72	0.82	0.82
3	0.62	0.74	0.76	0.53	0.74	0.75
2	0.49	0.67	0.71	0.38	0.67	0.71
1.5	0.45	0.63	0.67	0.34	0.61	0.67
1	0.32	–	–	0.26	–	–

C, P, and S represent measurement positions at the centre, periphery (1 cm deep), and surface of the CTDI phantoms.

14.8.3 Diagnostic reference levels (DRLs)

It is important that the quantities used for DRLs give a meaningful indication of patient exposure, yet at the same time are relatively easy to measure. Two quantities have been developed for this purpose, which are known as the weighted CTDI (CTDI_w) and the dose–length product (DLP).

$$\text{CTDI}_\text{w} = 1/3\ \text{CTDI}_{100,\text{c}} + 2/3\ \text{CTDI}_{100,\text{p}}\ \text{mGy}$$

where $\text{CTDI}_{100,\text{c}}$ is the CTDI measured with a 100 mm long pencil ionisation chamber at the centre of the standard phantom (body or head), and $\text{CTDI}_{100,\text{p}}$ is a similar quantity, which is the average of four measurements made around the periphery (i.e. 10 mm below the surface) of the phantom. CTDI_w is expressed in terms of absorbed dose to air.

$$\text{DLP} = \sum_i {}_\text{n}\text{CTDI}_\text{w} \times T \times N \times C\ \text{mGy cm}$$

where ${}_\text{n}\text{CTDI}_\text{w}$ is the normalized weighted CTDI (CTDI_w per mAs), T is the slice thickness, N is the number of slices, C the mAs per slice, and the sum i is over all scan sequences forming part of the examination.

Preliminary DRLs for adult patients have been proposed by the European Commission [28] and are given in Table 14.6 along with typical effective doses for some CT examinations.

14.8.4 Spiral CT

CTDI is not strictly defined for spiral or helical CT; however, for dose calculations it can be assumed to be the same as the value obtained for the corresponding standard axial scan, allowing for any overscan in the standard mode. When using the NRPB program to estimate effective dose, one can either use contiguous slices and divide the result by the pitch or choose a packing factor equal to the inverse of the pitch; the results are essentially the same. Here the pitch is defined

Table 14.6 Typical patient doses and provisional diagnostic reference levels for computed tomography

Examination	Effective dose (mSv)	Diagnostic reference level $CTDI_w$ (mGy)	DLP (mGy cm)
Head	2	60	1050
Chest	8	30	650
Abdomen	10	35	800
Pelvis	10	35	600
Liver and spleen	10	35	900
HRCT lung	3.5	35	280
Vertebral trauma	7.5	70	460
Face and sinuses	0.6	35	360

as the distance travelled by the couch per tube revolution, divided by the product of the nominal slice thickness and number of sections produced in a single tube rotation. It should be noted that some manufacturers use a different definition of pitch, namely the distance travelled by the couch per rotation, divided by the single slice detector aperture. According to this definition the pitch for a scanner collecting data for four simultaneous slices would be four times greater. Usually, additional scanning is performed at the start and end of a run for interpolation purposes, although for normal scan lengths the additional dose is insignificant. For spiral CT the equation for DLP needs to be modified slightly:

$$\mathrm{DLP} = \sum_i {}_{\mathrm{n}}\mathrm{CTDI_w} \times T \times A \times t \text{ mGy cm}$$

where T is the nominal slice thickness, A is the tube current, and t is the total acquisition time for the sequence.

14.8.5 Scan projection radiography (SPR)

SPR may be used to aid alignment and select the region to be scanned in cross-sectional imaging. In such cases the contribution to the total dose from the examination is very small and is usually ignored. SPR may also be used as a very low dose technique where the diagnostic features do not depend on high image quality, e.g. pelvimetry. In such applications the usual techniques for measuring doses in conventional radiography can be used. The dose will depend on factors such as the mA, couch speed, and slice width.

14.9 Specialist radiographic techniques

14.9.1 Mammography

In mammography the only part of the body which receives a significant dose is the breast itself. It is therefore usually unnecessary and irrelevant to estimate effective dose. The ICRP has recommended that the mean absorbed dose to the glandular tissue (including the ductal and acinar epithelium) is the most relevant dose quantity. However, the term glandular tissue is imprecise and Bryant *et al.* [29] have indicated that the volume of tissue at risk is much lower than implied by the standard breast model.

Particularly since screening for breast cancer has become widespread, standard protocols for dose measurements have been developed [30]. Although suitably calibrated TLDs can be used with standard perspex or breast tissue equivalent phantoms, they will be visible on mammograms if used on patients, and there may be some uncertainty as to whether backscatter is fully detected. Instead, the method of choice is by calculation from recorded exposure factors and output measurements. The relationship between mean glandular dose (MGD) and incident air kerma has been derived from Monte Carlo calculations [31] and is a function of beam quality, i.e. half-value layer and anode–filter combination, breast thickness, and breast composition (Box 14.6). Incident air kerma is easily derived from output measurements, taking care to undertake these with the breast compression plate in position. Breast composition can be estimated by inspection of the mammograms, although, relative to the standard 50% glandular–50% adipose composition, the correction does not amount to more than about 20%. Factors to convert incident air kerma to MGD can be found in the aforementioned protocols.

Measurements on groups of women in the UK National Breast Screening Programme have indicated a median MGD for the mediolateral oblique view of 1.7 mGy, with an interquartile range of 1.2–2.4 mGy [32]. Corresponding figures for the craniocaudal view were 1.4 mGy for the median, and 1.1–2.0 mGy for the interquartile range. These figures should not be confused with the MGD for the standard breast (40 mm perspex), which is used for quality control purposes and tends to be somewhat lower than doses measured on real women.

14.9.2 Dental radiography

Although the effective dose from a dental exposure is small, the frequency of dental radiography is very high, resulting in an annual collective dose of about 200 manSv in the UK. Unfortunately, projections and exposure parameters relevant to dental radiography are not available in the commonly used software packages for estimating organ and effective doses.

A number of workers have used sectioned head phantoms with TLD inserts to estimate the absorbed dose to the different organs in the head, and hence the effective dose. Doses are usually small and multiple exposures are generally needed. The estimation of effective dose needs careful consideration in view of the fact that much of the dose is to 'remainder' organs.

Dose estimation in panoral radiography raises two further problems, namely the narrow slit shape of the X-ray beam makes it difficult to make measurements of output or kV, and also the dose distribution inside the head is very non-uniform, making it difficult to estimate dose to organs. Figure 14.4 shows a typical dose distribution as measured by a film inserted between slices of a Rando head phantom. Together with a TLD, this can give a more complete picture of the dose. It is interesting to note the hot spot at the salivary glands, which is neither an ICRP organ with a specified weighting factor nor one of the named remainder organs. Frederiksen *et al.* [33] have considered the implications for effective dose including the salivary glands in the calculation and concluded that they contribute 61% of the total effective dose.

Box 14.6 Calculation of mean glandular tissue dose in mammography

The mean glandular tissue dose (MGD) can be calculated from the incident air kerma (K) at the breast surface. A 40-mm-thick perspex phantom with the same cross-sectional area as the standard breast is used in the UK [30] and European protocols to check and compare the dose performance of mammography units. The standard phantom equates to a 45-mm-thick breast and it is assumed that the composition is 50% glandular tissue and 50% adipose tissue for calculation of MGD using the equation:

$$\text{MGD} = K\,p\,g\,s$$

where the factor p converts air kerma for the perspex phantom to that for the standard breast and g converts air kerma for the standard breast to the mean glandular tissue dose for X-ray spectra obtained from a molybdenum target used with a molybdenum filter characterized by the half-value layer (HVL) in aluminium (Table B14.1) [30]. The factor s corrects for X-ray spectral differences arising from the use of alternative target/filter combinations (Table B14.2) [31].

Table B14.1 Conversion factors p and g for calculating the mean glandular tissue dose to the standard 40-mm-thick perspex phantom for different beam HVLs

HVL (mm Al)	0.30	0.35	0.40	0.45	0.50
p	1.10	1.10	1.09	1.09	1.09
g (mGy/mGy)	0.183	0.208	0.232	0.258	0.285

Table B14.2 s-factors for X-ray spectra used clinically

Anode/filter materials	s-factor
Mo/Mo	1.00
Mo/Rh	1.017
Rh/Rh	1.061
Rh/Al	1.044
W/Rh	1.042

Determination of MGDs for individual patients requires account to be taken of different breast thicknesses and the percentage of glandular tissue. The assumption of 50% glandularity is approximately correct for breast thicknesses of 40–60 mm, but not for thinner or thicker ones. For this an equation of the form:

$$\text{MGD} = \text{K g c s}$$

can be used, which includes an additional factor c related to the glandularity of the tissue. Values for the g-factor for a range of breast thicknesses have been derived from Monte Carlo simulation and are given in Table B14.3.

For intra-oral radiography, the DRL is most conveniently given in terms of the patient entrance dose per film, without backscatter, or in other words the dose in air at the end of the spacer cone. For panoramic radiography a different reference dose quantity is required because of the difficulty in defining a simple method for measuring patient dose resulting from the rotation of the X-ray tube. Dose detectors which are sufficiently narrow to lie entirely within the X-ray beam are now available for measuring the output from these units. The method proposed for dose assessment is based on the dose–width product, that is the product of the total dose per exposure cycle at the slot at the cassette carriage faceplate and the beam width at that position. The NRPB has recommended DRLs of 4 mGy for an adult mandibular molar intra-oral radiograph, and 65 mGy mm for a standard adult panoramic radiograph [34] (Table 14.7). However, in the future DAP is likely to be the dose quantity of choice in panoramic radiography.

14.9.3 Paediatric radiography

Paediatric doses can vary tremendously due to the great variation in the size of patients, from neonates to adult-sized teenagers. Because the risk of harmful radiation effects is higher than in adults, the need to minimize doses is of paramount importance. Also, the smaller body size means that precise collimation can be more difficult,

Box 14.6 *(continued)*

There is a close relationship between glandularity and breast thickness for women within particular age groups, which enables standard values to be assumed [31]. The percentage glandularity for women with different breast thicknesses in age groups examined frequently are given in Table B14.4, together with values for the c-factor for different beam HVLs and these values can be substituted directly into the above equation. Data for a wider range of HVLs and breast thicknesses can be found in [31]. If more than one film is required, because of the size of the breast, the MGD will be approximately proportional to the number of films, because the region of overlap is usually quite large.

Table B14.3 g-factors (mGy/mGy) as a function of compressed breast thickness for different X-ray beam HVLs

Breast thickness	HVL (mm Al)			
(mm)	0.30	0.35	0.40	0.45
20	0.390	0.433	0.473	0.509
30	0.274	0.309	0.342	0.374
40	0.207	0.235	0.261	0.289
50	0.164	0.187	0.209	0.232
60	0.135	0.154	0.172	0.192
70	0.114	0.130	0.145	0.163
80	0.098	0.112	0.126	0.140

Table B14.4 Average breast composition and values for c-factors for average breasts for women in two age groups, as a function of compressed breast thickness

	Women aged 40-49 years					Women aged 50-64 years				
Breast thickness	Gland ularity	c-factors for various unit HVLs (mm Al)				Gland ularity	c-factors for various unit HVLs (mm Al)			
(mm)	(%)	0.30	0.35	0.40	0.45	(%)	0.30	0.35	0.40	0.45
20	100	0.885	0.891	0.900	0.905	100	0.885	0.891	0.900	0.905
30	82	0.894	0.898	0.903	0.906	72	0.925	0.929	0.931	0.933
40	65	0.940	0.943	0.945	0.947	50	1.000	1.000	1.000	1.000
50	49	1.005	1.005	1.005	1.004	33	1.086	1.082	1.081	1.078
60	35	1.080	1.078	1.074	1.074	21	1.164	1.160	1.151	1.150
70	24	1.152	1.147	1.141	1.138	12	1.232	1.225	1.214	1.208
80	14	1.220	1.213	1.206	1.205	7	1.275	1.265	1.257	1.254

and more organs are likely to be within, or close to, the direct beam.

In general, the same techniques as described for adults can be used for estimating radiation dose, the main difference being that the doses are usually much less. For example, ESDs are typically in the range 0.1–0.5 mGy, and down to 0.02 mGy for chest examinations. Similarly, DAP readings may be only a few mGy cm^2. As indicated in §14.6.2, Monte Carlo generated data are available for estimating organ and effective doses for a range of paediatric examinations, although CT is a notable exception.

Typical figures for ESD and DAP can be ascertained by surveying the literature, although fewer large-scale paediatric studies have been performed compared with those undertaken on adults. DRLs for simple radiographic examinations have been proposed by the European Commission [35] and are reproduced in Table 14.8 along with typical doses. Insufficient data are currently available to enable corresponding reference levels to be developed for the more complex procedures involving fluoroscopy. Clearly, further work is also required to develop a framework for dealing with patients of different sizes. One possibility might be to derive a relationship between patient dose and size, and then use this to normalize doses to a fixed patient size. For instance, Martin *et al.* [36] have proposed the use of an 'equivalent diameter', calculated from patient weight and height, which could allow doses for children of different ages to be compared with the appropriate reference levels.

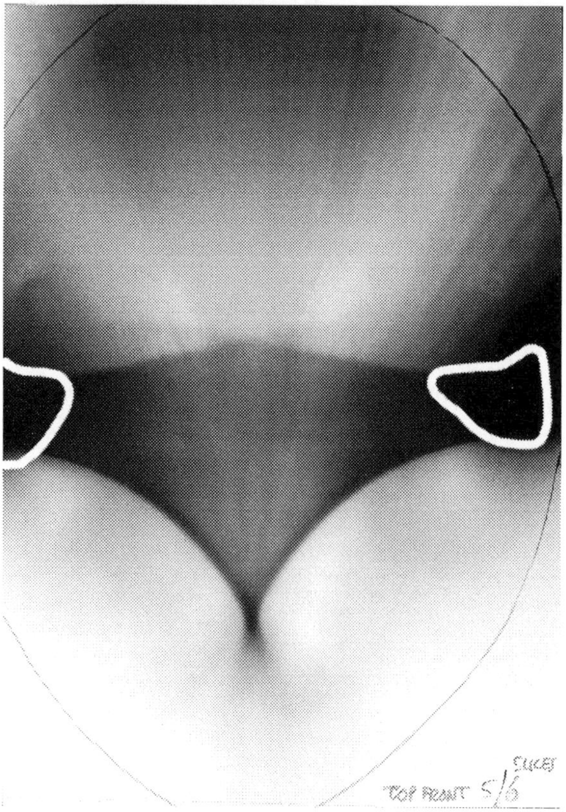

Figure 14.4 The dose distribution from a Planmeca Proline panoramic dental unit, obtained by exposing a non-screen film inserted between sections 5 and 6 of a Rando head phantom. The positions of the parotid glands are outlined in white. The effective rotating centre of the X-ray beam starts just outside the head, alongside the parotid gland, and follows a curved path coinciding with the lower edge of the most exposed area of the film.

14.10 Bone mineral densitometry

Bone density measurements can be made using a variety of techniques, such as radiographic absorptiometry (RA), single X-ray absorptiometry (SXA), dual X-ray absorptiometry (DXA), and quantitative computed tomography

Table 14.7 Typical patient doses and provisional diagnostic reference levels for dental radiography

Examination	Effective dose (μSv)	Entrance surface dose (mGy)	Diagnostic reference level[a] (mGy)
Bitewing, rectangular collimation, E speed film,[b] 70 kV, 200 mm FSD	1	1.8[c]	4
Bitewing, round collimation, E speed film,[b] 70 kV, 200 mm FSD	2	1.8[c]	4
Bitewing, round collimation, E speed film,[b] 50–60 kV, 100 mm FSD	4	4.1	4
Panoramic radiography	7		65 mGy mm[d]

[a]Dose in air at the end of the cone.
[b]The use of D speed film would double the dose from the intra-oral films.
[c]The figure of 1.8 mGy is an average for a survey which included both types of collimation.
[d]Product of total dose and slit width.

Table 14.8 Typical patient doses and provisional diagnostic reference levels for paediatric procedures

Examination	Age (years)	ESD (μGy)	Effective dose (μSv)	Diagnostic reference level[a] (μGy)
Abdomen AP/PA	1	329	69	400
Abdomen AP/PA	5	479	70	500
Abdomen AP/PA	10	756	103	800
Abdomen AP/PA	15	1287	122	1200
Chest AP	0	59	15	50
Chest AP/PA	1	44	5.5	50
Chest AP/PA	5	55	6.6	70
Chest AP/PA	10	88	6.3	120
Chest LAT	5			200
Pelvis AP (no grid)	0	49	5.8	200
Pelvis AP	1	388	45	500
Pelvis AP	5	445	63	600
Pelvis AP	10	713	50	700
Pelvis AP	15	1577	142	2000
Skull AP/PA	1	736	14	800
Skull AP/PA	5	910	11	1100
Skull LAT	1	476	8.5	500
Skull LAT	5	573	8	800

[a]Entrance surface dose.
DRLs based on European Commission [34] adapted to the UK.

(QCT). The most common techniques are probably DXA and QCT, although the other methods are gaining in popularity due to recent technical developments. With the exception of QCT, specialized equipment is needed. In the case of DXA, a pencil or fan beam of X-rays scans the area of interest, commonly the lumbar spine, proximal femur, or whole body. The energy of the beam is rapidly switched, either by changing the filtration or by changing the kV, resulting in a relatively hard beam compared with general radiography. This, together with the scanning geometry and size of the X-ray beam, will need to be considered when making measurements of patient dose.

Most dose estimations reported in the literature have been based on ESD measurements or scans of anthropomorphic phantoms loaded with TLDs. In order to determine effective dose, ESD measurements can be combined with depth dose data and anatomical information to derive organ doses, and hence effective dose. The doses are, however, very low and many scans will be needed to give measurable readings with TLDs in a phantom. Standard techniques, already described, can be used for estimating the dose from QCT.

As can be seen from Table 14.9, patient doses can vary considerably, depending on equipment design, scanning mode, and area of the body, but are generally very much lower than those arising from general radiography. Similarly, the doses from QCT are much lower than those from imaging CT. For further details the reader is referred to a review of techniques and doses,

Table 14.9 Typical patient doses in bone densitometry

	Entrance surface dose (μGy)	Effective dose (μSv)
DXA pencil beam		
spine	10–60	0.2–0.5
femur	10–60	0.02–0.1
whole body	10–20	4
DXA fan beam		
spine	60–900	0.4–75
femur	140–900	0.3–18
whole body	10–900	2.7–41
QCT spine	3000	60–500

The large differences are mainly due to differences in equipment design.
The above effective doses exclude the contribution from the ovaries, as may apply in postmenopausal women. In many instances it is not clear whether the ovaries will be in the X-ray beam or not.

including relevant references, published by Njeh *et al.* [37]. DRLs have not yet been developed for bone mineral densitometry.

14.11 Pregnancy and the estimation of fetal dose

Occasions arise where pregnant patients undergo X-ray examinations, either intentionally because the examination is required urgently for the management of the patient or inadvertently because the patient was unaware that she was pregnant at the time of the examination. Advice is available to clinical radiology departments on exposure to ionising radiation during pregnancy for dealing with such situations and this is summarized in Box 11.3.

Two common reasons for estimates of fetal dose to be required are as follows. First, individual X-ray departments need to know which of their procedures and techniques would give a dose to the fetus of tens of mGy (Box 11.3) and therefore require an examination to be scheduled in the first 10 days of the menstrual cycle. Second, whenever a pregnant patient is X-rayed it is usually necessary to estimate the fetal dose 'for the record', even though it is extremely unlikely that the dose would pose a significant risk or require any change in the management of the patient. The only routine examinations for which rescheduling is likely to be required are CT of the pelvis and abdomen and possibly barium enemas.

In the circumstances described above, in early pregnancy, it is relatively straightforward to estimate the dose to the fetus, since it can be assumed that the dose to the uterus will be a good estimate of the fetal dose, and the techniques already described for organ doses can be used. In later pregnancy the mean depth dose of the fetus will be greater and the ratio between effective dose and ESD or DAP will decrease accordingly. Adjustments may be made to the fetal dose based on depth dose data.

14.12 References

1 Hart, D., Jones, D. G., and Wall, B. F. (1994). *Estimation of effective dose in diagnostic radiology from entrance surface dose and dose–area product measurements.* NRPB-R262. NRPB, Chilton.

2 Hart, D., Jones, D. G., and Wall, B. F. (1996). *Coefficients for estimating effective doses from paediatric X-ray examinations.* NRPB-R279. NRPB, Chilton (and CHILDOSE program).

3 Harrison, R. M. (1982). Backscatter factors for diagnostic radiology (1–4 mm Al HVL). *Phys. Med. Biol.*, **27**, 1465–73.

4 Harrison, R. M. (1981). Central-axis depth–dose data for diagnostic radiology. *Phys. Med. Biol.*, **26**, 657–70.

5 Harrison, R. M. (1983). Tissue–air and scatter–air ratios for diagnostic radiology (1–4 mm Al HVL). *Phys. Med. Biol.*, **28**, 1–18.

6 ICRP (1996). Radiological protection and safety in medicine. ICRP Publication 73. *Ann. ICRP*, **26** (2).

7 European Commission (1997). Council Directive 97/43/ Euratom of 30 June 1997 on health protection of individuals against the dangers of ionising radiation in relation to medical exposure, and repealing Directive 84/466/Euratom. *Off. J. Eur. Communities*, No. L180/22. EC, Luxembourg.

8 Health and Safety Executive (1999). *The Ionising Radiations Regulations 1999.* SI 1999 No. 3232. HMSO, London.

9 Department of Health (2000). *The Ionising Radiation (Medical Exposure) Regulations 2000.* SI 2000 No. 1059. HMSO, London.

10 Health and Safety Executive (1998). *Fitness of equipment used for medical exposure to ionising radiation.* Guidance Note PM77 (2nd edn) (under revision). HMSO, London.

11 International Commission on Radiation Units and Measurements (1989). *Tissue substitutes in radiation dosimetry and measurement.* Report 44. ICRU, Bethesda, MD, USA.

12 International Commission on Radiation Units and Measurements (1992). *Phantoms and computational models in therapy, diagnosis and protection.* Report 48. ICRU, Bethesda, MD, USA.

13 International Electrotechnical Commission (1994). *Medical diagnostic X-ray equipment–radiation conditions for use in determination of characteristics.* IEC 61267 (1994-10). IEC, Geneva.

14 Wagner, L. K., Fontenia, D. P., Kimme-Smith, C., Rothenberg, L. N., Shepherd, J., and Boone, J. M. (1992). Recommendations on performance characteristics of diagnostic exposure meters: report of AAPM Diagnostic X-ray Imaging Task Group No. 6. *Med. Phys.*, **19**, 231–41.

15 Burke, K. and Sutton, D. (1997). Optimisation and deconvolution of lithium fluoride TLD-100 in diagnostic radiology. *Br. J. Radiol.*, **70**, 261–71.

16 Andreo, P. (1991). Monte Carlo techniques in medical radiation physics. *Phys. Med. Biol.*, **36**, 861–920.

17 Morin, R. (1988). *Monte Carlo simulation in the radiological sciences.* CRC Press, Florida.

18 Jones, D. G. and Wall, B. F. (1985). *Organ doses from medical X-ray examinations calculated using Monte Carlo techniques.* NRPB-R186. NRPB, Chilton.

19 Hart, D., Jones, D. G., and Wall, B. F. (1994). *Normalised organ doses for medical X-ray examinations calculated using Monte Carlo techniques.* NRPB-SR262. NRPB, Chilton. The XDOSE program, available from J. C. Le Heron, National Radiation laboratory, Ministry of Health, Christchurch, New Zealand, utilizes the NRPB data to calculate organ doses and effective doses.

20 Jones, D. G. and Shrimpton, P. C. (1991). *Survey of CT practice in the UK Part 3: normalised organ doses calculated using Monte Carlo techniques.* NRPB-R250. NRPB, Chilton.

21 Spiers, F. W. (1988). Bone and bone marrow dosimetry. In: *Patient dosimetry in diagnostic radiology*, Chapter 5. IPSM Report No. 53. IPSM, York.

22 IPSM/NRPB/CoR (1992). *National protocol for patient dose measurements in diagnostic radiology.* NRPB, Chilton.

23 Rosenstein, M., Suleiman, O. H., Burkhart, R. L., Stern, S. H., and Williams, G. (1992). *Handbook of selected tissue doses for the upper gastrointestinal fluoroscopic examination.* HHS

Publication FDA 92–8282. US Department of Health Education and Welfare, Rockville, MD, USA.

24 Stern, S. H., Rosenstein, M., Renaud, L., and Zankl, M. (1995). *Handbook of selected tissue doses for fluoroscopic and cineangiographic examination of the coronary arteries*. HHS Publication FDA 95–8289. US Department of Health Education and Welfare, Rockville, MD, USA.

25 Edyvean, S. (1998). *Type testing of CT scanners: methods and methodology for assessing imaging performance and dosimetry*. MDA Evaluation Report MDA/98/25. Department of Health, London.

26 Jones, D. G. and Shrimpton, P. C. (1991). *Normalised organ doses for X-ray computed tomography calculated using Monte Carlo techniques*. NRPB-SR250. NRPB, Chilton. The CTDOSE program, available from J. C. Le Heron, National Radiation laboratory, Ministry of Health, Christchurch, New Zealand, utilizes the NRPB data to calculate organ doses and effective doses.

27 ImPACT (1999). *Imaging performance assessment of CT scanners*. Medical Physics Department, St George's Hospital, London. http://www.impactscan.org/scannermatching.htm.

28 European Commission (1999). *European guidelines on quality criteria for computed tomography*. EUR 16262 EN. EC, Luxembourg.

29 Bryant, R. J., Underwood, A. C., Robinson, A., Stephenson, T. J., and Underwood, J. C. E. (1998). Determination of breast tissue composition for improved accuracy in estimating radiation doses and risks in mammographic screening. *The Breast*, **7**, 95–8.

30 IPSM (1994). *The commissioning and routine testing of mammographic X-ray systems*. Report No. 59 (2nd edn) (under revision). IPSM, York.

31 Dance, D. R., Skinner, C. L., Young, K. C., Beckett, J. R., and Kotre, C. J. (2000). Additional factors for the estimation of mean glandular breast dose using the UK mammography dosimetry protocol. *Phys. Med. Biol.*, **45**, 3225–40.

32 Burch, A. and Goodman, D. A. (1998). A pilot survey of radiation doses received in the United Kingdom Breast Screening Programme. *Br. J. Radiol.*, **71**, 517–27.

33 Frederiksen, N. L., Benson, B. W., and Sokolowski, T. W. (1994). Effective dose and risk assessment from film tomography used for dental implant diagnostics. *Dentomaxillofac. Radiol.*, **23**, 123–7.

34 Napier, I. D. (1999). Reference doses for dental radiography. *Br. Dent. J.*, **186**, 392–6.

35 European Commission (1996). *European guidelines on quality criteria for diagnostic radiographic images in paediatrics*. EUR 16261 EN. EC, Luxembourg.

36 Martin, C. J., Farquhar, B., Stockdale, E., and Macdonald, S. (1994). A study of the relationship between patient dose and size in paediatric radiology. *Br. J. Radiol.*, **67**, 864–71.

37 Njeh, C. F., Fuerst, T., Hans, D., Blake, G. M., and Genant, H. K. (1999). Radiation exposure in bone mineral density assessment. *Appl. Radiat. Isot.*, **50**, 215–36.

Chapter 15

Nuclear medicine and radionuclide laboratories

S. Batchelor

15.1 Nuclides used in nuclear medicine and radionuclide laboratories

A variety of radionuclides find application in nuclear medicine *in vivo* tests and *in vitro* assays. The use of radionuclides in laboratory work is confined for the most part to *in vitro* procedures. The principles and methods for radiation protection in both areas are similar. This chapter will attempt to address the issues that face the radiation protection practitioner working with unsealed sources in either field.

Table 15.1 gives the pertinent radiological data for the most commonly encountered radionuclides used in nuclear medicine and positron emission tomography (PET) imaging centres. Table 15.2 gives the same data for radionuclides encountered in radionuclide laboratories. The half-lives of the radionuclides employed range from seconds (^{15}O) to thousands of years (^{14}C).

Table 15.1 Radiological data for radionuclides used in nuclear medicine and positron emission tomography centres

Radionuclide	Decay mode	Principal emission energy (MeV) (beta energies are maximum energies)	Half-life (hours, h days, d months, m)	1st tenth-value layer (mm Pb)[a]	Annual limit of intake[b] (MBq)
Nuclear medicine					
^{57}Co	EC	E_β 0.122, 0.136	271 d	0.7	21
^{58}Co	β^+	E_β 0.475, E_γ 0.811	70.8 d	28	10
^{67}Ga	EC	E_γ 0.093, 0.185, 0.300	78.3 h	5.3	71
^{89}Sr	β	E_β 1.463	50.5 d	range 5000 air 5.5 perspex	3.6
^{99}Mo	β	E_β 1.232, E_γ 0.740, 0.141	66.0 h	20	17
^{99m}Tc	IT	E_γ 0.141	6.02 h	0.9	690
^{111}In	EC	E_γ 0.171, 0.245	2.83 d	2.5	65
^{123}I	EC	E_γ 0.027, 0.159	13.2 h	1.2	95
^{131}I	β	E_β 0.606, E_γ 0.364	8.04 d	11	1.8
^{127}Xe	EC	E_γ 0.172, 0.203, 0.375	36.4 d	–	–
^{133}Xe	β	E_β 0.346, E_γ 0.081, 0.033	5.25 d	0.7	–
^{201}Tl	EC	$E_{X/\gamma}$ 0.075 ave, E_γ 0.167	73.1 h	<0.9	211
Positron emission tomography					
^{11}C	β^+, EC	$E_{\beta+}$ 0.960, E_γ 0.511	20.4 m	13.5	880
^{13}N	β^+, EC	$E_{\beta+}$ 1.198, E_γ 0.511	9.97 m	13.5	not listed
^{15}O	β^+, EC	$E_{\beta+}$ 1.732, E_γ 0.511	2.03 m	13.5	not listed
^{18}F	β^+, EC	$E_{\beta+}$ 0.633, E_γ 0.511	110 m	13.5	215

[a]These data are taken from tables published from multiple sources; they may not take into account low-energy (20 keV) X- or gamma-emissions. Where a radionuclide is a pure beta-emitter the range in air is given.
[b]Data from [1]. These values are minimum values giving the most pessimistic case. Radionuclides in certain forms, or taken in through a different route, may have a higher annual limit of intake (ALI) than that shown.

Table 15.2 Radiological data for radionuclides encountered in laboratories

Radionuclide	Decay mode	Principal emission energy (MeV) (beta energies are maximum energies)	Half-life (hours, h days, d years, y)	1st tenth-value layer (mm Pb)[a]	Annual limit of intake[b] (MBq)
^{32}P	β	E_β 1.71	14.3 d	range 6000 air 6.5 mm perspex	6
^{33}P	β	E_β 0.249	25.4 d	range 460 air 0.5 mm perspex	14
^{22}Na	β^+, EC	E_β 0.546, E_γ 1.275, 0.511	2.60 y	37	6
^{24}Na	β	E_β 1.392, E_γ 1.369, 2.754	15.0 h	59	38
^{45}Ca	β	E_β 0.257	163 d	range 480 air 0.5 mm perspex	7
^{35}S	β	E_β 0.167	87.4 d	range 240 air 0.3 mm perspex	142
^{125}I	EC	E_γ 0.035, $E_{X/\gamma}$ 0.030 ave.	60.1d	0.06	1.3
^{3}H	β	E_β 0.0186	12.4 y	range 47 air <1 mm perspex	1111
^{14}C	β	E_β 0.156	5730 y	range 220 air 0.3 mm perspex	34
^{51}Cr	EC	E_β 0.320, E_X 0.005	27.7 d	7	526
^{59}Fe	β	E_β 0.467, E_γ 1.099, 1.292	44.5 d	44	6
^{65}Zn	β^+, EC	E_γ 1.115 (chiefly)	244 d	42	5
^{36}Cl	β β^+, EC	E_β 0.710 (chiefly)	3 x 10^5 y	range 2000 air 2.2 mm perspex	3

[a,b]Footnotes as in Table 15.1.

Those of the PET tracers tend to be the shortest in the group, those in nuclear medicine are intermediate, and those used in the laboratories are frequently the longest. This is a consequence of the work in laboratories tending to be either *in vitro* tests or basic/applied research frequently not involving human administration whereas the other two areas generally involve *in vivo* work and in these situations a shorter half-life often means a lower patient dose. There are of course exceptions to every rule, as there are some tests involving tritiated steroids that result in effective doses of the order of one microsievert, despite the long half-life of tritium (^3H). The half-life, decay mode, and energy of emitted radiations affect aspects of the environment in which the radionuclide is used, such as shielding and decontamination requirements.

15.2 Guidance on the degree of the hazard from the use of unsealed radioactive sources

Guidance on the facilities required for the use of unsealed radionuclides in hospital and medical research establishments is available from the International Commission on Radiological Protection (ICRP) [2] and elsewhere [3, 4]. The role of the radiation protection adviser (RPA) is to give the employer advice on the use of radiation which, of course, includes facilities associated with the use of radioactive materials. No new facilities or significant modification of existing facilities should be designed and brought into use without expert advice from the RPA, as the facilities required will depend on the nature of the hazard involved.

ICRP 57 [2] classifies laboratories in which radioactive materials are used as being of low, medium, or high hazard. This designation depends on the radionuclide identity and activity being handled (Table 15.3) and the type of operation being performed (Table 15.4) which takes account of the risks of contamination for the various procedures [2, 5]. In order to determine which hazard category a given procedure comes into, a 'weighted activity' is calculated. This is the activity encountered multiplied by two modification factors—one for the radionuclide (Table 15.3) and one for the type of operation to be carried out (Table 15.4). The 'weighted activity' is then compared with the values given in Table 15.5 from which the hazard category of the laboratory is determined (see Box 15.1).

15.3 Design of rooms for using unsealed radioactive sources

15.3.1 Requirements for different types of laboratory

The standards required in low-, medium-, and high-hazard laboratories are summarized below [2].

Table 15.3 Weighting factors for different radionuclides

Radionuclide	Weighting factor
^{36}Cl, ^{89}Sr, ^{125}I, ^{131}I	100
^{11}C, ^{13}N, ^{15}O, ^{18}F, ^{22}Na, ^{24}Na, ^{32}P, ^{33}P, ^{35}S, ^{45}Ca, ^{51}Cr, ^{57}Co, ^{58}Co, ^{59}Fe, ^{65}Zn, ^{67}Ga, ^{99}Mo, ^{99m}Tc, ^{123}I, ^{111}In, ^{201}Tl	1.0
^{3}H, ^{14}C, ^{81m}Kr, ^{127}Xe, ^{133}Xe	0.01

Table 15.4 Weighting factors for different activities performed

Operation performed	Weighting factor
Simple storage area	0.01
Radioactive waste: decay storage or storage prior to consignment	0.01–0.1
Diagnostic procedures (scans, sample counting), radioactive patients (diagnosis) in a waiting room or on wards	0.1
Dispensing and administering radionuclides, ward therapy patients, normal chemical operations	1
Complex operations, radiopharmaceutical preparation	10

- A low-hazard laboratory requires no structural shielding, cleanable floor and bench surfaces, no fume cupboard for radiation work activities, standard ventilation and plumbing, and simple handwash facilities.
- Upgrading this to a medium-hazard laboratory requires a continuous cleanable flooring, good room ventilation, a fume cupboard, and some decontamination facilities. This room is likely to be a supervised or might be a controlled area.

Table 15.5 Hazard category depending on weighted activity

Weighted activity (MBq)	Category
Less than 50	Low hazard
50–50 000	Medium hazard
Greater than 50 000	High hazard

- A high-hazard laboratory may require structural shielding, floor surface as before but covered to walls, special plumbing, forced ventilation, and enhanced fume cupboard facility–depending on the nature of the hazard. This room is likely to be a controlled radiation area.

15.3.2 Laboratory features

Security

Security of radiation sources necessitates locks on refrigerators and other stores containing stock and devices containing sources, etc. Stores may require built-in shielding to reduce external radiation dose rates to acceptable levels.

Shielding

Local shielding is often required, which will depend on the radionuclides and activities being handled (§15.4.4

Box 15.1 Examples of laboratory hazard classification

Suppose a radiopharmacy preparation involves a procedure using 74 MBq of the radionuclide ^{131}I. What type of laboratory is required to perform this work in?

- Weighting factor for ^{131}I is 100 (from Table 15.3). Multiplying the 74 MBq used by 100 gives 7400 MBq.
- A radiopharmacy preparation operation has a procedural weighting factor of 10 (from Table 15.4). Multiplying the figure above by 10 gives 74 000 MBq.
- Looking up in Table 15.5 shows that this should be a high-hazard laboratory.

Conversely, a simple storage facility for the decay of radioactive waste bags of ^{32}P (maximum activity 37 MBq) may have a weighted activity as low as 0.37 MBq (the radionuclide weighting factor is 1 and the procedure weighting factor is between 0.1 and 0.01; allowing judgement by the RPA considering local factors). This area will be a low-hazard category room, even if the higher value of 0.1 were to be used.

and §15.6.1). When designing shielding it is prudent to remember that long-handled forceps or tongs may need access around the side of the shielding in order to carry out manipulations.

Ventilation

Ventilation systems should be designed so that they do not extract radioactivity from one room and expel it into another room either by design (i.e. using part of the extracted air to mix with external air) or by the nature of the exhaust duct outlet position. Checks should be made at commissioning, using a smoke candle or similar, to ensure that recirculation does not occur. In some cases a fumehood operating at a negative pressure is indicated for protection of the worker, whereas in other cases, such as sterile production, it is appropriate to have a fully exhausted laminar vertical flow system under positive pressure.

Space

It is essential that the amount of space in work areas in rooms where radionuclides are handled is adequate for workers to safely perform their tasks without risk of collision and subsequent spills. Pressure on the availability of workbench area or rooms must not be allowed to cause a conflict between different requirements for work with radiation. For example, low-activity assay work areas must be separated from higher-activity work. Sensitive counting or imaging equipment, such as γ/β or whole-body counters, should not be sited physically close to high-energy sources such as molybdenum/technetium generators or stock amounts of positron-emitting radionuclides. The interference between such high- and low-activity work can invalidate results or significantly restrict the use of the facility for either purpose.

Washing facilities

It is usually best to site handwashing facilities close to the exit of the room. It should be possible to operate the taps without using the hands. Disposable towels for drying are preferred and a mains-operated monitor should be located next to the sink. The monitor should be left turned on so that staff are able and encouraged to use it without touching the controls. In addition, a log book should be kept with the monitor (preferably mounted on a dedicated small inclined shelf under the monitor) and a pen attached so that record keeping is made as easy as possible.

Designated sinks

In higher hazard areas the designated sink for aqueous waste disposal should be connected as directly as possible to a main sewer. This is not always possible, but in all situations the route of such a drainpipe should be traced back to determine whether there are any problems that can be foreseen as a consequence of the disposal. Examples that have been encountered (not infrequently) are:

- lengths of pipe that do not empty due to insufficient downward gradient on the pipe
- handwash basins situated further down the pipe run which are lower than the designated sink, so that if a blockage did occur waste would come into the handwash basin before appearing in the bottom of the designated sink
- large-volume 'traps' on the waste outlet that are designed for holding materials to encourage dilutions. These result in a delay in complete discharge of radioactive materials and therefore cause unnecessary irradiation to staff in the laboratory.

Solid waste

Provision should be made for the storage of solid radioactive waste that may eventually be sent off-site for disposal. This may need shielding unless it is very low level. If there is even a moderately low dose rate exposing staff or public, it is normally in accordance with the ALARA (as low as reasonably achievable) principle to reduce this with shielding.

Benching

It is preferable for medium- and high-hazard category laboratories to have a bench design with a raised lip at the front and coved at the back onto the wall to contain spills. These features should be either an integral part of the benching or mouldings that are sealed with appropriate material so that there is no absorption of radioactive contamination into the joins. It is recommended that these features are still employed even if the worker employs a spill tray covered with disposable liner. The benching should be resistant to corrosion by chemicals and should be easily decontaminated. Consideration should also be given to the ability of the bench to withstand the loading of lead shields.

15.4 Radiation protection requirements in nuclear medicine

15.4.1 Area designation

In nuclear medicine departments, areas such as the radiopharmacy, therapy rooms, and injection and scanning areas will usually need to be designated as controlled areas. The injection and scanning areas could be deemed to be supervised areas in departments with low workloads, which only perform low-activity patient investigations. The patient toilet and waiting area are more likely to be supervised areas. In nuclear medicine, the source will not be confined to a single room. In many cases the corridor adjoining rooms where activity is present will need to be a supervised or even a controlled area. It is important that such areas do not form a public thoroughfare to other parts of the hospital. The status of all areas must be clearly identified using signs and they should be fully described in local rules. It is generally convenient to control an entire room rather than declare only part of it to be controlled. The clear exception to this is an area behind a shield or in a fume cupboard, where only the hands can enter. In this case that area alone may be controlled on the basis of the dose limit for an extremity being likely to be exceeded. Rooms that are controlled radiation areas due to their potential for contamination (as well as direct radiation), such as a radiopharmacy, may require the entrance to be via a 'stepover' barrier. This not only serves to act as a convenient point at which to put on disposable overshoes and use monitoring facilities but also draws attention to the special nature of the area being entered.

Patient waiting areas should have their own toilets that should *not* be used by members of staff. If a receptionist *has* to be based within a waiting area then it is important that they are placed in a position such that they are not very close to patients who may have each received up to 0.9 GBq of ^{99m}Tc-labelled radiopharmaceutical. A distance of 2 to 3 metres should be sufficient in a situation like this. The waiting area for patients who have been injected with radiopharmaceuticals should not be shared by obstetric patients, e.g. waiting for ultrasound imaging.

Technetium-labelled aerosols are commonly used for lung ventilation imaging and these areas should ideally have suitable extraction systems to reduce the radioactive contamination. The used aerosol equipment may well need to be shielded.

15.4.2 Liquid waste disposal

Depending on the result of the assessment of the environmental impact from liquid waste disposal from a nuclear medicine therapy facility (§9.4), the regulatory body may require drainage from a facility to pass into a 'holding tank' under the ALARA principle. Here liquid radioactive waste is held to decay before it is discharged into the sewage system. Significant levels of ^{131}I have been detected in public watercourses in some areas in the UK. These may arise from discharges from several hospitals and nuclear medicine installations in such locations may be required to install holding tanks in newly designed premises. The tanks would generally work on the principle of there being two tanks: one holds back waste for decay (notably iodine in the urine of therapy doses from patients with cancer of the thyroid) while the other is being filled up. The tank containing decayed waste is discharged when the second tank is nearly full and is then filled while waste in the second tank is left to decay.

15.4.3 Wall shielding

Purpose-designed shielding of rooms for the radionuclides used in nuclear medicine imaging is often unnecessary. However, the same principles employed for X-ray rooms should be applied to assess the requirements (§13.3). A dose constraint of 0.3 mSv year^{-1} should be applied to staff and members of the public in adjacent departments and corridors to determine whether additional protection will be required for the walls of the department. Higher dose constraints may be applied to areas within the department where all staff are radiation workers, but the 0.3 mSv year^{-1} constraint may be appropriate for a receptionist.

The source may be a patient or a vial or syringe containing radioactive material. When assessing shielding requirements, a patient containing 'A' GBq of ^{99m}Tc may be regarded as a source giving a dose rate of 17A μSv h^{-1} at 1 m (Table 7.1). A source with an average activity derived from a weighted mean for the range of more common examinations performed can be used for the assessment with a representative position in the room for the source location (e.g. the gamma-camera for patients being scanned). Dose rates at room boundaries can then be calculated using the inverse square law. Reasonable assumptions based on the times patients spend in the department after injection, lengths of scans, and numbers of patients may be used to estimate the proportion of the time for which radiation sources are present in particular rooms in order to derive time-averaged dose rates. Occupancy factors can be applied to groups of exposed individuals, as for X-ray facilities, to ensure that they do not exceed dose constraints (Table 13.2). Since most of the emission of ^{99m}Tc is at 140 keV, a simple half-value layer (HVL) relationship is adequate for calculation of the amount of shielding required to reduce the dose rate to the required level. Data for other radionuclides are given in Table 7.3.

Shielding may also be required to prevent degradation of nuclear medicine images from radiation emitted from a patient in an adjoining room. This can occur between patients in two adjoining scanning rooms or from an injected patient waiting in an adjoining room. The severity of the problem will vary with the orientation of the camera. As an approximate rule of thumb, the dose rate at the camera from a patient in an adjacent area with the largest activity administered should be less than 1% of the dose rate from a patient being scanned with the smallest activity administered, at a distance of about 200 mm from the detector. Two millimetres of lead should reduce any such effect more than 100 times and this is often an appropriate solution in nuclear medicine. However, the use of leaded doors in nuclear medicine is not usually appropriate, except in therapy.

15.4.4 Local shielding

The term 'local shielding' refers to a shield applied to reduce the radiation dose from a specific source as opposed to shielding a large area such as an entire wall. Local shielding should be applied wherever a significant reduction in dose may be possible. Obvious examples of sources for which local shielding is appropriate are ^{99}Mo/^{99m}Tc generators, multidose vials for patient administrations, diagnostic and therapeutic patient doses, and flood sources for gamma-camera quality control. Multidose vials containing ^{99m}Tc-labelled products are easily shielded using 2 to 4 mm thickness of lead pot (Table 15.1). ^{131}I therapy doses need much more protection (tenth-value thickness is 11 mm) and additional shielding to the pot used for transit may be deemed necessary with the sources being locked away in a shielded store or safe. Distance can also be usefully employed to reduce the dose rate as well as time by storing the source in a room that has close to zero occupancy.

For operational procedures other shielding solutions are employed. Manipulation of activity must take place behind a body and eye shield often termed an 'L shield' (Figure 15.1). Note that there is a bottom to the shield to protect the worker's lower body and to make the shield more stable. It is essential that the benching is able to safely accommodate the weight of the shielding. Commercial benching can be specified to take various loads. Note that the shield acts both to attenuate radiation and as a splash guard to stop the operator becoming contaminated.

Flood sources for quality control of gamma-camera uniformity are best deployed utilizing a shield that protects the worker's hands from exposure during handling. The surface dose rates of these sources are significant and such protection is again warranted under the ALARA principle.

Radioactive waste, whether solid or liquid, must not be overlooked when it comes to shielding. For bulky items, such as sacks of clinical radioactive waste, it is often more convenient to use distance to reduce dose than to provide large shielded containers. When this is considered appropriate, it can be accomplished by the use of an entire dedicated room or by depositing the waste in the institution's central radioactive waste store. Such areas should be well ventilated.

15.4.5 Radionuclide manipulation and administration

Vials and syringes used either for formulation, dispensing, or administration will need protection by using syringe and vial shields. For γ-emitters, tungsten is generally used in commercial products as it has a higher atomic number and a higher density than lead thereby providing more attenuation for the same thickness. Some lead glass shields can provide better visibility. If β-emitters are being manipulated, other than ^{14}C or ^{3}H, perspex syringe shields are generally used as they attenuate the β-particles and minimize the bremsstrahlung radiation that can be significant if a high atomic number shield is used on high-energy radiation. However, if the thickness of lead is sufficient, the attenuation will predominate over bremsstrahlung production [4]. Thus a shield with 0.5 mm lead or more is suitable for use with ^{32}P. The operator must not become complacent

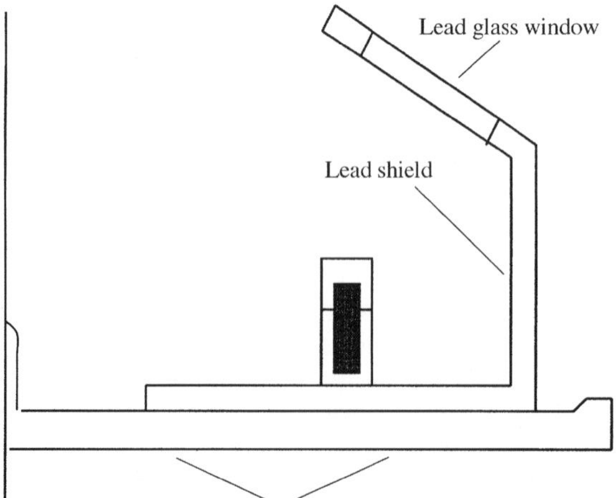

Figure 15.1 Typical shield for operational shielding of sources.

when using syringe shields, since the radiation emitted from the ends of the shield results in a far lower protection in practice than might be expected from the thickness of lead in the shield [6].

Preplacing a butterfly cannula in a vein before handling the radioactive syringe can aid in dose reduction. A short (95 mm) cannula has been shown to reduce doses to the left and right hands by 50% and 70%, respectively [7]. However, consideration must be given to other clinical implications. For example, 'clumping' of particles in lung perfusion imaging may occur if blood is pulled back into the line and premixes with the macroaggregated albumin. An unnecessarily long catheter may increase the exposure of the operator from activity in the tubing.

15.4.6 Radiopharmacy

Although the ^{99}Mo/^{99m}Tc generator comes with its own primary shield, it is normal for this to be placed within a secondary shield for operational use. This is because the application of ALARA to the shielding requirements for the transport of radioactive material does not necessarily equate to its application during storage and use. For example, upon installation within the radiopharmacy, the generator needs to be moved without lifting equipment and hence the weight of the primary shield has to take this into account. The primary shield may be depleted uranium as this offers more attenuation than lead (thickness for thickness) due to its higher atomic number and density. Dose rates around the secondary shield should be measured. Adjoining rooms should not be overlooked if the generator is placed in proximity to a dividing wall and further shielding added if required. Typically, with a tenth-value layer of 20 mm for lead and activities of the order of tens of GBq, total shielding of the order of 80–100 mm lead may be needed. All shielding within the radiopharmacy must be easily cleanable—this generally means that exposed lead surfaces are coated with paint or some other material.

There has been significant interest in whether the formulation of radiopharmaceuticals can be automated through the use of robotics and thereby considerably reduce hand doses of radiopharmacists. Despite optimism in the early assessment of some systems [8], the need for operator intervention and the concern over local contamination have been factors in such units not being more widely adopted. More simple automated 'syringe fill stations' are being developed to aid in manual manipulations. An example of such a device is shown in Figure 15.2. This, at least, may reduce the significant radiation dose that is received from the unshielded ends of syringe shields.

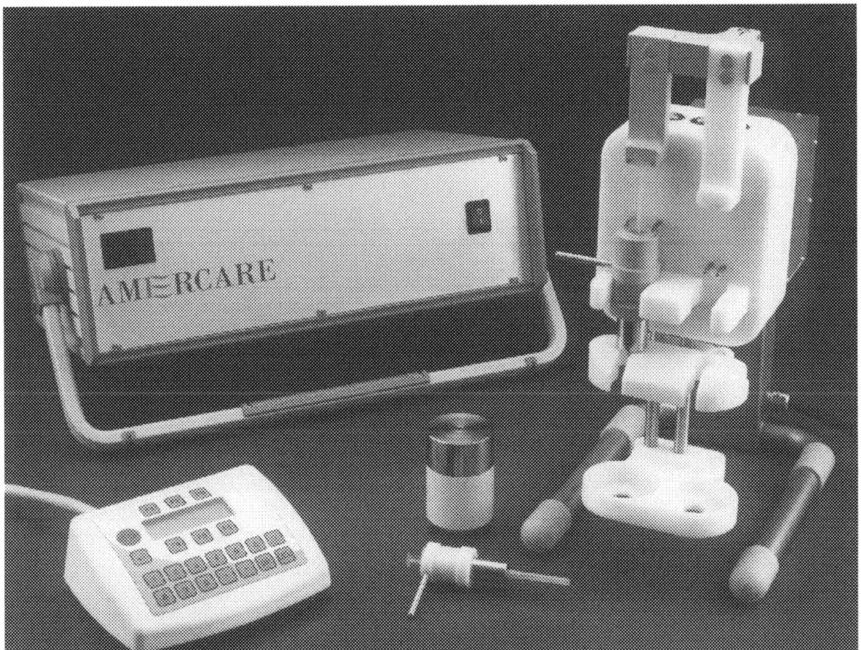

Figure 15.2 Automated 'syringe fill station'. (Photograph provided courtesy of Amercare Ltd.)

15.5 Special considerations in PET departments

PET procedures have the potential to give a higher dose to the operator. This is because:

- each disintegration is accompanied by the emission of positrons which, if unshielded, result in a high skin dose
- each emission results in *two* γ-ray photons (annihilation photons from the decay of the positrons)

Box 15.2 Example of assessment of protection for a PET suite

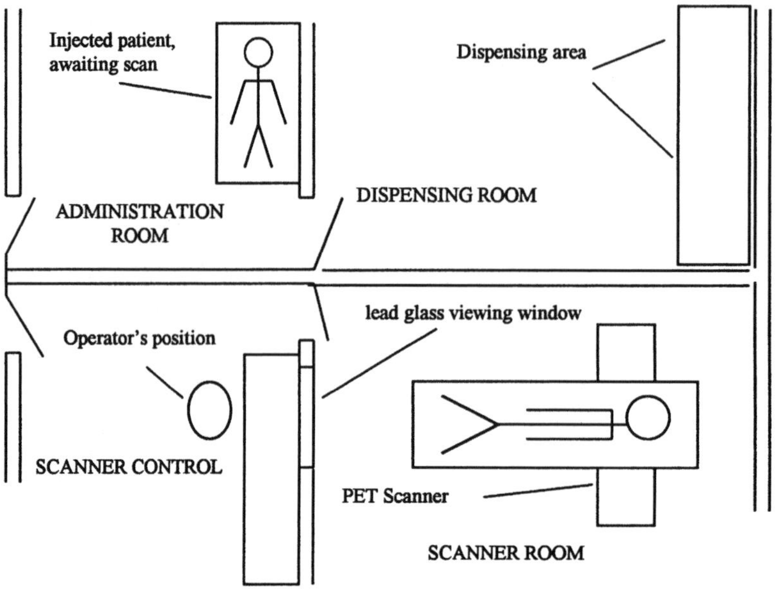

Figure B15.1 Possible layout for a PET scanning suite.

The plan in Figure B15.1 shows a patient on the scanning couch and another who has been injected and is awaiting uptake. Assume these are the only radioactive patients in the PET unit.

Assume the following:

Activity in each patient: 350 MBq in waiting patient, 240 MBq in patient being scanned (due to decay).

The dose rate from a PET patient containing 350 MBq is 15 μSv h^{-1} at 1 m from the patient.

Design dose constraint for radiation workers in the suite: 1.0 mSv per year (this is the dose that the employer intends not to be exceeded due to being in proximity to these patients, e.g. by sitting at the console, etc.) In reality, to this may be added the extra dose for other activities, e.g. injecting the patient, being closer to the patient before, during, and after the scan, drawing up the dose, quality control procedures, etc.

Design dose constraint to the public (or other workers in adjoining rooms whose work does not involve radiation): 0.3 mSv per year.

Each scan takes an hour and each patient waits an hour in the administration room (while the tracer, FDG, is being taken up).

The distance from the waiting patient to the scanning technologist is 3.0 m and from the scanning patient to the same member of staff is 3.5 m.

The process is continuous with 7 h exposure per day.

What shielding is required in the walls and glass panel?

Dose per day to scanning technologist is calculated from each patient component:

$$(15 \times 1/3^2 \times 350/350 \times 7) + (15 \times 1/3.5^2 \times 240/350 \times 7) = 11.7 + 5.9 = 17.6\ \mu\text{Sv day}^{-1}.$$

- these photons have energies of 511 keV which are harder to shield than the 140 keV photons from ^{99m}Tc.

This has implications for the design and operation of PET facilities.

The specific γ-ray constant for PET nuclides (i.e. ^{18}F, ^{15}O, ^{13}N, ^{11}C) is an order of magnitude higher than that for ^{99m}Tc and this does not allow for the skin dose that would be received from the positrons. The tenth-value thickness in lead is 15 times greater for the PET 511 keV

Box 15.2 (*continued*)

Hence in 1 year of 250 working days, the annual dose will be 4400 μSv or 4.4 mSv. This exceeds the design criteria by approximately a factor of 4 and hence protection of two half-value layer at 511 keV needs to be incorporated into the walls and window between these patients and the scanning technologist. This can be achieved using a 200 mm thick concrete-equivalent wall and a 11 mm lead-equivalent lead glass window.

Note that the activity in the patient decreases as time progresses due to physical decay—this means that the effective activity can be decreased by about 83% of the value at the start, although this step has been omitted from the shielding assessment above.

One can go through this procedure again—this time perhaps to allow for another member of staff from another department (e.g. a medical secretary sitting at her desk on the other side of the wall). Suppose the distances concerned from each of the patients were both 6 m.

What shielding would be necessary?

Dose per day:

$$(15 \times 1/6^2 \times 350/350 \times 7) + (15 \times 1/6^2 \times 240/350 \times 7) = 2.9 + 2.1 = 5\ \mu\text{Sv day}^{-1}.$$

Hence in 1 year the dose received from 250 working days would be 1.25 mSv.

Not only is this above the dose constraint of 0.3 mSv per annum but it is above the public dose limit of 1 mSv per annum. To reduce this to 0.3 mSv the wall would need to provide shielding to give a reduction by a factor of 4, i.e. about 2 half-value layers. This could be accomplished with two courses of concrete-equivalent bricks or 11 mm of lead in a dry wall or approximately 25 mm of steel.

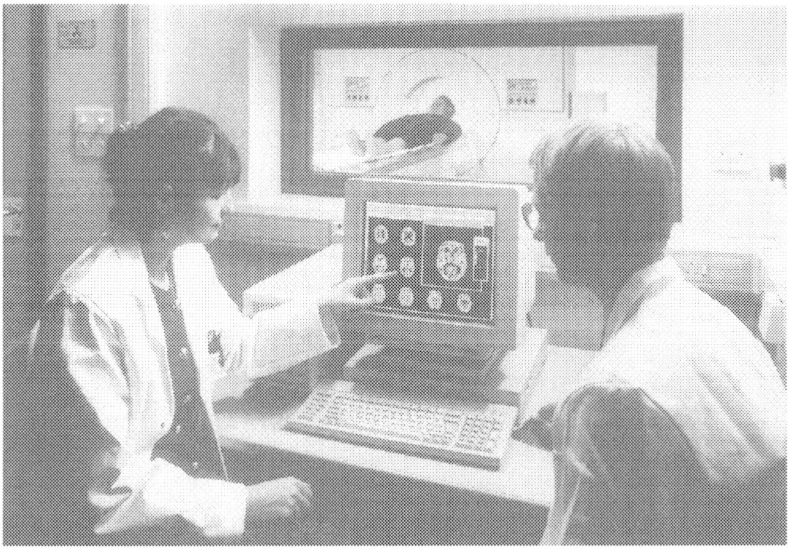

Figure B15.2 View of a PET scanning room through a lead glass window. (Photograph provided courtesy of M. Dakin, Clinical PET Centre at Guy's and St Thomas' Hospital Trust.)

γ-ray photons compared to those from ^{99m}Tc. Therefore unless rooms are large and distance is used to reduce dose rates, it is consistent with ALARA to utilize shielding in the structure of a PET scanning department. Concrete density-equivalent bricks are available and a two-course wall (approximately 200 mm) gives an attenuation of just under 10, a single course 2.

In a PET facility, there is frequently a cyclotron to consider unless two PET centres are nearby and one supplies the other with PET tracers. These cyclotrons may be relatively small machines operating at 10–11 MeV or a larger multipurpose machine used also for radiotherapy. A PET cyclotron will usually have its own shield which is hydraulically operated to allow access to targetry. These machines do not have to be sited in a vault but this may still be the option chosen so that further shielding is gained. There are neutrons released outside the manufacturers shield which have to be shielded as they have a high radiation weighting factor. If work needs to be carried out on the targetry, it is necessary for a delay of several hours, if not a day, to occur since the end of the last bombardment, as the induced activity on some of the components within the machine will mean that radiation levels are very high. This induced activity has to be stated on the operator's 'site licence' (in England and Wales, this is the Environment Agency). There is generally some degree of automated chemistry to facilitate the production of the more routine PET tracers (e.g. ^{18}F-labelled fluorodeoxyglucose, FDG). The chemistry may result in release of volatile by-products during synthesis and this has to be allowed for in the arrangements agreed with the regulatory bodies. It may be prudent to fit a monitoring system on the extract from the cyclotron room, chemistry unit, and any shielded fume cupboards ('hot cells') so that data can be logged continuously and emissions recorded automatically.

Hand doses in PET, whether in the radiochemistry or the patient scanning area, have the potential to be high and so it is advisable to monitor hand doses and to employ devices to reduce doses received as much as possible.

Possible dose-saving measures are the following.

- Use of large perspex syringe shields protects the skin from positrons and distance can be employed to reduce dose.
- Preplacement of butterfly cannulae reduces time of exposure to radiation during administration.
- Arrangement for assaying each patient dose with the $H_2{}^{15}O$ tracer remaining in the lead transit pot can avoid direct unshielded manipulation [9]. Because of the short half-life of ^{15}O (2 min) it is necessary for high activities to be administered to patients. This can lead to high operator doses if the syringe of $H_2{}^{15}O$ is removed from its shield and assayed in a radionuclide calibrator in the normal way. To avoid this, the tracer, inside its shielded pot, is placed at a defined point alongside the exterior shield of a radionuclide calibrator ionisation chamber and an appropriate modified activity calibration factor employed.
- Possible modifications can be made to delivery systems for the automated chemistry, so that tracers are delivered straight into a vial within a radionuclide calibrator [10].

15.6 Radiation protection requirements for a radionuclide laboratory

15.6.1 Local shielding for work activities

The activities handled in radionuclide laboratories are frequently lower than in nuclear medicine. However, the use of certain radionuclides (e.g. ^{131}I, ^{32}P) and the specific activities handled require high standards of safety in technique and in the laboratory environment. The information given earlier in this chapter will be used by the RPA to determine which hazard category a laboratory belongs to. In general, an iodination suite would be expected to be a high-hazard area, ^{32}P cell hybridization may be a high- or medium-hazard area, and areas where bactec vials or commercial radioimmunoassay are involved will require a low-hazard area.

Structural shielding is seldom necessary in many laboratories although this will need to be assessed by the RPA. Radionuclides that are difficult to shield adequately are ^{22}Na, ^{24}Na, and ^{65}Zn. These all require local shields of several tens of millimetres of lead to significantly reduce dose rates. As stated above, it is important to ensure that benching can take the weight of shielding being used. It is sometimes more effective to designate a small lockable room for their storage. Lead bricks can still be used as well as the (concrete) floor. Distance, however, may be the most effective factor in reducing dose to other personnel.

There are situations where it may be reasonable *not* to employ shielding. For example, the doses received from handling during certain critical procedures may be relatively low and the disadvantage of using shielding, in terms of loss of sensitivity to the operation being performed, may outweigh the benefit obtained by further dose reduction. Self-attenuation in the container is another aid in dose reduction when handling β-emitters such as tritium and even ^{14}C and ^{35}S. Most β-emitters can be shielded effectively by 10 mm of perspex or less.

However, the range of β-particles in air must not be underestimated (Tables 15.1 and 15.2). Energetic β-emitters such as ^{32}P and ^{90}Y and many positron-emitting radionuclides have a range that means organs such as the eye could be significantly exposed during open manipulations.

15.6.2 General procedures

The access allowed to the laboratory for cleaning staff and service personnel must take into account the hazards that such staff may be exposed to. Staff must follow a written system of work if the area remains controlled when they need access. Bins used for the accumulation of solid radioactive waste must be marked clearly with an appropriate radiation trefoil warning symbol as well as a clear written message stating the nature of their contents and that they must not be removed by cleaning staff. Radioactive waste leaving the premises as ordinary or clinical waste can result in prosecution of the employer under radioactive substances legislation due to the failure to keep waste secure and disposal via an appropriate waste stream.

15.6.3 Special techniques for specific radionuclides

Phosphorous-32

The potential hazard in handling ^{32}P is illustrated in Table 15.2 in that it has the third lowest annual limit of intake (ALI) in the listing. It is particularly hazardous as sodium phosphate since in this form it can irradiate important cells related to the blood–indeed it is used in this form to treat polycythaemia vera. A potential side-effect is the induction of leukaemia. Therapeutic amounts are only of the order of 200 MBq and so the ingestion of any amount is of significant concern. For dosimetry purposes phosphorous is assumed to be deposited in the skeleton and retained on the bone surfaces (endosteal cells) so there is also a risk of bone cancer. Details of a model used to describe the whole-body retention of phosphorous are given by Jackson and Dolphin [11]. Phosphorous can be ingested in aerosol droplets, which can be formed inadvertently in processes such as centrifuging, blending, or transference of liquids using syringes. Skin doses from bodily contamination of ^{32}P can cause concern and hence regular monitoring is very important. Gloves should be changed whenever they are found to be contaminated, and decontamination of any contaminated skin should be carried out according to the instructions given in §15.10. When a shipping container is opened, either from the supplier or from a former user, it is wise to perform a simple wipe test, using a 'ready turned on' contamination monitor. This enables contamination to be detected at source from a previous, perhaps undetected, incident. Such an incident could leave a dried residue on the surface of the vial creating an invisible, insidious hazard.

Staff should be aware that Eppendorf tubes have an attenuation for the β-particles from ^{32}P of a third to a half that for average glass vials. Indeed the surface dose rate from such tubes containing tens of MBq of ^{32}P can be several mSv per minute. An operator handling a few tens of these tubes a day, each for less than a minute, could receive more than the dose limit to the skin of the fingers (500 mSv per year). Eppendorf tubes should be placed behind a 10 mm thick perspex shield or in perspex sample blocks which are obtainable commercially. Balance *et al.* [12] have shown that a 1 MBq spot of ^{32}P contamination, spread over one square centimetre, can give a skin dose 1.82 Sv per hour. This is consistent with a value of 2 Sv per hour obtained by Curran [13], who also provides calculations for contamination which has penetrated the skin.

An alternative to ^{32}P is ^{33}P which decays by beta-emission but of a much lower energy and with a 25-day half-life. The ALI is therefore much higher (Table 15.2).

Iodine radionuclides

^{125}I and ^{131}I have the two lowest ALIs in Tables 15.1 and 15.2 reflecting the danger of ingestion. The thyroid gland is well known to be avid for iodine which is also found in the salivary and pituitary glands, ovaries, muscle, and bile [14]. As an approximation the committed dose equivalent from thyroidal ingestion of either ^{125}I or ^{131}I is 1 mSv per kBq in the gland. Prevention of uptake of iodine in the thyroid gland after an episode of contamination can be accomplished by blocking the thyroid using stable iodine. There are a number of possible methods of achieving this, but one must beware of potential side-effects and it is recommended that a medical adviser is consulted. Potassium iodate has been considered the simplest method and the daily dose has been reported to be from '>5 mg' [15] to 100 mg [16]. Effectiveness depends on the delay in administration. A 100 mg dose given within 3–4 hours after ingestion will reduce uptake by more than 50% [17]. The mechanism by which this ionic blocking works is the Wolff–Chaikoff block. Excess stable iodine should not be taken routinely prior to iodination procedures.

Manipulating iodine inside fume cupboards is essential when there is a possibility of volatility and advisable in most other situations as volatility can be induced by deviation from recommended procedures. An exception to the use of fume cupboards could be the manipulation of the very small amounts used in individual radio-immunoassay procedures. Connor and McLintock [4] suggest the wearing of two pairs of gloves, possibly of different materials, when handling iodine as there is evidence that iodine-labelled materials penetrate gloves. They also suggest that if it is necessary to store liquid radioactive waste, this should be done by preparing a solution of 25 g sodium thiosulphate and 2 g sodium iodide in 1 litre of 1 M sodium hydroxide, and then adding the waste to this solution as it arises. Similarly treat spills of iodine radionuclides by adding a solution of 5% sodium thiosulphate before carrying out the decontamination.

Workers handling MBq quantities of iodines should check their thyroid regularly; good practice would be to check at least weekly or preferably a few hours after a procedure using 10s of MBq of ^{125}I or ^{131}I. Although this can be done elegantly on a dedicated thyroid uptake probe system, a contamination monitor with a scintillation crystal a few millimetres thick will suffice. Data on the fraction of ^{125}I remaining for up to 60 days after ingestion with normal thyroid function are given in appendix 3 of Prime [15].

Lassmann *et al.* [18] reported that up to 0.1% of ^{131}I activity administered to patients is released into the air from a therapy ward. This reinforces the need for all such areas to be well ventilated. Wellner *et al.* [19] calculated that patients returning home after being hospitalized for 2 days following radioiodine therapy may give up to 0.2 kBq to thyroids of family members, resulting in an equivalent dose to the thyroid of up to 4.7 mSv for adults and 20 mSv for children.

15.7 Personnel monitoring

Most staff in radionuclide laboratories or nuclear medicine will not be designated as classified workers but a few in large busy departments will require classification because relevant extremity or body dose limits are exceeded. Two groups whose dose to the hands may be high enough to warrant their classification are radiopharmacy staff, who provide radiopharmaceuticals for a busy department and to nuclear medicine departments in other hospitals, and PET radiochemistry staff, if they perform a certain amount of 'manual radiochemistry', which is not uncommon if new tracers are being developed. Facilities for routine production of materials such as ^{18}F-FDG often have automated chemistry units thus saving on handling of large activities of radionuclides. Both classified and non-classified staff working with radioactive patients or radiopharmaceuticals wear a personal dosemeter to give an estimate of effective dose and many wear a dosemeter on an extremity to monitor their skin/extremity dose (§8.4).

The activities handled in laboratories are generally lower than in nuclear medicine and frequently may involve β-emitting radionuclides. The use of a whole-body monitor may not therefore be the best use of resources in all situations and it may be more appropriate, as in the nuclear medicine situation above, to wear finger monitors under gloves. Most work with MBq quantities of ^{35}S and ^{14}C is unlikely to justify the use of finger dosemeters. However, it is prudent to monitor all staff starting to use MBq quantities of ^{32}P to obtain an initial dose assessment of the technique being used.

15.7.1 Wearing extremity dosemeters

Most dosemeters for extremity monitoring are made from thermoluminescent material (§4.12.2). They should be worn routinely by staff who may receive a significant dose. They are also of value in assessing new techniques and in checking that ALARA is being followed when a member of staff starts a new work activity. Wearing the dosemeter for a transient period can be useful in optimising techniques and demonstrating that doses are low. The dose received from the manipulation of radiopharmaceuticals is not uniform across the hand. Under legislation which is consistent with the recommendations of ICRP 60, the dose to the skin can only be averaged over 1 cm^2. Whereas it may not be crucial as to exactly where on a hand dosemeters are worn if the dose received is less than 10% of a dose limit, it does become important when the dose starts to approach the limit. Ideally a dosemeter should be used to monitor the part of the finger receiving the highest dose, which is usually the tip. If this is impractical, it may be necessary to monitor a different part of the finger or an adjacent finger, in which case a factor may be employed to ensure dose limits are not being exceeded. There have been several articles [7, 8, 10, 20, 21] dealing with the variation in dose across the hand for exposure during different work activities. These have shown that in dispensing, injecting, and formulating in nuclear medicine and clinical PET, doses to different parts of the hand where dosemeters may be worn can vary by a factor of six [7, 10, 21]. If the procedures performed are similar to those in published work, the dose to the fingertip may be estimated from the dose measured on a thermoluminescence detector ring.

It is important that the hands are checked for contamination regularly for two reasons:

1. The dose to the skin and possible subsequent ingestion are particular hazards that can be reduced if decontamination measures are taken as soon as contamination is detected.
2. A contaminated dosemeter will show a very high dose if the contamination remains on the surface of the dosemeter. The actual skin dose received will usually be lower as the TLD shields the skin and irradiation of the dosemeter will continue after work with radiation has ceased. This can lead to a dose

limit apparently being exceeded and an incorrect report to a regulatory body.

Dosemeters must not be kept in an area where the radiation level is above background while not being used. This may sound obvious advice but it is not rare for film badges or TLDs to be found inside investigation rooms. Similarly it is important that the hands of the person distributing or collecting these devices are not contaminated with radioactivity.

15.7.2 Communication of results to individuals wearing dosemeters

It is imperative that individuals are informed of their results as soon as possible after their dosemeters are returned for processing. Where an external service is used, this may be 1 to 2 months after the end of the monitoring period. If people are aware of their doses and can compare them with those received by others then there is a general tendency for their dose to decrease over time. If the system is such that viewing their dose is not made easy then the reverse is true. Similarly a policy of telling workers their dose only when there is a problem tends to encourage complacency in the workers attitude to the ALARA principle. A radiation protection supervisor (RPS) who undertakes their duties conscientiously fulfils an invaluable role in ensuring that doses to staff are kept as low as possible.

15.7.3 Electronic personal dosemeters

Electronic personal dosemeters (EPDs) are becoming increasingly popular because of their ability to instantly tell the user the dose that they have received (§8.3.5). Some have the ability to log dose against time so that an analysis of when a dose was received can be made. Their prime use is either as a quick way of monitoring received dose when worn together with an approved dosemeter or as an aid to reassure staff or visitors when they enter radiation areas. Some have even been produced the size of a credit card and have a barcode on to provide area access. It is important that due consideration for energy response is made so that the instrument is suitable for its intended use.

15.8 Monitoring for contamination

Levels of contamination should always be kept as low as practicable (Box 15.3). In order to achieve this, monitoring for contamination must be carried out in all areas where radioactivity is handled. This includes the monitoring of people who enter an area where radioactive materials are used. It is mandatory that such monitoring is documented and available for inspection by regulatory inspectors. Unsurprisingly, they may take the attitude that if it is not recorded it is not being performed. Discussion of the choice of instrument is given in §4.4.2. For detecting β-radiation from ^{14}C, ^{35}S, ^{32}P, etc., a thin end-window Geiger or a proportional counter is required (§4.8), while for low-energy γ-radiation a scintillation detector is superior to a Geiger as it has a much higher attenuation for γ-rays (§4.9).

15.8.1 Monitoring technique

Monitoring may be routine or may follow a suspected spill. In both cases the monitor must not be moved across the area too quickly or else a false negative result is obtained. Where the level is significantly elevated an assessment of activity (Bq cm^{-2}) may be required, in which case the monitor must also be held away from the surface at the distance at which the calibration was performed. It is important to be aware that the nature of a surface can significantly affect the measurement. Radionuclides emit many different particles and photons and these can be partially or totally absorbed in the surface material, thereby affecting the reading obtained. Apart from checking the area of benching or flooring where the work is carried out, it is good practice to check certain items that are likely to have been touched by a contaminated glove, such as telephones, door handles, and communal pens. Monitoring of staff clothing and hands should be performed to the same frequency.

It is important that regular checks of the monitor are carried out as well as the annual traceable calibration. These checks should include a battery check every time the monitor is used and a go/no-go field-check at intervals specified in the local rules. When a battery is checked it is important that the instrument is left on in the 'battery check' mode for at least 30 seconds as batteries can appear to have useful life within them but this quickly drops when they are 'on load'. This might then result in an unnoticed, decreased, sensitivity of the monitor.

In areas of high ambient background (e.g. the radiopharmacy adjacent to the $^{99}Mo/^{99m}Tc$ generator) or when tritium is being monitored, monitoring may still be accomplished by wipe testing the environment. A wipe test consists of wiping the area with a material that is moistened with a liquid in which the suspected compound is soluble. The area wiped is noted (this should be part of a standard specified protocol) and the activity is measured using a γ-counter, or for a soft β-emitter, liquid scintillation counter. It is standard practice to assume that 10% of the activity from the surface has been transferred to the material. After correcting the result for the efficiency of the counter to determine the radionuclide activity on the wipe, multiply by 10 (to allow for the fact that only 10% of the activity has been

Box 15.3 Surface contamination action levels and operational levels

Contamination levels should be kept as low as reasonably practicable and any contamination cleaned up as soon as it occurs. The setting of upper action levels above which the amount of contamination is considered to be unacceptable can provide a guide as to whether further action or reporting is required, while the setting of levels based on monitor sensitivity, here called 'operational levels', can be used to indicate when no further decontamination is necessary.

Upper action levels

The NRPB produced derived levels of surface contamination that could result in dose limits under ICRP 77 being exceeded [22]. These derived levels have not been revised to take account of changes in dose limits and ALIs, but nevertheless are considered to represent reasonable values for use in evaluation of contamination [23]. Using the NRPB model, upper action levels, which are based on a conservative approach, have been proposed for three types of surface and these are given in Table B15.1 [23]. The radionuclides are grouped into five classes according to their toxicity. The upper action levels represent an upper limit when further action is required and are in no way an ALARP solution. They may be translated into readings in counts per second for particular meters to facilitate their use. The practical application will depend on the sensitivity of the contamination monitor available for use and it may be necessary to make some adjustments to the upper action level set in order to ensure that its use is practicable.

Table B15.1 Levels of contamination that should not be exceeded (Bq cm^{-2}): 'upper limit' action levels

Surface	Class I	Class II	Class III	Class IV	Class V
Controlled areas	3	30	30	300	3000
Supervised or public areas, personal clothing, or hospital bedding/skin	3	3	30*	300	3000

*For α-emitters use one-tenth of this value for the skin.

Class I	Th natural, ^{231}Pa, ^{234}U, α-emitters with $Z > 92$
Class II	^{147}Sm, ^{210}Pb, ^{235}U, ^{238}U, U natural, U depleted
Class III	^{22}Na, ^{32}P, ^{33}P, ^{45}Ca, ^{86}Rb, ^{111}In, ^{131}I
Class IV	^{14}C, ^{35}S, ^{54}Mn, ^{57}Co, ^{65}Zn, ^{67}Ga, ^{75}Se, ^{99m}Tc, ^{109}Cd, ^{123}I, ^{125}I, ^{201}Tl
Class V	^{3}H, ^{51}Cr, ^{55}Fe, ^{63}Ni

Notes on the derivation of levels in Table B15.1 and their application

Comments on application of the data

The condition for public areas is similar to that for the skin, so these two are considered together. The contamination level may be averaged over an area of up to 1 m^2 for general surfaces, while an area of 1 cm^2 is recommended for skin contamination to link with the area over which the skin dose limit is applied. The action level set can be applied directly to skin monitoring with a small-area probe, but should be reduced by a factor of 10 when a 300 cm^2 probe is employed.

assumed to be removed) and divide by the area wiped to give the value of contamination in Bq cm^{-2}. A quench correction may be allowed for in liquid scintillation counting by using a glass fibre disc 'wipe' as these wet more effectively, thus allowing the liquid scintillator to absorb more fully onto the fibres of the disc and thereby giving a higher counting efficiency [4]. HHSC Handbook 14 [4] contains a wealth of information on responses of commercially available monitors to different laboratory-based radionuclides. Clearly these assumptions apply to removable contamination and are not appropriate for fixed contamination.

15.8.2 Monitoring records

Typical environmental monitoring records are shown in Figure 15.3. It may be effective for an organization to adopt a comprehensive, standardized system for keeping these records (and those of radioactive stock/waste) and then enforce its adoption throughout the many depart-

Box 15.3 (*continued*)

Operational levels

Methods of defining operational levels which provide an indication of the point at which the decontamination process may be halted are somewhat more arbitrary. Most tend to be linked to the sensitivity of the contamination monitor. This may involve the setting of a level based on a multiple of background or on a more sophisticated approach, which takes monitor sensitivity and radionuclide into account. The operational levels are attempts to define an ALARP approach to contamination monitoring and define a point at which it is reasonable to stop trying to remove further contamination. The simplistic approach in which a multiple of background is used as the operational level has its appeal but in practice may present problems. The levels are very low and, depending on the monitor, may be difficult to distinguish from background and result in reduced compliance with the contamination monitoring regime. The Association of University Radiation Protection Officers (AURPO) have produced guidance for levels based on monitor sensitivity [23]. A summary is presented in Table B15.2 along with corresponding contamination concentrations for some relevant radionuclides.

Table B15.2 Operational levels based on ALARP considerations

Monitor type	Action level (cps)	Effective contamination level (Bq cm^{-2})				
		^{14}C	^{35}S	^{32}P	^{125}I	^{51}Cr
Mini E[a]	40	60	60	21	–	
MiniEL/EP15[a]	100	71	71	19		
Mini 5.44A[b]	100	–	–	–	27	–
Mini 5.44B[b,c]	100	–			27	360

[a]All betas except ^{3}H.
[b] ^{125}I and electron capture radionuclides.
[c] ^{51}Cr (β-probe only).

Model used to derive levels in Table B15.1

Contaminated surfaces in controlled area

- External dose: the skin is in contact with the surface throughout the working year
- Inhalation: resuspension from a contaminated area of 10 m^2 at a rate of 5×10^{-5} Bq m^{-3} $(Bqm^{-2})^{-1}$

Contaminated surfaces in supervised or public areas

- External dose: the skin is in contact with the surface throughout the working year
- Ingestion of activity from 10 cm^2 of contaminated surface is ingested each day

Contaminated skin

- External dose: radionuclide remains on skin throughout the year
- Ingestion of activity from 10 cm^2 of skin each day

ments within the organization. This speeds up auditing by the RPA and by external regulatory bodies and ensures that an adequate quality of record is maintained.

15.9 Spills and decontamination

The first important point to make on the subject of handling spills and decontamination is that most, if not all, situations should have been thought about and planned for, with a contingency plan in place in the local rules. Contingency plans must have local input from the RPS as well as the RPA and must be approved by the RPA. Any contingency plans should be on display in the areas where the incidents are likely to occur. There should thus be available information on:

- immediate action to be taken
- who to contact (RPA, RPS, phone numbers, etc.)

Details:

Main User:____________________ Department:____________________

Floor:____________________ Lab / Room No:____________________

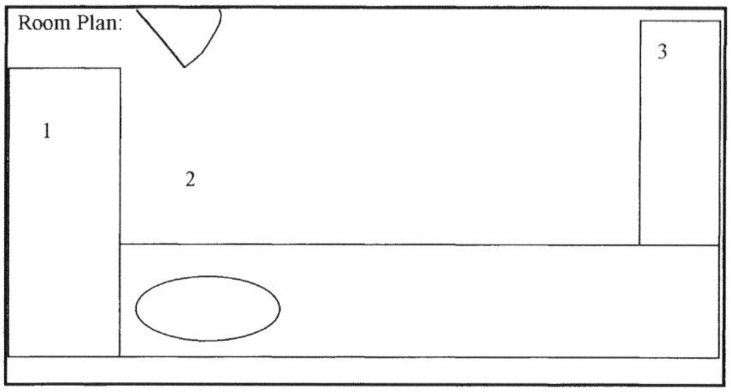

Location Index:

1: Benching
2:Floor near designated sink
3:Inside store
4:etc
5:
6:
7:
8:

Date	Init:	R/N:	Meter Model:	Bkd	Detected Count Rate (cps - Bkd)								Equivalent Max. Bq/cm^2	Result:
					1:	2:	3:	4:	5:	6:	7:	8:		

Figure 15.3 Surface contamination monitoring log.

- spill kit location.

The first question that needs to be asked is what radionuclide is involved and the second is how much can be spilt. In this section it will be assumed that α-emitters are not being dealt with.

15.9.1 Spills: general procedure

The contingency plan should cover issues such as:

- what to do with non-removable contamination—either cover to decay or remove surface. This depends on the quantity remaining, half-life, and type of emission.
- whether it is necessary to notify regulatory bodies.

Staff should have received training in dealing with spills before one occurs. Part of the local training should cover the location and use of the departmental spill kit. Table 15.6 gives a typical list of the contents of a spill kit.

Immediate action after a spill:

- warn others in the area that may be affected and summon assistance (preferably from the RPS)
- make safe any apparatus that may exacerbate the situation (e.g. pumps, disconnected tubing, etc.)
- turn off ventilation and close windows and doors if appropriate
- evacuate uncontaminated staff and restrict access to contaminated area (e.g. rope off area, erect warning signs—all this should be in spill kit)

After this:

- try and make a realistic assessment of the hazard
- those dealing with the incident need to use protective clothing (gloves, overshoes, labcoat, and masks, if appropriate)
- release potentially contaminated people only after checking for contamination
- if decontamination is not simple to effect, it may be appropriate to move individuals to a new area for more complex treatment (§15.10).

15.9.2 Dealing with the spill

Absorbent material such as tissue should be dropped on to the spill to absorb the bulk of the liquid. Remove these materials carefully so as not to drip liquid onto new areas and place in a heavy-duty plastic bag which has a radiation trefoil warning sign on it. Using further absorbent material wipe up the rest of the free liquid by wiping towards the centre of the spill. Monitor the

Table 15.6 Decontamination spill kit

Object	Comments
Protective clothing	
Overalls/labcoat	Overalls are more appropriate if the spill presents a very serious hazard to clean-up staff
Gloves	Different pairs may be indicated for different situations
Face masks	
Wellington-type boots	These may be heavy duty or lightweight
Disposable overshoes	These should not be absorbent the whole way through from outside to inside onto shoe/sock
Decontamination agents	
Soap	As a liquid to quickly make into solution and as a bar
Cetrimide solution	Concentration should be written on container
'Swarfega'	
Potassium permanganate	
Sodium bisulphite	
Saline, sterile water	Several sealed containers each of 500 ml
Calamine lotion	
Potassium iodate/iodide	Tablets or solution (monitor expiry date)
Other proprietary agents (Decon, Lipsol, Camtox, Countoff, RBSA 350)	
Miscellaneous equipment	
Large warning sign capable of standing up on ground	Trefoil plus worded warning—'Do Not Enter, Radioactive Contamination'
Contamination monitor	Keep one monitor with kit for speed of access in emergency (remember to keep within calibration)
Radiation hazard adhesive tape	
Coloured rope to control access	
Impermeable material to cover floor	To be used with adhesive tape to keep in place
Absorbent tissue, large/small rolls	
Polythene waste bags with radiation warning symbol	
Plastic bucket	Minimum size: 2 litres
Tweezers and tongs (various sizes)	
Notebook, pen	
Scissors	1 pair, medium size (e.g. blades about 125 mm long)
Soft brush	
Marker pen	

surface, with a colleague recording results and working out the contamination levels from the readings where necessary. It is most likely that the surface will need washing first with water and then with a decontaminating agent. A prewash with water means further radioactivity can be removed whereas a decontaminating agent will also remove activity and the protective layer of wax finish on the surface, making it more likely that activity will be chemically absorbed into the surface. This process may have to be repeated or different decontaminating agents tried as they may work in different ways.

A dry spill is dealt with in a similar way after adding a decontaminating agent to the surface so that the dry material may be mopped up with less hazard of ingestion through lungs and stomach.

15.9.3 Decontamination of clothing

Decontamination can only be effected by the removal of contaminated clothing. Protective clothing should always be worn and would in most cases be the only clothing affected. While removing contaminated clothing take care to ensure that the contamination has not spread to other parts of the body and other clothing. Assess the activity on the clothes and store them in a sealed bag. The decision as to whether to decay store or decontaminate has to be made. If decontamination is the required route (e.g. long half-life radionuclide) the clothing must not be washed with other clothes. If a non-dedicated washing machine is used (which is likely) then it must be checked to be free of contamination before being put back into communal use. Serious consideration should be

Table 15.7 Decontamination procedures for polythene, plastics, glassware, trays, sinks, metal tools

Object	Procedure
Paintwork, polished lino, epoxy resin floor coverings	Clean with detergent and water, in severe cases if long half-life contaminant, remove paint with paint stripper or consider physical removal of surface. If half-life short, covering with impermeably coated paper or strong polythene sheeting may be appropriate. For all removals of radioactive contamination consider disposal before creation of the waste
Glassware	Clean immediately with detergent. Ammonium citrate or chelating agents such as EDTA may be useful
Plastics	Dilute nitric acid may be useful since it usually does not attack plastics. Care if using ketonic solvents and certain chlorinated hydrocarbons that dissolve plastics. Note that no organic solvents have any effect on polythene
Metal tools, trays, workbenches, and sinks	Use a heavy-duty detergent followed if necessary by specific chelating agents. If lipids are involved 1,1,1-trichloroethane or EDTA mixed with swarfega may be used. An abrasive cleaner can be used as a last resort

given to careful handwashing (pre-soaking and draining several times) or to disposal as solid radioactive waste.

15.9.4 Decontamination of equipment

Where possible follow the procedure as for decontamination of a surface. Useful advice on the decontamination of polythene, plastics, glassware, trays, sinks, metal tools, etc., is summarized in Table 15.7.

15.10 Decontamination of personnel

This section describes procedures appropriate for dealing with varying degrees of personal contamination from hospital staff who have been splashed with radioactive liquid to a casualty admitted to an accident and emergency department following a major contamination incident. The decontamination process is split into three stages:

- decontamination of the body
- reduction in absorption of radionuclide
- speeding up of excretion from absorbed contamination.

15.10.1 Decontamination of body areas

Showering is rarely a warranted decontamination method as it is likely to spread contamination to other parts of the body or to the rest of the environment. Methods for dealing with contamination to different parts of the body are given below.

Skin

The affected area should be scrubbed gently employing a soft brush and warm water with mild soap. One should work towards the centre of the contamination so as to avoid making the area contaminated larger. The area should be dried using disposable tissues and then monitored to assess the efficacy of the procedure. This should be repeated until the area shows no significant fall in radiation level. Any wounds that are not contaminated must be covered to prevent rapid entry of contamination into the blood. Particular attention needs to be paid to creases of skin, fingernails, and interdigital spaces.

If the contamination does not reduce to an acceptably low level, the skin can be swabbed with a solution of 1% cetrimide and rinsed with water. Another further measure that may be adopted is the application of 4% potassium permanganate which, after drying, is then removed with a 5% sodium bisulphite solution. Finally one can try 'sweating' the contamination out by covering with a non-porous plaster and removing it a few hours later.

Ear

Trained medical staff should be asked to syringe out ears if the contamination has entered the ear. The water used should be at body temperature and care should be taken with the flushed water so that the patient or operator does not contaminate themselves.

Nasal system

The nose should be blown into a disposable tissue and the waste carefully collected in a cup. If this does not reduce the contamination down to an acceptably low level then nasal irrigation under medical supervision should be carried out. The head must be tilted forwards so that the bridge of the nasal septum is almost vertical. This is to encourage the flushings of contaminated liquid to flow out of the nostrils rather than into the nasopharynx or the nasal sinuses. Saline or sterile water should be used and the individual should be in the sitting position with a waterproof cover and absorbent material over their front and lap. The irrigation tube needs to be just inside the nostril and waste again needs to be collected and monitored. The nose should again be blown and the effectiveness of the procedure assessed via monitoring. The whole process should be repeated and a decision made according to whether either the level has been reduced as far as possible or the method is not proving at all beneficial in reducing contamination.

Hair

The hair should be shampooed carefully, first with soap, and then, if necessary, with cetrimide solution. Care must be taken not to allow the contamination to enter the nose, mouth, ears, or eyes. It may be necessary to trim off hair if the contamination cannot be reduced significantly.

Fingernails

The affected nail should be cut away as much as possible. The treatment of the nail should be as for skin but also calamine lotion may be applied, dried, and then carefully brushed off and monitored to check the effectiveness of the method.

Eyes

The eyes can be irrigated with normal saline or sterile water but care must be taken to ensure that the contaminated washings do not run into other orifices.

Mouth

First remove dentures (if appropriate). Warn the subject not to swallow and ask them to wash out their mouth, then brush the teeth away from the gums, and carefully spit out the water.

Wound decontamination

The surrounding skin should be cleaned carefully. The wound may be encouraged to bleed moderately (provided the blood loss is not life-threatening) as this encourages dispersal of the contamination. Bleeding can be increased by the use of a torniquet so that venous return is inhibited but arterial supply is not. Applying the torniquet too tightly will not achieve this objective and may also cut off the supply of blood to the limb. The wound can be irrigated with sterile water or saline but the washings must be collected carefully. The area should be dried by wiping away the liquid from the edges of the wound. Small skin tags can be cut away and, if large amounts of β-activity are present, the wound may need excision of tissue. This must be done by a medically qualified professional under the supervision of a competent radiation safety person (e. g. an RPA, a medical radiation physicist, or a nuclear medicine physician, as long as they feel competent to supervise the procedure).

15.10.2 Reduction in absorption

Material can be removed from the gut by

- using a stomach pump, i.e. physically pumping out the stomach contents thereby removing contamination
- administration of competitive ions so that the body takes in non-radioactive material as well (e.g. potassium iodate for radioiodine ingestion)
- administering an emetic which will cause the individual to be sick
- giving an enema thereby speeding up transit through the last stages of the gastrointestinal tract and preventing further absorption.

All the above procedures require the supervision of medically trained individuals.

Material can be removed from the lungs by carrying out pulmonary lavage. This is, however, a specialist procedure, only to be carried out by a specialist when the potential benefit outweighs the risk involved.

15.10.3 Speeding up excretion from absorption of contamination

The following actions, which are specific for particular radionuclides, can help in eliminating these materials:

- give potassium iodate/iodide for thyroid ingestion of radioiodine; there may be stable isotopes which can displace other radioactive ones
- increase liquid intake to speed up tritium excretion
- administer potassium ferric cyanoferrate (prussian blue) to reduce thallium or caesium from the gut
- administer chelating compounds such as EDTA and DTPA which scavenge radiometals from the body and excrete them through the kidneys and bladder.

In all these cases the toxicity of the administered materials must be weighed against the hazard from the radioactive material ingested.

Mountford [24] gives further details of the handling of decontamination.

15.11 Radioactive waste management

Waste disposal routes and the environmental aspects of radioactive waste disposal are dealt with in §9.3 and only the management aspects are covered in this section. An excellent reference to which the reader is referred for more detail is the HHSC Handbook No. 19 [25].

The national policy for the management of radioactive waste is based on the principal of 'sustainable development' from which the following principles are developed:

- decisions must be based on the best scientific information and the analysis of subsequent risks
- precautions must be taken where there may be potential serious risks
- environmental assessment must be made
- the *polluter pays* principle is used to bring home to users the consequences of their activities.

According to these principles radioactive waste should not be created unnecessarily, should be managed in a safe manner, and appropriate arrangements made for disposal. Before a procedure is implemented and waste is created, departments should have costed and analysed their disposal options and applied dose constraints to the disposal procedure. Procedures relevant to radioactive waste disposal should either be included, or referred to, in the local rules, e.g. in an appendix. Someone should have formal responsibility both at department level (e.g. the RPS) and at organizational level to manage the waste.

15.11.1 Management of radioactive waste

Prior to commencement of work, consideration should be given to minimization of both the volume and total activity of the radioactive waste generated.

- Use of alternative non-radioactive methods should be promoted where possible.
- Decay can be used to full effect by separation of radionuclides of significantly different half-lives. Longer half-life radionuclides will not be significantly reduced in activity by decay storage and if no shorter half-life materials are mixed in, they may be disposed of as soon as is practicable.
- Waste should be 'streamed' according to its activity level. Very low-level waste may go out with normal refuse to landfill provided that special conditions are met (Table 9.3); these include the conditions that it does not contain any material that is defined as clinical or special waste and that any labels bearing the warning that it is radioactive are removed. Higher activity waste may be incinerated in an authorized disposal facility.
- For radioactive waste that is also clinical waste, the biological hazards need to be taken into account as well as the radiological ones (see [26]).
- Long half-life or higher activity solid sources (particularly sealed sources) may go to an external organization for special disposal (this may require a special authorization from the regulator).
- Waste can be collected most readily in a thick polythene bag, which may be placed within a rigid outer container. Both of these should be labelled as radioactive and with the radiation trefoil sign.
- Care should be taken that waste which is non-active (e.g. packaging after checking for contamination) is clearly identified and not put into a bin with radioactive waste.
- The radioactive waste store should have adequate space, be secure, be easily decontaminated, and be adequately ventilated and shielded (Box 9.2).
- A system must be in place to record the amount of waste being stored. This can be done by means of a spreadsheet or database, including automatic correction for decay.
- Hard copy records of disposals should be available together with copies of consignment notes.

15.11.2 Transport of radioactive waste

Radioactive waste will need to be transported within the organization to a central store or collection point, which should be in a secure location. It will also need to be taken from the central store to the waste contractor's disposal facility. It is important that the waste is moved in a manner that minimizes the risk of spillage or contamination of adjacent areas. The method of 'double containment', usually within two strong bags, may be used. If a clear polythene bag with a radiation trefoil is used, a copy of the documentation can be placed inside the outer clear bag to facilitate auditing or bag identification at a later stage. It is advisable to place bags of waste in a rigid outer container so that any spillage is contained should a bag be torn. If the rigid container is lined with absorbent material this will help to prevent the spread of any contamination. Containers should have appropriate labels describing their contents as well as the radiation trefoil. The transport of waste off-site by a contractor does not remove the responsibility from the waste producer to ensure that legal criteria are met. Transport outside the user's premises is dealt with in §9.5. Generally radioactive waste from laboratories and hospitals will come within the category of excepted packages, which are exempt from certain regulatory requirements (§9.5.1).

15.12 Pregnancy and work with radionuclides

The dose to the fetus should be as low as reasonably practicable. The recommendation of ICRP 60 is that a fetus should receive no more radiation than a member of the public and so should not receive more than 1 mSv during the declared term of pregnancy. This gives a risk of 3.0×10^{-5} or about 1 in 33 000 of developing a fatal malignancy up until the age of 15 years, which compares with the natural risk of 1 in 1300 (§3.6.2). A fetal dose of 1 mSv can be interpreted as broadly equivalent to a dose at the surface of the abdomen of a pregnant woman of about 2 mSv for X-rays, but a lower level, possibly 1.3, for higher energy radiation from radionuclides such as ^{99m}Tc and ^{131}I (§16.7.3), and here advice from the RPA will be required. Most of the routine activities performed by technologists in nuclear medicine would not result in a dose of this magnitude. There are a few higher risk activities in which this dose may be approached or exceeded, such as where a technologist is dealing with potential or actual contamination (including volatility/aerosol droplets), is in the presence of a high radiation field, or may be close to patients for prolonged times. Hence, Harding and Mountford [27] advise that it is probably wise for staff known to be pregnant who are working in nuclear medicine to avoid the following tasks:

- dealing with radioactive spills
- using aerosols or unshielded krypton generators
- imaging very ill patients
- preparing radionuclide therapy doses.

Because of the potential for an incident to occur, it would seem prudent that a radiopharmacist working alone does not continue working with radioactivity while pregnant. The radiopharmacist may still be involved in supervising the work of a colleague, as being several metres away from the formulation process should reduce risks to an acceptable level. The anxiety that an expectant mother may have in this situation, even after being given reassurance, should be considered. It is often possible for the person to change duties with a colleague and work in a non-radiation area, where the source of the anxiety can be removed entirely.

In assessing potential fetal doses it may be helpful to consult the *Notes for guidance on the clinical administration of radiopharmaceuticals and the use of sealed radioactive sources* [28] where in parts A and B is given the dose to the uterus from the administration of commonly encountered forms of radiopharmaceuticals. Note that these doses do not include any contribution from cross-placental transfer of radiopharmaceuticals but they do give a rough guide to the relative seriousness of ingestion between the different radiopharmaceuticals.

15.13 References

1 International Commission on Radiological Protection (1994). Dose coefficients for intakes of radionuclides by workers. ICRP Publication 68. *Ann. ICRP*, **24** (4).

2 International Commission on Radiological Protection (1989). Radiological protection of the worker in medicine and dentistry. ICRP Publication 57. *Ann. ICRP*, **20** (3).

3 Goldstone, K. E., Jackson, P. C., Myers, M. J., and Simpson, A. E. (ed.) (1991). *Radiation protection in nuclear medicine and pathology*. IPSM Report No. 63. IPSM (now IPEM), York.

4 Connor, K. J. and McLintock, I. S. (1997). *Practical radiation protection. Radiation protection handbook for laboratory workers*, No. 14 (2nd edn), pp. 17–22, HHSC, Leeds.

5 International Commission on Radiological Protection (1977). The handling, storage, use and disposal of unsealed radionuclides in hospitals and medical research establishments. ICRP Publication 25. *Ann. ICRP*, **20** (1).

6 Harding, L. K., Hesselwood, S., Ghose, S. K., and Thompson, W. H. (1985). The value of syringe shields in a nuclear medicine department. *Nucl. Med. Commun.*, **6**, 449–54.

7 Batchelor, S., Penfold, A., Aric, I., and Huggins, R. (1991). Radiation dose to the hands in nuclear medicine. *Nucl. Med. Commun.*, **12**, 439–44.

8 Allen, S., Mackenzie, A., Stark, G., Inwards, G., Lazarus, C., and Batchelor, S. (1997). Comparison of radiation safety aspects between robotic and manual systems for the preparation of radiopharmaceuticals. *Nucl. Med. Commun.* (abstract), **18**, 295.

9 Marsden, P. K., Gee, A. D., Batchelor, S., and Maisey, M. N. (1994). A system for measuring and injecting PET radiopharmaceuticals. *Nucl. Med. Commun.* (abstract), **15**, 259.

10 Batchelor, S., Marsden, P. K., Saunders, J. E., and Gee, A. D. (1994). Staff and patient dosimetry issues in clinical positron emission tomography. Abstracts of the World Congress on Medical Physics and Biomedical Engineering. *Phys. Med. Biol.*, **39a** (Part 2) (abstract OS32-3.4), 820.

11 Jackson, S. and Dolphin, G. W. (1966). The estimation of internal radiation dose from metabolic and urinary excretion data for a number of important radionuclides. *Health Phys.*, **12**, 481–500.

12 Ballance, P. E., Day, L. R., and Morgan, J. (1992). *Phosphorous 32: practical radiation protection*. HHSC Handbook No. 9. HHSC, Leeds.

13 Curran, A. R. (1986). Calculation of the dose to the basal layer of the skin from beta/gamma contamination. *J. Soc. Radiol. Prot.*, **1**, 23–32.

14 Underwood, E. J. (1977). *Trace elements in human and animal metabolism* (4th edn). Academic Press, New York.

15 Prime, D. (1985). *Health physics aspects of the use of radioiodines*. Science Reviews Occupational Hygiene Monograph No. 13. HHSC, Leeds.

16 Bolton, A. E. (1985). *Radioiodination techniques: review 18*. Amersham International plc.

17 National Council on Radiation Protection and Measurement (1977). *Protection of the thyroid gland in the event of release of radionuclide*. Report No. 55. NCRP, Washington, DC.

18 Lassmann, M., Hanscheid, H., Alt, P., and Borner, W. (1994). Measurement of ^{131}I-activity to air emitted from a radioiodine therapy ward. In: *Strahlenshultz: Physik und Messtechnik* (ed. W. Koelzer and R. Maushart) pp. 719–22. TUV Rheinland, Koln.

19 Wellner, U., Eschner, W., Hilger, W., and Schicha, H. (1998). The exposure of relatives to patients of a nuclear medical ward after radioiodine therapy by inhalation of ^{131}I in their home. *Nuklearmedizin*, **37**, 113–19.

20 Williams, E. D., Laird, E. E., and Forster, E. (1987). Monitoring radiation dose to the hands. *Nucl. Med.* Commun., **8**, 499–503.

21 Batchelor, S., Baldock, C., and Weber, D. (1991). Radiation dose distribution to the hands of a radiopharmacist. *Pharm. J., Hosp. Pharm. Suppl.*, **247**, 38–9.

22 National Radiological Protection Board (1979). *Derived limits for surface contamination.* NRPB-DL2 and Supplement (1982). HMSO, London.

23 Association of University Radiation Protection Officers. *AURPO guidance on working with ionising radiations in research and teaching*. (In press).

24 Mountford, P. J. (1991). Techniques for radioactive decontamination in nuclear medicine, *Nucl. Med. Commun.*, **21**, 82–9.

25 McLintoch, I. S. (1996). *The management of radioactive waste in laboratories.* Handbook No. 19. HHSC, Leeds.

26 Health and Safety Commission; Health Services Advisory Committee (1992). *Safe disposal of clinical wastes.* HMSO, London.

27 Harding, L. K. and Mountford, P. J. (1993). Pregnant employees in a nuclear medicine department. [Editorial.] *Nucl. Med. Commun.*, **14**, 345–6.

28 National Radiation Protection Board (1998). *Notes for guidance on the clinical administration of radiopharmaceuticals and the use of sealed radioactive sources.* NRPB, Oxon.

Chapter 16
The nuclear medicine patient

P. J. Mountford

16.1 Introduction

There are two categories of radiation risk presented after a radiopharmaceutical has been administered to a patient. First, there is the risk to the patient due to the self-absorbed radiation. Second, the patient acts as a mobile source of radiation presenting a risk to other critical groups. This second risk can be subdivided into two types: contact with radioactive tissue from the patient, and exposure to radiation emitted from radioactivity retained by the patient. Critical groups inside a hospital comprise certain members of staff (particularly imaging technologists and nurses), other patients, and members of the public. After discharge from hospital, the critical groups are fellow travellers on the journey home, family members, and colleagues at work.

An important distinction between the risk to hospital staff and the risk to patients and to critical groups outside the hospital is that the exposure of staff can be quasi-continuous, particularly for those working in the nuclear medicine department. Therefore, the energy of the principal emissions will usually have a greater impact on the dose to nuclear medicine staff than the effective half-life, whereas for patients and critical groups outside the hospital, the reverse may be true.

Practical procedures to minimize any risk depend partly on the magnitude of the radiation dose. The first part of this chapter explains the methodology used for assessing the doses to patients and to critical groups and reviews its limitations. The remainder of the chapter follows the 'patient journey' through the nuclear medicine process, and describes the relevant dosimetry data available and the practical procedures to minimize the risks.

16.2 Internal dosimetry

The Medical Internal Radiation Dose Committee (MIRD) of the American Society of Nuclear Medicine has developed a method of estimating organ absorbed dose after radiopharmaceutical administration which is referred to as the MIRD schema [1]. Organ absorbed doses can then be used to derive the organ equivalent doses followed by the effective dose which allows an estimate of the associated risk (see Chapter 11) [2].

Effective doses for a wide range of radiopharmaceuticals are given in publications produced by the International Commission on Radiological Protection (ICRP) [3, 4] and the Administration of Radioactive Substances Advisory Committee (ARSAC) [5]. The ICRP compendia also list the organ absorbed doses and effective doses for these radiopharmaceuticals for the adult, and for children aged 15, 10, 5, and 1 year. If individual estimates of organ absorbed dose or effective dose are required, such as for novel radiopharmaceuticals or for unusual biokinetic data, then they can be calculated using the computer program MIRDOSE3 [6]. The software requires organ residence times to be entered, and it will provide tables of dose estimates for one or more anthropomorphic mathematical phantoms representing standard man, children at different ages, and the pregnant female at different stages of gestation, as well as tables of S-values (§16.2.1).

A worked example showing the calculation of organ absorbed doses and effective dose for a radiopharmaceutical is given in Box 16.1, based on the MIRD schema and the other methods described in the ICRP compendia [3, 4].

16.2.1 Calculation of organ absorbed dose

In the MIRD schema [1, 6–9], the body is considered to consist of source organs which accumulate radioactivity, and target organs which are irradiated by activity in the source organs. The mean absorbed dose to a target organ r_k from its exposure to a source organ r_h is given by:

$$\bar{D}\,(r_k \leftarrow r_h) = \tilde{A}_h S(r_k \leftarrow r_h) \qquad (16.1)$$

where $\tilde{A}_h$ is the source organ cumulated activity and represents the total number of radioactive disintegrations which have occurred in the source organ. It is measured in terms of the activity time product (i.e. MBq s). The term $S(r_k \rightarrow r_h)$ is usually referred to as the S-value [6, 9], and is the mean dose in the target organ per unit cumulated activity in the source organ, and can include the situation of a target organ and a source organ being the same.

When the cumulated activity in a source organ is normalized to the activity administered A_o, it is described as the residence time τ_h:

$$\tau_h = \tilde{A}_h/A_o. \quad (16.2)$$

Therefore, the absorbed dose per unit administered activity, from its exposure to a particular source organ, is given simply by the product of the source organ residence time and the appropriate S-value (see Box 16.1). The total mean absorbed dose to the target organ from its exposure to all source organs, per unit administered activity, is given by:

$$\bar{D}(r_k)/A_o = \sum_h \tau_h S(r_k \leftarrow r_h). \quad (16.3)$$

If the residence time is not available, then it can be calculated from equation (16.2) by equating the cumulated

Box 16.1 *An example of the calculation of organ absorbed doses and the effective dose*

A male adult has a fractional uptake of 65% in the liver, 15% in the spleen, and 20% in the red marrow after administration of 400 MBq of a ^{99m}Tc-labelled small colloid for bone marrow imaging. Following administration, the uptake is immediate, and there is no biological elimination. The activity in all other organs and tissues is assumed to be negligible.

(i) *Calculate the residence time for each source organ*
Because there is no biological elimination, the effective half-life of the decay in each source organ activity = the physical half-life of ^{99m}Tc = 6.02 h = 21 672 s.

Therefore, the residence time t_h in each source organ is given by the simplified case described by equation (16.6):

$t_{liver} = 0.65 \times 21\,672/\ln\{2\} = 2.03 \times 10^4$ s
$t_{spleen} = 0.15 \times 21\,672/\ln\{2\} = 4.69 \times 10^3$ s
$t_{red\ marrow} = 0.20 \times 21\,672/\ln\{2\} = 6.25 \times 10^3$ s

(ii) *Calculate the absorbed dose in each target per unit administered activity*
For a particular target organ T, multiply a source organ residence time by the appropriate S-value (tabulated in columns 2–4 below) to give the absorbed dose D_T (per unit administered activity) from its exposure to that source organ (equation 16.3). The tabulated S-values are those listed by the computer program MIRDOSE3 [6] for the reference adult.

The total absorbed dose (per unit administered activity) to the target organ is given by adding the contribution from each of the three source organs (equation 16.3), and is tabulated in column 5 below. For instance:

$D_{adrenals} = [(2.03 \times 10^4) \times (4.34 \times 10^{-7})] + [(4.69 \times 10^3) \times (4.56 \times 10^{-7})] + [(6.25 \times 10^3) \times (2.41 \times 10^{-7})]$
$= 1.3 \times 10^{-2}$ mGy MBq^{-1}

(iii) *Calculate the equivalent dose to each target organ per unit administered activity*
Multiply the total absorbed dose (per unit administered activity) to each target organ by the radiation weighting factor w_R (= 1.0 for the radiations emitted by ^{99m}Tc) to give the corresponding equivalent dose H_T (per unit administered activity). As the values of the latter doses are numerically equal to the former, they have been omitted from the table below.

(iv) *Calculate the effective dose*
Multiply the values in the fourth column by their respective tissue weighting factor w_T [2] tabulated in column 6 below, to give $H_T w_T$ in column 7. For instance:

$H_{liver} w_{liver} = 6.6 \times 10^{-2} \times 0.05 = 3.3 \times 10^{-3}$ Sv MBq^{-1}

The effective dose per unit administered activity is given by the summation of the $H_T w_T$ values listed for 13 target organs in column 7, which is then added to the value of $H^* w^*$, where H^* is the mass weighted average equivalent dose to the other eight 'remainder' organs (marked with an asterisk in column 7)—see the last row to the table and its footnotes:

Effective dose per unit administered activity $= \Sigma H_T w_T + H^* w^* = (10.1 \times 10^{-3}) + (2.87 \times 10^{-3} \times 0.025)$
$= 1.02 \times 10^{-2}$ mSv MBq^{-1}

Effective dose = 1.02 × 10^{-2} × 400 = 4.1 mSv

activity to the area under the source organ time–activity curve. This area can be derived from sequential gamma camera images of the organ activity taken over a period of time which is dependent on the rate of clearance of the radioactivity. A common method is to derive the geometric mean of the background subtracted region-of-interest count-rates taken from anterior and posterior gamma-camera images of the organ, and convert to absolute activity by correcting for attenuation with a transmission image and an appropriate system sensitivity factor. SPECT images can also be used to generate a three-dimensional count-rate distribution, and the organ activity derived by correcting for attenuation, scatter, and collimator response [8]. Other more indirect methods include whole-body, blood, and urine clearance measurements.

Alternatively, if the source organ time–activity curve can be described by a mathematical function $A_h(t)$, then the cumulated activity is given by:

$$\tilde{A}_{\rm h} = \int_0^\infty A_{\rm h}(t). \tag{16.4}$$

In the simple case of a source organ activity which decreases monoexponentially with a decay constant λ after a rate of uptake which can be regarded as instantaneous, the cumulated activity is given by:

Box 16.1 *(continued)*

Target organ	S-value ($\times 10^{-8}$ mGy MBq^{-1} s^{-1}) of source organ					
	Liver	Spleen	Red marrow	D_T ($\times 10^{-3}$ mGy MBq^{-1})	w_T[a]	H_Tw_T ($\times 10^{-3}$ mSv MBq^{-1})
Adrenals	43.4	45.6	24.1	13	*	
Bladder	1.16	0.802	9.16	0.85	0.05	0.043
Bone surfaces	12.3	12.6	107	9.8	0.01	0.098
Brain	0.0081	0.0052	8.05	5.2	*	
Breasts	6.80	4.36	5.11	1.9	0.05	0.095
Gall bladder	86.7	13.5	11.4	19		
Stomach	14.8	77.3	8.21	7.1	0.12	0.85
Small intestine	11.6	10.1	18.5	4.0	*	
Colon[b]				3.8	0.12	0.46
Upper large intestine	18.8	10.6	15.5	5.3		
Lower large intestine	1.44	4.64	19.8	1.7		
Heart	23.2	16.7	10.9	6.2		
Kidneys	29.3	66.1	16.9	10	*	
Liver	323	7.2	8.93	66	0.05	3.3
Lungs	20.8	16.4	10.9	5.7	0.12	0.68
Muscle	7.49	10.3	9.04	2.6	*	
Oesophagus[b]				1.9	0.05	0.095
Ovaries	3.80	3.84	21.2	2.3		
Pancreas	38.5	128	14.7	15	*	
Red marrow	8.29	8.41	174	13	0.12	1.6
Skin	3.61	3.49	4.19	1.2	0.01	0.012
Spleen	7.20	2330	9.17	110	0.025	2.8
Testes	0.157	0.217	3.08	0.23	0.20	0.046
Thymus	5.92	3.88	8.42	1.9	*	
Thyroid	0.862	0.781	7.52	0.68	0.05	0.034
Uterus	3.28	2.56	15.4	1.7	*	
$H^* = \Sigma D^* w_R m^*/\Sigma m^* = 2.87 \times 10^{-3}$ mGy MBq^{-1}				$\Sigma H_T w_T = 10.1 \times 10^{-3}$ mSv MBq^{-1}		

[a]ICRP recommends an individual tissue weighting factor w_T to 12 organs, and a weighting factor of 0.05 to some 'remainder' organs [2]. The spleen is one of these 'remainder' organs and in this example, it has an equivalent dose greater than the highest dose for any of the 12 organs with an individual weighting factor. In these circumstances, ICRP recommends that it is assigned a weighting factor of 0.025, and that for the eight other 'remainder' organs (marked with an asterisk in column 7), a weighting factor w^* of 0.025 is applied to the mass weighted average equivalent dose H^*. The masses m^* of these eight 'remainder' organs are given in the footnote to the table in Box 11.1 [28].

[b]Following the method used in ICRP Publication 80 [4]:

(i) The tissue weighting factor for the colon is applied to the mass average of the equivalent dose to the walls of the upper and lower large intestine (ULI, LLI), and this mass average dose is given by $D_{\rm colon} = 0.57D_{\rm ULI} + 0.43D_{\rm LLI}$.

(ii) S-values for the oesophagus are not listed by MIRDOSE3, and the dose to the thymus is used as a surrogate for the dose to the oesophagus.

$$\tilde{A}_h = \int_0^\infty A_s\, e^{-\lambda t}\, dt = F_s A_0 t_{1/2}/\ln 2 \qquad (16.5)$$

where A_s is the initial source organ activity, F_s is the fraction of the administered activity which would arrive in the source organ over all time if there was no radioactive decay, and $t_{1/2}$ is the effective half-life [3]. Hence by substituting in equation (16.2), the residence time is given by:

$$\tau_h = F_s t_{1/2}/\ln 2. \qquad (16.6)$$

The term $S(r_k \rightarrow r_h)$ is given by the equation:

$$S(r_k \leftarrow r_h) = \textstyle\sum_i \Delta_i \phi_i(r_k \leftarrow r_h)/m_k \qquad (16.7)$$

where Δ_i is the mean energy emitted per nuclear decay for emission type i (the equilibrium absorbed dose constant), $\phi_i(r_k \rightarrow r_h)$ is the fraction of energy emitted in the source organ which is absorbed in the target organ (the absorbed fraction), and m_k is the mass of the target organ [10]. For non-penetrating radiation such as β-particles, the absorbed fraction has a value of one where the source organ is the target organ, and zero where the two organs differ.

16.2.2 Limitations

The accuracy of absorbed dose estimates will depend on uncertainties in the cumulated activities and S-values. Cumulated activities may be affected by factors such as disease, age, sex, diet, and drugs. There are very few data to describe these effects, although the ICRP dosimetry compendia does include some estimates based on biokinetic data for different imaging techniques (e.g. cardiac rest and exercise) and for abnormal physiology [3, 4]. However, not all disease states are represented, and in some cases, values of organ absorbed dose are even based on animal data. The MIRDOSE3 software includes S-values for the shape, size, and separation of organs in different anthropomorphic mathematical phantoms [6]. However, these values will vary with body stature and weight, and with disease. Uncertainties in the radioactivity decay parameters and in the energy absorption are insignificant compared to the uncertainties in the biokinetic data and in the S-values, particularly organ mass. Estimates of organ absorbed doses will agree with actual patient doses within a factor of three [11]. This factor will reduce for short-lived radionuclides, and for estimates of effective dose because it is less sensitive to variations in the radiopharmaceutical distribution.

Although the methodology exemplified in Box 16.1 is appropriate for routine dosimetric estimations, it should be noted that if a radionuclide emits low-energy Auger and Coster–Kronig electrons (e.g. ^{99m}Tc) whose ranges vary from subcellular to multicellular dimensions, then the assumption in the MIRD schema of a uniform source is not strictly correct. Any non-uniformity in activity distribution can lead to a large variation in the dose to individual cells, and even in the dose to the cell nucleus. The radiobiological effect of these low-energy electrons is enhanced if the radionuclide is near or bound to DNA, or even just contained within the cell nucleus. Two developments have addressed these issues: S-values for source–target combinations at the sub-organ, cellular, and subcellular level [11], and the application of microautoradiography to identify the cellular and subcellular distributions of radiopharmaceuticals [12].

16.3 External dosimetry

There are two methods for determining the dose to an individual in a critical group: first by an integrating dosimeter, and second, from measurements of the time-averaged dose rate at different distances from the patient multiplied by the time spent by the individual at each distance, and then summing the separate contributions at each distance [13].

16.3.1 Integral dose method

Wearing a small radiation detector which will record the total dose received during the period of exposure has the advantage of allowing for any decrease in dose rate with time. However, instructions have to be issued to the individual in the critical group, such as the length of time and where on the body the detector is to be worn, and it may be necessary for the individual to record data such as times and instrument readings. Therefore, this method has the practical disadvantage of relying on the individual complying with instructions for an extended period of time. It also assumes that the measured dose represents the actual dose received by the individual, which may not be the case if he or she has not complied with the instructions. A further significant disadvantage is that the recorded dose is specific to the conditions under which it was measured, and it may be impossible to infer the dose which would have resulted from a different set of circumstances.

Direct measurements of the integral dose received by an individual from a single procedure have been made possible by the development of the electronic personal dosimeter (§8.3.5). Characteristics such as its threshold dose, energy and angular response, and battery life may have an important bearing when selecting the most appropriate model. If the aim is to record the integral dose to an individual from a series of patients, then it may be acceptable to use a less sensitive detector such as a thermoluminescence dosimeter (TLD) (§8.3.3) or a film badge.

16.3.2 Dose-rate method

The total dose D to the individual is given by adding the separate doses received at n positions, each at a different

Table 16.1 Maximum dose rates per unit activity administered for nuclear medicine procedures, recorded at different distances from the anterior mid-trunk of adult patients at the time of departure from the nuclear medicine department [13–16]

Procedure	Radionuclide	Maximum dose rate per unit activity (μSv h^{-1} MBq^{-1})		
		0.1 m	0.5 m	1.0 m
Diagnosis				
Fluorodeoxyglucose	^{18}F	0.5	0.3	0.1
Gallium	^{67}Ga	0.2	0.03	0.01
Static renal	^{99m}Tc	0.1	0.02	0.01
Dynamic renal	^{99m}Tc	0.3	0.08	0.02
Bone	^{99m}Tc	0.2	0.06	0.01
Lung	^{99m}Tc	0.2	0.04	0.02
Thyroid	^{99m}Tc	0.3	0.06	0.02
Liver	^{99m}Tc	0.3	0.07	0.02
Marrow	^{99m}Tc	0.4	0.07	0.02
Brain	^{99m}Tc	0.2	0.06	0.01
Bile reflux	^{99m}Tc	0.2	0.02	0.01
MUGA	^{99m}Tc	0.4	0.06	0.02
Cardiac (1-day)	^{99m}Tc	0.5	0.05	0.02
Cardiac (2-day)	^{99m}Tc	0.3	0.05	0.02
Lymphoscintigraphy	^{99m}Tc	0.09	0.2	0.01
Thyroid	^{123}I	0.6	0.1	0.03
Leucocyte	^{111}In	1.6	0.2	0.06
Somatostatin receptor	^{111}In	0.7	0.2	0.06
Cardiac	^{201}Tl	0.2	0.07	0.02
Treatment[a]				
Thyrotoxicosis	^{131}I	1.5	0.2	0.06
Thyroid cancer ablation	^{131}I	1.42	0.15	0.07
Thyroid cancer follow-up	^{131}I	1.44	0.25	0.07

[a]Ninety-fifth percentile dose rate values.

distance from the patient:

$$D = {}_{i=1}\sum_{i=1,n} d_i t_i \tag{16.8}$$

where d_i is the average dose rate over the exposure time t_i spent at each ith position. Published values of the maximum dose rate (per unit activity administered) measured at the time of departure from a nuclear medicine department at different distances from the anterior mid-trunk of adult patients who have undergone diagnostic procedures are listed in Table 16.1 [13–16], and for paediatric patients in Table 16.2 [14]. Published values of the dose rate per unit activity (95% upper confidence limit of the mean) of sodium ^{131}I-iodide administered for the treatment of thyrotoxicosis are also listed in Table 16.1 together with ninety-fifth percentile values found in patients receiving ^{131}I for ablation of thyroid cancer after surgery, or for follow-up treatment of thyroid cancer (i.e. second or more administration to treat residual, recurrent, or metastatic disease). The equivalent values at the same distances from other sides of the patient may differ depending on the radiopharmaceutical distribution and the patient's size.

The dose-rate method has several advantages: it requires only the patient's cooperation, the dose rates can be used to assess any type of critical group exposure, and it is a simple procedure to infer the dose for any behaviour pattern. Special circumstances can be modelled using computer programs or programs incorporating spreadsheets, which are available for general use [17, 18]. They allow for the effect of variations in parameters to be assessed, such as contact times and distances, the dose rate at the time of departure, and dose-rate decay.

This method also has a number of potential disadvantages: it assumes that the total dose to the critical

Table 16.2 Maximum departure dose rates per unit activity administered for common ^{99m}Tc nuclear medicine procedures, recorded at three distances from the anterior mid-trunk of paediatric patients at the time of departure from the nuclear medicine department [14]

Procedure	Maximum dose rate per unit activity ($\mu Sv\ h^{-1}\ MBq^{-1}$)		
	0.1 m	0.5 m	1.0 m
Static renal	0.3	0.2	0.1
Dynamic renal			
(i) pre-micturition	0.5	0.2	0.09
(ii) post-micturition	0.2	0.08	0.03
Bone	0.3	0.1	0.02
Lung	0.2	0.05	0.02
Thyroid	0.1	0.05	0.02
Meckel's	0.4	0.05	0.02
Biliary	0.3	0.07	0.06
Gastric	0.02	0.04	0.03
Lymphatic	0.03	0.03	0.03
Erythrocytes	0.1	0.02	0.01

group can be based on a constant period or a repetitive sequence of exposures at certain distances from the patient. Its accuracy depends on the validity of the times and distances used to describe the pattern of behaviour, of the half-life used to describe the rate of decrease of dose rate with time, and of any dose rates which have to be deduced from data available at other distances.

The decrease of dose rate with time will depend on the radiopharmaceutical and on the patient's pathology. For instance, the dose rate decreases biexponentially with time at distances of 0.1, 0.5, and 1.0 m from patients receiving ^{131}I for ablation of thyroid cancer after surgery (typically 80%, 0.5 days; 20%, 3.6 days) [14]. However, a monoexponential decrease has been found at each distance from patients receiving follow-up ^{131}I treatment of thyroid cancer when there is very little residual thyroid tissue. If the relevant data are not available, the decline in dose rate can be estimated from the rate of clearance of the whole-body radioactivity, and for short-lived radionuclides, it may be acceptable to use the physical half-life.

The variation of dose rate with distance from a patient will depend on the size of the patient, and on the anatomical distribution of the radioactivity (and hence on the type of radiopharmaceutical administered and possibly on the pathology). As the cross-sectional area of the radioactivity increases, the dose rate decreases with distance at a slower rate. TLD measurements and Monte Carlo calculations have shown that the inverse square law can be applied beyond a certain distance which depends on the area of the source (e.g. 0.5 m for $0.09\ m^2$; 1.5 m for $0.14\ m^2$) [14].

16.4 Patient safety

16.4.1 Justification and optimisation

Every nuclear medicine examination must be justified by a qualified practitioner and sufficient information must be provided by the referring clinician to enable this decision to be taken. This is discussed in more detail in §11.4. The methodology used for the examination must be optimised to ensure a satisfactory outcome is obtained with the dose to the patient and the risk of any error being kept to the minimum. The main components of the optimisation process are dealt with in §11.5, but aspects relating specifically to nuclear medicine are discussed in this section.

As part of the optimisation process, it is necessary to consider whether it is clinically acceptable to use an alternative radiopharmaceutical which results in a reduced dose (Table 16.3), and whether the administered activity is as low as reasonably practicable. This will depend on the type of detection system available (e.g. single- or multi-headed gamma-camera) and the type of data acquisition required, such as a dynamic study (i.e. the rate of image acquisition), SPECT images, delayed static images, etc. Diagnostic reference levels (in units of administered activity) (§11.5.2) have been recommended by ARSAC for all routine procedures [5]. Values of the effective dose to adult patients corresponding to these levels are given in Table 16.3 for common procedures [3–5]. However, clinical conditions may justify an increase in this activity on an individual basis, such as for a patient who is exceptionally obese, or is in extreme pain and cannot keep still for the usual imaging time.

Table 16.3 Effective doses to adult patients and uterine absorbed doses corresponding to the diagnostic reference levels of administered activity recommended by ARSAC [3–5]

Radiopharmaceutical	Diagnostic reference level (MBq)	Effective dose (mSv)	Uterine absorbed dose (mGy)
^{18}F-fluorodeoxyglucose	400	8	8
^{67}Ga-citrate	150	15	9
^{75}Se-selenonorcholesterol	8	12	14
^{99m}Tc-diphosphonates	600	3	3
^{99m}Tc-DMSA	80	0.7	0.4
^{99m}Tc-DTPA	300	2	2
^{99m}Tc-DTPA (aerosol)	80	0.5	0.5
^{99m}Tc-erythrocytes	800	6	3
^{99m}Tc-IDA derivatives	150	3	2
^{99m}Tc-HIG	200	1	0.9
^{99m}Tc-HMPAO	500	5	3
^{99m}Tc-leucocytes	200	2	0.7
^{99m}Tc-MAA	100	1	0.2
^{99m}Tc-MAG3	100	0.7	1
^{99m}Tc-MIBI (resting)	400	4	3
^{99m}Tc-MIBI (exercise)	400	3	3
^{99m}Tc-pertechnetate	80	1	0.6
^{99m}Tc-sulesomab	750	6	4
^{99m}Tc-tetrofosmin (resting)	400	3	3
^{99m}Tc-tetrofosmin (exercise)	400	3	3
^{111}In-leucocytes	20	7	2
^{123}I-iodide (35% thyroid uptake)	20	4	0.3
^{123}I-MIBG	400	5	4
^{131}I-iodide (0% thyroid uptake)	400	24	22
^{201}Tl-chloride	80	18	4

Any potential change in effective dose to a patient must always be balanced against any corresponding change in benefit (e.g. patient discomfort, accuracy of the investigation, etc.). In addition, doses to other organs should be minimized by administration of thyroid-blocking agents where appropriate when using radio-iodide-labelled compounds, and encouraging the patient to drink plenty of fluids and to empty their bladder frequently after the procedure is completed in order to hasten excretion of the radioactivity.

16.4.2 Patient exposure incidents

Operational procedures must be specifically designed to avoid incidents arising from incorrect administration of a radiopharmaceutical. The most likely patient-related incidents are misadministrations and maladministrations. The management of such incidents may well involve senior hospital managers as well as nuclear medicine staff (§11.5.5 and §10.5.1).

A misadministration is when all or part of a radiopharmaceutical injection has been extravasated. There have been a few reports of deterministic effects such as pruritus, erythema, and ulceration. The dose will be greater for radiopharmaceuticals which linger at the site of extravasation, due to a long physical half-life or slow biological clearance, and which emit short-range radiations (e.g. β-particles or Auger electrons). Detailed practical advice has been published for avoiding and dealing with misadministrations of diagnostic and therapeutic radiopharmaceuticals [19].

A maladministration is when the incorrect activity or the wrong radiopharmaceutical has been administered to the patient [20]. When this occurs the procedure should be halted immediately and an estimate made of the dose to the patient. This type of incident can cause alarm, and may attract criticism as well as adverse publicity and should be dealt with as described in §11.5.5. Maladministrations are most likely to be caused by dispensing or patient identification errors, and it is vitally important that as much as possible should be learnt from the incident and corrective action taken. Checks should be incorporated into the procedures for vetting request forms, dispensing radiopharmaceuticals, identifying patients, and administering radiopharmaceuticals in order to minimize the possibility of maladministration. The exact form of these checks will depend on the procedures and resources available, but they must be carried out independently by a second identified member of staff.

16.4.3 Avoidance of conception

In certain circumstances there may be a need to avoid conception for a period after administration of a radiopharmaceutical. This is determined by the potential risk resulting from the irradiation of the parent's (male or female) germ cells, from the appearance of long half-life radionuclides in ejaculate or sperm of the father, and from irradiation of the embryo by a long half-life radionuclide retained by the mother. The possible genetic effects from gonadal irradiation during diagnostic or therapeutic procedures can be considered against the results of long-term follow-up studies of children, adolescents, and adults treated with multiple doses of ^{131}I for hyperthyroidism or cancer. No significant differences have been found in fertility rate, complications in subsequent pregnancies, prematurity, and abnormalities in their progeny including stillbirth, birth weight, congenital malformation, and death during the first year of life [21].

ARSAC recommends that male patients undergoing routine diagnostic procedures do not need to be given any advice about avoiding conception [5]. For female patients, no restriction is recommended for a diagnostic procedure using a radionuclide with a physical half-life of less than 7 days. Periods of time have been recommended for which a female patient should avoid conception following administration of a long-lived diagnostic or therapeutic radionuclide in order that the dose to the fetus does not exceed 1 mGy (Table 16.4). It is recommended that male patients should avoid fathering a child for 4 months after treatment with ^{131}I-iodide, ^{32}P-phosphate, or ^{89}Sr-chloride, as this period is greater than the life of a sperm cell. For a male or female patient being treated for thyroid cancer with ^{131}I-iodide, it may be advisable to recommend that conception should be avoided until there is no intention of administering any follow-up ^{131}I treatment.

16.5 Pregnant and breastfeeding patients

16.5.1 Patients who may be pregnant

The administration of a radiopharmaceutical to a pregnant woman will result in exposure of the fetus to radiation emitted from adjacent maternal organs and from any radioactivity transferred across the placenta.

Table 16.4 Periods of time recommended by ARSAC for female patients to avoid conception following a diagnostic or therapeutic administration of a radiopharmaceutical [5]

Radiopharmaceutical	Activity (MBq)[a]	Period (months)
Diagnosis		
Any procedure using a radionuclide with a physical $T_{1/2}$ < 7 days	Up to the diagnostic reference level	0
^{59}Fe	4	3
^{75}Se-selenonorcholesterol	8	12
^{131}I-iodide	30–400	4
^{131}I-MIBG	20	2
Treatment		
^{131}I-iodide	800	4
^{131}I-iodide	6000	4
^{131}I-MIBG	7500	3
^{32}P-phosphate	200	3
^{89}Sr-chloride	150	24
^{90}Y-colloid	400	0
^{90}Y-colloid	4000	1
^{169}Er-colloid	400	0

[a]For all activities up to the value tabulated.

The types of procedure which should be adopted for female patients to avoid the potential hazard of administering a radiopharmaceutical without realizing that the patient is pregnant are outlined in Box 11.4. Only ^{67}Ga-citrate, ^{75}Se-selenonorcholesterol, and ^{131}I-iodide scans may produce a dose to the embryo of greater than 10 mGy (see Table 16.3) and so may require restriction of exposure to the first 10 days of the menstrual cycle [22]. However, any procedure resulting in an absorbed dose to the fetus of more than 1.0 mGy requires particular justification [5]. Risks of inducing radiation effects in a fetus are set out in Box 11.2 and advice which might be given to a pregnant patient is discussed in §11.6.2, §11.6.3, and Box 11.5. However, before advice can be given, an estimate must be made of the fetal dose.

Procedures involving the administration of ^{131}I for therapy or imaging are of particular concern because of uptake by the fetal thyroid. There are some empirical data to describe the risk following inadvertent administration of ^{131}I to pregnant patients for the treatment of hyperthyroidism [21]. No increased risk of spontaneous abortion or fetal abnormalities has been observed in children born to mothers treated during the first trimester of pregnancy. For administration during the later stages

Box 16.2 An example of the derivation of a period to interrupt breastfeeding.

A mother breastfeeding a 4 kg infant was administered 400 MBq of ^{123}I-MIBG at 11.00 a.m. She was advised not to feed her infant for a period of time which was to be decided the following morning on the basis of milk sample measurements, and not to cuddle her infant until 9.00 a.m. the next morning. She was asked to express milk at her usual feeding times, and to record the time of expression. By 9.00 a.m. the following morning, she had expressed five milk samples, with the last sample expressed at 8.00 a.m., and the dose rate measured at 0.1 m from her anterior chest surface was 30 μSv h^{-1}.

When can she resume breastfeeding to ensure the total dose to the infant from ingested activity and from cuddling does not exceed 1 mSv?

The activity concentration had reached a peak value by the second sample. A monoexponential curve fitted to the decrease in activity concentration with time after radiopharmaceutical administration for the last four samples gave an effective half-life of 7.5 h. The measured activity concentration in the last sample was 1.0 kBq ml^{-1}.

(i) *Calculate the dose due to ingested activity if feeding had been resumed at the time of the last sample*
Any appropriate value of volume per feed and time between feeds can be used. For this example, it is assumed that the infant ingests 850 ml of milk per day [28], and there is an average time of 4 h between feeds, giving a volume per feed of 142 ml. Therefore combining equations (16.9) and (16.10) gives:

$$\text{Ingested activity} = 1.0 \times 10^{-3} \times 142 \times [1 - \exp\{-(\ln\{2\}/7.5) \times 4\}]^{-1} = 0.46 \text{ MBq}$$

ICRP 61 gives a value of 0.22 mSv MBq^{-1} to an adult ingesting ionic ^{123}I [27].

The dose to the infant if feeding had been resumed at 8.00 a.m. (i.e. 21 h after radiopharmaceutical administration) is given by equation (16.11):

$$\text{Dose} = 0.46 \times 0.22 \times (70/4) = 1.8 \text{ mSv}$$

(ii) *Calculate the close contact dose from resuming cuddling at 9.00 a.m.*
The dose from resuming close contact as soon as she left the department after the scan (see §16.9), using an effective exposure time for ^{123}I-MIBG of 4.4 h (Table 16.8), is given by:

$$\begin{aligned}\text{Close contact dose} &= \text{dose rate at 0.1 m} \times \text{effective exposure time} \\ &= 30 \times 10^{-3} \times 4.4 = 0.13 \text{ mSv}\end{aligned}$$

(iii) *Calculate the additional period of time before breastfeeding can be resumed*
To ensure the total dose to the infant does not exceed 1 mSv, the dose from breastfeeding needs to be limited to 1–0.13 = 0.87 mSv.

Therefore, the total period after radiopharmaceutical administration to interrupt breastfeeding is given by equation (16.12):

$$\begin{aligned}\text{Period} &= 7.5 \times (\ln\{1.8/0.87\}/\ln\{2\}) + 21 \\ &= 29 \text{ h after radiopharmaceutical administration} \\ &= 8 \text{ h after the last milk sample was expressed at 8.00 a.m.}\end{aligned}$$

Therefore, to restrict the infant's total dose to 1 mSv, breastfeeding can be resumed at 4.00 p.m. on the day after administration if close contact had been resumed earlier that morning at 9.00 a.m.

Table 16.5 Recommendations for interrupting breastfeeding after administration of radiopharmaceuticals in routine use [14, 21, 26]

Category	Recommendation	Radiopharmaceutical
I	Interruption not essential (up to the activity given; if an activity limit is omitted, it is much greater than the ARSAC diagnostic reference level)	^{51}Cr-EDTA, ^{99m}Tc-DISIDA, ^{99m}Tc-DMSA, ^{99m}Tc-DTPA, ^{99m}Tc-diphosphonates, ^{99m}Tc-glucoheptonate, ^{99m}Tc-gluconate, ^{99m}Tc-HMPAO, ^{99m}Tc-MAG3 (100 MBq), ^{99m}Tc-MIBI, ^{99m}Tc-sulphur colloid, ^{111}In-leucocytes (10 MBq),[a] ^{201}Tl-chloride (80 MBq)
II	Interruption for a definite period (period: corresponding maximum administered activity)	^{99m}Tc-MAA (13 h, 100 MBq) ^{99m}Tc-pertechnetate (47 h, 800 MBq; 25 h, 80 MBq)
III	Interruption with measurement	^{99m}Tc-erythrocytes, ^{99m}Tc-technegas, ^{99m}Tc-MAG3 (>100 MBq), ^{99m}Tc-microspheres, 99mTc-pyrophosphate, ^{111}In-leucocytes (>10 MBq),[a] ^{123}I-iodide, ^{123}I-MIBG, ^{123}I-hippuran, ^{201}Tl-chloride (>80 MBq)
IV	Cessation	Sodium ^{32}P-phosphate, ^{67}Ga-citrate, ^{125}I-HSA, ^{131}I-iodide

[a]The limit for ^{111}In-leucocytes is set at 10 MBq for nursing mothers because of the close contact dose received from cuddling the infant (see §16.8.1).

of pregnancy, there is an increased risk of hypothyroidism in the infant with the possibility of mental deficiency if the hypothyroidism is not detected. Inadvertent ^{131}I treatment for hyperthyroidism in the later stages of pregnancy is unlikely to justify termination of pregnancy [23].

16.5.2 Fetal dosimetry

In the MIRD schema for internal dosimetry [1, 6–9], there are three factors specific to the pregnant patient which will affect the fetal dose according to the age of the fetus: first, the shape, size, and position of the maternal abdominal organs (i.e. *S*-values); second, the uptake and clearance of radioactivity in the placenta and fetus; and third (perhaps of less importance), the effect of pregnancy on the cumulated activity in the maternal organs. During the early stages of pregnancy, it can be assumed that the abdominal organs have not yet been displaced or changed in shape, and the embryo dose is taken to be the same as the dose to the uterus (Table 16.3) [3–5].

Two developments have sought to improve the accuracy of fetal dose estimations. First, the latest version of the MIRD dosimetry software (MIRDOSE3) contains *S*-values for the non-pregnant female adult, and for the female adult at 3, 6, and 9 months pregnancy [6]. The calculated absorbed fractions also include values for the fetal skeleton, fetal soft tissue, and the fetal whole body. Second, extensive studies of the placental transfer and fetal uptake of radiopharmaceuticals have been carried out in the guinea pig whose placental structure has certain similarities to the human [24]. Fetal dose estimates based on these two developments tend to decrease through pregnancy because the increase in fetal mass is greater than the increase in the absorbed fraction for the fetus irradiated by the maternal organs [25]. The lack of human data including the uptake and clearance from the fetus remains the main limitation to the accuracy of fetal radiopharmaceutical dosimetry.

16.5.3 Breastfeeding patients

When a radiopharmaceutical is administered to a breastfeeding mother, radioactivity will be secreted in her milk, and her infant will be exposed to the radiation emitted by the ingested radioactivity. Procedures of a similar type to those outlined in Box 11.4 for pregnant patients should be adopted to ensure that patients who are breastfeeding are identified and consideration given to whether the examination could be postponed. If the effective dose to the infant from breastfeeding is too high, then it should be reduced to an acceptable level by an interruption in feeding. If the radioactivity has a relatively slow rate of clearance in milk, then it may be necessary to cease feeding. As well as issuing appropriate advice to a breastfeeding patient, good radiation practice should include prevention of the uncontrolled exposure of the infant, justification and optimisation of the exposure, and ensuring a member of staff is available to explain the recommendations to the patient and, where appropriate, the referring clinician.

16.5.4 Advice to a breastfeeding patient

Before arriving at the nuclear medicine department for her appointment, the mother should be issued with the following advice [5]:

(1) express some breast milk and store it in a refrigerator;
(2) breastfeed her infant immediately before attending the department;
(3) interrupt feeding according to the recommendations in Table 16.5 [14, 21, 26];
(4) feed her infant with the stored milk during the period of interruption.

If she follows this advice, then the effective dose to her infant will be no more than 1 mSv, and in many cases, much less than this value.

If an interruption to breastfeeding is not essential (category I in Table 16.5), the mother can be reassured by advising a short interruption (e.g. 4 h) and then to express and discard her milk before resuming breastfeeding. If a definite period of interruption can be recommended (category II), then breast milk should be expressed and discarded at normal feeding times during this period. If the recommendation is to interrupt with measurement (category III), then the mother should be instructed to express milk samples. The inclusion of this category III in Table 16.5 represents a more cautious approach for radiopharmaceuticals where the available data are sparse [26] than that recommended by the ARSAC which assign an interruption period to these agents [5]. This recommendation should also be applied to the radiopharmaceuticals listed under category I in Table 16.5 (interruption not essential) if their administered activity exceeds the value given. The method in §16.5.5 can be used to estimate the dose if feeding had been resumed when a particular sample was expressed, and to derive the interruption time to reduce this dose to the desired value (see Box 16.2).

If the patient is still producing colostrum, then because the rate of secretion of radioactivity appears to follow a different pattern, the mother should be advised to interrupt with measurement (category III), unless the radiopharmaceutical falls into category IV (cease breastfeeding). An additional dose will be incurred if the administered radiopharmaceutical has an unusually high quantity of free pertechnetate, free iodide, free ^{111}In (with labelled leucocytes), or ^{124}I and ^{125}I contamination of ^{123}I [26]. Appropriate quality control measurements of the radiopharmaceutical should be made to assess these quantities.

16.5.5 Calculation of a period to interrupt breastfeeding

The activity I which would be ingested if feeding was resumed on the occasion that the last milk sample was expressed can be calculated from:

$$I = cK \qquad (16.9)$$

where c is the concentration of activity in the last sample. K is a constant representing a single effective ingested volume which accounts for the progressively decreasing importance of each feed with time after administration because of the corresponding decrease in the concentration of activity. It is given by [26]:

$$K = V\{[1 - \exp[-(\ln 2/t_{1/2})\tau]\}^{-1} \qquad (16.10)$$

where V is the volume of milk ingested per feed, $t_{1/2}$ is the effective half-life of the radioactivity in milk, and τ is the time between feeds.

If feeding had been resumed when the last sample had been expressed, then assuming an adult weighs 70 kg, the effective dose D to the infant is given by:

$$D = IE(70/w) \qquad (16.11)$$

where E is the effective dose to an adult per unit activity ingested in ionic form [27] (available data indicate secreted activities are in ionic form) and w is the infant's body weight (kg). This simple weight correction of the adult dose per unit activity ingested is used because of the lack of data to describe the equivalent value for young infants.

The period P after the time of administration for feeding to be interrupted in order to reduce the infant's effective dose from D to x can be calculated from:

$$P = t_{1/2}[\ln(D/x)/\ln 2] + t_c \qquad (16.12)$$

where t_c is the time after administration when a resumption of feeding gives a dose D. The effective half-life, $t_{1/2}$, can be obtained from the decrease in the activity concentrations measured in the milk samples. If it is appropriate to use the physical half-life for the radionuclide administered, or if there is sufficient confidence in published data to describe the effective half-life, then the patient only needs to express one milk sample. Appropriate values of V, τ, and w can be selected to suit individual circumstances. The recommendations in Table 16.5 are based on 850 ml of milk ingested per day [28] by a 4 kg infant fed six times per day (i.e. $V = 142$ ml, $t = 4$ h). Selection of the value of x should allow for the contribution of the close contact dose from cuddling the infant (Table 16.8). An example of the use of this method to calculate a period to interrupt breastfeeding is given in Box 16.2.

16.6 Paediatric patients

16.6.1 Administered activity

The requirement to reduce the administered activity compared to the usual adult value has to be balanced against the criteria of maintaining the image information density for any age of child. Reduction of administered activity according to the child's body surface area rather than methods based on age, height, or weight is the best method for maintaining the same count density. ARSAC recommends that paediatric administered activities should be calculated by reducing the adult diagnostic reference level by a schedule of factors produced by the Task Group on Paediatrics of the European Association of Nuclear Medicine [5, 29]. These factors are listed in Table 16.6 against body weight, where each value is derived from the ratio of the child's body surface area to that of an adult. If an individual factor is required for a particular child, then the body surface area B (m^2) for the child's height h (cm) and body weight w (kg) can be obtained from a formula given by Haycock *et al.* [30]:

$$B = w^{0.5378} \times h^{0.3964} \times 0.024265. \qquad (16.13)$$

ARSAC also recommends that the administered activity for each type of procedure should not be less than 10% of the adult activity [5].

Table 16.6 Schedule of factors to reduce the adult administered activity for a diagnostic procedure in a child according to the child's body weight [5, 29]

Weight (kg)	Factor	Weight (kg)	Factor
3	0.1	32	0.65
4	0.14	34	0.68
6	0.19	36	0.71
8	0.23	38	0.73
10	0.27	40	0.76
12	0.32	42	0.78
14	0.36	44	0.80
16	0.40	46	0.82
18	0.44	48	0.85
20	0.46	50	0.88
22	0.50	52–54	0.90
24	0.53	56–58	0.92
26	0.58	60–62	0.96
28	0.58	64–66	0.98
30	0.62	68	0.99

This method assumes for each organ that the ratio of its mass to the total body weight and its fractional uptake of the administered activity remain constant throughout the paediatric age range. Examples of where the first assumption is not valid are the brain, which reaches 70% of its adult weight by the age of 1 year, and the testes, which barely increase their weight until the onset of puberty. Examples of where the second assumption is not valid are the concentration of ^{99m}Tc-phosphonates and ^{67}Ga-citrate in the growing regions of bone.

16.6.2 Dosimetry

S-values have been derived for paediatric mathematical phantoms representing children at different ages, and are included in the MIRDOSE3 software [6]. Organ absorbed doses in the ICRP compendia are based on adult biokinetic data, with the exception of ^{99m}Tc-hexamethylpropyleneamine oxime (HMPAO) and an age-related bladder voiding model for other ^{99m}Tc-labelled radiopharmaceuticals in routine use [3, 4].

Effective doses for children at these ages are given in Table 16.7 for radiopharmaceuticals used in common procedures. They are based on the adult diagnostic reference levels, and on the administered activity scaling factors recommended by ARSAC (Table 16.6) [5], and on ICRP values of effective dose per unit activity administered at each age [3, 4]. For ^{99m}Tc-radiopharmaceuticals, the effective doses lie within the range 0.5–8 mSv, and with the exception of ^{67}Ga-citrate and ^{123}I-iodide, the effective dose is more or less independent of body weight for each radiopharmaceutical listed. In younger children, effective dose tends to be higher than the value produced by a factor based directly on body weight ratio. Effective doses based on organ and tissue weighting factors derived for children (0–9 years) and for adolescents (10–19 years) differ from those derived from the whole population weighting factors by less than the uncertainties in the organ absorbed doses, even for radiopharmaceuticals where age-specific biokinetic data are available [31]. Therefore, whole-population weighting factors should continue to be used for estimates of effective dose to children.

16.7 The hospital environment

Individuals will be exposed to radiation from radioactivity in patients or in tissue samples from patients. Potential doses and methods for assessing these doses will be considered for different groups within a hospital in this section.

16.7.1 The waiting room

Concerns about the exposure of accompanying relatives, nurse escorts, and other patients in the waiting room are

Table 16.7 Effective doses to paediatric patients for common diagnostic procedures [3–5]

Radiopharmaceutical	Adult diagnostic reference level (MBq)	Effective dose (mSv)[a] 15/55[b]	10/35	5/18	1/10
^{67}Ga-citrate	150	18	21	22	26
^{99m}Tc-diphosphonates	600	4	5	4	4
^{99m}Tc-DMSA	80	0.8	0.8	0.7	0.8
^{99m}Tc-DTPA (normal renal function)	300	2	2	1	1
^{99m}Tc-erythrocytes	800	6	8	7	8
^{99m}Tc-IDA derivatives (normal biliary function)	150	3	3	3	4
^{99m}Tc-HIG	200	2	3	3	3
^{99m}Tc-HMPAO	500	5	6	6	7
^{99m}Tc-leucocytes	200	3	3	4	3
^{99m}Tc-MAG3 (normal renal function)	100	0.8	0.8	0.5	0.6
^{99m}Tc-MAG3 (abnormal renal function)	100	0.7	0.7	0.5	0.5
^{99m}Tc-MAG3 (acute unilateral renal blockage)	100	1	1	1	1
^{99m}Tc-MIBI (resting)	400	4	5	5	6
^{99m}Tc-MIBI (exercise)	400	4	4	4	5
^{99m}Tc-pertechnetate (no thyroid block)	80	1	1	1	2
^{99m}Tc-tetrofosmin (resting)	400	4	4	4	5
^{99m}Tc-tetrofosmin (exercise)	400	3	3	3	4
^{123}I-iodide (55 % thyroid uptake)	20	10	12	16	19
^{123}I-iodide (total thyroid block)	20	0.3	0.3	0.3	0.3
^{123}I-MIBG	400	6	7	7	7

[a]Effective doses based on an administered activity given by the ARSAC adult diagnostic reference level reduced by the scaling factor given in Table 16.6 [5].
[b]Age (years)/weight (kg).

unwarranted. In a busy department carrying out a wide range of routine procedures and with a dedicated waiting room, a dose-rate study found a median and a maximum dose of 2.0 and 33.0 μSv, respectively, to accompanying relatives, 2.3 and 17.0 μSv, respectively, to accompanying nurses, and 0.2 and 5.0 μSv, respectively, to other patients [32]. However, results from a dedicated positron emission tomography (PET) centre indicate that a member of the public accompanying a patient could exceed a dose of 0.3 mSv [33].

Dosimetry studies have also shown that a second waiting room brings no dose reduction benefit to these accompanying individuals [34]. Changes in the ambient dose in the waiting room can be monitored by attaching integrating dosemeters such as a film badge or a TLD to the wall.

16.7.2 Imaging staff

The annual exposure of nuclear medicine staff is not insignificant, and can reach a value of typically up to 2–3 mSv. There are obvious sources of high exposure such as radiopharmaceutical dispensing and aerosol generator preparation. However, the quasi-continual exposure to patients can be significant. If technologists dispense and inject radiopharmaceuticals as well as operate the imaging equipment, then the radiation dose from the patient during injection and imaging will exceed that from the contents of the syringe while dispensing and injecting. In the imaging area of a dedicated PET facility the patient will provide the largest contribution to non-extremity doses to personnel.

Box 16.3 Parameters affecting the doses to imaging technologists

Administered activity
Time between injection and scan
Imaging time
Attenuating material around imaging bed (e.g. number of gamma-camera heads)
Patient size (e.g. children, obese patients)
Critically ill patients
Patient cooperation
Technologist's individual technique
Variations in anatomical distribution (e.g. due to pathological effects, patient age, etc.)
Camera–console distance
Shielding between console and patient
Note: Some of these parameters can be used to optimise the exposure of these members of staff. All can be used to reconcile the results of different dosimetry studies.

There are many factors which affect the doses to imaging technologists (see Box 16.3), and an evaluation of their contribution in the local working environment can be used to minimize exposure. Although the effects of some of these factors are obvious, they may have more than one effect. For instance, a double-headed gamma-camera will reduce the imaging time but may also place more radiation-absorbent material between the technologist and the patient for some of this time. A paediatric patient will require less administered activity than an adult, but will not self-absorb as much of the gamma radiation and will probably require the technologist to spend a longer time in close proximity. The technologist's individual technique and the level of difficulty experienced in handling a patient can significantly increase their exposure. Consequently, the dose to imaging staff from different ^{99m}Tc procedures can vary over a wide range (typically 0.5×10^{-3} to 10×10^{-3} μSv MBq^{-1}) even for the same procedure. For a dedicated PET centre, technologists have recorded an average daily dose of 14 μSv [33]. Separating the console from the camera head/imaging bed with lead shielding or a wall with a lead-glass screen has been found necessary by some departments. The replacement of ^{201}Tl-chloride for myocardial perfusion imaging with ^{99m}Tc-radiopharmaceuticals is an example of where a development resulting in a lower dose to the patient (and better quality images) has had the opposite effect of increasing the dose to imaging staff. Another development in nuclear medicine with the potential for increasing the exposure of imaging staff is the use of multiple studies on the same patient which may require accurate repositioning.

16.7.3 Pregnant staff

Exposure to sources of potentially high exposure (e.g. dispensing, generators, aerosol equipment, therapy patients, etc.) can probably be avoided without disrupting the clinical service. However, unless a department has a large number of staff, it will be impossible for a pregnant member of staff to avoid exposure to radioactive patients undergoing diagnostic procedures.

The fetus of a pregnant employee is required to be treated as a member of the public, and should not exceed a dose of 1 mSv during the declared term of pregnancy. Although a limit of 2 mSv to the maternal abdominal surface may be appropriate for restricting the exposure of the fetus to 1 mSv for pregnant staff exposed to patient scatter in diagnostic radiology, radioactive patients emit higher photon energies and have a larger cross-sectional area. These factors will lead to a greater tissue penetration, and it has been shown that a limit of 1.3 mSv to the maternal abdominal surface is required to restrict the fetal dose to 1 mSv if the patient has been administered ^{99m}Tc or ^{131}I [14, 21].

The dose to imaging staff for any particular investigation varies greatly between departments (see §16.8.2), and individual departments will need to assess the impact of this limit in terms of their local dosimetry. However, it could have a significant impact, corresponding typically to a maximum of six ^{99m}Tc studies per day or one ^{131}I study per day for a declared term of pregnancy of 7 months. For practical purposes of enforcement, it may be advisable to set this abdominal dose limit for pregnant nuclear medicine staff to 1 mSv (rather than 1.3 mSv), particularly in a PET centre. However, whichever limit is applied, it must be appreciated that compliance will only be achieved if a more sensitive personal dosemeter than a film badge is worn. Active monitoring of a pregnant member of staff's dose with an electronic personal dosimeter may be advisable (§8.3.5), and prior risk assessment of the potential exposure should enable plans to be drawn up to maintain the clinical service during the term of pregnancy.

16.7.4 Porters

A greater exposure will occur where the nuclear medicine department has its own porter for taking in-patients back to their ward. However, even for this situation, on the basis of dosimetry estimates, no special precautions are required: from dose rates measured at 0.5 m from the patient in a hospital where the journey time between the ward and the department is greater than average, the dose to the porter is only about 0.1 mSv per month [32].

16.7.5 Ward staff

Nursing staff will be exposed to radiation emitted from diagnostic nuclear medicine patients when they return to their ward. The magnitude of these doses will increase according to the level of nursing care required, with nursing procedures requiring close contact with the patient (e.g. feeding, insertion and/or removal of catheters) causing higher doses. A nurse will not exceed 24 μSv in an 8-hour working day (the daily limit equivalent to an annual occupational limit of 6 mSv) even when providing the highest level of nursing care for an adult patient who has undergone a low-activity ^{99m}Tc procedure such as a lung scan [14]. A dose of 24 μSv may be exceeded when nursing a chairfast/bedfast adult patient after a high-activity planar or SPECT ^{99m}Tc scan, a partially helpless adult patient after an ^{111}In-octreotide or ^{18}F-FDG scan, a partially helpless paediatric patient after any ^{99m}Tc procedure, or a totally helpless adult patient after an ^{111}In-leucocyte or ^{201}Tl-chloride scan [14, 15, 21].

However, these findings are based on maximum values of measured dose rates, and to reach the annual limit of 6 mSv would be most unlikely because a nurse would have to attend to nuclear medicine patients requiring these high levels of care (or higher) on almost a daily basis. Such exposures can in any case be reduced by minimizing close nursing activities and by placing the patient under the care of more than one nurse. If a patient is incontinent, then adequate protection against radioactive contamination will be given by the nursing staff following the normal hygiene precautions for dealing with urine and soiled linen.

Sodium ^{131}I-iodide and ^{131}I-MIBG administered for the treatment of thyroid cancer and neural crest tumours, respectively, are the most common in-patient therapy procedures. They present a much greater potential hazard to nursing staff on wards, and the administrations should be carried out in specifically designed shielded rooms, and the patients kept in these rooms until the retained activity has declined to the level allowed for the patient to leave hospital. These rooms should be constructed to the appropriate specification for handling radionuclides (see Chapter 15) to allow for the possibility of spills and other contamination, and they should have their own separate toilet, washing, and waste disposal facilities. Nursing staff and visitors must be given specific instructions designed to minimize their exposure. Patients who are severely immobile with marked discomfort from secondary malignancies may require high-dependency nursing care. Measurements of instantaneous dose rates coupled with likely exposure times and published values of effective half-lives can be used to calculate the potential doses to nursing staff and to draw up duty rotas.

16.7.6 Pathology staff

Although pathology staff will receive a dose from analysing radioactive tissue samples from nuclear medicine patients, the total exposure is likely to be shared among different members of staff, and will be reduced if the analysis of the samples can be delayed (e. g. for batch processing). Estimates have shown the monthly whole-body doses in a large busy acute hospital to be small: 20 and 2 μSv for urine and blood samples, respectively, taken from patients administered ^{99m}Tc [32]. Contamination and external dose-rate hazards following Sentinel Node procedures are low provided that appropriate activities are administered to the patient and normal precautions for handling biological specimens are followed. Although the dose to staff per specimen will be greater if the patient has been administered ^{131}I, the number of such radioactive samples handled per month by pathology laboratory staff will be very much lower.

16.7.7 Ultrasonographers

An ultrasonographer is required to sit close to a patient when carrying out an examination, and will be exposed to radiation when scanning a patient who has recently undergone a nuclear medicine investigation or has been administered a radiopharmaceutical for a nuclear medicine imaging procedure to be performed later. Maximum doses of 0.33 and 0.06 mSv to the hands and gonads, respectively, have been estimated for an ultrasonographer carrying out an examination of the upper abdomen, the pelvis, or upper abdomen and pelvis, and the thyroid of patients on the same day or on the days following the administration of activities of up to 555 MBq of ^{99m}Tc, 178 MBq of ^{67}Ga, or 19 kBq of ^{131}I [35].

Avoiding an ultrasound examination on the same day as a nuclear medicine procedure will minimize this exposure. However, it is an issue which has to be considered in the context of 'one-stop' out-patient clinics. Risk assessment requires a knowledge of the number of patients requiring both types of investigation and the number of ultrasonography staff involved, as well as the potential dose per examination. The ultrasonography service should be notified if a patient has recently undergone a nuclear medicine investigation in order to allow any practical precautions to be implemented.

16.8 Discharge from hospital

Before discharge from hospital, it is necessary to consider whether a nuclear medicine patient needs to restrict their contact with critical groups in order to reduce their exposure. Potential hazards arise from external radiation and from radioactive contamination, and advice should be based on a generic or an individual risk assessment as appropriate. Where it is necessary to restrict the contact between a patient and a critical group, then not only should the advice be discussed with the patient, and/or accompanying members of the family or other carers, but also written instructions should be issued giving details of the radiopharmaceutical administered, hospital contact name(s), as well as the restrictions to be followed.

Special considerations may also be required if a patient dies following administration of a radiopharmaceutical. Precautions are unlikely after a diagnostic administration, and the appropriate precautions following a therapeutic procedure will depend on the method used for the disposal of the body as well as on the radiopharmaceutical and administered activity.

The greatest risk from contact with radioactive tissue is presented by a patient undergoing radioiodine (^{131}I) therapy. Although radioiodine will appear in sweat, saliva, and urine, this potential risk of contamination is very much lower and easier to manage than the potential hazard presented by the emitted radiation [14]. In general, normal hygiene precautions will provide adequate protection to the hazards of radioactive contamination excreted from the body.

The recommendations discussed below for patients following discharge from hospital refer to the external radiation hazard, and have been derived from critical group dosimetry studies [14, 36–38]. They apply to the exposure from a patient receiving a single radiopharmaceutical administration under conventional circumstances for each of the situations described. When an individual in a critical group will be exposed to more than one patient or to the same patient receiving more than one administration, or where the circumstances of the exposure are unusual, then it should be possible to derive appropriate recommendations from the dose-rate data given in Tables 16.1 and 16.2 or from individual measurements. If necessary, appropriate exposure parameters can be applied to the computer software which is available to model contact between a patient and an individual in a critical group [17, 18].

Members of the public sitting close to a nuclear medicine patient on their journey away from hospital will receive a dose from the emitted radiation. When considering the exposure of fellow travellers, individual recommendations should take into account the likely seating distances and journey times which may differ, for instance, between private and public transport. Any patient who has received an oral administration of a radiopharmaceutical should not use public transport if there is a risk of vomiting.

The children of a parent who has undergone a nuclear medicine procedure will be exposed to the emitted radiation after the parent has returned home. The critical group will be the infants young enough to be held for prolonged repetitive periods in close contact with the parent. A simple estimation of a close-contact dose to a young infant in these circumstances can be obtained by multiplying the initial surface dose rate (Table 16.1) by an effective exposure time (Table 16.8) which accounts for the intermittency of close contact and for the decay in the dose rate [14, 21].

The partner of a nuclear medicine patient will also be exposed to emitted radiation. Dosimetry studies have shown that the greatest component of this exposure is caused by the partner sleeping in the same bed as the patient [36]. Members of the family of a young child who has undergone a nuclear medicine procedure will receive an emitted radiation dose from the radioactivity retained by the child's organs. The critical group will be parents of young infants who require extended periods of close contact, and therefore the close-contact dose to the parent can be derived by applying the concept of the effective exposure time in reverse: individual dose estimations can be derived from the paediatric dose-rate data in Table 16.2 or from a single surface dose-rate measurement, multiplied by the effective exposure times listed in Table 16.8.

If a patient to whom a radiopharmaceutical has recently been administered sits near to a colleague at work, then the colleague will receive a dose from the emitted radiation. This dose can also be estimated using the type of dose-rate data given in Tables 16.1 and 16.2 together with estimated values of working time and distance from the patient.

16.8.1 Diagnostic patients

In general, a patient administered no more than the ARSAC diagnostic reference level of activity for planar or SPECT imaging [5] does not need to adhere to any restrictions with regard to their travel home, contact with any member of their family, or with a colleague at work. These recommendations apply to all routine diagnostic procedures including the administration of ^{18}F-FDG as long as a child did not accompany the patient to the PET

Table 16.8 Effective exposure times for estimating close contact doses to young infants [14, 15, 22]

Radiopharmaceutical	Effective exposure time[a] (h)
^{67}Ga-citrate	32.8
^{111}In-leucocytes	35.9
^{111}In-octreotide	10.9
^{99m}Tc (all compounds)	3.9
^{123}I-iodide (euthyroid)	4.2
^{123}I-iodide (hyperthyroid)	5.5
^{123}I-MIBG	4.4
^{131}I-iodide (euthyroid)	27.4
^{131}I-iodide (hyperthyroid)	32.2
^{131}I-MIBG	11.5
^{201}Tl-chloride	30.2
^{32}P-phosphate	82.5
^{90}Y-colloid	34.3
^{89}Sr-chloride	638

[a]Assuming that a total close-contact time of 9 h in a 24-h period consisted of 35 min in close contact at the start of each hour for the first 8 h after radiopharmaceutical administration, 35 min at the start of each fourth hour for the next 12 h (i.e. feeding times overnight), and 35 min at the start of each hour for the remaining 4 h.

centre [16]. The exceptions are where the parent of a small child has been administered more than 10 MBq of ^{111}In-leucocytes, 200 MBq of ^{67}Ga-citrate (e.g. for a high-activity lymphoma scan), 150 MBq of ^{201}Tl-chloride (e.g. for a non-specific tumour scan), or 120 MBq of ^{111}In-octreotide, or has been administered a total of 800 MBq of ^{99m}Tc for a rest–exercise myocardial perfusion scan (carried out over 1 or 2 days) [13–15, 21]. In these cases, initial restrictions in the close contact with an infant are necessary to restrict their dose to 1 mSv. For instance, a 30% reduction in the dose to the infant after administration of ^{111}In-leucocytes to the parent can be achieved by restricting close contact to 35 min every fourth hour for the first 3 days, compared to that received from the close-contact sequence used to calculate the effective exposure times (see footnote to Table 16.8).

The recommendations for close contact with a young infant are based on a close-contact time of 9 h in every 24-h period, and maximum published values of dose rate per unit activity at 0.1 m. Therefore, it may also be necessary to advise a short restriction if the duration of close contact is likely to be even greater, or if the administered activity is to exceed the ARSAC diagnostic reference level. In practice, activities exceeding the appropriate diagnostic reference level which would cause a close-contact dose of more than 1 mSv are only likely to be administered for certain individual SPECT studies. In all cases, the need for a restriction can be determined from an individual prediction of the close-contact dose given by multiplying the patient's surface dose rate by the effective exposure time.

16.8.2 Patients administered ^{131}I

To comply with statutory requirements, patients have to restrict their contact with critical groups after leaving hospital following administration of ^{131}I for a whole-body scan for thyroid metastases, or for the treatment of hyperthyroidism or thyroid cancer. Unless there are unusual circumstances, for instance, regarding their

Table 16.9 Restrictions for patients administered ^{131}I for hyperthyroidism after discharge from hospital [14, 37–39]

Restriction	Time after discharge to comply with restriction (days)						
Retained activity (MBq)	*200*	*300*	*400*	*500*	*600*	*700*	*800*
Arrange care elsewhere for children aged under 3 years	15	19	21	23	25	26	27
Stay at least 1 m away from children aged 3–5 years	11	14	16	18	20	21	22
Stay at least 1 m away from children aged over 5 years and from adults who are not 'comforters and carers'	5	8	11	12	14	15	16
Sleep separately from 'comforters and carers'	0	0	0	0	4	6	8
Avoid prolonged close contact (more than 3 h at < 1 m) with other adults	0	0	0	0	0	0	1

Box 16.4 An example of the recommendations to be followed by a patient after administration of ^{131}I

A female married patient with one child at home (aged 3 years) is to be administered 600 MBq of ^{131}I to treat her thyrotoxicosis. Her clinician does not rule out the possibility of further treatment during the next couple of years. If necessary, her husband is able to take some time off work to look after their child. Her full-time occupation is to teach the entry class in a primary school, and her child attends a nursery during school hours. The family has only just moved into the area, the treatment is to be given during term time, and there are no close relatives or friends living nearby. They own their own car, and they live about 10 miles from the hospital.

How should the patient modify her behaviour?

1. There is no restriction on the journey home from hospital after treatment and on prolonged contact with other persons, such as visiting a place of entertainment.
2. The patient should stay off work for 20 days because of the impossibility of avoiding any form of close contact with young children as part of her routine duties.
3. The patient should refrain from all close contact with her child (a minimum distance of 1 m) for the next 20 days. The child should not sleep in the same bed as the mother for this period of time.
4. In the absence of any other support, the husband will need to take the next 20 days off work even with the child continuing to attend their nursery.
5. With the husband acting as a 'comforter and carer', the parents need only sleep in separate beds for the next 4 days.

ability to comply with the restrictions, patients need only be hospitalized if they have been administered ^{131}I for the treatment of thyroid cancer.

In the UK, the recommendations for patients administered ^{131}I for hyperthyroidism to follow after leaving hospital have been revised [39], based on recent measurements [14, 21, 36–38] and modelling data [17] (Table 16.9). They aim to ensure that the dose to a critical group is unlikely to exceed the following values:

(1) a member of the public at a place of potential contact—1 mSv per year, 0.3 mSv per procedure
(2) a 'comforter and carer' [2, 39]—no annual limit, 5 mSv per procedure
(3) adult and child members of the household—5 mSv in 5 years, 1 mSv per procedure.

These recommendations are based on the assumptions that the patient is to be discharged to a private dwelling where they will only come into close contact with a 'comforter and carer', other adult or child members of the household, and that arrangements can be made for any children under 3 years old to be cared for elsewhere. If the latter requirement is impossible, then treatment as an in-patient should be considered. It is also assumed that ^{131}I is administered only once in a year, and that the patient will not provide a significant risk of contamination. Patients who vomit or are incontinent of urine within 24 h after discharge should be recommended to contact the hospital for advice which will depend on the patient's personal circumstances and the nature of the incident. An example of the formulation of recommendations for a patient to follow after treatment with ^{131}I for thyrotoxicosis is given in Box 16.4.

However, the patient's circumstances may differ from those on which the recommendations are based; for instance, the patient may have to be discharged with more than 800 MBq of retained activity or the patient may be unable to comply with their recommendations. In cases such as these, an individual risk assessment should be made, based on dose-rate measurements and perhaps using the modelling software [17, 18]. Appropriate instructions should be derived to satisfy the above restrictions to the exposure of critical groups.

The dose rate at a distance from a patient receiving ^{131}I for ablation of thyroid cancer decreases with time at a different rate to that from a patient administered ^{131}I for follow-up treatment (§16.3.2), and in both cases it decreases more rapidly than that from a patient administered ^{131}I for hyperthyroidism. Recommendations for restricting close contact between critical groups and a patient treated with ^{131}I for thyroid cancer have been derived from dose-rate data and the modelling software [40], and the same method can be used on an individual basis. However, unlike the restrictions for hyperthyroidism, these published recommendations for thyroid cancer patients have not been validated with integral dose studies.

The only restriction for travel is that a patient retaining up to 800 MBq of ^{131}I should not sit immediately adjacent to another person on public and private transport for more than 1 and 6 h, respectively, on the day of discharge from hospital, in order to restrict their dose to no more than 0.3 mSv. A patient with a retained activity of up to 800 MBq of ^{131}I can be advised to return to work on the day after discharge as long as they do not spend more than 8 h per day at a distance of less than 2 m from the same colleague. Special precautions at work may be necessary to avoid the possibility of food contamination, or if the patient's duties involve proximity to materials or alarms sensitive to ionising radiation. If the patient's occupation entails extended close contact with another adult or child, then the patient should not return to work until after the periods of time given in Table 16.9.

Patients should be advised about the likely restrictions to their behaviour at least a day before the treatment is administered. This will give them time to consider the consequences of the advice, and they must be allowed to discuss it with hospital staff who in turn must ensure the patient has understood it. The detailed recommendations should be emphasized to them immediately after administration and they should be issued with a card carrying the written instructions and details of the treatment. They can be advised that if they follow this advice, then the dose to anyone acting as a 'comforter or carer' will be less than 5 mSv, and the dose to any other individual (including young children) will be less than 1 mSv. They should be instructed to show the card to medical staff if they have to attend a health centre or hospital during their periods of restriction.

They may receive some preliminary advice about restrictions at an earlier stage, for instance from their referring clinician as part of the consent procedure. Consequently, the advice will often be issued by more than one member of the hospital staff. It is essential that the recommendations received by the patient from each source are consistent. Otherwise, the patient may lose confidence in the advice, a consequence of which may be a failure to comply with the restrictions.

16.8.3 Other radionuclide therapies

For other therapeutic radionuclides whose values of effective half-life are not very different to ^{131}I (about 6 days), it has been recommended that the appropriate restrictions can be formulated by deriving the 'equivalent activity of ^{131}I', A_{eq} (MBq), from the equation [37]:

$$A_{eq} = D_1/0.05 \times T_{eff}/6 \qquad (16.14)$$

where D_1 is the measured dose rate at 1 m from the trunk of the patient (μSv h^{-1}) and T_{eff} is the effective half-life of the retained radioactivity (days). This equation was derived from the assumptions that the radiation dose to another individual is proportional to the effective half-life of the retained activity, the effective half-life for sodium ^{131}I-iodide is about 6 days, and the dose rate per unit activity at 1 m from the trunk of a patient administered ^{131}I is about 0.05 μSv h^{-1} MBq^{-1}. The recommendations above for ^{131}I corresponding to the derived value of A_{eq} can then be used as an indication for the appropriate restrictions.

If the radionuclide has an effective half-life which is different from that of ^{131}I, then the restrictions can be derived from applying the appropriate individual exposure parameters to computer modelling software [17, 18], or in the case of a young infant, by estimating the close-contact dose from a calculation of the effective exposure time [14, 21]. It should be noted that beta-particle emitting radionuclides administered to a patient may produce a significant external dose rate from bremsstrahlung radiation (typically 0.03 μSv h^{-1} MBq^{-1} at 1 m, after administration of ^{89}Sr). Another potential hazard with beta-emitting therapeutic radionuclides is the possibility of urine contamination.

16.8.4 Disposal of a radioactive corpse

Potential risks will be presented to various critical groups if a patient dies following a radionuclide therapeutic procedure. For post-mortem, embalming, burial, and cremation, there is a risk from radiation emitted from the corpse, and from handling radioactive tissue. Critical groups include ward staff, mortuary staff, undertakers, crematorium staff, and family members. If a patient dies following a diagnostic procedure, no precautions are necessary in addition to those normally followed during a post-mortem or embalming unless death occurs within 48 h after administration. For therapeutic radionuclides, the appropriate precautions can be decided on an individual basis, which may include taking dose-rate measurements at the appropriate distances from the corpse, and identifying the relevant occupancy factors from discussions with the individuals involved. Advice about whole-body dose and extremity dose monitoring, contamination monitoring and radioactive waste disposal may also be needed. Other more general precautions and advice specific to each of the above processes have been published [39].

For cremation, members of the public who may be exposed to the radioactive discharge from the crematorium chimney represent another critical group. The risk of death in patients undergoing routine radionuclide therapy is probably greatest for those receiving palliative treatment with ^{89}Sr for bone metastases. The UK Health and Safety Executive have advised that there is no cause for concern for the cremation of a body containing up to 500 MBq of ^{89}Sr. This advice was based on an environmental impact assessment which estimated a resulting inhalation and skin dose of 0.1 and 2 μSv, respectively, to an adult member of the public, and a maximum inhalation and ingestion dose of about 0.3 and 0.4 μSv, respectively, to a crematorium worker [21].

16.9 Summary

The internal dose from a radiopharmaceutical and its associated risk can only be regarded as an estimate because of the many uncertainties involved in the calculation. These uncertainties arise from the lack of data which have been pointed out in relevant parts of this chapter–for instance, biokinetic data in disease, in children, and in pregnancy, particularly placental transfer. It is the responsibility of the nuclear medicine practitioner to rectify this deficiency in data whenever a practical opportunity arises.

In the past, the patient has often been overlooked as a mobile source of radiation. However, the recent efforts to measure the doses to critical groups have been rewarded by the acquisition of sound data on which appropriate restrictions have been based. Moreover, these studies have shown that the downward pressure on dose limits need not place any restrictions on the growth and development of clinical nuclear medicine, despite the significantly greater potential exposure associated with many of these developments. However, there will be a continuing need for such dosimetry measurements–as part of novel clinical research and in the implementation of service developments or other changes which will affect the radiation exposure of critical groups.

16.10 References

1 Loevinger, R., Budinger, T. F., and Watson, E. E. (ed.) (1989). *MIRD primer for absorbed dose calculations*. Society of Nuclear Medicine, New York.

2 International Commission on Radiological Protection (1991). 1990 Recommendations of the International Commission on Radiological Protection. ICRP Publication 60. *Ann. ICRP.*, **21** (1–3).

3 International Commission on Radiological Protection (1994). Radiation dose to patients from radiopharmaceuticals (including Addendum 1). ICRP Publication 53 (2nd edn). *Ann. ICRP*, **18** (1–4).

4 International Commission on Radiological Protection (1999). Radiation dose to patients from radiopharmaceuticals. Addendum to ICRP53. ICRP Publication 80. *Ann. ICRP*, **28** (3).

5 Administration of Radioactive Substances Advisory Committee (1998). *Notes for guidance on the clinical administration of radiopharmaceuticals and use of sealed radioactive sources*. Department of Health, London.

6 Stabin, M. G. (1996). MIRDOSE: personal computer software for internal dose assessment in nuclear medicine. *J. Nucl. Med.*, **37**, 538–46. MIRDOSE is available from the Radiation Internal Dose Information Center, Oak Ridge Institute for Science and Education, PO Box 117, Oak Ridge, TN 37831-0117, USA.

7 Watson, E. E., Stabin, M. G., and Siegel, J. A. (1993). MIRD formulation. *Med. Phys.*, **20**, 511–14.

8 Stabin, M. G., Tagesson, M., Thomas, S. R., Ljungberg, M., and Strand, S. E. (1999). Radiation dosimetry in nuclear medicine. *Appl. Radiat. Isot.*, **50**, 73–87.

9 Snyder, W. S., Ford, M. R., Warner, G. G., and Watson, S. B. (1975). *'S,' absorbed dose per unit accumulated activity for selected radionuclides and organs*. MIRD Pamphlet No. 11. Society of Nuclear Medicine, New York.

10 Cristy, M. and Eckerman, K. (1987). *Specific absorbed fractions of energy at various ages from internal photon sources*. Report ORNL/TM-8381/V1-7. Office of Science and Technical Information, Oak Ridge, TN.

11 Mountford, P. J. (1996). Internal dosimetry: developments and limitations. *Eur. J. Nucl. Med.*, **23**, 491–3.

12 Blower, P. J. and Gardin, I. (1997). A place for cellular dosimetry in risk assessment. *Nucl. Med. Commun.*, **18**, 989–91.

13 Harding L. K., Mostafa, A. B., Roden, L., and Williams, N. (1985). Dose rates from patients having nuclear medicine investigations. *Nucl. Med. Commun.*, **6**, 191–4.

14 Mountford, P. J. and O'Doherty, M. J. (1999). Exposure of critical groups to nuclear medicine patients. *Appl. Radiat. Isot.*, **50**, 89–111.

15 Greaves, C. D. and Tindale, W. B. (1999). Dose rate measurements from radiopharmaceuticals: implications for nuclear medicine staff and for children with radioactive parents. *Nucl. Med. Commun.*, **20**, 179–87.

16 Cronin, B., Marsden, P. K., and O'Doherty, M. J. (1999). Are restrictions to behaviour of patients required following fluorine-18 fluorodeoxyglucose positron emission tomographic studies? *Eur. J. Nucl. Med.*, **26**, 121–8.

17 Kettle, A. G., Barrington, S. F., and O'Doherty, M. J. (1997). Radiation dose rates post ^{131}I therapy and advice to patients on discharge from hospital. *Health Phys.*, **73**, 711.

18 Cormack, J. and Shearer, J. (1998). Calculation of radiation exposures from patients to whom radioactive materials have been administered. *Phys. Med. Biol.*, **43**, 501–16.

19 Keeling, D. H. and Maltby, P. (1994). Maladministrations and misadministrations. *Nucl. Med. Commun.*, **15**, 63–5.

20 William, E. D. and Harding, L. K. (1995). Radiopharmaceutical maladministration: what action is required? *Nucl. Med. Commun.*, **16**, 721–3.

21 Mountford, P. J. (1997). Risk assessment of the nuclear medicine patient. *Br. J. Radiol.* **70**, 671–84.

22 National Radiological Protection Board (1993). Board statement on diagnostic medical exposures to ionising radiation during pregnancy. *Doc. NRPB*, **4** (4).

23 Berg, G. E. B., Nystrom, E. H., Jacobsson, L., Lindberg, S., Lindstedt, G., Mattsson, S., *et al.* (1998). Radioiodine treatment of hyperthyroidism in a pregnant woman. *J. Nucl. Med.*, **39**, 357–61.

24 Palmer, A. M. and Preece, A. W. (1993). Placental transfer of technetium labelled radiopharmaceuticals in the guinea pig. *J. Nucl. Med.*, **34**, 159P.

25 Russell, J. R., Stabin, M. G., Sparks, R. B., and Watson, E. (1997). Radiation absorbed dose to the embryo/fetus from radiopharmaceuticals. *Health Phys.*, **73**, 756–69.

26 Mountford, P. J., Lazarus, C. R., and Edwards, S. (1996). Radiopharmaceuticals. In: *Drugs and human lactation* (2nd edn) (ed. P. N. Bennett), Chapter 8, pp. 609–77. Elsevier Science, Amsterdam.

27 International Commission on Radiological Protection (1991). Annual limits on intake of radionuclides by workers based on the 1990 recommendations. ICRP Publication 61. *Ann. ICRP*, **21** (4).

28 International Commission on Radiological Protection (1975). *Report of the task group on reference man.* ICRP Publication 23. Pergamon Press, Oxford.

29 The Paediatric Task Group of the European Association of Nuclear Medicine (1990). A radiopharmaceutical schedule for imaging in paediatrics. *Eur. J. Nucl. Med.*, **17**, 127–9.

30 Haycock, G. B., Schwartz, G. J., and Wisotsky, D. H. (1978). Geometric method for measuring body surface area: a height–weight formula validated in infants, children, and adults. *J. Pediatr.*, **93**, 62–6.

31 Gadd, R., Mountford, P. J., and Oxtoby, J. W. (1999). Effective dose to children and adolescents from radiopharmaceuticals. *Nucl. Med. Commun.*, **20**, 569–73.

32 Harding, L. K., Mostafa, A. B., and Thomson, W. H. (1990). Staff radiation doses associated with nuclear medicine procedures–a review of some recent measurements. *Nucl. Med. Commun.*, **11**, 271–7.

33 Benetar, N. A., Cronin, B. F., and O'Doherty, M. J. (2000). Radiation dose rates from patients undergoing PET: implications for technologists and waiting areas. *Eur. J. Nucl. Med.*, **27**, 583–9.

34 Harding, L. K., Bossuyt, A., Pellet, S., and Talbot, J. (1994). Radiation doses to those accompanying nuclear medicine department patients: a waiting room survey. *Eur. J. Nucl. Med.*, **21**, 1223–6.

35 Brateman, L., Shawker, T. H., and Conca, D. M. (1980). Potential hazard to ultrasonographers from previously administered radionuclides. *Radiology*, **134**, 479–82.

36 Thomson, W. H. and Harding, L. K. (1995). Radiation protection issues associated with nuclear medicine out-patients. *Nucl. Med. Commun.*, **16**, 879–92.

37 Working Party of the Radiation Protection Committee of the British Institute of Radiology (1999). Patients leaving hospital after administration of radioactive substances. *Br. J. Radiol.*, **72**, 121–5.

38 Barrington, S. F., O'Doherty, M. J., Kettle, A. G., Thomson, W. H., Mountford, P. J., Burrell, D. N., *et al.* (1999). Radiation exposure of the families of outpatients treated with radioiodine (iodine-131). for hyperthyroidism. *Eur. J. Nucl. Med.*, **26**, 686–92.

39 Institute of Physics and Engineering in Medicine (2002). *Medical and dental guidance notes.* IPEM, York.

40 Barrington, S. F., Kettle, A. G., O'Doherty, M. J., Wells, C. P., Somer, E. J. R., and Coakley, A. J. (1996). Radiation dose rates from patients receiving iodine-131 therapy for carcinoma of the thyroid. *Eur. J. Nucl. Med.*, **23**, 123–30.

Chapter 17
Radiotherapy: external beam therapy

R. M. Harrison and G. D. Lambert

17.1 Radiotherapy in perspective

Approximately one-third of the population will develop cancer during their lifetime and about half of these are cured. Of all cancer patients, 22% are cured by surgery, 18% by radiotherapy, and 5% by chemotherapy alone or in combination with either of the other two modalities [1].

Radiotherapy therefore plays a major role in cancer treatment and is given with either curative or palliative intent. Curative (radical) treatment aims to remove all tumour cells and effectively destroy the tumour. Palliative treatment is intended to relieve symptoms and is appropriate for the treatment of widespread primary tumours and the treatment of metastases.

Typically, around 95% of radiation treatments are delivered by external beam radiation sources.

High-energy X-ray beams in the range 4–25 MV from linear accelerators and cobalt-60 γ-rays are the most common sources of therapy. These machines are usually 'isocentrically mounted' so that irrespective of the radiation beam direction, the central axis of the beam always passes through a single point in space: 'the isocentre'. By positioning the patient so that this point coincides with the tumour, beams may be applied from different directions so that they are additive at the tumour. This is important because the dose required to kill the tumour is often extremely close to the dose that would result in irreparable damage to adjacent normal tissue.

The increasing likelihood of normal tissue damage with increasing dose sets a practical limit to the dose which can be delivered to the tumour. Some therapeutic benefit is gained by dividing the overall dose into daily subunits or 'fractions' because normal tissue tends to recover better than tumour from lower doses of radiation. Typically 5–35 daily fractions are used, the lower numbers being associated with palliative treatment which also typically receive a lower overall dose. Tumour doses are typically in the range 20–75 Gy.

In approximately 15–20% of treatments and for more superficial tumours, lower energy X-rays from kilovoltage X-ray units (50–300 kV) and electrons (3–25 MeV) from dual mode linear accelerators are used in preference. Generally, the latter produce no practical shielding problems because any shielding designed for the linear accelerator X-ray mode is likely to be adequate for electrons. However, consideration should be given to cases in which a low-megavolt accelerator can produce high-energy electrons [2]. The delivery of fractional doses of the order of a few gray, in exposures of approximately 1 minute duration, precludes the presence of staff and persons other than the patient in the treatment room during the exposure. The room structure must therefore provide sufficient shielding for adequate protection of staff and members of the public outside the room. The principles of dose limitation by design of appropriate shielding are explained in this chapter.

17.2 General objectives

17.2.1 *Design criteria*

The mandatory objective of treatment room design is to ensure that statutory dose limits for staff and the public are not exceeded. In practice, annual doses to medical and dental staff from external beam radiotherapy should be considerably less than current dose limits. Thus the application of the ALARP (as low as reasonably practicable) principle will lead to the choice of a realistic annual design dose for staff and/or the public. For example, in the UK, the National Radiological Protection Board (NRPB) have recommended a dose constraint of 0.3 mSv year^{-1} for the public from a single source [3]. This constraint could reasonably be applied also to radiotherapy staff who are not radiation workers.

From a practical point of view, it is convenient to confine the controlled area to the interior of the treatment

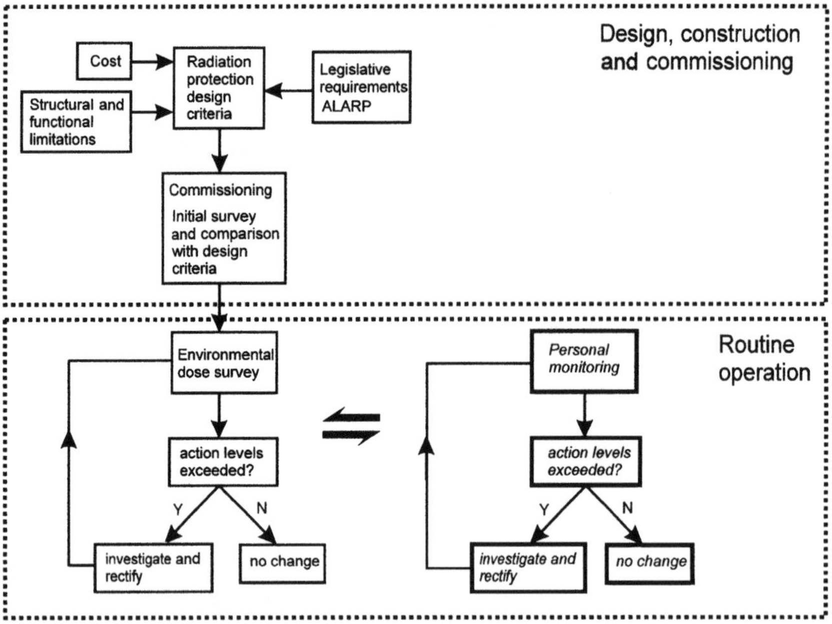

Figure 17.1 Simplified description of the management of radiation protection for staff and the public in external beam radiotherapy facilities.

room. This can be accomplished by restricting the time-averaged dose rate (TADR—averaged over 8 h) to less than 0.5 μSv h^{-1} and the instantaneous dose rate (IDR—averaged over 1 min) to less than or equal to 7.5 μSv h^{-1}. The conditions outside the treatment room are then compatible with an unsupervised or public area.

Areas where 0.5 μSv $h^{-1} \leq$ TADR < 7.5 μSv h^{-1} or 7.5 μSv h^{-1} < IDR $\leq$ 500 μSv h^{-1} should be designated as supervised, provided that only employees trained in radiation protection can enter the area.

Two comprehensive texts on radiation protection in radiotherapy are particularly recommended for further reading [2, 4].

17.2.2 Protection of staff and the public

Some general principles for the design and operation of external beam radiotherapy facilities to ensure the safety of members of staff and the general public are shown in Figure 17.1.

Design, construction, and commissioning

The upper box in Figure 17.1 shows the processes of design and construction, leading to the commissioning exercise. The design of the facility should take into account current legislation and good professional practice. At this stage, structural and functional limitations may necessitate a departure from the ideal case, and the benefits of protection measures may need to be weighed against their cost. As part of the commissioning procedure, an environmental dose survey should be carried out, the results compared with the design objectives, and any differences reconciled. These measurements form the baseline data set against which future regular environmental dose survey results are compared. Action levels should be set which invoke remedial action if results depart significantly from the baseline values.

Routine operation

Two complementary dose-monitoring aspects to routine operation of the facility are shown in the lower box in Figure 17.1. In routine use and in parallel with regular environmental surveys, staff whose duties require them to work directly with treatment equipment or who are in close proximity to treatment facilities should be monitored regularly. Even if there is no legal requirement to monitor staff, it is essential in external beam radiotherapy because of the potentially high doses which could result from an incident (e.g. if the X-ray beam is inadvertently switched on while a member of staff is still inside the treatment room). Action levels should be set which invoke remedial action if either personal dosimetry or environmental monitoring results depart significantly from those expected.

The procedures outlined in Figure 17.1 may be included under quality management systems such as

ISO9000 [5, 6]. Note that ISO9000 does not set absolute standards but provides a procedural and audit structure to ensure objectives are met.

17.2.3 Protection of the patient

Radiation protection of the patient in the context of external beam radiotherapy involves the assurance that the prescribed dose is delivered to the correct patient at the correct time, with acceptable geometric and dosimetric accuracy. It is beyond the scope of this chapter to discuss in detail all the factors which could contribute to this objective, since it involves the entire dosimetry chain and all the radiographic procedures for both planning and treatment. It is important, however, to ensure that procedures exist for identifying and rectifying incidents or errors which may affect a patient's treatment. Figure 17.2 outlines a procedure in which action is taken if an error due to equipment failure occurs. The nature of the action depends upon the magnitude of the error and whether correction is possible within the constraints of the treatment schedule.

In addition, errors of more than 5% may lead to key staff, management, outside agencies, and the patient being informed. The action levels of more than +10% (or more than +20% for any fraction) are requirements of the UK Health and Safety Executive [7]. A similar diagram may be devised to describe the procedure in the event of human or procedural error.

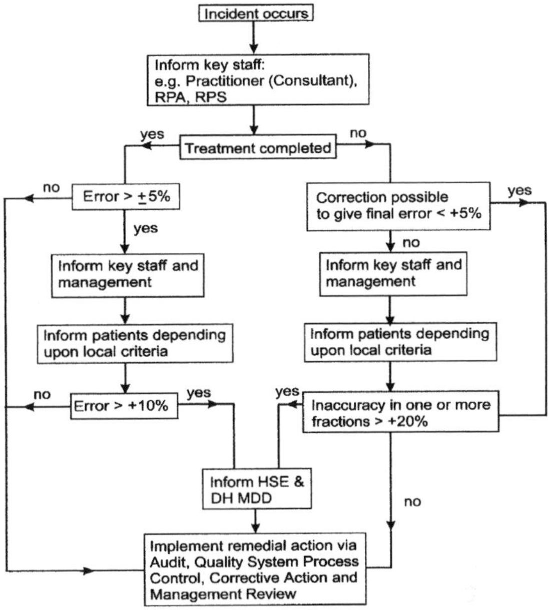

Figure 17.2 A procedure for investigating a possible incident caused by failure of radiotherapy equipment. HSE, Health and Safety Executive; DH MDD, Department of Health Equipment Devices Directorate.

17.3 Megavoltage and ^{60}Co equipment

17.3.1 General features of linear accelerators

Linear accelerators (linacs) producing X-ray beams with maximum energies in the range 4–25 MV are available from a number of manufacturers and are the most common devices currently used for delivering external beam radiotherapy. X-rays are produced from a high-energy electron beam utilizing bremsstrahlung interactions in a transmission-type metal target. Some accelerators also feature an alternative electron treatment mode, essentially by withdrawing the target from the electron beam path, inserting one or more scattering foils, and making a number of other adjustments for safe and practical usage. Because of their limited range in tissue, electron beams tend to be used for single-field superficial treatments whereas the X-ray beam is highly penetrating and is used in multiple-beam arrangements to treat deep-seated targets (e.g. pelvic tumours). Overall, the relative usage of megavoltage X-rays to electrons is of the order of 10:1.

For any accelerator, a maximum energy limit is set by the waveguide design and input power. On some accelerators, alternative (lower) energy beams are available by, for example, varying either the input power or effectively utilizing less of the available power to accelerate the electrons in the waveguide. Corresponding alterations to other running parameters and calibrations are also required.

Linear accelerators are usually mounted isocentrically on a 'C'-shaped gantry. The isocentre corresponds with the rotational axes of the collimating system, gantry, and treatment couch. By positioning the centre of the tumour at the isocentre, multiple-beam treatments are effected by simple rotational (as opposed to translational and rotational) movements of the treatment unit around the patient. The distance from X-ray source to the isocentre (SID) is usually set to 1 m. From the perspective of radiation protection, the significance of this mounting arrangement is that there is a strictly limited solid angle of possible direct beam incidence on the walls, floor, and ceiling of the treatment room. These are correspondingly designed as primary barriers as distinct from secondary barriers which cannot be intercepted by the primary beam.

At megavoltage energies, the predominant direction of the bremsstrahlung produced by the interacting electron is in the forward direction of the incident electron. Despite this, considerable radiation shielding is required around the target area of the radiation head to avoid high levels of unwanted stray radiation (leakage). The leakage dose rate must be less than 0.5% of the main beam isocentre dose rate at 1 metre from the path of electrons from the gun to the target (averaged over an area of 100 cm^2) [8–12]. However, in practice, commercial linac manufacturers frequently quote leakage levels less than 0.1%. The maximum possible dimension of the primary beam is determined by the divergence of the circular aperture in the radiation shielding close to the target which is known as the primary collimator. Appropriately dimensioned fields for treatment are achieved by a system of orthogonally mounted secondary collimators downstream of the primary collimator and closer to the patient.

Beam performance is monitored and exposure controlled by an integrating dosemeter (transmission-type ionisation chamber) in the radiation head which requires periodic calibration against an external reference standard. A redundant secondary chamber and exposure timer are provided as a back-up in case of failure of the primary dosemeter. Exposures are initiated by setting a predetermined number of 'monitor' units (mu) at the linac control console. The exposure is terminated when this number is reached. It is usual to adjust the sensitivity of the integrating dose monitors to correspond to a convenient delivered dose at the isocentre under reference conditions–usually 0.01 Gy per mu.

Typically, X-ray dose rates of the order of 2–5 Gy min^{-1} in the photon mode are available depending on equipment and running parameters. Potentially higher rates are available in the electron mode but dose rates are usually restricted to be comparable to those in the X-ray mode. Ozone formed by irradiation of the air should be removed by a ventilation system which should ensure that concentrations are below 0.1 ppm.

Above 10 MV, the potential exists for production of neutrons as a result of photonuclear interactions (see §2.5.5). Neutrons can also be emitted from elements heavier than bismuth by photon- or electron-induced fission, an interaction process which has no lower energy threshold but which is usually negligible, even in uranium.

The practical consequences of both types of interaction are the following.

- There may be induced activity in the walls of the room and the radiation head of a linear accelerator operating at above 10 MV, due to the decay of the products of (γ, n) reactions and subsequent neutron capture. This requires consideration and appropriate working arrangements, particularly during maintenance procedures on the radiation head.

  For example, both experiment and theory have demonstrated dose rates of 10 μSv h^{-1} (persisting for 40 min) at the walls of the room following a 30-min irradiation with 18 MV photons [2, appendix III.6]. There are relatively few experimental data available but it is likely that ^{28}Al ($T_{\frac{1}{2}} = 2.3$ min), ^{49}Ca ($T_{\frac{1}{2}} = 8.8$ min), and ^{24}Na ($T_{\frac{1}{2}} = 2.3$ min), due to thermal neutron capture, are significant components. In practice, irradiation times will be much shorter than 30 min and there should be no significant enhancement of personal doses to radiographic staff undertaking normal duties.
- Induced activity in the treatment head (target, collimators, flattening filter) poses a potentially more serious problem, particularly if maintenance of the head is needed immediately following irradiation, with dose rates of up to 300 μSv h^{-1} within the collimator jaws, 35 μSv h^{-1} near the surface of the head, and 18 μSv h^{-1} at the treatment couch following a 30-min irradiation at 18 MV [2, appendix III.6]. These dose rates reduced to 100, 10, and 3 μSv h^{-1}, respectively, after 35 min. Dose rates will be lower for more typical treatment times but should nevertheless be considered for the safety of maintenance staff.
- Small quantities of radioactive gases are produced in the air which can be mitigated by provision of adequate ventilation.
- There is a very small (< 0.4%) neutron dose equivalent contribution in the useful beam and some negligible induced activity in the patient.
- Neutron (and associated photon) dose equivalents at maze exits and treatment room doors may require specific consideration because of the general incompatibility of neutron and photon protection design requirements (see §17.4.4 Maze design: neutrons).

17.3.2 General features of cobalt-60 units

^{60}Co teletherapy units are an alternative source of high-energy photons for external beam radiotherapy but their relative popularity is diminishing. They offer high reliability and relatively low operating costs. They are less satisfactory than low-energy linacs in respect of beam penetration, penumbra width, and available dose rate. The latter is usually no greater than 2 Gy min^{-1} at the isocentre and diminishes exponentially as the activity decreases over the working lifetime until the source is replaced.

Like a linear accelerator, modern ^{60}Co units are mounted isocentrically. The source container is situated within a highly protected radiation shield, within which an aperture provides the primary collimation. Exposure is initiated either by movement of a shielded shutter which exposes the aperture or by movement of the source so that it is aligned with the aperture. Secondary collimation required for the production of treatment fields is achieved by an additional pair of orthogonally mounted secondary collimators similar to a linear accelerator.

Duration of exposure is controlled by means of a presettable primary and back-up timer system. The signals for initiating timer function are activated by movement of the shutter or source. In its standby (beam off) state, allowable head leakage is 0.02 mGy h^{-1} at 1 m from the source. During an exposure, the maximum allowable leakage is 0.2% of the primary beam dose rate under geometric conditions specified in BS5724 [13]. Departments should have contingency plans to cover circumstances when the exposed source is unable to be secured in the 'safe' position due to mechanical and/or electrical failure. These plans should cover the action to be taken to manoeuvre manually the source or shutter, usually by means of a wheel or lever on the treatment head, and to assist the patient from the room. The gantry should be rotated if possible so that the primary beam points away from those carrying out these operations.

17.4 Megavoltage and ^{60}Co room design

As indicated above, the isocentric mounting of linear accelerators and cobalt units means that there is a strictly limited solid angle of primary beam confinement. This means that a primary/secondary barrier approach may be usefully employed in designing the protection features.

The most commonly used barrier material is concrete (density 2350 kg m^{-3}). Steel plates may be used to supplement a concrete barrier (usually at increased cost) where space is limited. An alternative high atomic number material manufactured in the form of interlocking bricks (Ledite^{TM}) is available commercially and may also be used to reduce the linear barrier thickness and thus save space.

The general principles of barrier thickness design may be described in the following stages:

1. Estimation of the acceptable TADR on the 'safe' side of the barrier, in accordance with the ALARP principle and national regulations.
2. Estimation of the workload and duty cycle (see Box 17.1–17.3 for definitions), based on departmental working practices.
3. Estimation, from 1 and 2, of the acceptable instantaneous dose rate on the 'safe' side of the barrier.
4. Calculation of the instantaneous unattenuated dose rate at the same point as in 3 and the generation of an attenuation factor.
5. Calculation of the barrier thickness in terms of numbers of tenth-value (TVL) or half-value (HVL) layers and translation into a thickness of the shielding material of choice.

Some typical minimum barrier thicknesses, which should be used only as planning guidelines, are given in Table 17.2 (§17.8). TVL values for concrete, concrete/steel, and concrete/lead thickness ratios are given as a function of X-ray energy in Table 17.2 (§17.8).

17.4.1 Primary barriers

The application of these steps for a primary barrier is illustrated in Figure 17.3 and Boxes 17.1–17.6. The barrier thickness thus calculated should be entirely adequate for protection against leakage and scattered radiation. It is advisable to provide a margin to the distal lateral extent of the barrier, *l*, shown in Figure 17.3, based on the maximum field size. Thus:

$$l > d_{\mathrm{prim}}\, L_{\mathrm{diag}}/\mathrm{SID} \qquad (17.1)$$

where L_{diag} is the maximum field diagonal at the source–isocentre distance (SID) and d_{prim} is as shown in the diagram. A rough guide is that $l \approx 2d_{\mathrm{prim}}/3$ for a 40 × 40 cm field at an SID of 100 cm.

17.4.2 Secondary barriers

Regions of the walls, ceiling, and floor which are not irradiated directly by the primary beam are termed secondary barriers and must be designed to provide sufficient attenuation of leakage and scattered radiation.

Standards for acceptable leakage dose rates have been given in §17.3.1. Monte Carlo calculations suggest that scattering in the treatment head leads to a reduced leakage radiation energy compared with the primary beam [14], with a corresponding reduction in TVL (Table 17.3; §17.8).

Scatter dose rates are of the order of 0.1% of the incident dose rate (per 100 cm^2 irradiated). Thus wall thicknesses calculated for leakage radiation will be sufficient to provide adequate shielding for scatter also [15], although care should be taken when dealing with small-angle forward scatter, which may be similar in energy to the primary beam.

For both scatter and leakage radiation, it is possible to allow for the obliquity of the incident radiation on a barrier, but this is scarcely worthwhile in practice and normal incidence is usually assumed. This will, of course, introduce an overestimate of the dose rate on the 'safe' side of the secondary barrier. The stages in the calculation follow those given previously up to the estimation of the acceptable unattenuated dose rate on the safe side of the barrier. The secondary barrier thickness may then be calculated if the leakage dose rate is known.

Box 17.1 Estimation of the acceptable time-averaged dose rate on the 'safe' side of a primary barrier

Starting from a decision to adopt an acceptable maximum annual dose for a particular staff group, we can estimate, for the purposes of room design, the time-averaged dose rate (TADR), D'_{av}, due to primary radiation on the 'safe' side of a primary barrier for megavoltage installations (please note units):

The TADR (D'_{av}) for the working day in μSv h^{-1} is given by:

$$D'_{av} = \frac{D_{acc} \,.\, 10^3}{(w \,.\, d \,.\, h)} \qquad (17.2)$$

where:

D_{acc} is the acceptable maximum annual dose (mSv $year^{-1}$) for a particular group
w is the number of treatment weeks per year
d is the number of treatment days per week
h is the number of hours in a working day.

Box 17.2 Estimation of the workload

The workload (W_L) in Gy $week^{-1}$ is given by:

$$W_L = D_{presc} \,.\, N \,.\, d \qquad (17.3)$$

where:

N is the number of patients treated per day
D_{presc} is the mean or typical prescribed dose at the isocentre (Gy) per patient.

Box 17.3 Estimation of the duty cycle

The duty cycle C (i.e. the fraction of the time that the beam is on, $C \leq 1$) is given by:

$$C = \frac{W_L}{(D'_0 \,.\, 60 \,.\, h \,.\, d)} \qquad (17.4)$$

where D'_0 is the dose rate at the isocentre (Gy min^{-1}).

Box 17.4 Estimation of the acceptable instantaneous dose rate on the 'safe' side of a primary barrier

Using the results from Boxes 17.1–17.3, for a given TADR, D'_{av}, the acceptable instantaneous dose rate (IDR) D'_{inst} due to primary radiation on the 'safe' side of a primary barrier may be estimated as follows:

$$D'_{inst} = \frac{D'_{av}}{(C \,.\, f_0 \,.\, \Omega_f)} \qquad (17.5)$$

where:

f_0 is the beam orientation factor (i.e. the fraction of time that the beam irradiates a particular barrier)
Ω_f is the occupancy factor, i.e. the fraction of the working week spent by an individual in the area to be protected.

Box 17.5 Example estimation of TADR and IDR

Suppose:

- Acceptable maximum annual dose (D_{acc}) = 0.5 mSv year^{-1}
- Dose rate at the isocentre (D'_0) = 3 Gy min^{-1}
- Number of treatment weeks per year (w) = 50
- Prescribed dose at the isocentre (D_{presc}) = 4 Gy
- Number of patients treated per day (N) = 50
- Number of treatment days per week (d) = 5
- Number of hours in a working day (h) = 8
- Beam orientation factor (f_0) = 0.25
- Occupancy factor (Ω_f) = 1.0

Then:
The TADR is 0.25 μSv h^{-1}, the duty cycle is 0.14, and the IDR is 7.1 μSv h^{-1}. This area would be neither controlled nor supervised.

Box 17.6 Calculation of barrier thickness

The unattenuated dose rate D'_A at point A in Figure 17.3 is given by:

$$D'_A = \frac{D'_0}{d^2_{prim}} \qquad (17.6)$$

The attenuation factor η is given by:

$$\eta = \frac{D_{inst}'}{D_A'} \qquad (17.7)$$

and the thickness of the barrier in TVLs, n_{TVL}, is given by

$$n_{TVL} = -log_{10}\eta \qquad (17.8)$$

or, in terms of the number of HVLs, n_{HVL}

$$n_{HVL} = \frac{-ln\ \eta}{0.693} \qquad (17.9)$$

Some TVLs for concrete, lead, and steel are given in Table 17.8.2 (§17.8).

An example calculation is given in Boxes 17.7 and 17.8, with reference to Figure 17.3, which, for this room configuration, also indicates the need to take transmitted leakage and scattered radiation into account—in addition to radiation scattered down the maze—when estimating the dose rate at the maze entrance. Calculations should be based on the minimum distance between the source of leakage radiation and a point such as B, depending on the orientation of the gantry.

Typical attenuation values for primary and secondary barriers are of the order of 10^{-6} and 10^{-3}, respectively.

17.4.3 Roof and skyshine

Roof thickness may be calculated as outlined in §17.4.1 and §17.4.2. It is usually possible to allow higher IDRs from the upward-pointing primary beam than from other beam orientations if access to the roof is prohibited during linac operation. The roof area will then be a controlled area. However, the ease with which roof access can be subsequently controlled or prohibited during routine operation should be considered at an early stage in the design. IDRs of up to 2 mSv h^{-1} are usually acceptable, unless surrounding buildings encroach or the resulting skyshine (see below) is excessive. Obviously, if occupied premises are built above the treatment room,

Box 17.7 Calculation of secondary barrier thickness for leakage radiation

The determination of the acceptable instantaneous dose rate D'_{inst} follows the procedures outlined in Boxes 17.1–17.4, but with an orientation factor of unity, to allow for the emission of leakage radiation in all directions.
The actual unattenuated instantaneous dose rate D'_B in μSv h^{-1} at point B in Figure 17.3 is given by:

$$D'_B = \frac{D'_0 \,.\, \varepsilon \,.\, 60 \,.\, 10^6}{d_{leak}^{\;2}} \qquad (17.10)$$

where:
D'_0 is the dose rate at the isocentre (Gy min^{-1})
ε is the leakage dose rate (expressed as a fraction of D'_0) at 1 m from the gun–target electron path
d_{leak} is the minimum distance from the gun–target electron path to the point B in Figure 17.3

The attenuation factor η is given by:

$$\eta = \frac{D_{inst}{}'}{D_B{}'} \qquad (17.11)$$

and, as before, the thickness of the barrier in TVLs, n_{TVL}, is given by

$$n_{TVL} = -log_{10}\eta$$

or, in terms of the number of HVLs, n_{HVL}

$$n_{HVL} = \frac{-ln\ \eta}{0.693}$$

Box 17.8 Example of maze dose-rate calculation

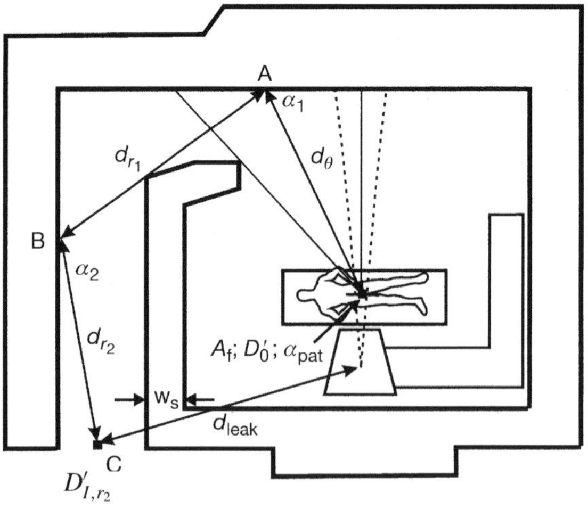

Figure B17.1 Room layout illustrating an empirical formula for maze exit dose rate.

For the case shown in Figure B17.1:

$$D'_{total} = D'_{I,r_2} = \frac{D'_0}{d_\theta^2} \cdot \frac{\alpha_1 A}{d_{r_1}^2} \cdot \frac{\alpha_2 A}{d_{r_2}^2} \cdot [\alpha_{pat} \cdot (A_f/400) + \epsilon] + \frac{\epsilon D'_0}{d_{leak}{}^2} \cdot \eta(\mathrm{w_s}) \qquad (17.17)$$

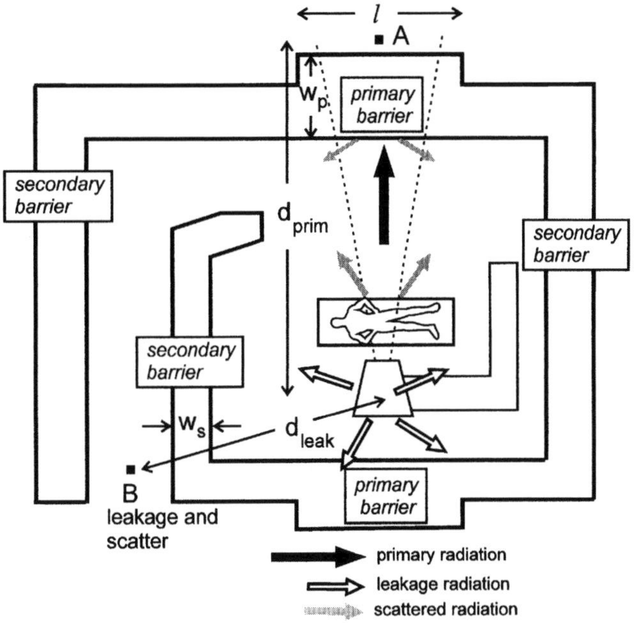

Figure 17.3 Plan of a linear accelerator suite showing design considerations for primary and secondary barrier shielding.

then the primary barrier thickness should be increased accordingly to provide acceptable dose rates.

An X-ray beam pointing upwards through a roof may lead to a measurable dose rate at ground level outside the building due to scatter from the air. This is known as skyshine.

An expression for skyshine is given in [16]. In the radiotherapy treatment room context, this may be expressed as

$$D'_{\text{sky}}/D'_1 = (2.5 \times 10^{-2})\Omega^{1.3}\eta_{\text{roof}}/d_s^{\,2} \qquad (17.12)$$

where:

D'_{sky} is the dose rate at point P in Figure 17.4;

D'_1 is the dose rate at 1 m from the source (same units as D'_{sky});

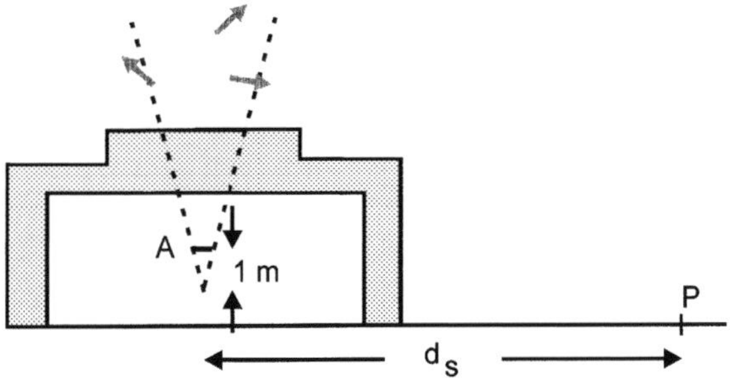

Figure 17.4 Calculation of skyshine.

Ω is the solid angle (in steradians) subtended by the X-ray source and the collimation. This may be approximated by A, the area of the beam (in m^2) at 1 m from the source;

η_{roof} is the attenuation provided by the roof;

d_s is the horizontal distance from the source to the point P in metres.

Monte Carlo calculations and measurements at 10 MV [2] suggest that this expression overestimates D_{sky} by a factor between 5 and 30, in particular close to the wall of the building where attenuation by the building itself is ignored in the expression. Moreover, equation (17.12) is based on ^{60}Co and ^{137}Cs γ-rays rather than megavoltage X-ray spectra. Although equation (17.12) may be used, with caution, for planning purposes, supplementary measurements are recommended in practice.

17.4.4 Room entry design

Principles

Entry design needs to take into account ease of access for staff and patients (including those on trolleys or beds) both in routine use and in emergencies, while simultaneously providing acceptable radiation protection. Access for equipment is clearly also important. At initial installation and on subsequent replacement, the largest items will be the components of the machine itself. It

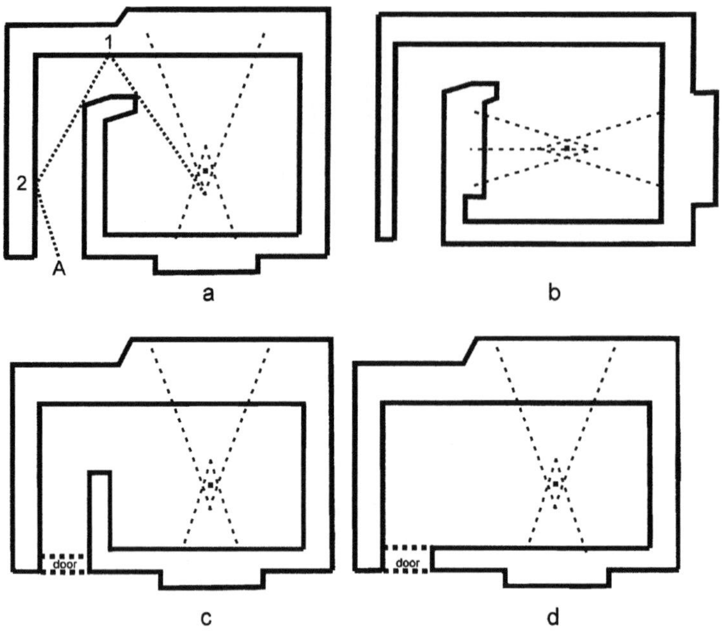

Figure 17.5 Four general designs for entry to a treatment room: (a) maze only; (b) maze incorporating primary barrier; (c) shortened maze with shielded door, giving smaller room area; (d) no maze, with shielded door acting as a full secondary barrier.

may be possible to remove part of a wall or roof temporarily for these infrequent but disruptive tasks.

Mazes

Mazes of various lengths and complexity are almost always used as the means of access to radiotherapy treatment rooms. However, their design may be modified by the addition of a shielded door, a practice more common outside the UK. Relatively long mazes may be designed so that multiple scattering and absorption along the length of the maze reduces the dose rate to acceptable design levels at the exit, thus dispensing with shielded doors, or indeed doors of any kind, allowing access to be controlled by visible light or infrared beams. The advantage of ease of entry to a door-less maze must be balanced by the increased floor area of the whole room and the distance that patients and staff need to travel down the maze.

The critical point of interest is usually at the entrance to the maze from outside the room. There may be several components to the dose rate at this point:

- X-rays scattered from primary beam interactions with the patient
- X-rays from primary beam and scatter interactions with the room surfaces
- Leakage X-rays scattered down the maze from the treatment head
- Leakage X-rays transmitted through the interior maze wall
- Neutrons scattered down the maze (for accelerators operating above 10 MV)
- Capture γ-rays generated at or near the maze entrance by scattered neutrons (average γ-ray energy 3.6 MeV for neutrons on concrete).

Shielded doors

Motorized shielded doors are available commercially and their use means that the maze may be considerably shortened, leading to advantages in floor area and a shorter route to the treatment couch. This is offset to some extent by the extra time needed to open and close a heavy shielded door, especially in the event of an emergency. There is always the possibility of mechanical or electrical failure of a motorized door, so that fail-safe devices will be required. Shielded doors for 15 MV are typically constructed from layers of lead (~6 mm) and borated polyethylene (~80 mm) sandwiched between steel sheets (each ~6 mm).

Maze design: photons

One of the problems with measuring maze dose-rate data is that the experimental conditions (e.g. room dimensions and geometry) cannot easily be varied systematically. Thus empirical formulae have been developed and tested on a relatively small range of room sizes and designs.

However, the increasing utilization of Monte Carlo simulations may allow a wider range of designs to be explored, at least theoretically.

Four general examples of maze design are given in Figure 17.5(a–d). In Figure 17.5(a), a maze is used without a shielded door to attenuate scatter from the patient and the primary barrier. In Figure 17.5(b), the central axis is rotated so that the maze wall acts as one of the primary barriers. In this case, scatter at the maze exit is supplemented by transmitted radiation when the beam points to the left in the diagram. In Figure 17.5(c), the shortened maze requires a shielded door, and in Figure 17.5(d), with no maze, the door shielding would be equivalent to a secondary barrier. The designs shown in Figures 17.5(a) and 17.5(c) and their variants are probably the most common.

As a rule of thumb, for a maze without a shielded door, an observer positioned at the maze exit (point C in the figure in Box 17.8) should see two 'reflections' (A and B in the figure) and should not be able to see any area of the room's interior surface which is intercepted by the primary beam.

Several empirical methods for the calculation of scatter down a treatment room maze have been described in the literature [16–19]. The method described here assumes that scatter from the patient and leakage radiation, rather than radiation scattered from the first reflecting surface (the primary barrier), are the main contributions to the dose rate at the treatment room end of the maze. Furthermore, there are several ways in which the contribution of scattered radiation from irradiated areas of walls, floor, and ceiling may be calculated. These include calculating the areas irradiated at each 'reflection' or simply using the cross-sectional area of the maze (assumed constant) as an approximation. The latter method is used here. The contribution from primary barrier scatter may be reduced by positioning the primary barrier as far as possible from the maze entrance. For designs where the primary barrier is close to the maze entrance, an additional calculation of scatter from this surface may be required.

With reference to the figure in Box 17.8, the scattered component of the instantaneous dose rate at the maze exit $D'_{\mathrm{I},n,\mathrm{scatter}}$, after n 'reflections', is given by

$$D'_{1,n,scatter} \cong \frac{D'_0.(\alpha_{pat}(MV,\theta)[A_f/400]}{d_\theta^2} \cdot \prod_{j=1}^{n} \frac{\alpha_j(E_{eff},\phi).A}{d_{rj}^2} \tag{17.13}$$

where:

D'_0 is the dose rate at the isocentre (assumed 1 m from the source), on the central axis, in the absence of scattering material;

α_{pat} is the dimensionless scatter coefficient, defined as the dose rate measured at 1 m from the phantom or patient when the field area is 400 cm^2 at the phantom surface, expressed as a fraction of the incident dose rate at the centre of the field 1 m from the source but without the phantom (i.e. D'_0). α_{pat} is a function of effective accelerating potential (MV) and scattering angle θ. Data for α_{pat} are reproduced in Table 17.4 (§17.8).

A_f is the field area at the phantom surface in cm^2;

d_θ is the distance in metres from the isocentre to the back wall of the maze along the direction of scatter indicated by the angle θ. The convention adopted here is to take d_θ as the distance from the isocentre to a point on the wall midway between the intersection of the central axis with the wall and a point corresponding to the line of maximum angle θ which grazes the nib of the maze (Box 17.8).

α_j are reflection coefficients given as functions of the effective photon energy E_{eff} and angle of incidence ϕ. It is often assumed that $E_{\mathrm{eff}} \approx 0.5$ MeV for all reflections apart from the first interaction of the beam with the primary barrier, although Numark and Kase [20] have suggested $E_{\mathrm{eff}} \approx 0.3$ MeV. Reflection coefficients are given in Figure 17.9 (§17.8) and related data may be found in [2].

For most common maze configurations and photon energies, order-of-magnitude dose-rate estimates may be obtained by using a value of $\alpha_j = 2 \times 10^{-2}$.

A is the cross-sectional area of the maze (assumed constant) in m^2;

d_{rj} are distances in metres between successive reflections as indicated in Box 17.8. Definitions of these distances in the literature may vary.

The expression for the instantaneous dose rate due to leakage radiation scattered down the maze, $D'_{\mathrm{I},n,\mathrm{leakage}}$ is

$$D'_{\mathrm{I,\ n,\ leakage}} \cong \frac{\varepsilon D'_0}{d_\theta^2} \cdot \prod_{j=1}^{n} \frac{\alpha_j(E_{\mathrm{eff}},\phi)\ .\ A}{d_{rj}^2} \tag{17.14}$$

where:

ϵ is the dose rate due to head leakage at 1 m from the source expressed as a fraction of the dose rate D'_0 at the isocentre.

Other symbols are as defined above.

The contribution to the point C (figure in Box 17.8) of leakage radiation transmitted through the secondary barrier, D_{trans}, is given by

$$D_{\mathrm{trans}} = \varepsilon D'_0/d_{\mathrm{leak}}{}^2 \eta(w_{\mathrm{s}}) \tag{17.15}$$

where:

d_{leak} is the distance defined in Box 17.8;

$\eta(w_{\mathrm{s}})$ is the attenuation of the secondary barrier (maze wall) using a normal thickness w_{s}, shown in Box 17.8.

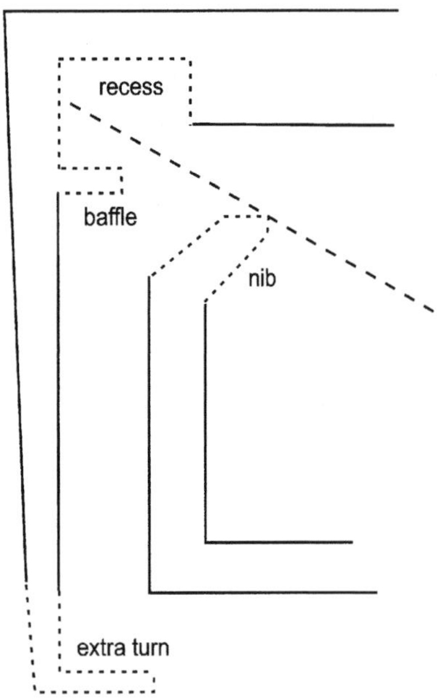

Figure 17.6 Scatter reduction features in maze design.

The total X-ray dose rate D'_{total} at C is given by

$$D'_{\text{total}} = D'_{\text{I, n, scatter}} + D'_{\text{I, }n\text{, leakage}} + D'_{\text{trans}}. \qquad (17.16)$$

More detailed examples of case studies and worked designs are given in [2]. These formulae are usually sufficiently accurate for most purposes and it is unreasonable, given the many assumptions and approximations, to expect empirical estimates and measurements to agree to better than a factor of two, particularly when the dose-rate reduction from the isocentre to the maze entrance amounts to seven orders of magnitude. If the maze is of an unusual configuration, however, Monte Carlo techniques may be employed to model photon transport down the maze using, for example, the MCNP code whose applications are reviewed in chapter 7 of [2].

Some modifications to the maze design are illustrated in Figure 17.6. A nib is commonly employed to reduce scatter and leakage reaching the treatment room end of the maze. In addition, a recess and baffle will further reduce the scatter down the maze. It may be possible to taper the outside wall of the maze, since the dose rate is progressively diminishing towards the exit. Ceiling lintels may be used to restrict the effective cross-sectional area of the maze. If the dose rate is still unacceptably high at the exit, a further turn may be employed. This will usually only be necessary for adequate neutron, rather than photon, protection.

Ducts to carry cables from the interior of the treatment room to the control console will be required for dosimetry purposes. These should not be sited within an area intercepted by the primary beam and should be angled to prevent direct transmission of scatter from the patient or leakage from the treatment head.

Maze design: neutrons

Above approximately 10 MeV, photonuclear (γ,n) reactions lead to near-isotropic fast neutron production at the target and other high atomic number components of the treatment head. These neutrons lose energy within the head by inelastic and (n,2n) reactions and emerge with an average energy typically of the order of 0.5 MeV and are subsequently scattered from the room surfaces. In general, maze design for an installation with a significant neutron component should favour turns and baffles as means of increasing the number of scattering events. As these neutrons scatter down the maze, the proportion of thermal neutrons increases. Several methods have been developed to estimate the neutron dose at the maze exit and these are summarized in [21]. One empirical method [22] assumes a tenth-value distance (TVD) of 5 m (i.e. the distance along the centreline of the maze over which the neutron intensity falls by a factor of 10). A first TVD of 3 m and a modified formula has been recommended in [2]:

$$D'_n = \frac{D'_0.R_{n.\gamma}.A}{d_\theta{}^2.10^{[1+(\Sigma\, d_{rj}-3)/5]}.S_0} \qquad (17.18)$$

where:

D'_n is the neutron absorbed dose rate at the maze entrance;

$R_{n,\gamma}$ is the neutron absorbed dose rate at the isocentre per unit photon absorbed dose rate, also at the isocentre. This will vary from 3×10^{-5} to 3×10^{-4} [2] and is subject to limits imposed by BS5724 [11].

S_0 is an area constant (6 m^2).

Other symbols have their previously defined meanings, although the distances d_{rj} in equation (17.18) are defined in references [2] and [22] as centreline distances.

This formula does not include the use of boron- or lithium-loaded polyethylene which may be used further to attenuate neutrons by the (n,γ) reaction, making use of the high neutron capture cross-sections for these elements. The ends of mazes may be lined with such material, although it may be more convenient to line a door if one is used. It should be noted that energetic γ-rays are produced in these reactions (0.48 MeV for boron capture and up to 10 MeV for concrete) and for installations with a relatively short maze, a door may need to incorporate lead or steel to reduce the γ-component. The dose equivalent rate due to capture γ-rays at the end of the maze may be taken as approximately 20% of the neutron absorbed dose rate at the same point, with a radiation weighting factor of unity [2] (§6.5).

For protection purposes, when combining X-ray and neutron contributions, the neutron equivalent dose should be calculated using radiation weighting factors given by ICRP [23] (see also Table 3.1). Measurement or estimation of the neutron spectrum at the maze exit is not trivial and in the absence of data, a worst-case radiation weighting factor of 20 could be used. However, for a maze with two or more turns and with lintels and baffles, the proportion of neutrons with energies greater than 100 keV is likely to be small, so that a radiation weighting factor of 10 may be justified.

Example calculation and measurement

Figure 17.7 illustrates a treatment room designed to accommodate a linear accelerator operating at 6, 15, and 25 MV at Newcastle upon Tyne. Examples of shielding calculations for this facility have been given in [2] but are reworked here (for 15 MV) to demonstrate the method described in this chapter (Table 17.1).

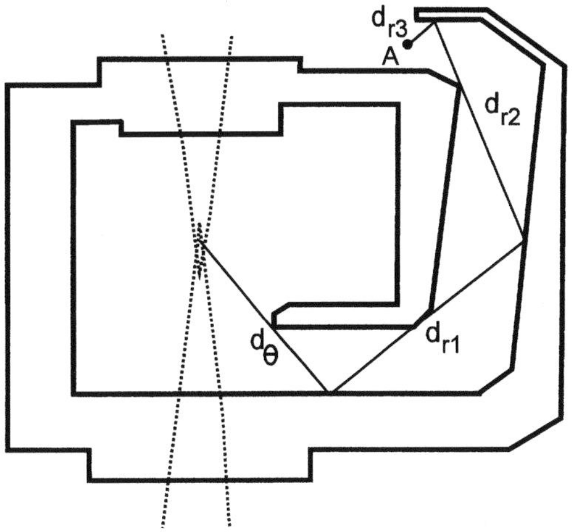

Figure 17.7 A treatment room designed to accommodate a linear accelerator operating at 6, 15, and 25 MV (not to scale).

Table 17.1 Calculated and measured dose rates at the maze exit for the 15 MV installation shown in Figure 17.7 with the beam pointing horizontally towards the treatment room end of the maze

Quantity	Data	Instantaneous dose rate at maze entrance (μSv h^{-1}) (Point A in Figure 17.7)		Comments
		Calculated	Measured	
X-ray scatter ($D'_{l,n,\text{ scatter}}$) + scattered leakage ($D'_{l,n,\text{ leakage}}$)	D'_0 = 4 Gy min^{-1} d_θ = 5.3 m d_{r1} = 5.9 m d_{r2} = 7.7 m d_{r3} = 2.0 m α_{pat} = 0.004 $\alpha_1 = \alpha_2 = \alpha_3 = 2 \times 10^{-2}$ A_f = 1600 cm^2 A = 6.8 m^2	0.05[a]		[a]Assuming (i) 0.5 MeV scatter from concrete (ii) α_{pat} (15 MV) α_{pat} (6 MV) at 30° (iii) 0.2% leakage
Transmitted leakage (D'_{trans})		0.56		
Prompt gammas		0.06[b]		[b]Assuming 0.2 x D'_n [2]
Total photon dose rate		0.67	0.5; 1.5[c]	[c] Measured for two nominally identical rooms
Neutron scatter (D'_n)	D'_0 = 4 Gy min^{-1} $R_{n,\gamma} = 10^{-4}$ Gy(n) Gy^{-1} (photon) A = 6.8 m^2 d_θ = 5.3 m $\sum d_{rj}$ = 15.6 m S_0 = 6 m	2.9[d]	<4	[d] Incorporating a radiation weighting factor = 10
Total equivalent dose rate		3.6	⩽5.5	

17.5 Protection for kilovoltage facilities

17.5.1 Kilovoltage X-ray equipment

For kilovoltage installations, design criteria may often need a different approach. This is because, unlike megavoltage installations which are purpose-built, kilovoltage installations are frequently adaptations of existing rooms and the shielding requirements to ensure consistent application of design criteria for occupational staff and the public may need to be supplemented by a restriction of beam direction detailed in the local rules.

Therapy X-ray equipment with peak-generating potentials between 50 and 150 kV (e.g. 1.0–8.0 mm Al HVL) are often described as 'superficial' X-ray units and those generating X-rays in the range 150–300 kV (e.g. 0.5–4.0 mm Cu HVL) as 'orthovoltage' units. These are not rigorous definitions and single treatment units spanning the entire range, i.e. 50–300 kV, are currently supplied by at least two manufacturers.

The use of superficial X-rays for the treatment of some forms of skin cancer is commonplace. The use of orthovoltage X-rays for the treatment of advanced skin cancer and other relatively superficial targets has become less common with the widespread availability of electron beams from linear accelerators which are an alternative treatment modality.

Orthovoltage and superficial X-ray equipment share some common features:

- The X-ray beam emerges from an aperture in a protected X-ray tube housing which acts as a primary collimator.
- Secondary collimation is provided by a number of individual demountable treatment applicators which define both the lateral extent of the beam and the treatment distance relative to the radiation source. The patient is positioned in contact with the proximal end of the applicator
- The X-ray tube is supported by a floor- or ceiling-mounted stand. The tube mounting is such that commonly there is no restriction in primary beam direction which is particularly significant in determining protection requirements.
- Focus–skin distance (FSD) for treatment usually lies in the range 15–50 cm and is determined by the applicator geometry. The lower values are associated with small-field size applicators and superficial units and the upper value with larger-field higher-energy treatments.
- The use of beam-hardening filters uniquely interlocked to selected tube voltage.

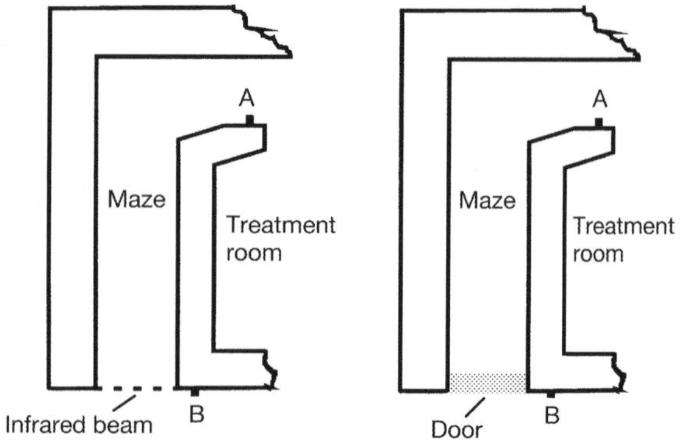

Figure 17.8 Safety interlock systems for a megavoltage treatment room.

- Surface dose rates for treatment vary widely. For short FSDs and low added filtration, dose rates of the order of 20 Gy min^{-1} may be available at maximum available tube currents but electively tube currents are often reduced to avoid very short treatment times. Conversely, for 50 cm FSD treatments and heavily filtered beams, dose rates may be as low as 0.5 Gy min^{-1}.

Depending on the maximum tube voltage, there are a number of differences in the specification standards of treatment units:

- The allowable leakage through the tube housing at a distance of 1 m is 10 mGy h^{-1} for orthovoltage units (>150 kV) and 1 mGy h^{-1} for superficial units (<150 kV) [12].
- For generating potentials greater than 150 kV, radiation exposure must be controlled by an integrated dose monitor system similar to a linear accelerator with back-up timer. Below 150 kV, exposure control can be by means of a dual timer system provided the tube potential and current are stabilized to within ±2% of preset values [24].

17.5.2 Kilovoltage X-ray room design

The X-ray tube mounting of kilovoltage X-ray units may allow direct irradiation of all walls, floor, and ceiling of the treatment room which would require their designation as primary barriers with corresponding levels of protection. In practice, it may be possible either mechanically or electrically to confine the range of possible beam directions without adversely restricting clinical usage. Alternatively, it might be possible to define working procedures in local rules which restrict operational usage in particular directions. This would enable financial savings to be made in the correspondingly less stringent shielding requirements.

Particularly above 150 kV, concrete is likely to be the lowest cost option for building room protection. Alternatives are brick or stud walls lined with lead ply or barytes plaster. Where space or building weight are at a premium, the high atomic number materials (lead, barytes plaster) may be preferred. Doors are likely to give direct entry to the treatment room and to be lead lined. Careful attention needs to be paid to closure overlaps and the frame construction. Viewing windows have traditionally been of lead glass but a modern CCTV system may be an acceptable lower cost option. Typical primary and secondary barrier thicknesses for orthovoltage radiation quantities are given in Table 17.5, §17.8.

17.6 Interlocks and warning systems

Several systems need to be implemented to ensure that access to the treatment room is prevented while the radiation beam is on.

Warning signs are required by legislation and should consist of four components: (i) the radiation trefoil; (ii) an indication of the nature of the hazard; (iii) an indication that entry is prohibited except for unauthorized personnel; and (iv) an indication that the interior of the treatment room is a controlled area when a warning light is on. The specification for signs is given in BS 5378 Part 1 [25].

Warning lights should indicate the imminent start of a radiation exposure and be illuminated continuously during the emission of radiation. They are required both at the entrance to the room and within the room. Both warning signs and lights should be positioned close to head height in a prominent position.

A parallel audible signal of radiation exposure should sound both inside and outside the room, together with a radiation monitor inside the room which emits a visible and/or audible indication of radiation and which is ideally powered independently from the radiotherapy equipment.

The maze entrance should be interlocked so that an exposure may only be initiated when the door or other barrier (e.g. made by an infrared beam) is closed. Closing the door should not in itself allow an exposure to be made. A suitable arrangement would be as follows: the last person to leave the room would activate a time-delay interlock (at A, in Figure 17.8) which allows just sufficient time to leave the room and operate switch B which makes operational the infrared beam or the door closure mechanism.

Interlock circuitry (e.g. for the detection of door closure) must be designed to be fail-safe.

Observation of the patient must be possible from the control console. This may be conveniently achieved by closed circuit television. Further patient protection measures include interlocks which control various aspects of the treatment, for example the correct set-up parameters as checked against a reference data set plan and aspects of machine operation such as dose rate and beam flatness.

17.7 Environmental monitoring

17.7.1 Requirements for environmental monitoring

In external beam radiotherapy, the primary objective is to ensure that the restriction of personal exposures remains adequate in areas immediately adjacent to the treatment room. Two kinds of dosimetry survey are required.

A commissioning survey should be carried out after a new installation has been built or whenever modifications have been made which may change the environmental dose rates in the vicinity of the treatment room. This should be a comprehensive survey based on design dose rates and is described in §17.7.3.

On a regular basis, a simplified survey should be carried out which is sufficient to demonstrate that the design dose rates continue to apply. This is necessary to cover increases in workload, such as the more frequent use of the highest energy beam from a dual-energy linear accelerator, increased patient throughput, or, very unusually, structural deterioration of shielding. Such surveys may be complemented by the results of a personal monitoring programme.

17.7.2 Commissioning survey

Primary barriers

Primary barriers should be tested by pointing the maximum energy X-ray beam at each primary barrier in turn with no intervening material and scanning the 'safe' side over its entire area with a suitable survey meter, investigating unusual or significant variations from the design dose rates. Both typical and maximum field sizes should be investigated. Contributions due to small-angle scatter just outside the primary barrier should be investigated by directing the beam into a full-scatter water or water-equivalent phantom positioned at the normal treatment distance.

Secondary barriers

The X-ray beam should be directed into a full-scatter water phantom. Several orientations of the beam may be required. For example, the beam should be directed horizontally through the phantom towards a given primary barrier to generate scatter incident on the adjacent secondary barrier as well as vertically into the phantom. The angular orientation of the gantry should also be varied to minimize the distance between the X-ray target and the measuring point and to maximize the contribution to an external point from leakage radiation. As for the primary barrier case, the barrier should be scanned over its entire area and unusual or significant variations from the design dose rates investigated. The exercise should be repeated for all available X-ray energies and for both typical and maximum field sizes.

Mazes

The critical dose rate is usually at the maze entrance. Dose rates should be measured at this point for worst-case beam direction (normally the maximum field size pointing at the wall at the treatment end of the maze, with and without scatterer in place). Unusual results may require dose rates at other points along the maze to be made. These should be carried out using a remote camera to observe the monitoring instrument when the beam is on.

Control area

Actual and design dose rates at this location should be measured for worst-case beam orientations, usually the unattenuated beam pointing in the direction of the control area or conditions of maximum scatter down the maze. Several measurement points may be necessary, depending on the size of the control area and occupancy patterns. These should include the points at which subsequent routine environmental monitoring is to take place.

Some texts advise against a room design which allows the primary beam to point directly at the control console, even when adequately shielded. Although this arrangement should be avoided if possible, the authors' view is that such an arrangement is acceptable provided that a comprehensive commissioning survey is carried out, followed by regular personal and environmental monitoring.

17.7.3 Routine environmental monitoring

Personal monitoring dosimeters (TLD or film badge) may be used. A small number of critical points around the installation should have been chosen at the design stage and dose rates at these points under specified conditions measured at commissioning. The choice of these points will depend on the design of the room but should include at least one location within the control area and the maze entrance and any adjoining areas of public occupancy or offices, on the same level, above or below. It is suggested that an annual survey is appropriate. Dosimeters should be mounted on walls or other locations where they will not be disturbed or damaged. Approximately three control dosimeters should be stored in a location where they will be exposed only to natural background radiation. Dosimeters should be left in place for a maximum of 8 weeks and the results after processing compared with those of previous surveys and initial commissioning tests. The integrated dose over this period should reflect both the integrity of the barriers and workload changes. IDR measurements may also be useful at these locations, particularly in the investigation of anomalous survey results.

17.8 Useful data

The purpose of this section is to draw together some previously published data for shielding calculations.

Table 17.2 Typical minimum barrier thicknesses (mm) of concrete (density 2355 kg m^{-3}) (*Note: For initial estimation purposes only*)

Type of shielding	4 MV	6 MV	10 MV	15 MV	18 MV	20 MV	24 MV
Primary (general: 100% occupancy)	1675	1980	2185	2390	2440	2490	2540
Primary (exterior: 10% occupancy)	1320	1575	1830	1980	2030	2085	2135
Secondary (general: 100% occupancy)	840	915	1065	1065	1065	1145	1220
Secondary (exterior: 10% occupancy)	610	610	760	915	915	915	1065
Door shielding							
lead	3	3	6	6	19	19	19
wood	51	51	76	n/a	n/a	n/a	n/a
2% borated polyethylene	n/a	n/a	n/a	76	102	102	102
steel—both sides	n/a	n/a	n/a	6	6	6	6

Courtesy Varian Associates, Inc. (1992).

Table 17.3 TVLs in mm for concrete (density 2355 kg m^{-3}), with concrete/steel and concrete/lead ratios

	4 MV	6 MV	10 MV	15 MV	18 MV	20 MV	24 MV
Leakage X-rays (90)	254	279	305	330	330	343	356
Primary beam	290	343	389	432	445	457	470
Concrete to lead and steel ratios (mm of concrete equivalent to mm of lead or steel)							
Steel: primary	3.2	3.5	3.7	4.0	4.0	4.1	4.4
Steel: secondary	3.2	3.5	3.6	3.8	3.8	3.9	4.0
Lead: primary	5.4	6.2	7.0	7.6	8.0	8.3	9.0
Lead: secondary	5.4	6.2	6.6	7.0	7.0	7.0	7.0

Courtesy Varian Associates, Inc. (1992).

Table 17.4 Scatter coefficients, α_{pat} (dose rates measured at 1 m from the patient when the field area is 400 cm^2, as a fraction of D_0')

Source	Scattering angle (from central ray)					
	30	45	60	90	120	135
X-rays						
50 kV	0.0005	0.0002	0.00025	0.00035	0.0008	0.0010
70 kV	0.00065	0.00035	0.00035	0.0005	0.0010	0.0013
100 kV	0.0015	0.0012	0.0012	0.0013	0.0020	0.0022
125 kV	0.0018	0.0015	0.0015	0.0015	0.0023	0.0025
150 kV	0.0020	0.0016	0.0016	0.0016	0.0024	0.0026
4 MV	–	0.0027	–	–	–	–
6 MV	0.004	0.0018	0.0011	0.0006	–	0.0004
Gamma rays						
^{137}Cs	0.0065	0.0050	0.0041	0.0028	–	0.0019
^{60}Co	0.0060	0.0036	0.0023	0.0009	–	0.0006

Reproduced from NCRP Report 49 (1976), table B2, by permission of the National Council on Radiation Protection and Measurements, USA.

Table 17.5 Typical primary and secondary barrier thicknesses for orthovoltage radiation quantities

Radiation source	Attenuation factor	Thickness (mm)	
		Lead	Concrete (2350 kg m^{-3})
Primary			
100 kV	10^{-3}	2.4	165
300 kV		17	460
Secondary			
100 kV	10^{-1}	1	60
300 kV		7	260

Reproduced from IPEM Report 75, table 5.2, with permission of the Institute of Physics and Engineering in Medicine.

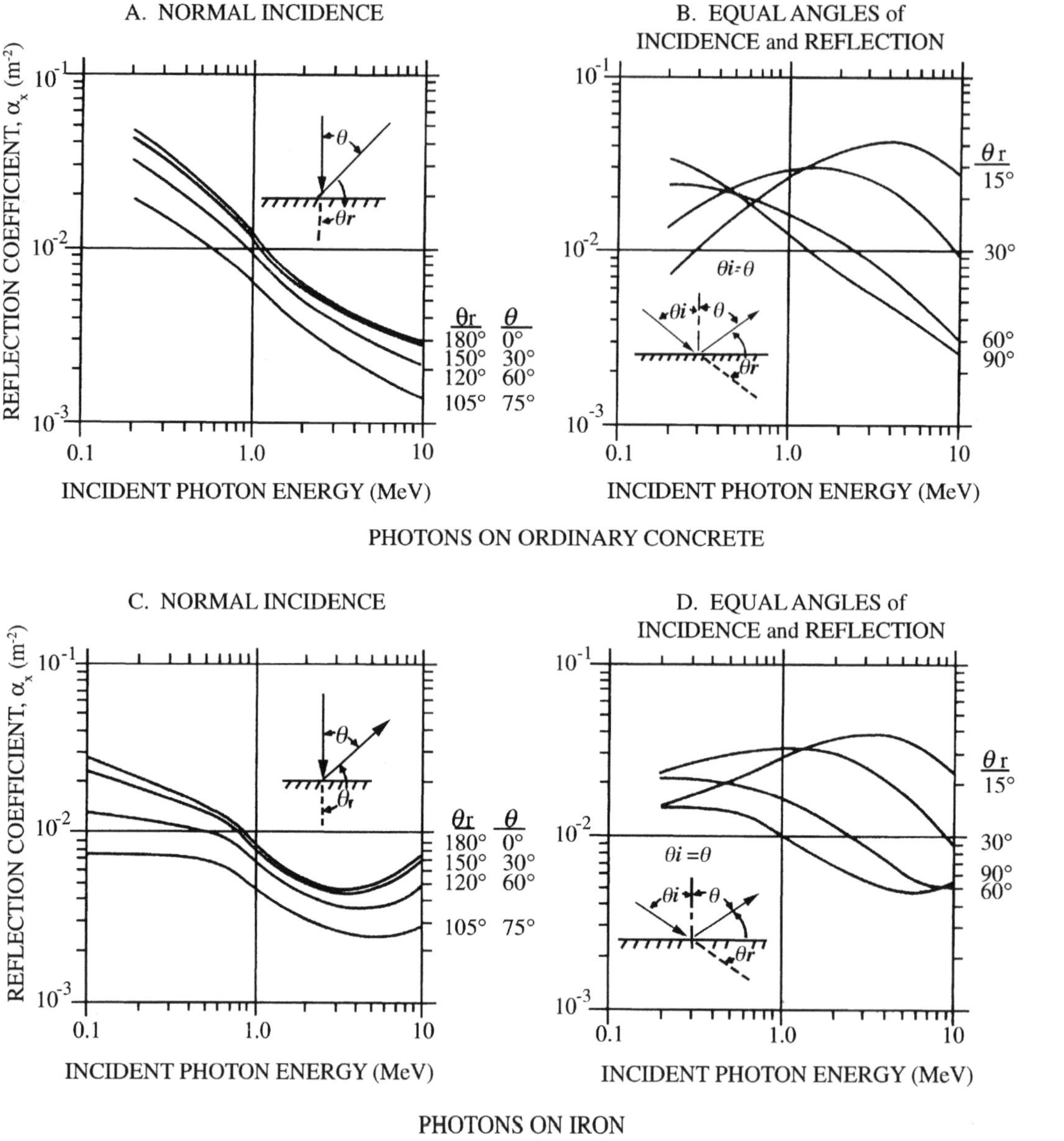

Figure 17.9 Reflection coefficients, α_x, for monoenergetic X-rays on concrete and iron as a function of photon energy for normal incidence (A and C) and equal angles of incidence and reflection (C and D). For photon energies greater than 10 MeV, in the absence of other data, the values of α_x for 10 MeV should be used. For photons incident on lead, a conservative upper limit of $\alpha_x = 5 \times 10^{-3}$ for any energy and scattering angle should be used. (Reproduced by permission of the National Council on Radiation Protection and Measurements, USA, from NCRP Report 51 [16], appendix E, figure E15.)

17.9 References

1 Royal College of Radiologists (1999). Clinical Oncology Information Network (COIN): guidance for external beam radiotherapy. *Clin. Oncol., R. Coll. Radiol.*, **11**, 5135–72.

2 Institute of Physics and Engineering in Medicine (1997). *The design of radiotherapy treatment room facilities*. IPEM Report 75. IPEM, York.

3 National Radiological Protection Board (1993). 1990 Recommendations of the International Commission on Radiological Protection. Recommendations for the practical application of the board's statement. *Doc. NRPB*, **4** (1), 9–22.

4 Institute of Physics and Engineering in Medicine (1986). *Radiation protection in radiotherapy*. Report No. 46. Institute of Physical Sciences in Medicine.

5 British Standards Institution (1994). *Quality systems–specification for design, development, production, installation and servicing*. BS EN ISO 9001. BSI, London.

6 British Standards Institution (1994). *Quality systems–model for quality assurance in production, installation and servicing*. BS EN ISO 9002. BSI, London

7 Health and Safety Executive (1992). *Fitness of equipment used for medical exposure to ionising radiation*. Guidance note PM77.

8 National Council on Radiation Protection and Measurements (1989). *Medical X-ray, electron beam and gamma ray protection for energies up to 50 MeV*. NCRP Report 102. NCRP, Bethesda, MD.

9 International Commission on Radiological Protection (1984). *Protection of the patient in radiation therapy*. ICRP Publication 44. ICRP, Pergamon Press.

10 British Standards Institution (1988, 1989, 1991). BS 5724. Medical Electrical Equipment. Part 1 IEC 601-1 (1988) *General requirements for safety*. Part 2 Section 2.1 (1989) *Particular requirements for safety. Specification for medical electron accelerators in the range 1 MeV to 50 MeV*. Part 2 Section 2.1 Suppl. 1 (1991) *Particular requirements for safety. Specification for medical electron accelerators in the range 1 MeV to 50 MeV*. BSI, London.

11 British Standards Institution (1991). BS 5724. Medical Electrical Equipment. Part 2 Section 2.1 *Particular requirements for safety. Specification for medical electron accelerators in the range 1 MeV to 50 MeV*. BSI, London.

12 British Standards Institution (1987). BS 5724 Section 2.8 (IEC 601-2-8:1987). *Specification for therapeutic X-ray generators*. BSI, London.

13 British Standards Institution (1989). BS 5724. Medical Electrical Equipment. Part 2 Section 2.11. *Specification for gamma beam therapy equipment*. BSI, London.

14 Nelson, W. R. and LaRiviere, P. D. (1984). Primary and leakage radiation calculations at 6, 10 and 25 MeV. *Health Phys.*, **47**, 811–18.

15 Almen, A., Ahlgren, L., and Mattsson, S. (1994). Leakage photon radiation around accelerators used for radiotherapy. *J. Radiat. Prot.*, **14**, 349–57.

16 National Council on Radiation Protection and Measurements (1977). *Radiation protection design guidelines for 0.1–100 MeV particle accelerator facilities*. NCRP Report 51. NCRP, Bethesda, MD.

17 McGinley, P. H. and James, J. L. (1997). Maze design methods for 6- and 10-MeV accelerators. *Radiat. Prot. Manage.*, January/February, 14(1), 59–64.

18 Morgan, S., Morgan, H. M., and Lillicrap, S. C. (1995). Dose rates and energy spectra in the maze of a linear accelerator treatment room. *Br. J. Radiol.*, **68**, 1237–41.

19 Morgan, S., Morgan, H. M., and Lillicrap, S. C. (1996). Dose rates and energy spectra in the maze of a linear accelerator treatment room (addendum). *Br. J. Radiol.*, **69**, 977.

20 Numark, N. J. and Kase, K. R. (1985). Radiation transmission and scattering for medical linacs producing X-rays of 6 and 15 MV: comparison of calculations with measurements. *Health Phys.*, **48** (3), 289–95.

21 National Council on Radiation Protection and Measurements (1984). *Neutron contamination from medical accelerators*. NCRP Report No. 79. NCRP, Bethesda, MD.

22 Kersey, R. W. (1979). Estimation of neutron and gamma radiation doses in the entrance mazes of SL75-20 linear accelerator treatment rooms. *Medicamundi*, **24**, 151–5.

23 International Commission on Radiological Protection (1990). Recommendations of the International Commission on Radiological Protection. ICRP Publication 60. *Ann. ICRP*, **21**.

24 Department of Health and Social Security (1975). *Recommendations of the radiotherapy apparatus safety measures panel*. Document RASMP/75.

25 British Standards Institution (1980). BS 5378 Part 1: *Safety signs and colours. Specification for colour and design*. BSI, London.

Chapter 18

Radiotherapy: brachytherapy

J. M. Parry, T. Kehoe, and D. G. Sutton

18.1 Introduction

Two situations are discussed in this chapter, the use of sealed sources, where high-energy photon radiation is the main protection hazard, and the use of unsealed sources, where contamination is the major hazard but the external hazard may also need to be considered.

Sealed-source techniques vary enormously from surface moulds, through intracavitary, intraluminal, interstitial, to intraoperative. Sometimes radioactive sources are placed permanently *in situ* but most are temporary. These sources may be loaded directly in theatre or loaded on the ward in one of two ways: by 'hand'—termed manual afterloading; or automatically—termed remote afterloading. The techniques employed will depend on the patient's presentation, the oncologist's and support staff's expertise, and the facilities available. Although local situations vary, wherever possible investment in a remote afterloading machine will minimize potential dose to staff. Excellent guidance on the requirements of sealed-source brachytherapy can be found in Glasgow [1].

Unsealed sources may be administered directly into a cavity but are usually applied systemically, relying on preferential uptake at the target site. The interested reader is directed to Flower and Chittenden [2] for more information.

The following sections present a description of:

- the clinical applications of brachytherapy sources
- the facilities and resources required to deliver brachytherapy treatments
- work practices for receiving, storing, using, and disposing of sources
- systems and controls to ensure that work practices comply with protection requirements
- precautions taken to minimize the doses received by patients, staff, and the general public
- contingency plans arising from risk assessments.

The common sources used in brachytherapy are listed in Table 18.1.

Table 18.1 The common sources used in brachytherapy

Radionuclide	T1/2	Max. photon energy (keV)^{a*}	Max. electron energy (keV)^{a**}	TVL mm lead
^{137}Cs	30 years	662^{b}	1170^{c}	22^{b}
^{192}Ir	74 days	610^{b}	670^{c}	15^{b}
^{125}I	60 days	35^{b}	none^{c}	0.1^{b}
^{198}Au	2.7 days	680^{b}	960	11^{b}
^{131}I	8 days	720	610	11^{d}
^{103}Pd	17 days	23^{c}	none^{c}	0.1^{b}
^{90}Sr–^{90}Y	28.9 years	none	2270	n/a
^{90}Y	2.7 days	none	2270	n/a
^{32}P	14.3 days	none	1710	n/a

*Contributions of 1% or greater included in table.
**Contributions of 5% or greater included in table.
[a] [3]. [b] [4], table 12.1. [c] [1], table 18.2. [d] [5].

18.2 Sealed-source therapy: manual insertions

18.2.1 Direct implantation

Caesium-137 tubes used for intracavitary gynaecological insertions and Caesium-137 needles used for interstitial implants require sources to be implanted directly into the body. For intracavitary treatment a combination of tubes with a nominal activity of 460–2300 MBq is used to deliver a dose rate of 50–70 cGy h^{-1} to the prescription point. Interstitial implants comprise a number of needles with a nominal activity of 55–333 MBq designed to deliver a dose rate of 30–90 cGy h^{-1} to the prescription point [4]. Both of these techniques involve the presence of radioactive sources throughout the whole treatment process and a number of staff groups will be exposed to radiation. The use of direct implantation techniques is now rare because of the radiation protection implications and the introduction of afterloading systems.

For each theatre session medical physics staff should prepare the sources required. This will usually take place in the sealed-source laboratory (SSL) using the appropriate shielding, as described in §18.6. Using mechanical handling/loading devices significantly reduces exposure. Finger doses should be monitored and audited to ensure consistency of handling techniques. Each source must be identifiable by type—normally achieved by attaching colour-coded silk threads. The prepared sources are then transported to theatre using a specially designed transport trolley.

A small shielded bench must be provided in the operating theatre and the source transferred to it on arrival. Only staff essential to the procedure should be in theatre while sources are present. Appropriate handling forceps will be contained in the sterilized instrument set for the procedure. For gynaecological implants, the trunk dose to the radiotherapist can be reduced if he or she sits on a stool with a shielded front. It is appropriate to monitor the dose to the radiotherapists' fingers. While attending to the patient in the recovery area, the nursing staff should stand as far away from the sources as practicable. Before the patient leaves theatre a radiation warning sign must be displayed along with a list of the sources inserted, e.g. on a clipboard at the end of the bed. It is good practice to attach a wrist-band to the patient showing the radiation symbol and listing of the sources inserted.

Following the implant, radiographs are required for dosimetry purposes. An X-ray facility in the theatre is ideal, but usually the patient has to be radiographed in the radiotherapy or diagnostic radiology department. A system should be in place where the patient can be dealt with on arrival and continue to the ward as soon as the images have been taken. Hospital porters moving the patient should be advised to stand at the end of the bed furthest away from the implanted sources and to transfer the patient as quickly as possible.

When nursing implant patients the ward staff are exposed during all nursing procedures which should only be carried out as necessary and as quickly as possible. To reduce the risk of losing sources the insertion site should be checked periodically by the nursing staff. Patients should not be allowed to use the toilet to avoid the risk of losing a source down the drain. Gynaecological implant patients are catheterized and given a low-residue diet to reduce bladder and bowel dose.

Monitors must be provided over ward entrances to indicate if a source is being taken out of the ward, e.g. if the patient leaves the ward. Monitors should also be provided in the sluice rooms. All laundry connected with implant patients should also be monitored before being sent away. Ward staff must take notice of and investigate any alarm that sounds.

The sources should be removed at the end of the treatment time by nursing or medical staff and returned to the SSL for cleaning and storage. A system should be in place to allow the sources to be returned to the store as soon as possible, including sources removed outside normal working hours. The patient and the treatment room must be monitored before the patient is allowed to leave the ward.

18.2.2 Afterloading

Afterloading techniques were developed to reduce the dose to staff. Inert applicators are inserted into the patient and the sources only introduced once the patient is on the ward where the treatment will take place. Theatre, medical, portering, and radiography staff do not come into contact with radiation and therefore the technique is of immediate benefit to them. Most systems allow the sources to be retracted temporarily for nursing procedures to be undertaken, thus reducing the dose to the nursing staff considerably. Afterloading is carried out either by manually loading sources into the applicators, as discussed in this section, or by attaching the applicators to a treatment unit which transfers the sources remotely, as discussed in §18.3.

Gynaecological manual afterloading

Miniature cylindrical sources with a nominal activity of 550–1300 MBq are used in source trains to deliver a dose rate of approximately 0.3 Gy h^{-1} to the prescription point [4]. The source trains should be stored in a permanent safe in the SSL and taken to the bedside as required, where they should be stored in a lead pot at the foot of the bed. The medical physics staff undertaking the preparation and transport will still be exposed to some radiation. The source trains are inserted into the applicators by the nurses and are then returned to the storage pot for nursing procedures to be carried out. Source trains are secured in place by locks on both the pot and the applicators. Nursing staff will still be exposed to the radiation sources during the removal and insertion of the trains, but the overall doses received will be dramatically reduced compared to nursing a patient with sources *in situ*. Sources may also be removed to allow visitors.

^{192}Ir *wire and pins*

Iridium wire is still used occasionally. It can be obtained as a coil of wire, usually 50 cm long, or as single-pin and hairpin shapes, approximately 6 cm long, with a nominal activity of 1.11–11.10 MBq mm^{-1}. Typical dose rates to the prescription point are 40 cGy h^{-1}.

Wire from a coil is most commonly used for breast implants, where a flexible source is desirable to conform to the curve of the chest wall. The wire is cut to provide sources of the length required for each implant. Sources are made up by inserting the required length of wire into small-diameter plastic tubing. A series of large-diameter flexible plastic tubes are implanted in the patient, under an anaesthetic in theatre. The sources are afterloaded into the outer tubing when the patient is in the treatment room. Once loaded, the sources are fixed in place and are not removed until the end of the treatment. Therefore, although this is an afterloading technique, activity is always present throughout the nursing phase. It may be possible to reuse the wire if the integrity of the source is good and the activity meets clinical needs, and this will involve stripping the plastic sleeve from the wire.

Iridium pins are supplied at a standard length and cut to the length required. Slotted stainless-steel guide needles are inserted into the patient, under an anaesthetic in theatre. The pins are inserted into the guide needles, sutured in place, and then the guide needles removed, leaving the pins 'directly implanted'. From the time of implant in the theatre the protection issues are the same as for direct implantation.

It is recommended that a shielded mechanical device is used for preparing the wires and suitable handling tools are used for preparing sources for disposal (or reuse) and cutting pins to length. ^{192}Ir wire is technically not classified as a sealed source. Iridium is covered by a thin platinum sheath to filter out β-emissions. The source is activated by neutron bombardment, which also activates the cladding. The activity of the cladding, however, is negligible and has little consequence in practice. It should be noted that the iridium core is exposed at the ends of a wire. Cutting instruments may become contaminated and should be monitored regularly.

Each length of wire cut from a coil becomes an individual source. A stock control and record-keeping system must be set up for source identification and traceability of movement, and appropriate storage provided, until disposal (§18.7). Discarded off-cuts must also be stored in labelled pots until disposal. It is good practice to keep the length of off-cuts at least 5 mm.

18.2.3 Permanent implants

Permanent insertions are always performed under anaesthetic in a theatre. The most favoured radionuclide is ^{125}I. ^{103}Pd (maximum energy 23 keV) is currently used most often in clinical trials as an alternative for ^{125}I, and has the same protection requirements as ^{125}I. ^{198}Au is still available but is rarely used. The characteristics of these radionuclides are outlined in Table 18.1.

^{125}I *seeds*

By far the largest use of ^{125}I seeds is for permanent implantation into prostate tumours, which appears to be on the threshold of a large expansion. Typical seed activity is 12 MBq with a minimum prescription dose from typically 100 seeds being 144 Gy delivered in some 2080 hours [4]. The fact that ^{125}I has a maximum photon energy of 35 keV means that shielding prior to insertion is not a particular issue, since lead or tin foil will suffice. It is good practice to monitor the theatre area following implantation to ensure that no seeds have been misplaced. Once the implant has been performed, the surface dose rate from a patient is generally insufficient to cause any restrictions on their movement [4]. Patients should, however, refrain from close contact with pregnant women and children for 2 months after treatment [7]. Garments for the patient to wear, with shielding incorporated, are available commercially, but are not essential and are unlikely to be comfortable for the patient. A common way of treating is to use multiple seeds in a fixed linear geometry, inside a rigid tubular suture. It is possible for seeds to become loose and migrate in the body. Because of their physical size they are most likely to be passed out through the urethra and so filtration of the urine by a fine mesh may be necessary. The risk of this occurrence will be minimized by good theatre technique. It is uncommon for seeds to be released well after implantation.

^{198}Au *grains*

Gold grains are cylindrical seeds encased in platinum and are available with a nominal activity of 50–1460 MBq. A 'gun' is used to deliver the sources. Pulling the trigger incrementally moves a stilette down the implant needle and deposits a grain at the tip of the needle. Gold is used in the mouth and for superficial lesions. The sources themselves are 'retained' only by the surrounding tissues and source migration is therefore possible. Radiographs of the clinical site are, therefore, not only essential for dosimetry but also for confirming the location of the grains. Monitoring of the theatre area post-insertion is essential. Occasionally a grain is swallowed. Under these circumstances, the faeces must be kept in a container until the source is located and recovered.

Beta applicators

The use of beta applicators is decreasing and will probably be encountered only as ^{90}Sr or possibly ^{106}Ru ophthalmic applicators. ^{90}Sr applicators contain a strontium compound incorporated in a rolled silver foil. The foil is covered by 0.1 mm silver to screen any bremsstrahlung radiation, so that the applicators can be considered to be pure β-emitters. It should be noted that some ophthalmic applicators have active foils on the back surface as well as the front. The surface dose rate in tissue is very high (up to 40 mGy s^{-1}) and poses a hazard to the operators skin and eyes, but is easily shielded by 7 mm perspex. Applicators should be kept shielded in a storage/transport container until used for treatment, handled at a distance from the body, preferably using a tool that incorporates a perspex shield, and the active surface(s) should never be looked at directly.

18.2.4 Source handling

When a source is purchased it will be delivered with a certificate, which includes a statement of its activity. All sources are purchased against specifications and must conform to a number of regulations:

- BS5288:1976 specification. Sealed radioactive sources [8]
- ISO/TR 2919:1999 Sealed radioactive sources classification [9]

Box 18.1 Leak testing of sealed sources

All sealed sources, both therapeutic and non-therapeutic, should be routinely checked for leakage. Typical therapy level sources that should be checked include sources used for brachytherapy, sources used for γ external therapy, and calibration sources. Non-therapeutic sources that should be checked include flood sources (for example ^{60}Co), marker sources, radionuclide calibrator check sources, check sources inside liquid scintillation counting equipment such as ^{226}Ra, ^{133}Ba, and ^{137}Cs and, sources in gas chromatographs such as ^{63}Ni-electrodeposited sources or ^{3}H-foil sources. Leak testing is not appropriate for smoke detectors or containment vessels for unsealed-source material. There is no need to leak test sources smaller than 5 mm, such as ^{198}Au grains, since they can effectively be treated as dispersible sources.

No new source should be used until a leakage test has been carried out unless a leakage certificate has been obtained from the manufacturer. A risk assessment should be made to determine the frequency of subsequent leak testing. The assessment should consider the potential for the source to leak and the consequences of any leakage. Factors which will be taken into account in the risk assessment should include:

- The nature of the radionuclide, e.g. its toxicity, dispersibility, chemical nature, and physical form
- The activity of the source, taking into account the ALI
- The purpose for which the source is intended.

It is normal practice to perform at least annual leak tests on sources that are in routine clinical use. Any sources suspected of leaking must also be tested. Any source found to be leaking should be placed in a separate container, labelled accordingly, and stored in an appropriate place in the sealed-sources laboratory. The frequency of testing should be increased if a source is used beyond its recommended life. In any event, in the UK, the interval between tests should not exceed 2 years. In the United States, regulation requires some sources to be checked every 6 months. There should be definite pass/fail criteria associated with the leak test, which would normally be the detection of 200 Bq contamination. In some cases, for example, where the contamination may conceivably come from another source, it would be prudent to decontaminate the source and retest before confirming a leak.

Records of leak tests should be maintained and should indicate [11]:

- Identification of the source being tested, the date of the test, and the name of the tester
- The reason for the test and the test method
- The test result (both numerical and pass or fail)
- The action taken if the source failed the test.

Manufacturers or suppliers will normally provide advice on methods of leak testing and include a description of the methods used for their quality control checks as part of the source certification documents. Test methods are also set out in ISO 9978 [10]. The following practical methods can be adopted.

- ISO/TR 9978:1992 Sealed radioactive sources—leakage test methods [10].

Source receipt and acceptance of new sources

The following procedure for accepting new sources is recommended:

- check the documentation supplied, to ensure consistency with the order
- check the leak test documentation supplied—confirm by monitoring the packaging using a Geiger–Müller (GM) counter, once all the sources have been removed
- leak test and visually inspect the sources for damage as soon as practicable (Box 18.1)
- amend source registers, etc.

Source sterilization

Many institutions use centralized sterilization. The transportation to and from these facilities is dealt with in the next section. It is highly unlikely that the usual sterilization equipment will have sufficient protection, hence suitable signs and methods of restricting access (local rules) are necessary. No other instruments should be sterilized at the same time in the oven. Sterilizing staff will also need training and education about radiation protection.

Source transportation

Within the hospital, sources are transferred between the SSL and places of use in specially designed shielded trolleys. The trolley should:

- have a long handle, so that the operator is kept at a distance from the sources

Box 18.1 (*continued*)

Routine wipe tests on permanent therapy source stock, external γ-therapy sources, laboratory, diagnostic, and other sealed sources

γ-sources should be wiped with a swab or tissue, moistened with ethanol or water. A proprietary pre-injection alcohol wipe is ideal for this purpose. All of the surfaces of the source should be wiped thoroughly but quickly, holding the swab with forceps. The activity of the swab should then be measured in a γ-counter. It should be assumed that 10% of any contamination has been transferred to the swab and a correction should be made to allow for the efficiency of the γ-counter for the radionuclide. β-sources should be wiped with a thin glass-fibre sheet, moistened in alcohol or water. Care should be taken to avoid damaging the window through which the radiation is emitted. The sheet should then be dissolved in a scintillant solution and the activity measured in a liquid scintillation counter. Again, it should be assumed that only 10% of any contamination has been transferred and in this case the efficiency of the counting process should be allowed for. A source is considered not to be leaking if the activity measured is below 200 Bq.

Routine leak tests on the permanent therapy source stock

The following immersion test for leakage is an appropriate test for routine checks for both ^{137}Cs tubes/needles and ^{90}Sr applicators. The source is immersed in water at 50°C for 4 h. For γ-sources the water is then monitored in a γ-counter and the activity level determined. With β-sources an aliquot of the water is added to a scintillant solution and the activity measured in a β-counter. If the activity measured is less than 200 Bq the source is considered not to be leaking. A standard method of testing a large quantity of sources is to test a batch of the same type in the first instance. If a batch fails the test, each needle from the batch is then tested individually.

Indirect leakage tests

Tests for leakage should, wherever possible, be performed on the sealed source itself or on its container. There are instances where this is not practical due to the inaccessibility of the source or possible because of the risk of a high dose being received by the person carrying out the test and in such cases indirect tests should be performed. When indirect checks are carried out it is important that they are performed on areas of the equipment that will have become contaminated in the event of leakage. Some examples are given below:

- For γ-ray teletherapy equipment, it will be necessary to wipe test the surface of the radiation head including the beam aperture.
- In the case of remote afterloading apparatus, the internal surfaces of the transit tubes should be wipe tested.
- The track of the source and any access points to the source should be wipe tested when blood and small specimen irradiators are being checked.

The entry point for the check source and all accessible points should be wiped when liquid scintillation counters and gas chromatographs are being tested.

- be labelled with a radioactive sign and an indication of the type and number of sources within, e.g. a white perspex square with information written in marker pen
- be accompanied by a written list of the sources, in case of accident and in case the sources need to be accounted for
- be designed so that the surface dose rate never exceeds 2 mSv per hour
- never be left unattended.

Because of familiarity with the hazard, transportation should be performed by physics staff. Ideally, the facilities should be designed such that only limited movement of sources is required. It is desirable that the sources are not transported in lifts. However, if this is necessary, there should not be any other person in the lift.

Source decontamination

Sources used for temporary implants are likely to be contaminated with blood and tissue products and must be cleaned following use. A suitable procedure is detailed in Godden [12]; however, it is recommended that guidance is also sought locally from the theatre staff and infection control officer. Clearly, cleaning must take place within appropriate shielding. Once cleaned and dried, the sources should be inspected for damage prior to disposal of the cleaning fluid. If damage is suspected, the cleaning fluid should be suitably packaged and sent for counting as outlined in Box 18.1. It is good practice to monitor the cleaning fluid prior to disposal, even if damage is not suspected.

18.2.5 Disposal of sources

The reader is referred to §9.3 for a general discussion of the principles and practical arrangements for the disposal of any radioactive waste. The disposal of all radioactive material must comply with the requirements of the hospital's authorization certificate and the local rules and a mechanism must be in place for any disposal to be authorized by an identified person given responsibility for source disposal.

Short half-life γ- and β-emitting sealed/solid therapy sources

Disposal of sources with half-lives of up to 10s of days (e.g. ^{198}Au, ^{192}Ir) are likely to be made through an authorized contractor, which may be the supplier, but in some circumstances disposal may be via special burial (§9.3.5).

Arrangements should be in place for a responsible person to review the sealed-source waste at suitable intervals to identify batches of radionuclides which have decayed to an agreed level at which they may be disposed of. Before a disposal can be made, the responsible person should:

- identify a company or site with appropriate authorization to dispose of the waste and make arrangements for the disposal
- arrange appropriate packaging for transportation
- measure surface dose rates and levels of surface contamination for the packages to ensure compliance with requirements of transport regulations
- ensure packages are appropriately labelled and prepare transport documentation (§9.5.2)
- complete appropriate disposal forms and ensure that records of the disposal are held within the department
- arrange for the packages containing the waste to be picked up at a suitable time and location.

Longer half-life sealed/solid therapy sources

Disposal will usually be by special arrangement, either by direct return to the supplier/manufacturer or by arrangement with an authorized radioactive waste disposal company. Requirements for such disposal are that the responsible person should:

- identify a company with appropriate registration and/or authorization to hold and/or dispose of the sources
- liaise with the company to arrange appropriate packaging for transportation (§9.5.1)
- list source numbers, activities, physical form
- have ready access to the sources on a prearranged date
- monitor surface dose rates and contamination levels of packages to ensure compliance with the transport regulations
- ensure packages are appropriately labelled and prepare transport documentation (§9.5.2)
- arrange for the packages containing the sources to be picked up at a suitable time and location when trained staff are available to supervise the handover
- ensure that a record of the source transfer is made, signed, and dated by a representative of the hospital and the company performing the disposal
- amend the source inventory to reflect the change in stock held.

18.2.7 Discharge of patients from hospital

Patients with temporary implants should not be discharged from hospital. Those patients with permanent implants should remain in hospital until there is no longer any risk that the source will move or be expelled from the body. As noted above, if ^{125}I seeds have been implanted, then it is a sensible precaution for the patient to refrain from close contact with pregnant women or children for up to 2 months post-insertion. Advice concerning the discharge of patients permanently implanted with other radionuclides such as ^{198}Au should be formulated on a case-by-case basis [7].

18.3 Sealed-source therapy: remote afterloading units

The introduction of remote afterloading (RAL) devices has almost reduced the dose to staff to zero, under normal operation. The source(s) are stored in a shielded safe, which usually forms part of the machine. There may be a slight surface dose rate when the sources are in the safe and a survey should be conducted, at the time of commissioning, to ascertain the best position from which to operate the unit. Source activities are normally higher than for directly loaded and manually afterloaded treatments. Patients are treated in a shielded room and the unit is operated from outside. Sources are only sent out to the applicators once all staff have left the room and are retracted when staff need to enter the room, e.g. for nursing procedures. The room door is interlocked (cf. external beam treatment rooms), so that the sources will retract if the door is opened while the sources are out of the safe. Another advantage of these units is that in normal operation the sources are contained within a closed system.

The machine display indicates whether the sources are in or out of the safe, or in transit. It is, however, necessary to have an independent radiation monitor in the room to indicate the presence of radiation in the room, in case of a machine fault. The worst protection issue for RAL machines arises when sources stick in transit. Contingency plans for this situation are detailed in §18.8.2 and it is appropriate for a physicist to be on-call when a unit is operating outside normal working hours. Good practice involves a sensible quality assurance programme, good facilities, training of the nursing staff, and appropriate information and guidance (education) of the patient.

18.3.1 Low-dose rate/medium-dose rate

The most widely used low-dose rate/medium-dose rate (LDR/MDR) afterloading machine is programmed to compose source trains made up of active sources and non-active spacers. Nominal source activities of 370–1480 MBq are used to deliver dose rates of 0.5–1.5 Gy h^{-1} for gynaecological treatments. The sources comprise ^{137}Cs-impregnated glass beads soldered into a small-diameter stainless-steel sphere. During each source train movement the pellets collide with the adjacent ones. The soldering process hardens the steel casing and over many collisions the pellets become progressively less spherical. In extreme cases, this shape distortion can lead to the pellets jamming in valves and therefore the pellets have a limited life, typically of 10 years. It is also important that the transport tubes and catheter ends are routinely checked for any damage that may cause the sources to become stuck during transit.

18.3.2 High-dose rate

High-dose rate (HDR) afterloading machines are becoming more widespread. The unit houses a single, small-diameter, cylindrical ^{192}Ir source incorporated into a drive cable. Dose distributions are built up by moving the source to a specified number of dwell positions for specified dwell times. The small diameter of the source means that it can be used for both gynaecological and interstitial implants. Sources with a nominal activity of up to 370 GBq are used, which deliver an average dose rate of 1–5 Gy min^{-1} to the prescription point and the total prescribed dose is delivered in a number of short fractions. When flexible applicators are used for interstitial implants there is a danger of the source becoming stuck in a part of the applicator that has a small radius of curvature. To reduce the risk of this happening, a dummy source is sent into the applicator(s) before the treatment begins. The motor drive units incorporate a force feedback system. If the dummy source meets any resistance in the applicator it is retracted, a warning given, and the source will not be sent into the applicator. During the movement of the active source the speed of the drive varies depending on the force required for it to travel through the applicator. In the curved parts of the applicator the drive speed decreases to 'ease' the source through. A source that becomes stuck is a major problem, because of the high-dose rate, and there is a risk that the source may become detached from the drive cable in the process of trying to retract the source back to the safe.

18.3.3 Pulsed-dose rate

Pulsed-dose rate (PDR) afterloading machines are a recent development. They are essentially a modified version of the HDR machines and can be used for the same treatment techniques. The design of the source is the same as for the HDR, but a source with a nominal activity of approximately 37 GBq is used. It is designed to give an hourly pulse of treatment, typically lasting 10 min, over a number of days, to deliver a treatment that is radiobiologically equivalent to a continuous low-dose rate treatment. The protection issues are the same as for HDR.

18.3.4 Working practice

LDR/PDRs are usually under the control of nursing staff who will be less familiar with radiotherapy equipment than physicists and radiographers. Nurses will need additional training and education in basic radiation protection matters. As many treatments extend beyond normal office hours, special arrangements are needed to cope with potential protection issues. It is essential that there are appropriately trained nurses and a radiation physicist able to respond within a short period of time.

Since HDR equipment is similar to external beam treatment equipment, expertly trained therapy radiographers operate these units. Treatments are given during regular office hours so the presence of at least the RPS (and in some cases the RPA) is common. Radiographers are familiar with this technology and associated written instructions guiding practice can be less explicit, with details reflecting the high level of staff competence involved.

18.3.5 Performance of remote afterloading units

The performance of RAL units is defined by the specification at the time of its purchase. It should be a requirement that the unit conforms to BS 5724:1991 Part 2.17: *The specification of remote afterloading equipment* [13]. This document details the criteria for source transport, door interlocks, warning signs, leakage radiation from the safe, and fail-safe features. A new installation must be subject to a critical examination before it is used clinically, to ensure that:

- all safety features operate correctly
- all warning devices operate correctly
- the radiation shielding provides sufficient protection.

A definitive calibration of the source(s) is also required before the unit is used clinically.

Following acceptance, the continuing performance should be monitored by a regular planned maintenance and quality control programme. There is extensive documentation on quality control and safety programmes, e.g. IPEM Report 81 [14] and AAPM Task Group 59 [15].

18.4 Therapy with unsealed sources

Unsealed sources used for both in- and out-patient therapies should be prepared in the radiopharmacy or dispensary prior to administration. Chapter 15 contains a detailed discussion of the radiation protection issues involved. The therapy relies on large-scale biochemical uptake and retention by the target area. Table 18.1 outlines the physical properties of the common radionuclides used. Treatment may be relatively simple, i.e. via an oral route, or more involved, e.g. by injection over a relatively long time period, and may be given as an out-patient or in-patient administration. Patient dosimetry can be performed using the MIRD scheme outlined in §16.2. See also [2] for a worked example.

18.4.1 Out-patient administrations

Intravenous injections

^{32}P and ^{89}S are both given to outpatients as intravenous injections. These nuclides are β-emitters and adequate protection can be provided by 6 mm of perspex. Contamination resulting from radionuclide spillages and loss of body fluids are the possible protection problems with these patients. Contingency plans are detailed in §18.8.3.

All preparatory actions should take place behind a perspex shield. 'Double gloving' is sensible practice. Provide a sharps bin for all suspected or contaminated materials, particularly syringes, swabs, and gloves, and use a dedicated sharps bin for each radionuclide. Leaving the activity vial inside its carrier and replacing the lid with a hemispherical perspex shield should help the operator in preparing an injection, while providing adequate shielding.

Oral therapies

^{131}I, in the form of NaI, can be supplied both as a capsule and as a liquid and is the most common oral therapy. From a radiation protection perspective there are great advantages to the capsular form, primarily because of the reduced contamination risk both before and after administration. Administration of the capsule is straightforward and is performed using an applicator provided by the supplier which is designed to reduce the radiation dose to the operator. When in liquid form, iodine is taken through a straw to reduce the uptake in the mouth, and thick paper tissues are provided in case the patient needs to cough while swallowing. Following administration, the patient should not leave for a further 30 min in case the therapy produces an emetic reaction. The patient should be provided with appropriate instructions to ensure that the radiation dose to other members of the public is kept as low as practicable. Full details can be found in §16.8.

18.4.2 In-patient administrations

Therapy administrations of ^{131}I can involve activities of between 2 and 12 GBq, depending on the disease being treated. NaI used for the treatment of thyroid cancer is administered orally as with treatment for thyrotoxicosis. mIBG is used in the treatment of neural crest tumours. Patients are hydrated during therapy and the mIBG is delivered by syringe pump, over many hours. In this latter case, intensive nursing is needed over the treatment period, particularly in the first few hours. For both treatments, if the patient is catheterized, some workers recommend that the collection bag should be placed inside a shield with a lid to reduce exposure to nursing staff.

Inpatients who have received doses of up to 10 GBq of higher energy radionuclides such as ^{131}I represent a significant radiation hazard since the dose rates in adjoining rooms where there are other staff or members of the public (this also includes other patients) can exceed 10 $\mu Sv\ h^{-1}$. The dose rates can be reduced using large shields placed around the patient's bed. However, it is essential that radiation surveys are performed to ensure that the shields are being used effectively. The patient must also be supervised to ensure that they are not moving outside the shielded area. It is therefore better for a shielded room to be available for these patients so that they have the freedom of movement within the room and do not suffer from the claustrophobic feeling of being 'penned in' by the shields. From a radiation safety perspective, the shielded room solution is more satisfactory as it is more 'dose control by design' rather than 'dose control by procedure' as with the use of bed shields. Dose control by design is preferred in current legislation (see Chapter 5). Such rooms should also provide the patient with their own washing and toilet facilities and must be decontaminated and monitored after use. Patients are advised to flush the toilet at least twice. Absorbent material, e.g. incontinence pads, should be laid around the toilet in case of spills.

All waste leaving the patient's room should be monitored for contamination. It may well be that the simplest approach to waste is to treat it all as potentially radioactive and dispose of it via the radioactive waste stream. If laundry is found to be contaminated then it should ideally be washed in a separate facility to the hospital laundry, for example a washing machine in the medical physics department, and then rechecked for contamination and decay stored if necessary. Patients are often advised not to wear their own clothes during the duration of a treatment since the clothing may well suffer the same fate should it be contaminated. It is good practice to ensure that the patient is provided with disposable crockery.

There is no reason why a patient should not be allowed visitors. However, the arrangements for visitors must be determined with a risk assessment that takes into account such factors as the layout of the patient's room and the dose rates involved. Restrictions will be placed on the length of time visitors can stay and on the type of visitor allowed—for example, extra consideration should be given to children and pregnant women. Should the visitors be treated as 'comforters and carers' then they must be provided with adequate information.

The protection measures adopted by staff depend on their degree of involvement with the patient and the complexity of the procedure. It is advisable for all staff who come into contact with the patient to wear plastic overshoes, aprons, and gloves, which should be discarded after a single use. A system should be set up for staff to monitor themselves for contamination after leaving the treatment room. There should be clear instruction on the course of action to be followed should contamination be identified. An elementary spill kit should be provided in case of unforeseen contamination and staff should be trained in its use and be aware of the appropriate personnel to contact following any 'incident'. It must be remembered that the patient should not be isolated for the duration of their stay and that for this to happen, the nursing staff should themselves feel confident in the protection measures adopted.

External dosimetry with a calibrated survey meter should be carried out at regular intervals to determine when the patient can be discharged. The procedures and arrangements following discharge are discussed in §16.8.

18.5 Treatment room design and controls

This section outlines the basic issues and practicalities that need to be considered when planning a brachytherapy treatment facility. Further discussion of the issues involved can be found in IPEM Report 75 [16]. Ideally, brachytherapy patients should be treated in a shielded single room, which has been specially designed for the treatment to be given. It is, however, not uncommon for two patients to be treated simultaneously in a double occupancy room using a remote afterloading unit.

18.5.1 Room location

Brachytherapy treatment rooms, other than HDR remote afterloading units, are most suitably located on a radiotherapy ward. This confines brachytherapy treatment to one ward that is staffed by nurses with the expertise and training to tend to these patients. It is also usual for source storage facilities and physics staff to be accommodated on or close to the radiotherapy ward.

The location of the treatment rooms must be considered with regard to surrounding rooms. From the radiation protection point of view, rooms should be sited next to low-occupancy areas, rather than next to a high-occupancy office. This implies positioning them in the remotest area of the ward, but this must be balanced against the fact that as the patients are being treated in isolation the room should be in proximity to the nurses station so that they can be monitored regularly. Monitoring can be helped by using a CCTV and intercom system. Attention must also be paid to the rooms above and below, as shielding may have to be provided in the roof or the floor and the building assessed structurally to ensure it could support the extra weight. A ward sited on the top or ground floor reduces this problem, but a ground floor may need to have an area around the window cordoned off to restrict access.

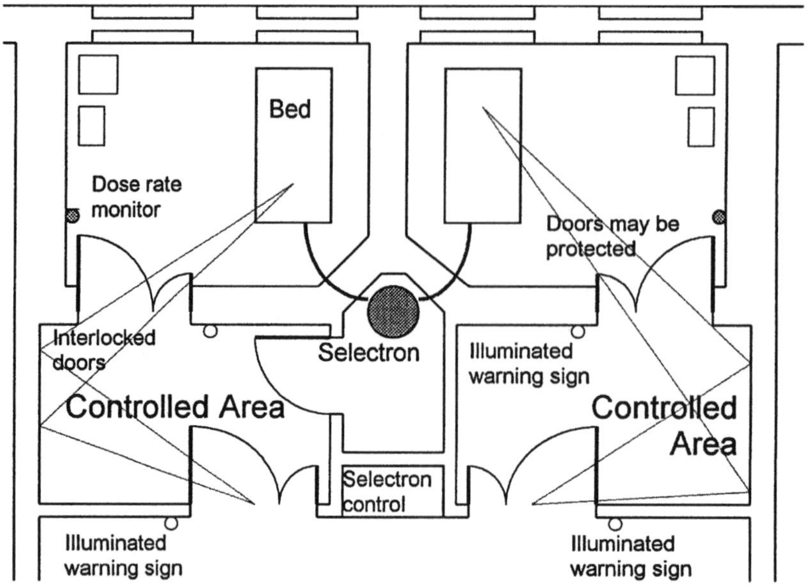

Figure 18.1 Example layout in which two remote afterloading units are situated in adjoining rooms.

If more than one treatment room is to be provided it may prove advantageous to locate them next to each other. This will reduce the overall shielding requirements, as the rooms will have common adjoining walls. It may also be possible for them to be served by a single anteroom, with a single entrance from the ward. In many cases, the brief will be to modify existing rooms and the choice of location will be limited.

18.5.2 Room layout

The room layout should allow the patient to be nursed safely, efficiently, and comfortably and, depending on the function of the room, provide space for:

- access for beds and trolleys
- access around both sides of the bed for nursing and domestic duties
- a locker and personnel effects
- a chair for iodine and interstitial patients who are not confined to bed
- mobile shielding (if in use) to be moved clear of the bed
- storage of a lead pot and handling tools for emergency use
- the afterloading unit and source transfer tubes
- visitors to sit at a reasonable distance from the patient
- *en suite* facilities for unsealed-source patients
- an anteroom, to prevent access directly into room.

The *en suite* facilities should include a shower unit to reduce the contamination from sweat. Siting the toilet facility at the opposite end of the room to the door reduces the possibility of spreading contamination from that area. Fitting a wall-mounted toilet makes it easier to lay absorbent material on the floor to reduce contamination. An anteroom can also be used to provide a handwashing facility and storage space for protective clothing, monitoring equipment, and a spill kit. For a remote afterloading unit an anteroom will act as the control area and may be used to house the unit if it is serving two adjacent rooms. Figure 18.1 shows a layout in which two remote afterloading units are situated in adjoining rooms.

18.5.3 Shielding design

The room shielding is designed for the proposed use of the room, taking account of the technique, radionuclide, activity, number of patients to be treated simultaneously, and occupancy of the room and surrounding areas. The most common design aims are to:

- reduce the dose and dose rate in all adjacent areas to below that which would require them to be designated as controlled areas
- ensure that the dose received by any member of the public in 1 year from this source does not exceed the public dose limit, or a submultiple of the limit when dose constraints (usually 0.3 mSv) are applied (see Chapter 13).

The inside of the room will be designated as a controlled area while treatment is being carried out and this designation may be extended to any anteroom.

It should be remembered that where controlled area status can be determined by dose rate criteria, then it is theoretically possible to design shielding which complies with the dose constraint but is insufficient because of dose rate considerations. This eventuality will be encountered in areas of very low use or where the maximum activity used is much greater than the average.

A number of factors should be taken into account when estimating shielding requirements.

Room usage

The brachytherapy room may not be fully utilized because:

- the number of patients requiring the treatment is lower than the capacity
- there may be a constraint on theatre sessions for sealed-source implants.

Thus, an estimation of the number of days the room is used per year (the number of patients × duration of treatment) should be used in the calculation.

Exposure time

During PDR afterloading treatments, the source is only exposed for a short time each hour, which can be expressed as a source exposure factor. Although sources are removed for nursing procedures during other afterloaded treatments, it is recommended that this is ignored. The length of time the sources are removed should be negligible and will vary between patients and may well be difficult to estimate.

Activity

The total activity used is individual to each patient so, where appropriate, the calculation should also reflect decay of the radionuclide. For unsealed-source therapy the activity will be decreasing continuously due to both radioactive decay and excretion of the source.

Occupancy

Realistic occupancy factors for surrounding areas should be employed and should ideally be based on actual rather than notional usage. Even when sources are continuously exposed is it reasonable to assume that:

- staff will only work an 8-hour day
- individual members of the public are unlikely to be on the ward for more than 2–3 hours in any one day
- the cumulative annual effective dose to a patient being nursed in an adjoining room is unlikely to exceed the dose constraints.

Before the shielding calculation is made, it is necessary to determine whether shielding to an annual dose constraint will ever result in dose rates being above the limit which signifies that an area is controlled. If this is the case, then the shielding must be designed for the maximum, rather than average, activity. One approach to making this decision is outlined below:

The average dose rate E_{ave} in μSv h^{-1} to a person in an adjoining room after transmission through the degree of shielding required to reduce the annual dose to the design limit (dose constraint) can be estimated from the following equation:

$$E_{ave} = D_{cons} \times 10^3 / p\, d\, h\, f \qquad (18.1)$$

and the maximum dose rate at any time in the adjoining room E_{max} from

$$E_{max} = D_{cons} \times 10^3 / p\, d\, h \quad A_{max}/A_{ave}$$

where:

D_{cons} = dose constraint (mSv year^{--1})
p = number of patients per year
d = average length of treatment (days)
h = number of hours per day the source is exposed
f = fraction of the day the adjoining area is occupied
A_{max} = maximum activity used for any one treatment
A_{ave} = average activity used per treatment.

The possible outcomes for the average and maximum dose rates are outlined below, along with the action associated with each combination.

Average dose rate	Maximum dose rate	Action
< dose rate limit	< dose rate limit	Design using average activity to dose constraint
	> dose rate limit	Design to dose rate limit using maximum activity

In the example of Box 18.2, the maximum dose rate will be 2.25 μSv h^{-1} and the average dose rate will be 0.47μSv h^{-1}. The dose rate limit is 7.5 μSv h^{-1} in the UK and 20 μSv h^{-1} in the USA. Neither limit is exceeded here and an average activity can be used in the calculation.

18.5.4 Calculation of barrier thickness

Brachytherapy sources are uncollimated and emit radiation isotropically. All barriers in direct 'line of sight' of

Box 18.2 Example 1

Estimate of the dose rate in an area adjacent to an LDR afterloading unit that will be used for gynaecological insertions.

If:

Appropriate dose constraint (D_{cons})	= 0.3 mSv year^{-1}
Number of patients per year (p)	= 40
Average length of treatment (d)	= 2 days
Number of hours per day the source is exposed (h)	= 24 h
Fraction of the day the adjoining area is occupied (f) (Assuming occupancy of 8 hours)	= 0.33
Maximum activity used for a treatment (A_{max}) (Unit contains 24 ^{137}Cs sources each of activity 1.48 GBq)	= 35.52 GBq
Average activity used per treatment (A_{ave}) (15 sources used in an average insertion)	= 22.20 GBq

Average dose rate = 0.47 μSv h^{-1}
Maximum dose rate = 2.25 μSv h^{-1}

the source must be shielded against the primary radiation. The primary component will be much bigger than the scatter component and hence scatter can be ignored when designing primary barriers. Other barriers, for example those permanently protected by mobile shielding or fixed design features, are considered to be secondary barriers and require shielding from scattered radiation.

Primary radiation

Calculation of the dose rate from the primary radiation to a point outside the room is relatively straightforward:

- Work with a scaled plan of the room.
- Define the position of the source in the room:
  - The positions of the sources used for a gynaecological implant are the easiest to estimate, as the patients are confined to bed and the sources situated in the pelvic area.
  - Patients receiving unsealed-source therapy and some with interstitial implants will have freedom to move about the room and it may be assumed that the source will not stay in one position.
- Unsealed sources may be concentrated in one part of the body or be distributed systemically.
- Determine the shortest distance from the source to a position, say 0.3 m, behind the barrier.
- Calculate the dose rate behind the barrier using the equation:

$$\dot{K}^{pr} = A_{des}\Gamma(1 - P_{att})1/d^2$$

where:

$\dot{K}^{pr}$ = air kerma rate at barrier from primary radiation
A_{des} = activity of source, either average or maximum, depending on the assessment described above
Γ = air kerma rate for a source of unit activity
d = distance from source to barrier
P_{att} = percentage patient attenuation, expressed as a decimal.

As in the case of shielding for diagnostic X-rays, it is usual to take the calculated quantity as being the easily measured quantity air kerma rather than the abstract effective dose (see §13.3.2).

The calculation allows for radiation attenuated within the patient to be taken into account. The attenuation will depend on the patient's dimensions, the radionuclide, and the position of the source within the patient. Patient attenuation factors of 10% have been used previously [16]. Estimates of patient attenuation should be conservative and if possible tested with low activity sources and tissue equivalent material.

Methods for determining the average activity per treatment depend on the type of therapy and the half-life of the radionuclide involved. For example, when the therapy is delivered with an unsealed ^{131}I source, it important that, if possible, both biological and physical half-lives are taken into account when estimating the average activity per treatment. Such considerations will not apply for therapy with long half-life radionuclides such as ^{137}Cs.

Scattered radiation

The dose to a point from scattered radiation is more difficult to estimate than for primary radiation. There is only a limited amount of published data available, particularly for the radionuclides used for brachytherapy (see for example IPEM 75 [16]).

One possible method, outlined below, assumes that there is no energy degradation with scatter and that the

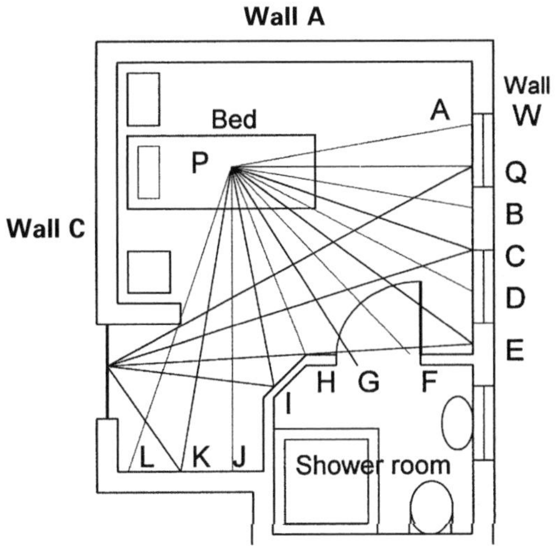

Figure 18.2 Example layout of a brachytherapy room with walls 3.5 m high. See text for meaning of points A–L, P, and Q.

inverse square law applies. The method is described using the example layout of Figure 18.2 which shows a brachytherapy room with walls 3.5 m high.

The patient is on the bed and the source is assumed to be at point P. No primary radiation is incident on the door but radiation scattered from two walls will be present. The total scattered radiation at the door will in effect be the integral of the scatter emanating from each point on the walls corrected for the distance to the door.

- Identify the point Q on wall W from which the first single scatter event can reach the centre of the door. The distance from the source to this point is r_1 and from this point to the door is r'_1.
- Define points A and B at 10° either side of point Q
- The scatter air kerma rate at the door is then given by

$$\dot{K}_1^{sc} = A_{des}\Gamma[1/(r_1^{\,2}.\ r'_1{}^2)]\alpha A_1$$

where:

A_1 = area defined by distance AB multiplied by the height of the room (m^2)

$\dot{K}_1^{sc}$ = air kerma rate from scattered radiation from area A_1

Γ = air kerma rate at 1 m from the source

A_{des} = design activity, either average or maximum

r_1 = distance from source to scatterer (m)

r'_1 = distance from scatterer to door (m)

α = reflection coefficient for scatter obtained from Figure 17.9 [17].

The process is repeated at 20° intervals as shown in Figure 18.2, resulting in an estimate of the scattered dose at the door being given by

$$\dot{K}^{sc} = A_{des}\Gamma\alpha\sum_i \frac{1}{(r_i^2\ .\ r'^2_i)}\cdot A_i$$

where A_i, r_i, and r'_i refer to irradiated areas and path lengths at subsequent 20° intervals.

Barrier thickness

To determine the thickness of barrier required:

- determine the required transmission by dividing the design dose rate by the primary or scattered dose rates as appropriate
- use either published transmission curves or the Archer equation (Chapters 7 and 13), and determine the thickness of shielding material required. Sources of transmission information are IPEM report 75 [16], NCRP publication 49 [18], and the Handbook of Radiological Protection [19].

An example calculation of primary and secondary barrier thickness is given in Box 18.3, again using the example layout of Figure 18.2. To simplify the example, it is assumed that the room layout is fixed. In practice, the layout of the room may well be at the discretion of designer, and if, as would appear to be the case from the example, the door could not be realistically shielded then the designer would be able to extend the length of the wall between the bed and the door. This would have the effect of reducing the area bounded by points HJ and JL which makes the greatest contribution to the scattered component. Ease of access to the patient would of course need to be taken into account. The example makes the assumption that the wall between the door and the bed extends to ceiling height–if this is not the case, there may be a scatter component from the ceiling which would need to be taken into account (see below). It can be inferred from the example that if the area adjacent to wall A were to house a patient, the maximum dose rate in that area would be 0.475/0.33 = 1.5 μSv h^{-1}. The patient would be very unlikely to exceed the annual dose constraint of 300 μSv.

18.5.5 Other considerations

Ceilings

It is important that if possible, shielding is provided to the full height of the roof slab and not just to the level of a suspended ceiling since radiation will be scattered into adjacent areas from the ceiling. If this is not the case, then considerable attention must be given to the magnitude of the secondary radiation scattered from the roof. It should be borne in mind that in this situation, use of a room which is adequately shielded for, say, ^{137}Cs may not prove possible with the lower energy ^{192}Ir or ^{131}I

Box 18.3 Example 2

Using the data of Example 1 and applying them to the layout shown in Figure 18.2, the following calculations can easily be made using a spreadsheet The assumption is made that wall A is adjacent to an area occupied for 8 h (i.e. $f = 0.33$ in Example 1), and wall C is adjacent to a corridor with occupancy factor 1/20 based on an 8-h day (i. e. $f = 0.0165$).

Primary barrier

Primary distance (m)		Dose rate (μGyh^{-1})	Transmission (full occupancy in 8-h day)	Data	
Wall adjacent to bed	1.5	7.70E+02	6.17E–04	AKR*	78
Wall behind bed	1.75	5.65E+02	8.40E–04	Activity (GBq)	22.2
Wall W	3.25	1.64E+02	2.90E–03	Design dose rate (μSv h^{-1})	0.475
Wall at point K	3.8	1.20E+02	3.96E–03		

A transmission of 6×10^{-4} can be achieved with 58 cm concrete. It may well be prudent to provide all of the walls with this degree of shielding. However, if appropriate, the shielding on the other walls can be reduced to reflect the decreased occupancy. Note, however, that shielding designed using an overall occupancy factor of 0.0165 for the corridor will result in a dose rate of nearly 30 μSv h^{-1} in the corridor, so if the 7.5 μSv h^{-1} dose rate limit is not to be exceeded the walls should be shielded to this limit (transmission = 9.7×10^{-3}, requires 40 cm concrete).

Secondary barrier

The shielding required for the secondary barrier, in this case the door, can also be determined quite easily using a spreadsheet. In this case the assumption is made that the door opens into the corridor, which has an occupancy of 1/20 based on an 8-h day ($f = 0.0165$). It is also assumed that the wall between the bed and the door extends to true ceiling height. Consequently, in this example, scatter from the ceiling can be ignored. Note that if the door were to be specified using the occupancy factor for the corridor, the dose rate limit would be exceeded since no protection would be required, so in the example, an instantaneous dose rate constraint of 7.5 μSv h^{-1} is applied.

Path	Primary distance (m)	Secondary distance (m)	Data	
r1	3	5	AKR*	78
r2	3	4.75	alpha	2.20E–02
r3	3.5	4.5	Activity (GB$_q$)	22.2
r4	2.75	3	Height (m)	3.0
r5	2.75	2		
r6	3.7	1.5		

Wall section	Dimension (m)	Contribution to total scatter dose (μGyh^{-1})	
AB	1	AB	0.508
BD	1	BD	0.563
DF	1.5	DF	0.691
FH	1.5	FH	2.519
HJ	1.95	HJ	7.367
JL	1.25	JL	4.638
		Total scatter dose rate (μGy h^{-1})	16.286
		Design dose rate (μSv h^{-1})	7.500
		Transmission	0.461

The desired degree of protection can only be provided by 6 mm lead [19].

* AKR is the air kerma rate constant in units of μGy m^2 GBq^{-1} h^{-1}

because of the increase in reflection coefficient with decreasing energy (Figure 17.9; [17]).

Mobile shielding

A mobile shield can be placed near to the patient to reduce the thickness of the external barrier it is shielding. Such shielding can be upright, placed at the side of the bed to shield reduce a wall or a door, or be curved so that it extends over the patient and also protects the ceiling. Mobile shields are normally constructed of lead and the size of the shield is dictated by the practicalities of manufacturing, manual handling, floor loading, and cost. They should be designed to be placed as close as possible to the bed to keep the height and width to a minimum. If there are potential problems shielding the room below, consideration should be given to placing lead under the bed.

If the mobile shield is to be used in the same position for every patient treatment, then it can be taken into account in the design process. The barrier thickness is calculated as above but the contribution from the primary radiation is reduced by attentuation in the mobile shield.

Anteroom and beyond

If an anteroom is present, it may well act as a type of maze, potentially reducing the shielding requirements on the door to the treatment room. In this circumstance, the anteroom must be declared a controlled area.

Multiple occupancy rooms

If the treatment room is designed for multiple occupancy, it will be necessary to provide shielding between patients. These shields should be designed in such a way as to ensure that the dose to patients in the adjacent areas does not exceed the design limit for members of the public.

HDR

The dose rates resulting from HDR treatment units can be as high as 5 Gy min^{-1}. As a result, the amount of primary shielding required will be greater than for conventional therapies. Scattered radiation will also have a greater magnitude and as a result the room will require either a maze or a heavy lead door. The substantial dose rates from HDR units make it extremely unlikely that a room designed for low- or medium-dose afterloading could be converted to HDR operation without considerable construction work being required. HDR units have, however, been housed in former radiotherapy treatment rooms [16]. A typical HDR layout is shown in Figure 18.3.

18.5.6 Controls

To ensure that the exposure to staff, visitors, and the general public is kept as low as reasonably achievable a

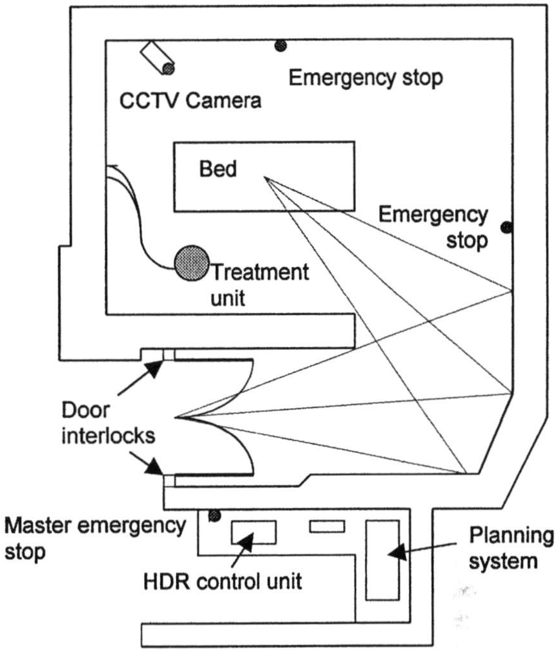

Figure 18.3 Layout of a typical high-dose rate (HDR) unit.

number of control measures can be employed:

- Signs must be displayed to indicate controlled areas. Illuminated signs are very effective at room entrances. An area on the roof or outside a treatment room that is designated as a controlled area must also be signed appropriately. Use of permits to work should be considered, see §6.6.2.
- Mobile shields that form part of the protection design must be used in the correct position during treatment.
- CCTV and intercom systems can be used for observation and communication, respectively. A telephone could also be provided for patients, although this should not replace personal visiting by visitors and comforters and carers.
- Door interlock systems must be provided on all rooms housing remote afterloading units.
- Protective clothing and emergency equipment, including monitoring devices, should be provided, as appropriate.
- Instructions for nursing staff should be available and unambiguous.
- Rooms should be monitored and decontaminated, as appropriate, at the end of a treatment.
- All waste from a room housing an unsealed-source therapy patient should be treated as radioactive waste and disposed of by physics staff.

18.6 Sealed-source laboratory: design and storage of sources

Sealed sources are usually stored and prepared for clinical use in a specialized room or area designed for the purpose, known as the sealed-source laboratory (SSL). The sources should be stored in a shielded safe, designed for the strength, quantity, and types of sources that it will hold. A good design is one that has several compartments. This allows sources of different types to be separated for ease of identification and stops the spread of contamination in the case of a source leaking. Each drawer should be designed to have suitable dimensions for the sources to be stored in it; it should be shielded at the front end and include an insert designed to ease access to the sources. For example, interstitial needles may be stored vertically in brass blocks drilled out to a depth that leaves the eye of the needle accessible to be picked up with a pair of forceps.

The safe is sited behind a protective lead bench so that the operator's trunk is protected when sources are removed from the drawers. The bench would ideally have built-in remote handling devices and a lead glass or mirror system so that sources are not viewed directly. Alternatively, a bench with a castellated top allows access for the operator's hands for source manipulation. A suitable bench can be constructed from interlocking lead bricks covered with a strong, scratch-resistant and waterproof material, such as linoleum. Any joints in the covering must be sealed. If a sink is incorporated into the bench it should be fitted with a suitable trap to prevent the loss of a source. The worksurface behind the shield should be large enough to allow all tasks to be carried out efficiently. Only necessary items of equipment should be behind the bench as this reduces the possibility of scattered radiation.

The SSL should be kept locked to restrict access and for general security. A separate lock on the safe may also be desirable. Arrangements for returning sources that have been removed from patients to the safe outside normal working hours and storing sources awaiting cleaning need to be considered. Ideally, the laboratory should be situated close to the area where the sources are to be used to reduce transportation distances. It is recommended that a warning notice is displayed outside the laboratory listing the principal contents or indicating the maximum activity of the principal radionuclides that will be stored in the room. Similarly, each safe drawer can be labelled to show the contents.

A custodian should be appointed with responsibility for the safe storage and control of the sealed-source stock. All aspects of storage, maintenance, and control of sources should be included in the local rules, for example:

- Only authorized personnel who have received appropriate training are allowed to work with sources.
- No source should be left out of the safe or storage area without good reason.

Sources should only leave the SSL for use in patients or for preparatory work prior to insertion, e.g. for sterilization.

18.7 Record keeping

Accounting for all sources at all times is an essential element of radiation protection practice in brachytherapy. This is achieved by maintaining detailed records within defined work practices set out in the local rules. Some of the record-keeping requirements are outlined below. A full discussion of the requirements for record keeping and the control of radioactive substances can be found in Chapter 9.

18.7.1 Sealed sources

The relevant documentation for sealed sources should include:

- a *source certificate file* containing all certificates supplied at purchase
- a *source record book* to record all the actions from preparation for use, through actual use until each source is finally disposed of off-site
- a *source ledger* to summarize the use of the sources on the patient
- a *source inventory* which contains records of periodic location checks, including radionuclide, type of source, source strength, calibration date, acceptance and leakage tests, the date of purchase, and serial number.

Inventory

The inventory in the SSL should be checked at least annually. All sources must be accounted for and checked against the safe contents diagram and other records. These checks should be signed and dated in the source inventory record.

Source use

When sources leave the SSL and when they are returned to the SSL, the patient's details should be entered into the source ledger and signed, and the safe contents diagram altered. When sources are made up specifically for individual patients, e.g. iridium wire, the details should be entered into the source record book. In the case of temporary insertions, the number and identity of sources are checked post-implant to ensure all activity has been returned. It is imperative that the whereabouts of the source be known at all times. The date of disposal or transfer of sources should be recorded.

18.7.2 Unsealed sources

Key records for unsealed-source therapy are:

- the date ordered
- the date received on-site
- the form of the source (liquid or capsule)
- the activity at the specified reference date
- the storage location
- the date of administration to the patient
- results of contamination monitoring after patient discharge
- disposal records (generally patient liquid waste—§9.3, Table 9.2).

18.8 Contingency plans

All hazards with the potential to cause a radiation accident should be identified and the risks arising from these hazards evaluated. Where the assessment shows that a risk exists, contingency plans must be drawn up and incorporated in the local rules. All staff who may become involved in an emergency must be aware of these contingency plans and be given suitable training, including rehearsals of the arrangements, if deemed appropriate. It is recommended that direct reading personal dosemeters, TL finger dosemeters, and a suitable hand-held radiation monitor are provided in an easily accessible place in the relevant area, to be used in addition to the normal whole-body monitor. A log book for recording doses from the direct reading dosemeters should be kept with them.

18.8.1 Sealed sources

Damage to a sealed source

Damage to a sealed source may cause the source to leak and pose a potential contamination hazard. Any source that is suspected of leaking should be leak tested Box 18.1. Damaged sources should not be reused, even if they are not leaking, as there is the potential for further damage once the encapsulation shows signs of weakness. Bent and broken sources should be kept isolated and sent for repair or disposal.

Loss of a sealed source

The loss of a sealed source creates an exposure hazard, which may be in an area where radiation is not normally expected and is a serious occurrence. When a source is lost or suspected to be lost, any actions which might cause the source to be moved further astray must stop immediately. This includes cleaning or disturbing the furniture in the area around the patient involved, disposal of waste, and movement of patients, and there should be minimal movement of staff. Use the nearest internal phone, i.e. least movement, to warn any persons or groups in other areas who may be affected, e.g. laundry, incinerator, those in neighbouring areas, as soon as possible. Physics department staff must be informed immediately and the head of department, the RPA, and the relevant RPS should also be informed. All movement of sources must be suspended so that an inventory may be taken to check which source is missing. The movement of the source up to the time it has been lost should also be traced from the source logging system. Do not discard anything from the area. These arrangements must remain in force until the RPA authorizes otherwise.

The RPA or responsible person should conduct a search for the source with a GM monitor, carrying out the following general sequence:

- Check the area immediately around the patient first. A visual inspection around the area, the bedclothes, and in the bed is a reasonable starting point. It may also be helpful to interview the patient.
- Survey the area with the monitor, paying particular attention to clothing, shoes, cracks in protection or flooring, suction apparatus, furniture, sinks, toilets, and soiled dressings. It will be difficult to find the source if other sources are in the vicinity, e.g. other implant patients, and they should therefore be moved temporarily while the search is being conducted.
- Progressively widen the search along transport routes and to other areas that it is likely that a source may have been lost in or carried to. These should be monitored in a sequence of decreasing likelihood of the source being present there.
- Extend the search to laundry skips, sluices, sinks, and drains in the area, and then if necessary to the laundry and further down the drain/sewer system.

If the source has not been found inform the hospital operational services manager and appropriate local and national regulatory bodies, e.g. police, local authority, HSE, Environmental Protection Agency.

When the source is found it can be returned to the store and examined for damage and leakage. If the source is leaking, check the areas where the source has been for contamination. It is recommended that a record of the incident be written, including the action taken by the RPA, and a copy held by the RPA.

18.8.2 Remote afterloading

Sources may become stuck in the applicators or transit tubes while being transferred back to the machine safe. As a minimum, a lead container constructed to accept the treatment catheters and long-handle forceps should be kept in the treatment room.

For an LDR unit, where the sources are transferred by compressed air, the first priority is to ascertain the location of the sources. A good plan would be to use a hand-held GM monitor to sweep along the entire length of the transit tubing, from the applicator to the base of the machine. If the sources are in the catheter, the coupling can be disconnected and the catheter placed into a shielded container. It may be possible to construct an uncoupling tool to keep the hands further away from the sources; however, this may increase the time taken to carry out the task. If the sources are in the transit tube, lead hemicylinders of suitable dimensions can be placed over the tubing to give the nursing staff some protection, and the patient uncoupled from the machine. Once the patient has been removed from the treatment room, time can be taken to assess the situation and plan the required action. If the sources are jammed in the transit tube and will not move, the tube will probably have to be cut and the sources transferred to a shielded container.

The problem is more serious for a unit that uses a single source on a drive cable, as the source activity is usually higher than that used in LDR machines. This is particularly the case for an HDR unit, where individual dwell times may only be 2–3 seconds and the patient will receive a significantly higher dose than anticipated. Action must be taken immediately and the source retracted into the safe using the manually operated system incorporated in the unit.

Whenever a problem with source transfer occurs, the machine manufacturer should be contacted for advice.

18.8.3 Unsealed sources

The major hazard from unsealed-source therapy is contamination, either from a spill of radionuclide or patient fluids. All spills should be dealt with promptly, using normal hygienic methods to ensure that the activity is contained. It is good practice to keep a spill kit in the vicinity of the treatment room. The person dealing with the spill must wear protective clothing, e.g. non-porous disposable gloves, a plastic apron, and overshoes, and it may be desirable to cover the GM probe with a polythene bag. Disposable towels are recommended for mopping up.

If contamination occurs as a result of a source spillage, establish the area affected and isolate it to prevent the spread of the contamination. The spill should be mopped up and the area then cleaned with soap and water or decontamination agent. If the contamination cannot be sufficiently removed, the affected area should be covered with polythene sheets for containment. If contamination affects a patient or member of staff, first remove contaminated clothing or bed linen and place it in a plastic bag. Allow the person to wash the affected areas with large quantities of water. If the face, hair, etc., is affected, take care not to contaminate the eyes, mouth, and nostrils. Continue to monitor until the residual activity is acceptable.

All radioactive material produced by the incident must be disposed of in the appropriate manner. Further information on dealing with contamination can be found in §15.9 and §15.10.

18.8.4 Fire

Fire potentially poses two hazards. First, there is the obvious external radiation hazard to fire-fighting staff if sources are in the region of the fire and the possibility of the fire causing the sources themselves to disintegrate and disperse. Second, patients with sources *in situ* may need to be evacuated into areas where radiation is not normally expected.

If a fire is found or suspected, the alarm should be raised and the normal hospital fire procedure followed. It is usual practice to ring the switchboard to confirm that the alarm is genuine and give the exact location. At this stage, the operator should also be informed that radiation sources are involved, so that the information can be passed on to the fire brigade. Any exposed sources should be replaced in a shielded container. If it becomes necessary to evacuate patients with sealed sources *in situ*, it is unlikely that there would be time to remove the sources, as it is more important to get the patients and staff to safety. Obviously, patients undergoing unsealed-source therapy will also be radioactive. Once evacuated, these patients must be isolated as much as practicable and arrangements made to continue the treatment in another area or to remove the sealed sources. The staff involved in the evacuation procedure could use a direct-reading personal dosemeter if one was easily available. Both the RPA and the RPS must be informed as soon as possible and make themselves available to give any advice required to the fire fighters.

It is advisable to discuss fire contingency plans with the local fire brigade officers. They should be made aware that there are sources on-site and informed of their location. A site visit by the fire brigade is also very worthwhile.

18.8.5 Cardiac arrest

The presence of sources must be considered as secondary to starting resuscitation, should this be necessary. For unsealed sources, a face mask with an oxygen bag is the preferred method to breathe for the patient, to avoid

Table 18.2 Maximum activities for post-mortem, burial and cremation of corpses without special precautions being necessary [7]

Radionuclide	Burial	Cremation
^{32}P	2000	30
^{89}Sr	2000	200
^{90}Y colloid	2000	70
^{125}I seeds	4000	4000
^{131}I	400	400
^{198}Au colloid or grains	400	100

contact with body fluids. Sealed sources may possibly be removed, once resuscitation has started. The staff resuscitating the patient could wear a direct-reading personal dosemeter if one was easily available. One piece of information often requested by resuscitation staff is the period of time basic life support has been given. This information is also valuable for the RPA to make an estimate of the dose received should no dosemeter be available.

18.8.6 Death of a radioactive patient

This subject is discussed with specific reference to unsealed-source therapy in §16.8.4. The same concepts apply to patients who have been administered permanent sealed-source implants and in this case the major concern will be prostate cancer patients with ^{125}I seed implants. Temporary sealed-source implants should be removed as soon as possible after death and certainly before the body is released from the ward.

Although it is preferable to assess the risks on a case-by-case basis, this may not always be possible and Table 18.2 shows the maximum activity of radionuclides permitted for burial and cremation of corpses without special precautions being necessary [7]. It is impossible to provide generic advice if a post-mortem is to be performed or the body is to be embalmed. In such cases individual risk assessments must be carried out.

18.8.7 Contingency rehearsal

It is good practice to organize regular rehearsals of contingency plans, particularly for nursing staff in case an incident occurs outside normal working hours. A 'stuck source' scenario can be simulated using a dedicated transport tube. The tube is modified so that activity can be introduced into defined places, in either the applicator area or the tubing or both. A small iridium wire, typically 5 mm long with a source strength of 2 MBq, is inserted into a holder and then positioned in the tubing. Staff are then requested to act out the 'stuck source' scenario. Videotaping the exercise is a useful training aid. The small amount of activity involved is a balance between ensuring the scenario is realistic while minimizing the exposure of the staff. The estimated dose at 1 metre from the activity is 0.004 μSv MBq^{-1} min^{-1} and such an exercise should only take 7–10 minutes maximum to perform.

18.9 References

1 Glasgow, G. P. (1999). Brachytherapy. In: *The modern technology of radiation oncology* (ed. J. V. Dyk), Chapter 18. Medical Physics, Madison.

2 Flower, M. A. and Chittenden, S. J. (2000). Unsealed source therapy. In: *Radiotherapy physics in practice* (2nd edn) (ed. J. R. Williams and D. I. Thwaites), Chapter 13. Oxford University Press.

3 *The radiochemical manual* (2nd edn) (1966). The Radiochemical Centre.

4 Aird, E. G., Williams, J. R., and Rembowska, A. (2000). Brachytherapy. In: *Radiotherapy physics in practice* (2nd edn) (ed. J. R. Williams and D. I. Thwaites), Chapter 12. Oxford University Press.

5 Goldstone, K. E., Jackson, P. C., Myers, M. J., and Simpson, A. E. (ed.) (1991). *Radiation protection in nuclear medicine and pathology.* IPEM Report 63. IPEM, York.

6 Institute of Physics and Engineering in Medicine (2002). *Medical and dental guidance notes.* IPEM, York.

7 British Standards Institution (1976). BS 5288: *Specification. Sealed radioactive sources.*

8 International Organization for Standardization (1999). *Radiation protection–Sealed radioactive sources–General requirements and classification.* ISO2919. ISO, Geneva.

9 International Organization for Standardization (1992). *Radiation protection–Sealed radioactive sources–Leakage test methods.* ISO9978. ISO, Geneva.

10 Health and Safety Executive (2000). *Work with ionising radiation. Approved code of practice and guidance.* HSE Books, Sudbury.

11 Godden, T. J. (1988). *Physical aspects of brachytherapy.* Section 9.4, Medical Physics Handbook 19. Adam Hilger, Bristol.

12 British Standards Institution (1990). BS 5724-2.17. *Medical electrical equipment. Particular requirements for safety. Specification of remote-controlled automatically-driven gamma-ray afterloading equipment.*

13 Institute of Physics and Engineering in Medicine (1999). *Physical aspects of quality control in radiotherapy.* IPEM Report 81. IPEM, York.

14 Kubo, H. D., Glasgow, G. P., Pethel, T. D., Thomadsen, B. R., and Williamson, J. F. (1998). AAPM Task Group 59. High dose rate brachytherapy delivery. *Med. Phys.*, **25**, 375–403.

15 Institute of Physics and Engineering in Medicine (1997). *The design of radiotherapy treatment room facilities.* IPEM Report 75. IPEM, York.

16 National Council on Radiation Protection and Measurements (1977). *Radiation protection design guidelines for 0.1–100 MeV particle accelerator facilities.* Report No. 51. NCRP, Washington.

17 National Council on Radiation Protection and Measurements (1976). Structural design and evaluation for medical use of

X-rays and gamma rays of energies up to 10 MeV. Report No. 49. NCRP, Washington.

18 The Radioactive Substances Advisory Committee (1971). *Handbook of radiological shielding, Part 1: Data prepared by a panel of the Radioactive Substances Advisory Committee.* HMSO, London.

Part IV

Non-ionising radiations

The radiation protection implications of non-ionising radiations in medical treatments are considered in the final part of the book. Requirements are not set out explicitly in legislation at the present time, but established good practice is given in standards and guidance documents and methods described are based on recommended practice. Chapter 19 on lasers covers mechanisms through which lasers can damage tissue, practical methodology for evaluating hazards, and general protection requirements. Chapter 20 deals with hazards and protection for non-coherent optical radiations. Electromagnetic fields covering a wide range of frequencies are encountered in a variety of areas, such as magnetic resonance imaging (MRI) systems, diathermy, and communication systems. Implications for safety of individuals from direct exposure and interference with electromedical devices are considered in Chapter 21. Exposure standards for ultrasound have only recently been established and Chapter 22 discusses the concept and application of protection to ultrasound techniques.

Symbols

angle of incidence	α, θ (degrees or radians)
angular frequency	ω (s^{-1})
area	a (m^2)
area	A (m^2)
atomic number	Z
blue-light hazard function	B_λ
current	I (A, mA)
current density	J (A m^{-2})
density	ρ (kg m^{-3})
effective irradiance	E_{eff} (W m^{-2})
electric charge	q (C) coulomb
electric field strength	E (V m^{-1})
electric conductivity	σ (S m^{-1}) (siemens m^{-1})
energy of photon	E (eV)
eye exposure (unprotected)	H (J)
divergence of laser beam	ϕ (degrees)
figure of merit (radiometer)	f_2 (%)
frequency	f (Hz)
gyromagnetic ratio	γ (MHz T^{-1})
intrinsic wave impedance	η (Ω)
irradiance	E (W m^{-2})
laser goggles (scale number)	L
linear attenuation coefficient	μ (m^{-1})
magnetic field strength	H (A m^{-1})
magnetic flux density	B (tesla)
maximum permitted exposure time	t_{max} (s)
maximum radiant dose	D_{max} (J m^{-2} sr^{-1})
permeability of free space	μ_o (H m^{-1})
permittivity of free space	ϵ_o (F m^{-1})
permittivity (complex)	ϵ (F m^{-1})
Planck constant	h (J s)
power	P (W or J)
power density	S (W m^{-2})
propagation constant	γ (m^{-1})
radiance	L (W m^{-2} sr^{-1})
radiant flux	ϕ (W)
radiant exposure	H (J m^{-2})
radiant intensity	I (W sr^{-1})
radiation force	F (mN)
retinal irradiance	E_r (W m^{-2})
specific heat	c (J kg^{-1})
spectral effectiveness factor	$S(\lambda)$
spectral irradiance	$E_s(\lambda)$ (W m^{-2} nm^{-1})
spectral radiance	L_λ (W m^{-2} sr^{-1} nm^{-1})
spectral thermal hazard function	R_λ
ultrasound absorption coefficient	α (dB cm^{-1} MHz^{-1})
ultrasound pulse-pressure-squared integral	p_i
ultrasound pressure	p
ultrasound spatial-peak temporal average intensity	I_{SPTA} (W m^{-2})
ultrasound time-averaged intensity	I_{TA} (W m^{-2})
total acoustic power	P (W)
velocity (of light or sound)	c (m s^{-1})
wavelength	λ (m)

Chapter 19

Lasers

H. Moseley

19.1 Introduction

Lasers are in widespread use in almost every clinical speciality. The use of the argon laser in ophthalmology dates back to the 1970s and the ability of the laser to deliver precise, targeted treatment with minimal collateral damage has driven the expansion into an ever-increasing variety of applications. Technological advances have also contributed enormously to the ongoing development. A major feature of modern laser systems using laser diodes is portability, a characteristic which has considerable safety implications. As well as their potential benefits, lasers also carry a risk of harm to any person accidentally exposed to the laser beam. The laser safety expert is tasked with the responsibility of ensuring that the risk is as low as reasonably achievable, within the context of a hospital environment. The purpose of this chapter is to equip the reader with some of the knowledge and understanding necessary to accomplish this. Basic laser physics is presented briefly in Box 19.1.

19.2 Laser–tissue interactions

There are four principal mechanisms whereby laser–tissue interactions take place. Photochemical effects are due to direct absorption of the laser beam by specific chemicals with little or no temperature rise. Photothermal effects are due to the temperature rise caused by absorption of the laser radiation. At higher powers, pressure waves and shock waves are generated, giving rise to photomechanical effects. If the photon energy of the laser beam is sufficiently high, this may cause direct breaking of molecular bonds, so-called photoablation. Characteristics of lasers commonly used in medicine, some of which are referred to in this section, are summarized in Box 19.2.

19.2.1 Photochemical effects

Photochemical effects refer to the type of reaction where there is a direct absorption of incident optical radiation by some specific chemical, known as a chromophore. The chemical may be endogenous (that is, present naturally) or exogenous (added by systemic or local administration). For an effect to be characterized as photochemical, there must be almost no increase in temperature. The conditions where such effects predominate are long exposure duration (10 seconds or more) and low power density. Photochemical effects are more likely to occur with short wavelength light since photon energy increases with decreasing wavelength. Photochemical effects occur naturally in the body. For example, different types of photoreceptors in the retina absorb light at different wavelengths. This produces a chemical reaction and the perception of vision. In the skin, vitamin D synthesis, tanning, and erythema (sunburn) are all the result of photochemical reactions.

The therapeutic procedure, photodynamic therapy (PDT), is an example of a photochemical reaction, where a chemical sensitizer is administered to the patient. The chemical is chosen such that it will tend to accumulate in cancer cells. Thereafter, the tumour is exposed to low-level irradiation from a light source of wavelength which matches the absorption characteristics of the chromophore. This then causes the release of a cytotoxic substance, with resultant tumour destruction.

Another example of a photochemical effect, this time with implications for laser safety, is the so-called blue-light hazard. Photoreceptors located within the retina are particularly sensitive to blue light, and photochemical damage may be caused by prolonged exposure of the eye to blue light [1]. Studies carried out in the Rhesus monkey showed that retinal lesions could be produced by irradiation with blue light of wavelength 441 nm at only 3 W m^{-2} although the temperature rise was less than 0.1°C [2].

Box 19.1 Basic laser physics

The word 'laser' is an acronym for light amplification by stimulated emission of radiation. A precondition for lasing is that the substance is in a condition whereby there is a greater occupation of higher than lower energy states. This is known as population inversion and requires input of energy from an external source, or pump. The pump may be a flash of light, an electrical discharge, or a chemical reaction. An incoming photon interacts with the excited atom, causing a second photon to be released which is identical to the original, stimulating, photon (Figure B19.1). The two identical photons continue to pass through the substance, interacting with more excited atoms, and eliciting the production of more photons, identical in frequency and phase. The photons are reflected back into the material from mirrors which are placed at opposite ends of the cavity. Light is amplified on each passage through the substance (Figure B19.2). One of the mirrors is totally reflecting while the other is only partially reflecting, thus allowing a small percentage of laser radiation to emerge from a small aperture in the centre. As a result of many reflections between the mirrors, light which emerges from the laser aperture is collimated, with very little divergence.

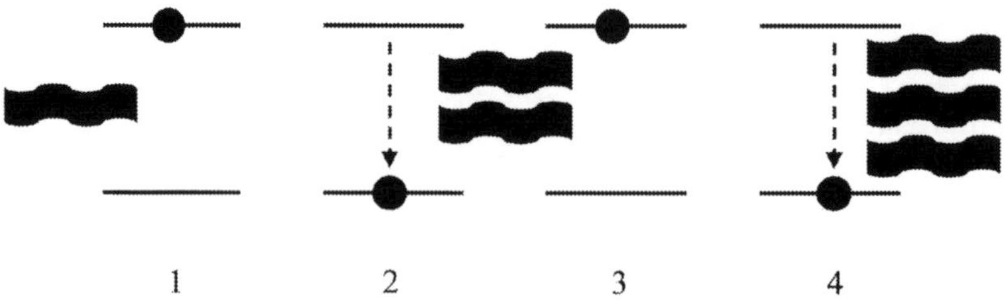

Figure B19.1 Diagram showing the basic laser process. 1. Incident photon interacts with excited atom. 2. Interaction stimulates the emission of identical photon as atom energy level drops to ground state. 3. Two identical photons travel through substance and interact with another excited atom. 4. Interaction stimulates the emission of identical photon as energy level drops to ground state, resulting in three identical photons.

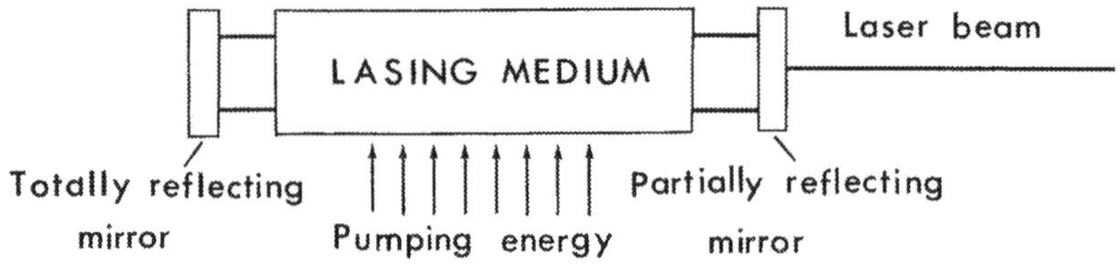

Figure B19.2 Components of a laser. The basic laser process takes place within the lasing medium, which is kept in a state of population inversion by pumping energy. Photons travel through the medium and are reflected off the mirrors, one of which is only partially reflecting and allows the emission of the laser beam.

A series of studies carried out on ophthalmologists showed that there was a reduction in colour discrimination in argon laser users [3]. Subjects who demonstrated this effect were unaware of its existence, and the clinical consequences are unknown. However, this caused concern among laser users. It was believed that it was due to prolonged exposure to the blue component in the low-power aiming beam, since when the treatment beam is on, the operator's eyes are protected by a filter. Most new argon lasers use a red aiming beam from a separate helium–neon or solid-state GaAs laser. Older lasers, which use an attenuated version of the blue–green argon laser beam, can be modified by the fitting of a 'green only' filter to the aiming beam.

Damage from blue light is linearly additive for exposure duration up to 3 hours [4]. There is even evidence to suggest that there is a cumulative effect for periods as long as 4 days [5]. The relative blue-light hazard of different wavelengths is contained in a published standard [4] which may be used to calculate the risk from non-laser sources. Standards devised for laser devices are described in §19.7 and these contain a hazard weighting towards the blue end of the spectrum.

Box 19.2 Characteristics of some common hospital lasers

The most common types of laser used in hospitals are given in the table below, with information on the applications. Laser diodes are increasing rapidly because of their small size and reliability.

Type of laser	Wavelength (nm)	Power/ energy	Application
Argon	488; 515	1 W	Retinal coagulation
Carbon dioxide	10 600	30 W	Cervical intra-epithelial neoplasia Laryngeal papillomata Vocal cord nodules
Diode	630 to 950 (fixed)	1.5 to 60 W	Laparoscopic surgery Prostatotomy PDT
Dye	400 to 700 (variable)	15 J	Port-wine stain Pigmented lesions
Excimer	193	450 mJ	Photorefractive keratectomy
HoYAG	2124	2 J	Endonasal surgery
KTP	532	10 W	Telangectasia
NdYAG (cw)	1064	100 W	Prostatotomy Endoscopic and bronchoscopic surgery Endometrial ablation
NdYAG (Q switch)	1064	10 mJ	Posterior lens capsulotomy Tattoo removal
Ruby	690	60 mJ	Tattoo removal

It has been shown that sensitivity to photochemical damage in the photoreceptors increases considerably with temperature rises of only a few degrees [6]. This is described as thermally-enhanced photochemical damage.

19.2.2 Photothermal effects

Most clinical applications of lasers rely on a photothermal reaction. The absorption of laser radiation causes a temperature rise. Protein denaturation takes place between 55 and 60C as the triple helical configuration of collagen is unwound. This causes blanching and contraction and the resultant coagulation seals small blood vessels. The NdYAG laser is particularly effective in this regard due to the deeper penetration of the beam through tissue [7]. It is well suited for photocoagulation of benign or malignant tumours in the gastrointestinal or respiratory tract. The argon laser and KTP laser radiation is absorbed by melanin pigmentation in the retinal pigment epithelium within the eye and by haemoglobin within the vasculature which leads to coagulation. Retinal photocoagulation is widely used in the treatment of diabetic retinopathy. There is a twofold mechanism by which photocoagulation seals small vessels—one is collagen shrinkage in and around vessel walls, the other is haemoglobin heating sufficient to cause blockage. Some laser techniques rely on coagulation to produce cellular necrosis. Cancers in solid organs, e.g. liver, are destroyed by interstitial laser photocoagulation using low-powered lasers in the near-infrared region. Coagulated tissue is eventually replaced by benign scar tissue.

Vaporization occurs when tissue temperature reaches 100°C, when intra- and extracellular water evaporates. Laser radiation from the CO_2 laser is in the far-infrared region where the absorption coefficient of water is very high. As a result, it is a very effective wavelength for vaporization with minimal subsurface damage, and tissue penetration is approximately 0.1 mm. The CO_2 laser has been widely used for vaporization in gynaecology, otorhinolaryngology (ENT), neurosurgery, dermatology, and general surgery. The CO_2 laser is primarily a cutting tool. One of its limitations is its poor coagulative properties. To produce generalized heating and achieve some thermal coagulation, the CO_2 laser may be used in a defocused manner. This spreads the beam over a larger area and thereby reduces the surface irradiance. Distances for absorption of 90% of the energy in lightly pigmented skin are 0.2, 0.5, and 2 mm for the CO_2, argon, and NdYAG lasers, respectively. This is referred to as the extinction length, namely the distance from the tissue surface at which the incident beam has been reduced to 10% of its initial intensity. A related parameter, the absorption coefficient, defines the distance within which the intensity is reduced to

1/e of the incident value. There are about 2.3 absorption lengths within each extinction length. At sufficiently high power (above 60 W) the NdYAG laser will also vaporize tissue. However, increased penetration of the NdYAG laser beam causes a greater zone of tissue necrosis and coagulation. It should be noted that penetration of the NdYAG laser beam is significantly reduced if carbonization takes place. In this case, the NdYAG laser becomes a predominantly surface absorber.

At higher temperatures, further thermal effects appear. Between 300 and 400°C carbonization occurs, with charring of tissue. At temperatures in excess of 500°C, carbonized tissue begins to burn.

The rate at which temperature rises in irradiated tissue depends on the rate at which energy is absorbed (laser power) and the rate at which cooling occurs. Within the body, cooling takes place by way of blood flow and also by conduction into surrounding tissue. For this reason smaller irradiated volumes can cool more rapidly than larger volumes. Also, tissues, such as the intraocular crystalline lens, which are situated far from blood vessels, are more susceptible to thermal damage.

The implications of the high rate of blood flow in the choroid, within the eye, for laser coagulation of the retina have been considered [8]. The choroid is a highly vascular tissue adjacent to the retinal pigment epithelium, where incident laser light is absorbed. Direct temperature measurement failed to demonstrate any differences in temperature readings during laser irradiation with or without choroidal circulation, indicating that the effect of circulation was negligible. A theoretical analysis showed that a cooling effect appeared when blood flow exceeded physiological values 10 times. However, calculations showed that blood flow was extremely effective in stabilizing retinal temperature in wide-area long exposure durations. Perfusion rates only a third of normal physiological values led to a reduction of more than 70% in the temperature rise caused by continuous large-area retinal irradiation (about 50 mm^2) within 10 minutes. Conditions such as this occur during illumination of the fundus with an indirect ophthalmoscope.

Photothermal effects can be restricted to absorbing chromophores within tissue where short laser pulses are used. The pulse length must be less than or comparable to the thermal relaxation time of the chromophore, which is the time for the raised temperature of the chromophore to have fallen by 50%, after the heat source has been removed. Vascular lesions such as port-wine stain are treated with pulsed dye lasers using a wavelength which is selectively absorbed in blood vessels. If the pulse is too long, heat is conducted to surrounding tissue and selectivity is lost.

19.2.3 Photomechanical effects

Photomechanical effects may arise when a very high-power, short-duration laser pulse is in use. Typical power density is about 10^{16} W m^{-2} and exposure time of the order of 10^{-9} seconds. This is a non-linear absorption phenomenon. If there is a sufficiently high concentration of power in a small volume, then a transient electrical plasma may be formed. This involves stripping electrons from the absorbing medium and producing a state of ionised matter. The collapse of the plasma produces a shock wave which is dissipated in the surrounding volume and is capable of disrupting tissue in close proximity. Although plasma temperature exceeds 10 000°C, there is no thermal effect on tissue because the exposure duration is too short. Mechanical forces may also be exerted on tissue as a result of very rapid heating even though there is not sufficient concentration of intensity to create a plasma.

The complex phenomena associated with laser-induced breakdown has been extensively studied and reviewed elsewhere [9]. Freshly extracted vitreous humour from the eye exhibits a threshold irradiance fairly close to that of distilled water or saline. As pulse duration increases, the threshold intensity for plasma breakdown decreases, and the threshold pulse energy increases. The occurrence of breakdown is thought to be due to avalanche ionisation initiated by so-called lucky electrons oscillating in phase with the electric field.

Short-duration nanosecond pulses can be produced using a technique called Q-switching. Energy stored within the lasing medium builds up and is released in the space of a few nanoseconds. A typical Q-switched NdYAG laser in ophthalmology has a pulse energy of 10 mJ and duration of 10 ns. The power level during the pulse is 1 MW. If focused into a small spot (25 to 50 mm) then a plasma is formed. Plasma breakdown threshold varies depending on the absorbing medium. In transparent targets, irradiance must be at least 10 TW m^{-2} [10]. In a liquid, threshold is lowered by the presence of impurities; in a solid it is reduced at a surface interface [11]. At such high irradiances the electric field associated with the laser emission is sufficiently high to overcome the dielectric strength of the target material and to create ion-electron pairs. A luminous spark may be seen and a cracking sound heard as the shock wave is transmitted. If the laser is being fired in air, the breakdown threshold depends on humidity. Blackened photographic paper provides a convenient target to check laser performance.

The Q-switched NdYAG laser is used in ophthalmology to carry out a procedure known as posterior lens capsulotomy. The lens in the eye is contained within a capsule. When the lens has been removed in the treatment of cataract, the posterior lens capsule is left in place. In some cases, this becomes opaque, thus limiting the effectiveness of the procedure. Fortunately, the posterior lens capsule may be opened without surgical intervention by focusing the laser beam from a

Q-switched NdYAG laser on this structure. The shock wave produced makes a hole in the capsule, which tears open because of the tension in which the membrane is held. This allows light transmission through to the retina. Sight is restored—and it only takes a few nanoseconds!

Once the plasma has been formed, the incident radiation will be effectively absorbed by the plasma. This effect, known as plasma shielding, is an important safety factor as it reduces the amount of energy delivered to the retina. In order to achieve very high irradiance, there is strong focusing of the laser beam. As the laser radiation approaches the focus, plasma breakdown may occur before the focal point is reached if the intensity is sufficiently great to initiate breakdown. This phenomenon, known as plasma wandering, may cause pitting of the intraocular lens implant, which has been inserted in the eye after removal of the natural lens.

19.2.4 Photoablative effects

In early laser literature, the term 'ablation' was used to describe vaporization of a large surface of tissue, e.g. the cervix, by making several passes over the area. Now, photoablation usually refers to the direct breaking of molecular bonds, using an excimer laser emitting short-wavelength ultraviolet radiation. Examples of excimer lasers are the argon fluoride and xenon chloride lasers, which emit laser radiation in the ultraviolet region. Pulse times are short, between 10^{-6} and 10^{-9} s. A purely photoablative reaction is non-thermal. Ultraviolet photons have sufficient energy to break molecular bonds directly. Clearly, for this to work, the photon energy must exceed that of the chemical bond.

Absorption of the short-wavelength excimer laser radiation principally occurs in protein in the cornea. Absorption peaks around 190 nm are thought to be due to absorption by the C–N peptide linkage. At longer wavelengths, there are absorption maxima around 260 nm, which correspond to absorption by nucleotide bases in nucleic acid. Ultraviolet radiation is known to have a number of undesirable effects on cells, including mutagenesis and carcinogenesis. This has raised concern regarding the use of the excimer laser in the cornea. However, it appears that at least at 193 nm, there is no clinically significant DNA damage [12].

The excimer laser is used to alter corneal curvature. In 1983, the first reported use of the excimer laser to achieve precise etching of the cornea was published [13]. Laser damage was localized to the zone of ablation with no sign of thermal effects. Photorefractive keratectomy (PRK) is a technique in which radial keratotomies are performed with the excimer laser. Two wavelengths, 193 and 248 nm, have been used. Differences in absorption result in damage zones of 0.1–0.3 μm for 193 nm and 2.5 μm wide at 248 nm, which may explain the superior performance achieved at 193 nm. Although still awaiting long-term follow-up, early results suggest that excimer laser PRK for mild to moderate myopia is predictable and successful but results are less encouraging for high myopia.

The XeCl excimer laser (wavelength 308 nm) has been used for angioplasty, particularly in the coronary arteries, but this has not become an established technique. Laser radiation is delivered via a multifibre catheter, consisting of about 100 fibres each of diameter 50 μm, arranged around a guidewire. Laser radiation emitted from the catheter cores out the plaque creating a lumen down the centre of the artery. Laser angioplasty is under investigation as an alternative to balloon angioplasty but, in practice, laser treatment is usually followed by balloon angioplasty. In addition, arterial wall injury remains a major risk.

19.3 Risks

Surgical lasers are not, and cannot be, zero-risk devices. They are capable of causing damage to biological tissue. If this were not so, they would be of no clinical value. The challenge is to minimize risk to patients and staff while still allowing the lasers to be used in an effective manner. An important principle is that all of the danger is contained within the beam, unlike X-rays where protection is required against scattered radiation during X-ray exposure. To avoid damage from accidental laser exposure, care must be taken to ensure that the laser beam does not accidentally strike anyone who may be present during laser surgery. With most surgical lasers the risk of damage is high if the beam strikes someone. The damage may be severe if the eye is the target.

19.4 Direct effects

The immediate hazard is a direct consequence of accidental exposure to the laser beam. Although a laser burn to the finger of the operator may be painful, it is unlikely to cause significant damage. It may even serve as a salutary reminder of the dangers of unintentional exposure to the laser beam. However, if the laser beam were to strike the unprotected eye, serious damage could occur which might even be sight-threatening. It is, therefore, useful to consider separately hazards to eyes and skin.

19.4.1 Hazards to eyes

Light must pass through the outer cornea, aqueous humour, lens, and vitreous humour before it reaches the retina. Hence, the susceptibility of the retina depends on the optical transmission through the ocular media, which

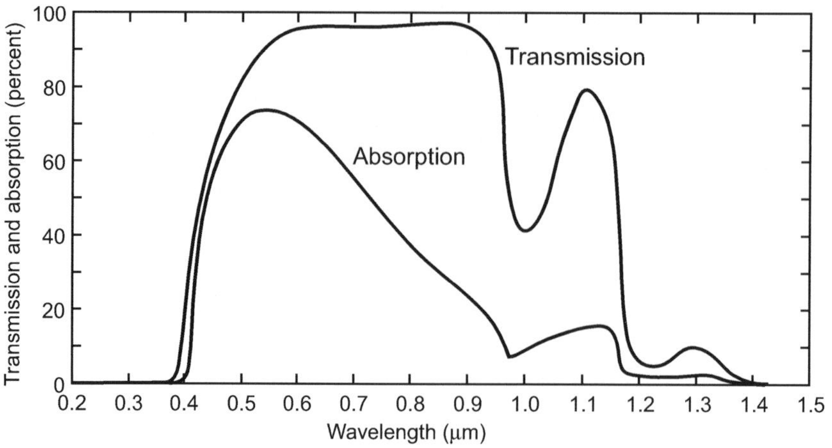

Figure 19.1 Transmission from the front of the eye through the cornea, anterior chamber, lens, and vitreous humour to the retina, and absorption in the retina. (From WHO 1982[13a].)

varies with wavelength (Figure 19.1). Wavelengths between 400 and 1200 nm pose a threat to the retina. This means that lasers which emit visible or near-infrared radiation are particularly dangerous. These cause photothermal damage to the retina, resulting in photocoagulation. The resultant visual impairment may be permanent.

The extent of the damage depends on which part of the retina is struck by the laser beam. If the beam enters the eye obliquely, it will strike some part of the peripheral retina. This is not catastrophic. Indeed, it is likely that it will not affect vision at all and will only be evident on ophthalmic examination. The reason is that the eye is moving continually and the image formed on any small portion of the peripheral retina is being continually refreshed. A critical area for retinal damage is the fovea, which is located in the centre of the macula (Figure 19.2). This is the region of the retina responsible for central vision. The visual angle subtended by the fovea is very small and is approximately equal to that subtended by the moon.

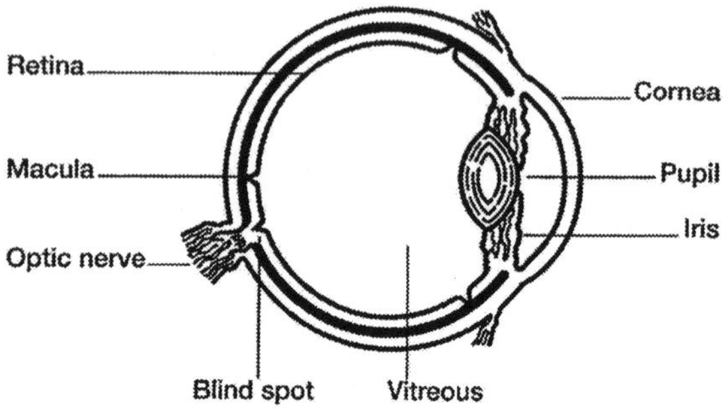

Figure 19.2 Cross-sectional diagram of the eye.

With respect to laser radiation in the visible and near-infrared region of the spectrum, the most important chromophore is melanin. This is located in the retinal pigment epithelium (RPE), adjacent to the rods and cones. Hence absorption of light in the RPE may cause damage to the retina by thermal conduction. Only about 5% of incident light is absorbed by the visual pigments in the rods and cones. Melanin is also located in the iris, uvea, and trabecular meshwork. Other absorbing substances include haemoglobin in blood vessels, and xanthophyll, which is found in the macular area. Xanthophyll absorbs blue light strongly and so use of the argon laser at a wavelength of 488 nm is inappropriate near the macula. Red light from the krypton laser is used in the macular area, but because of deeper penetration, red and near-infrared lasers cause increased patient discomfort and increased risk of choroidal haemorrhage. From theoretical considerations [14], yellow light would appear to be the most appropriate for retinal coagulation as it is at the peak of the oxyhaemoglobin absorption and is poorly absorbed by xanthophyll. As discussed in §19.2.1, the eye is especially sensitive to blue light. Prolonged exposure to blue light may cause photochemical damage leading to altered colour perception.

Ultraviolet (UV) and infrared (IR) radiation are absorbed in both the cornea and the lens. UV-A (315 to 400 nm) is absorbed principally in the lens. UV-B (280 to 315 nm), UV-C (100 to 280 nm), IR-B (1400 to 3000 nm), and IR-C (3000 nm to 1 mm) are all absorbed by the cornea. A damaged cornea may be treated effectively by a corneal graft but there is no treatment for laser-induced retinal damage.

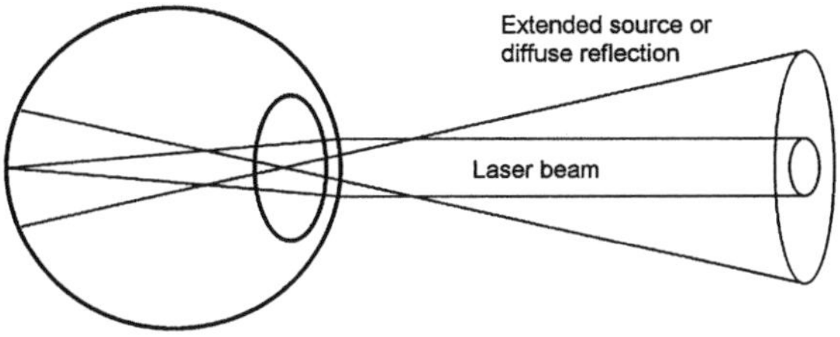

Figure 19.3 Schematic representation of the eye showing intrabeam viewing when a collimated beam is focused to a small spot on the retina, compared to viewing an extended source forming a larger image on the retina.

The eye has its own protective mechanisms. A bright light causes an aversion response, which comprises closure of the eyelids (the blink reflex) and rotation of the eyeball. This takes up to 0.25 seconds. So in terms of the hazard potential of a bright light, the question is whether sufficient light enters the eye in 0.25 seconds to cause damage. Many pulsed lasers are capable of delivering radiated power to the eye in a time which is too short to invoke the blink reflex. The pupil of the eye also adjusts in diameter according to ambient light levels but this is comparatively slow. It can alter in area by a factor of 30:1.

The eye focuses parallel light on to a very small spot on the retina (Figure 19.3). This is part of its normal functioning. Unfortunately, it increases the hazard to the retina from accidental ocular exposure to a laser beam. Most of the focusing power of the eye takes place at the cornea, the lens providing an additional variable focus element. If light enters the eye as a collimated beam (e.g. from a laser), the optical gain within the eye is 10 000 to 100 000. This is because the light, which passes through the pupil, diameter 7 mm, is focused to a spot on the retina of about 10 μm diameter. This produces an irradiance at the retina, which is at least 10 000 times greater than that incident on the cornea.

High-power, short-duration Q-switched laser pulses cause photoacoustic damage. Q-switched NdYAG lasers are widely used in ophthalmology. The beam has a high angle of convergence in order to achieve a high power density at the focal spot. This means that there is an equally high divergence beyond the focal spot. Since the laser is generally used to treat the area just behind the lens, the rapid divergence confers protection on the retina. In addition, the Q-switched NdYAG laser beam forms a plasma which enhances absorption and means that there is very little transmission beyond the focal spot (§19.2.3). Of course, this is only the case once the plasma has been formed. Paradoxically, the power transmitted to the back of the eye is greater when the power density is just below threshold for plasma formation.

A laser beam may induce a bright flash of light which, potentially, may constitute a hazard. A Q-switched NdYAG laser, when it is tightly focused, produces a plasma, which is seen as a bright flash of light. Viewing the flash inside the patient's eye is not considered hazardous to the ophthalmologist performing the treatment, but looking through the microscope at a plasma in air could be [15]. Another situation in which a flash of light is produced is laser-induced tissue incandescence. This is fairly common during CO_2 laser application. A combined theoretical and experimental study showed that viewing the incandescent flashes did not constitute a hazard at powers up to 100 W [16].

19.4.2 Evaluation of eye hazard

Intrabeam viewing

Maximum permissible exposure (MPE) levels have been set for viewing laser radiation in terms of energy incident on the cornea per unit area derived from measurements of thresholds to produce lesions. The standards current at the time of publication are given in Table 19.1 [17]. The MPEs depend on both the wavelength and duration of the exposure (Figure 19.4). When a person views a well-collimated laser beam in the wavelength range 400–1400 nm, all the power may be focused onto a single spot on the retina and the hazard may be almost independent of the distance. The MPEs for these wavelengths are orders of magnitude less than those for wavelengths absorbed in the cornea in most cases. Derived factors (C_1–C_4 and C_7) are used to change MPEs with wavelength in a manner linked to the hazard level. Hazard assessments are made by comparing the irradiance at the cornea with the relevant MPEs.

For wavelengths between 400 and 1400 nm, the radiation is averaged over a circle of diameter 7 mm, representing the limiting aperture and the worst-case condition, while for other wavelengths an aperture of 1 mm is used. MPEs depend on the length of the exposure, but for visible lasers the aversion response of 0.25 s can be used as the limiting time, unless the aversion response is inhibited, e.g. by anaesthesia. The MPEs are used in determining the optical density of goggles required to provide protection for each type of laser (§19.10) and the range of distances over which the laser presents an ocular hazard or nominal ocular hazard distance (§19.9.2) (see Box 19.3).

Extended sources

When viewing extended light sources (400–1400 nm), the image on the retina is larger (Figure 19.3) and so the radiated power is distributed over an increased area. Radiation diffusely reflected from a surface irradiated by a laser may represent an extended source. For all sources,

Table 19.1 Maximum permissible exposure (MPE) (J m^{-2}) at the cornea and on skin for ocular and skin exposure, respectively, to laser radiation for a range of exposure times [17]

Wavelength range (nm)	Eye 10^{-8} s to 1.8×10^{-5} s	Eye 1.8×10^{-5} s to 10^{-3} s	Eye 10^{-3} s to 10 s	Skin 10^{-7} s to 10 s
180–302.5	30	30	30	30
302.5–315	C_1 ($t < T_1$) C_2 ($t > T_1$)	C_1 ($t < T_1$) C_2 ($t > T_1$)	C_1 ($t < T_1$) C_2 ($t > T_1$)	C_1 ($t < T_1$) C_2 ($t > T_1$)
315–400	C_1	C_1	C_1	C_1
400–700	5×10^{-3} C_6	18 C_6 $t^{0.75}$	18 C_6 $t^{0.75}$	1.1×10^4 $t^{0.25}$
700–1050	5×10^{-3} C_4 C_6	18 C_4 C_6 $t^{0.75}$	18 C_4 C_6 $t^{0.75}$	1.1×10^4 C_4 $t^{0.25}$
1050–1400	5×10^{-2} C_6 C_7	5×10^{-2} C_6 C_7, $t < t_1$ 90 $t^{0.75}$ C_6 C_7, $t > t_1$	90 $t^{0.75}$ C_6 C_7	1.1×10^4 C_4 $t^{0.25}$
1400–1500	10^3	10^3	5600 $t^{0.25}$	5600 $t^{0.25}$
1500–1800	10^4	10^4	10^4	5600 $t^{0.25}$
1800–2600	10^3	10^3	5600 $t^{0.25}$	5600 $t^{0.25}$
2600–10^6	100, $t < 10^{-7}$ s 5600 $t^{0.25}$, $t > 10^{-7}$s	5600 $t^{0.25}$	5600 $t^{0.25}$	5600 $t^{0.25}$

$C_1 = 5.6 \times 10^3\ t^{0.25}$; $C_2 = 10^{0.2(\lambda-295)}$; $C_4 = 10^{(\lambda-700)/500}$; C_6 is given in §19.4.2; $C_7 = 1$ for λ = 1050–1150 nm, $C_7 = 10^{0.018(\lambda-1150)}$ for λ = 1150–1200 nm, and $C_7 = 8$ for λ = 1200 – 1400 nm; $T_1 = 10^{0.8(\lambda-295)} \times 10^{-15}$ s; and $t_1 = 5 \times 10^{-5}$ s. MPEs for other exposure times and wavelengths can be found in standards [17].

there comes a point as the source approaches the eye where it becomes an extended source. As the distance is further decreased, the hazard is reduced as the retinal image size increases. The MPEs applied to intrabeam viewing are increased by a factor C_6 if the angular subtense of the source (measured at the viewer's eye) is greater than an angle α_{min}, which varies with exposure time *t*.

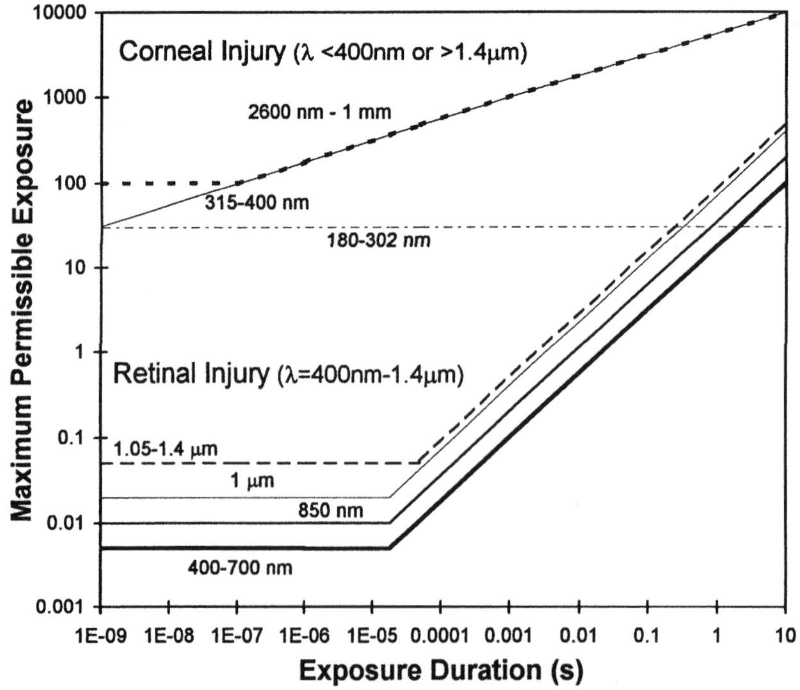

Figure 19.4 Plots of the variations in maximum permissible exposure (MPE) levels in J m^{-2} against duration of exposure. MPEs are shown for various wavelength ranges, with those relating to retinal injury from the visible and near-infrared (400 nm–1.4 μm) being lower than those for corneal injury from the ultraviolet (180–400 nm) and far-infrared (1550 nm–1 mm).

$$\alpha_{min} = 1.5 \text{ mrad} \qquad \text{for } t < 0.7 \text{ s}$$

$$\alpha_{min} = 2t^{0.75} \text{mrad} \qquad \text{for } 0.7\text{s} < t < 10 \text{ s}$$

$$\alpha_{min} = 11 \text{ mrad} \qquad \text{for } t > 10 \text{ s}$$

The correction factor C_6 is given by

$$C_6 = 1 \qquad \text{for } \alpha < \alpha_{min}$$

$$C_6 = \alpha/\alpha_{min} \qquad \text{for } \alpha_{min} < \alpha < \alpha_{max}$$

$$C_6 = \alpha_{max}/\alpha_{min} \qquad \text{for } \alpha > \alpha_{max}$$

where $\alpha_{max} = 0.1$ rad and is the angular subtense of the apparent source above which MPEs and accessible emission limits (AELs, §19.7) are calculated independently of the source size.

Pulsed lasers

Where a repetitively pulsed laser is used, additional restrictions are applied. In determining the MPE to the eye at wavelengths from 400nm to 10^6 nm, use the most restrictive of a), b) and c); for other wavelengths use the more restrictive of a) and b).

a) The exposure for any single pulse within a train must not exceed the MPE for a single pulse (MPE_{single}).
b) The average irradiance for a pulse train of a given duration must not exceed the MPE for a single pulse for the same duration.
c) When the exposure consists of N pulses, the MPE for any single pulse within the train (MPE_{train}) must not exceed $MPE_{single} \times N^{-\frac{1}{4}}$. The parameter $N^{-\frac{1}{4}}$ is identified as C_5 in standards (Table 19.1).

19.4.3 Hazard to skin

The hazards to skin are essentially akin to those in other soft tissues. With most surgical lasers, damage is thermal in nature. The result is vaporization of tissue with a surrounding zone of coagulation. This is painful but, provided there is no infection, it should prove to be a relatively minor problem. Naturally, if a large crater is formed, the damage will be more severe. Since the concentration of absorbing pigment is an important factor, dark-skinned persons will receive a more severe skin burn than fair-skinned. Some MPEs for skin exposure are given in Table 19.1. Assessments are based on a 3.5 mm aperture for the wavelength range 400–1400 nm and a 1 mm aperture for other wavelengths.

Absorption of laser radiation may alter the level of melanin pigmentation in the skin. Both hyper- and hypopigmentation may occur after laser treatment of vascular and pigmented lesions in the skin. Scarring may also follow laser irradiation when the heat is not limited to the upper layers of the skin but is conducted throughout the dermis.

19.5 Indirect effects

While attention is placed on the hazards from accidental exposure to the laser beam, it should also be recognized that there are indirect effects, which otherwise might be overlooked.

19.5.1 Fire

Since the laser beam is a concentrated energy source, there is the possibility of ignition if it is misdirected. Flammable preparations with an alcohol base should be avoided in order to prevent flash fires. There should be no flammable material near the laser beam. Cloth drapes are preferred to disposable paper items and flame-retardant drapes are most suitable. Gauze placed around the treatment site should be kept moist.

Prevention of fire through a misdirected laser beam is in the hands of the user. Apart from equipment malfunction, the laser beam will strike the drapes only if the user is careless. It is also the case that laser equipment carries a risk, as with any other electrical equipment, of developing a fault which might result in a fire. To prevent fire spreading in the operating theatre, there should be easy and quick access to a fire extinguisher (preferably a CO_2 type). Staff should know where this is located and know how to deal with a fire if one should start.

It is a good precaution to have a sizeable syringe loaded with sterile saline at hand so that the surgeon can easily extinguish a fire near the surgical field. This is particularly appropriate when there is a risk of ignition at the treatment site, for example laser surgery of the vocal cords with an endotracheal tube in place (§19.6). Ignition of the endotracheal tube during laser surgery has been recognized as a major hazard. Other materials (such as PTFE) may not ignite but produce toxic fumes when heated.

19.5.2 Plume emission

A plume of debris is emitted from tissue when laser-induced vaporization takes place. This obscures the vision of the surgeon and for this reason, if for none other, it needs to be evacuated. Moreover, the vapours have a noxious smell which is unpleasant for staff and off-putting for the patient if he or she is conscious. More seriously, it may represent an inhalation hazard. Although the high temperature (greater than 100°C) at the centre of the plume will ensure that there are no active particles in that region, there is concern that absorption of energy in deeper tissues may cause subsurface explosions and possibly disperse viable cells in the plume. Pathological changes have been observed in the rat lung following exposure to smoke produced by NdYAG lasers and electrosurgical devices [18]. There is also a possibility that active viruses may be present in the plume caused by irradiation with a CO_2 laser. However, contamination of the operator is unlikely during laser vaporization of infectious lesions of the lower genital tract provided a suitable smoke evacuator is used [19]. Laser treatment of laryngeal papillomas did not produce detectable HPV DNA [20]. However, viable bacteria have been found in *in vitro* studies [21, 22].

To minimize the risk, an efficient evacuation system containing a viral trap should be used. This should incorporate a filter capable of removing particles down to a diameter of 0.2 μm with an efficiency of 99.9% and a secondary carbon filter to remove odours.

19.5.3 Toxic fluids

Some of the fluids used in lasers are surface irritants and some are even carcinogenic. Gases used in excimer lasers and laser dyes may be hazardous. Halogen gases in excimer lasers are highly toxic, even at small concentrations. Dyes require periodic changing and so special precautions are required when replacing organic dyes in the laser. In all cases, a risk assessment must be carried out in accordance with the Control of Substances Hazardous to Health (COSHH) Regulations. Care should be taken with liquid which has leaked from a dye laser. Another type of laser which contains a hazardous gas is the He–Cd laser. If this does not have a sealed tube, the exhaust gases should be taken outside to avoid contaminating the room with cadmium vapour.

19.5.4 Electrical hazards

It is easy to forget that the risk from laser equipment is not restricted to the laser beam. There have been more fatalities from electrical accidents associated with lasers than from exposure to laser radiation. Some lasers utilize large capacitor banks which are capable of storing very high quantities of electrical charge. This charge may persist long after the equipment has been switched off and is capable of delivering a lethal current if there is direct human contact. It is always advisable to ensure that capacitors are discharged before working close to the terminals. Unfortunately, it is all too easy to forget about basic electrical safety precautions when attention is given to avoiding the obvious risks from the laser beam. This is particularly important when the covers are removed, thus exposing live connections and/or highly charged terminals. Panels are usually interlocked to prevent laser operation when they are removed but this facility may have to be overridden to allow work to be undertaken with the power on. This is of particular relevance during maintenance, or adjustment of mirrors.

As with any other item of electrical equipment, electrical safety checks should be carried out. Earth continuity and earth leakage are important parameters but there may be difficulties in performing the checks when a three-phase supply is used.

In the event of someone accidentally contacting an electrical terminal, the person must be safely removed from the electrical source before any resuscitation is attempted. Usually this means disconnecting the equipment from the electricity supply.

Some laser systems have water cooling and there is a potential risk from water spillage on to live contacts. Water-cooling hoses are liable to fail, and so the equipment should be designed to minimize any risk in the event of such an occurrence. Water and electricity should be physically separated.

19.6 Patient protection

It is easy to overlook the patient as the laser enthusiast concentrates on the technology. However, the concerns of patients about to undergo laser treatment should be appreciated. One study showed that, before treatment of cervical intra-epithelial neoplasia, 77% of patients expressed some concern about laser therapy but, afterwards, 78% described the laser procedure as just a bit uncomfortable [23].

If the power or energy density delivered to the patient differs from that which was intended, then damage may occur. Clearly, if either power or energy were too high then the exposure would have a greater impact than intended. The extent of the damage would depend on the site being treated. For example, perforation of the bowel would be a very serious consequence; also, when removing vocal cord nodules it is important not to cause damage to the underlying structure. It is also true that if the power delivered were significantly less than intended, then thermal damage would be inflicted on a greater volume of surrounding tissue. This would result in a poorer outcome. This situation can easily happen when an optical fibre is used after tissue has become burned on the distal end. Delivered power may be reduced by 50%. In addition, some optical fibres have tips made of sapphire or other material. There is a danger that they may become detached and put the patient at risk from burns or physical injury.

If the treatment beam is misdirected, then it may strike another area of tissue. This can happen if there is misalignment of the aiming beam and the therapy beam or if there is a fault in the beam delivery system, e.g. a break in the fibre or detachment of part of the articulated arm/focusing assembly. The user should be aware of the risk of reflection, and instruments with shiny surfaces should not be used near the laser beam. Instruments should have a matt finish, and if protection is required from visible laser radiation, they should have a blackened surface.

If there is a risk of the patient's eyes being accidentally exposed to the laser beam then they should be adequately protected. Wet eye pads or appropriate eye shields should be used with CO_2 or NdYAG lasers. For some types of laser procedures, e.g. KTP laser for facial telangectasia, tight-fitting goggles are suitable. For treatments on the eyelids, corneal shields should be used.

Areas around the treatment site should be adequately protected. In the case of laryngeal CO_2 laser surgery and a wide range of other surgical applications, the surrounding area should be protected by the use of damp gamgee. If it is allowed to dry out, the level of protection is minimal. The protective covers should be kept damp throughout the duration of the procedure.

Non-alcohol-based skin preparations should be used because of the risk of ignition of the flammable vapour (§19.5.1).

An accident with potentially fatal consequences is that of endotracheal tube ignition. This has been highlighted when CO_2 laser tracheobronchial surgery is being carried out. Incidents of ignition have occurred within the airways of the patient [24–26]. There has also been a case of tube ignition when an NdYAG laser was used [27]. There is a danger of death or at least very serious injury and so precautions must be taken to prevent such an incident occurring. Laser-safe endotracheal tubes are available commercially. Some are made of metal and these can withstand very high power density. Others are made of protective plastics but they have a much lower damage threshold; they should be used only if their specification is suitable.

19.7 Legislation, standards, and guidance

In most countries there is currently no specific legislation governing use of lasers. This is true for National Health Trust (NHS) hospitals in the UK, although the use of class 3B and class 4 lasers in independent healthcare establishments is included in the Registered Homes Act for England and Wales and in the new National Minimum Standards Regulations. The NHS, in common with all employers throughout the UK, is obliged to comply with the requirements of the Health and Safety at Work, etc. Act [28]. This places an onus on the employer to ensure that no persons (staff or public) are at risk of harm from its activities. The management of laser safety is covered by general health and safety legislation [29] and choice and use of laser goggles by personal protective equipment legislation [30].

A British/European standard [17] provides the basis for a considerable amount of safety advice on lasers and includes light-emitting diodes (LEDs). An important component is equipment classification which sets accessible emission limits (AELs). It is the responsibility of the manufacturer or their agent to provide correct classification of a laser product. The classification scheme at the time of publication is as follows.

- Class 1 lasers are safe under reasonably foreseeable conditions. They are either low-power lasers which are intrinsically safe or high-power devices rendered Class 1 by use of engineering control. The AEL depends on wavelength and exposure duration. For a continuous-wave HeNe laser operating at 633 nm the Class 1 limit is 7 μW.
- Class 2 lasers emit visible radiation in the wavelength range 400 to 700 nm. Eye protection is normally afforded by aversion responses including the blink reflex, which takes 0.25 seconds. For a continuous output laser, the limit is 1 mW.
- Class 3A lasers are safe for viewing with the unaided eye. For a laser emitting in the wavelength range 400 to 700 nm, protection is afforded by aversion responses including the blink reflex. For other wavelengths the hazard to the unaided eye is no greater than for Class 1. Direct intrabeam viewing of Class 3A lasers with optical aids (e.g. binoculars, telescopes, and microscopes) may be hazardous. For wavelengths between 400 and 700 nm and exposure duration greater than 0.25 seconds, the AEL has two criteria. Radiated power must be less than 5 mW and irradiance from the emitted beam must not exceed 25 W m^{-2} averaged over an area of diameter 7 mm. The latter condition is equivalent to 1 mW into a 7 mm diameter aperture. This class is being replaced in a revised scheme (see below).
- Class 3B lasers are always hazardous when the beam is viewed directly. Viewing diffuse reflections is normally safe. For continuous output lasers of wavelengths greater than 315 nm, the limit is 0.5 W. Class 3B lasers should only be operated in a controlled area and precautions taken to prevent accidental exposure. Eye protection may also be required.
- Class 4 lasers are also capable of producing hazardous diffuse reflections. They may cause skin injuries and could also cause a fire hazard. Their use requires extreme caution. Beam paths should be enclosed whenever practicable. Access to the laser controlled area should be limited to persons wearing suitable protective eyewear and clothing.

Amendments to this classification scheme are to be made in a revision of the standard. Under this system laser classes 1, 2, and 3A will be replaced by new classes 1, 1M, 2, and 2M, and a new class 3R created. The definitions of classes 1, 2, 3B, and 4 will be essentially unchanged. Classes 1M and 2M will apply to lasers or LEDs with divergent beams but will include products with wide collimated beams and there will be no cap on the total output of these laser products. The new classes introduced are the following.

- Class 1M lasers are safe under reasonably foreseeable conditions provided optical instruments (mainly magnifiers) are not used.
- Class 2M lasers are visible lasers which are safe provided no optical instruments are used and the aversion response operates.
- Class 3R lasers have accessible emissions exceeding the MPE level for 0.25 s exposures, if they are visible, or for 100 s exposures, if they are invisible. Their total output does not exceed the AEL for class 2 (visible) or class 1 (invisible) by more than a factor of five. The class does not include lasers emitting between 180 and 302.5 nm.

The standard also includes a user's guide which provides safety precautions and control measures that should be considered when a Class 3B or Class 4 laser is being used. These include:

- use of a remote interlock connector
- key control
- beam stop or attenuator
- warning signs
- beam paths
- specular reflections
- eye protection
- protective eyewear
- protective clothing
- training
- medical supervision.

Other standards are available for medical laser equipment [31] and protective eyewear [32, 33].

The Medical Devices Agency has published a document entitled *Guidance on the safe use of lasers in medical and dental practice* [34]. This is essential reading for everyone involved with medical lasers in the UK. It provides advice and guidance on safety requirements applicable to lasers in medical use. It outlines principles of laser safety management, user safety measures, and device features; it provides an example of local rules and a core of knowledge for laser users.

The American National Standards Institute has published a standard on safe use of lasers in healthcare facilities [35]. This is more detailed and prescriptive than the British guidance document. It is clearly relevant to practices in the United States and may also be cited by users from elsewhere. There is a significant difference in the criteria for Class 3A lasers between Europe and the United States. The irradiance limit of 25 W m^{-2} does not appear in the American standard. Thus some devices marked as Class 3A [36] have been imported into Europe where they are in fact Class 3B devices. Examples have included laser pointers which are potentially hazardous [37]. Misuse of these devices has resulted in prosecution of the offender.

The International Electrotechnical Commission has published guidelines for the safe use of medical laser equipment [38]. The publication of the guide as a technical report indicates that it is not intended to take precedence over national guidelines. However, where none exists, it should prove helpful.

19.8 Equipment features

Manufacturing requirements for laser equipment are specified in British/European Standards [17, 31]. Every medical device must carry a CE-mark, which means that it satisfies the requirements essential for it to be fit for its intended purpose. Some important safety features for Class 3B and 4 lasers are listed in the guidance [34] and these are summarized below.

- *Key control.* Operation should require the use of a key.
- *Laser ready warning.* There should be a visible 'laser ready' warning if the laser is capable of being fired when the footswitch is pressed or other firing mechanism activated.
- *Laser emission occurring warning.* There should be a visible or audible warning when laser radiation is being emitted.
- *Beam stop, shutters, or attenuators.* Lasers should be equipped with a beam stop. The position of a beam stop, shutter, or attenuator should be monitored. It is not sufficient to monitor the fixing mechanism. Beam stops, shutters, and attenuators should be attached using a secure fixing and should always fail to safety.
- *Remote interlock facility.* There should be a facility to connect a door interlock switch to disable the laser if the door is opened.
- *Target indicating device.* The laser should incorporate a target indicating device, which is usually an aiming beam, unless it is used in contact with or in close proximity to the target.
- *Aiming beam requirements.* The aiming beam should not normally exceed the Class 2 limit (1 mW). If the aiming beam spot cannot be easily seen then a 5 mW output is acceptable, but for ophthalmic procedures a deliberate and positive action by the operator is required to increase the power above 1 mW. The aiming beam and therapeutic beam should be concentric. Maximum allowable tolerance between the two centres is 50% of the larger diameter. It should not be possible to operate the laser without the

aiming beam first being present. If the aiming beam should fail during use, then it should be possible to continue the current exposure as it may be preferable to complete a treatment after it has been started, even without an aiming beam.

- *Output measurement systems.* The laser should incorporate a power or energy meter to measure the laser radiation output. A 20% tolerance is generally acceptable.
- *Exposure termination system.* There should be some means of monitoring the operation of a timed exposure to ensure that laser output is of the desired duration.
- *Emergency laser stop.* A readily accessible emergency stop switch should be provided.
- *Enable switch.* There should be a switch which has to be operated to place the laser in a 'ready to fire' mode. Until this switch is depressed, the laser firing switch is inactive.
- *Footswitches.* Footswitches should be waterproof and shrouded to prevent accidental operation. They should be checked regularly as they are a potential source of faults.
- *Beam transmission systems.* Disconnection of the articulated arm or optical fibre should either be interlocked to disable the laser or should require the use of a tool.
- *Protective filters and shutters.* Protective filters or shutters should be fitted to equipment if the beam may be reflected into the operator's eyes. CO_2 laser radiation is not transmitted through glass.
- *Labelling.* Labelling should be provided [17], showing laser classification, maximum output, wavelengths, output aperture, and warnings.
- *Electrical safety.* Appropriate electrical safety checks should be carried out.
- *Blue light.* The fitting of a green-only filter to the aiming beam of the ophthalmic argon laser should be considered (§19.2.1).

19.9 Laser safety management

The management of health and safety in the workplace is covered by legislation [28] and some important administrative aspects are listed [34].

- *Laser protection adviser.* There should be a laser protection adviser (LPA) appointed when a Class 3A, 3B, or 4 laser is installed. This person should be knowledgeable in the evaluation of laser hazards and should have responsibility for advising on their control.
- *Laser protection supervisor.* Each individual laser should have a designated laser protection supervisor (LPS) who will have overall responsibility for ensuring local implementation of local rules and guidelines. There should be good communication between the LPS and the LPA. The LPS will be someone closely involved with the laser, e.g. surgeon or nursing sister.
- *Local rules.* The use of lasers should be governed by local rules. These must be applicable to the type of laser, the particular laser procedures to be carried out, and the local situation.
- *Laser controlled area.* Controlled areas must be designated in which the laser may be used. Activity within these areas is restricted according to the local rules.
- *Authorized users.* There should be a register of individuals who are permitted to use the laser. This is to do with safety, not clinical competence. The user should sign a statement that he/she has read and understood the local rules. The procedure for authorization may vary. One method which has been found to be satisfactory in many situations is for the authorization to be administered by the LPS in consultation with the LPA.
- *Training.* Appropriate training should be given to all who are involved in the use of lasers in hospitals. This includes nursing and medical staff and others assisting in theatre. A core of knowledge for laser safety has been published [34] and it is recommended that all laser users should undergo training to acquire this.
- *Medical examination.* Regular medical examination is not necessary, but it is important that an eye examination is carried out within 24 hours of an alleged exposure incident. If the laser beam has caused retinal damage, this will show as a lesion on the retina. If this is followed over the next few days, it will change its appearance. This will show that it is a lesion of recent origin, which could have been caused by the laser.
- *Incident reports.* If an incident occurs, the LPA should carry out an investigation and prepare a report for the employer. Laser device defects should be reported to the Department of Health. Within the EU, incidents involving CE-marked devices resulting in serious injury or death must be notified to the appropriate competent authority (which is the Medical Devices Agency in the UK).
- *Equipment.* All medical lasers used in the EU must be CE-marked and comply with the necessary standards.
- *Equipment modification.* All laser equipment modifications should be reported to the LPA. Any modification carried out by the hospital may result in transfer of liability from the manufacturer.

- *Legislative health and safety requirements.* Employers are responsible to ensure, as far as is practicable, the health and safety of their employees and others who may be affected by their work. Employees also have a duty to take reasonable care of the health and safety of themselves and others.

19.9.1 Laser protection adviser

The role of the LPA is key to a sound, sensible, laser safety policy. The LPA should be able to make value judgements on necessary precautions to take during laser procedures. Basic to this is the idea of risk assessment. The LPA must be able to consider where the real risks to safety occur. This is often the most difficult aspect of the job of an LPA. There should always be a rational basis for the advice. This may be based on calculations of the nominal ocular hazard distance, which is the range over which the laser presents an ocular hazard. Other factors must also be taken into account, e.g. whether the laser is used in a closed or an open environment. Whatever the LPA recommends, he/she must be able to justify it. In an increasingly litigation-conscious society, it may also be necessary to defend the advice in court.

Other duties of the LPA include performing hazard analyses and risk assessments, ensuring that suitable local rules are drawn up and implemented, advising on equipment purchase, planning the installation, acceptance testing, and regular safety audit.

The term laser protection adviser is used in UK NHS hospitals and is analogous to the radiation protection adviser who advises on ionising radiation safety. Similarly, the laser protection supervisor (LPS) corresponds to the radiation protection supervisor in the ionising radiation field. Identification of the twin roles and responsibilities is extremely beneficial. By contrast, the term laser safety officer (LSO) appears in various documents and standards and sometimes equates with the LPA but at other times more closely resembles the LPS.

19.9.2 Controlled area

A controlled area should be specified within which the laser may be used. This is essentially the area within which there may be exposure to levels in excess of the MPE [17] (Table 19.1) (Figure 19.4). Control is exercised on activities undertaken within the area and entry to the area. It is preferable to designate the whole room or operating theatre as a controlled area rather than mark off parts of a room. Difficulties occur, for example, if there is a scrub with open access to the theatre. In this case, the scrub is part of the controlled area. The problem is that the local rules also apply to the scrub area. This may introduce some problems for the staff working in the area. Controlled areas should be specified in the local rules.

Appropriate notices should be placed at the points of entry to the controlled area. The wording may inform staff that the laser is in use and they should exercise caution. Alternatively, if there is an unacceptable risk of harm on entering the controlled area, staff must be instructed not to enter the area. It may be more appropriate to instruct staff to wear goggles, in which case protective eyewear must be available at each point of entry. In some cases, it may be necessary to fit a door interlock so that the laser cannot be fired if the door is opened. This should only be done if necessary, as it may interfere seriously with the successful outcome of the laser procedure. Exceptions may include skin laser applications and laser delivery via the indirect ophthalmoscope. There is also a difference between a laser room with direct public access and one within a theatre where there is access to staff only.

Nominal ocular hazard distance

A useful and relevant concept is that of the nominal ocular hazard distance (NOHD) [17]. Because a laser beam will diverge, the irradiance will decrease with distance and the NOHD is the distance at which the beam irradiance equals the appropriate MPE (Figure 19.5). If the beam from a laser diverges with angle ϕ, the NOHD will be determined from the position at which the irradiance from the laser power P equals the MPE. In terms of distances shown in Figure 19.5, assuming that ϕ is small so that $\phi = b/d$ radians, this will occur when

$$\text{MPE} = 4\,P/(\pi\, b^2) = 4\,P/(\pi\, d^2\, \phi^2) \qquad (19.1)$$

Thus

$$\text{NOHD} = d - (a/\phi) = (1/\phi)\,(\,[4\,P/(\pi\,\text{MPE})] - a) \qquad (19.2)$$

The NOHD should be taken into account when specifying the boundaries of the controlled area and the appropriate precautions to take at points of access. It is particularly useful when considering the need for door interlocks. If the door is more than 3 metres from the laser and the NOHD is less than 3 metres, then a door interlock is not required. An example of a calculation of the NOHD is given in Box 19.3.

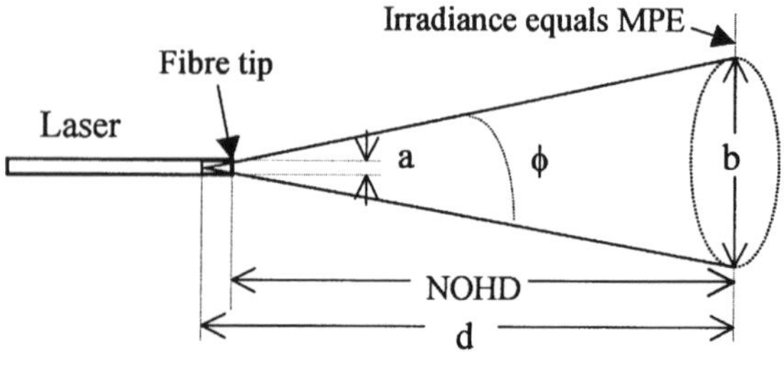

Figure 19.5 Configuration used in calculation of nominal ocular hazard distance (NOHD).

Box 19.3 Sample calculations

Calculate the nominal ocular hazard distance (NOHD) for a Laserscope AURA KTP laser used for treating facial vascular lesions. What is the required optical density (OD) for protective eyewear?

Maximum fluence is 18 J cm^{-2} and pulse duration is 10 ms at a repetition rate of 10 Hz. There are two delivery devices:

- a focused hand-piece (called a dermastat) producing a spot size of 2 mm; the beam itself has a divergence of 4° (0.07 rad)
- a scanner which directs a pulsed beam over a variable hexagonal area; the scanned pattern diverges at an angle of 38°; this is such that only a single pulse will enter the pupil of the eye in the event of accidental exposure. Thus, the scanner is less hazardous in use than the dermastat.

The laser beam is quasi-continuous, i.e. it looks continuous to the naked eye. The wavelength of the KTP laser is 532 nm. So exposure is limited by the blink reflex (0.25 s). During this time, the number of pulses emitted is three.

The maximum permissible exposure (MPE) for exposure times between 1.8×10^{-5} s and 10 s (Table 19.1) is given by:

$$\text{MPE} = 18\, t^{0.75}\ \text{J m}^{-2}$$

Note: a factor C_6 is included in MPE tables for viewing conditions which may be applied to extended sources, but in the present case $C_6 = 1.0$.

The NOHD may be calculated from equation (19.2):

$$\text{NOHD} = 1/\phi\ \{ [(4P) \ / \ (\pi\ \text{MPE})] - a\}$$

where ϕ is divergence, P is output of the laser, and a is diameter of the emergent laser beam. If MPE is given in J m^{-2} then P should be in J; if MPE is expressed in W m^{-2} then P should be in W. In this case, a is 0.002 m and may be ignored.

For a repetitively pulsed laser, the MPE is determined by using the most restrictive of requirements from those listed in §19.4.2.

(a) The exposure from any single pulse shall not exceed the corresponding MPE.

$$H_{\text{single}} = 18 \times \pi \times (0.1)^2 = 0.565\ \text{J}$$
$$\text{MPE}_{\text{single}} = 18 \times (10 \times 10^{-3})^{0.75} = 0.569\ \text{J m}^{-2}$$
$$\text{NOHD} = 1 \ / \ 0.07\ \{ [(4 \times 0.565) \ / \ (\pi \times 0.569)]\} = 16.1\ \text{m}.$$

(b) The average exposure for a pulse train of duration T shall not exceed the MPE for a single pulse of duration T. Since the laser emits visible light, use the blink response 0.25 s for the exposure time. Three pulses can lie within this time.

$$H_T = H_{\text{single}} \times 3 = 1.695\ \text{J}$$
$$\text{MPE}_T = 18 \times (0.25)^{0.75} = 6.36\ \text{J m}^{-2}$$
$$\text{NOHD} = 1 \ / \ 0.07\ \{ [(4 \times 1.695) \ / \ (\pi \times 6.36)]\} = 8.3\ \text{m}.$$

(c) The exposure from any single pulse within a train of N pulses shall not exceed $\text{MPE}_{\text{single}}\ N^{-1/4}$. In this case, $N = 3$ and $\text{MPE}_{\text{single}}$ was calculated to be 0.569 J m^{-2} in (a). Thus

$$\text{MPE}_{\text{train}} = 0.569 \times 3^{-0.25} = 0.432\ \text{J m}^{-2}$$
$$\text{NOHD} = 1 \ / \ 0.07\ \{ [(4 \times 0.565) \ / \ (\pi \times 0.432)]\} = 18.4\ \text{m}.$$

The most restrictive condition is (c) which gives an NOHD of 18.4 m.

The required OD of protective eyewear depends on exposure and MPE. It is given by the formula

$$\text{OD} = \log(H/\text{MPE}).$$

Taking exposure at the treatment site, $H = 18$ J cm^{-2}, and the lowest MPE for a single pulse,

$$\text{OD} = \log(18 \times 10^4/0.432) = 5.6.$$

19.9.3 Local rules

Local rules provide a set of written instructions which should be applied when a particular laser is in use. Their purpose is to ensure a safe working environment as far as is reasonably practicable. Inevitably, value judgements must be made. The local rules should reflect local circumstances, and the particular application and environment. Important issues which should be addressed in the local rules are listed [34]. An example set of rules is given in Box 19.4.

- *Nature of hazard to persons.* Local rules should not contain laser safety teaching, which should be carried

---

Box 19.4 Sample local rules

Local rules for the use of the ABC excimer laser in the eye department, XYZ hospital

The therapeutic laser beam is a class 4 device which can cause injury to unprotected skin and eyes from both direct and scattered beams. The aiming beams and fixation beams are class 2 devices. Class 2 devices are not intrinsically safe but eye protection is normally afforded by aversion responses including the blink reflex.

Safe use of the laser depends upon a strict adherence to the following rules:

1. The designated laser room (Appendix 1) is approved for laser use. This is designated a 'controlled area'. The laser shall be used only in an approved controlled area.
2. Suitable warning signs shall be fitted at the entrance to the controlled area (Appendix 1) and staff shall be instructed that they must not enter when the laser is in use.
3. A register shall be kept of personnel authorized to operate the equipment (Appendix 2). One authorized operator shall be designated laser protection supervisor (Appendix 3) to assume overall local control of the equipment and ensure that it is used in accordance with the local rules. The equipment shall only be used by an authorized operator who has signed a statement that he/she has read and understood the local rules. Copies of signed statements will be sent to the laser protection adviser. If the laser protection supervisor considers an individual to be unsuitable to use the laser, the laser protection adviser must be consulted and, if appropriate, authorization shall be denied or withdrawn.
4. It is the responsibility of the operator to be aware of the nature of the hazard and to be familiar with the manufacturer's operating instructions.
5. The operator shall ensure that the requirements for safety are being observed; the operator is responsible for the safety of the patient, staff, and visitors as well as for his/her own safety.
6. The operator shall ensure that anyone assisting with the procedures is adequately trained in the safe performance of their duties.
7. When the laser is in operation, the number of persons in the room shall be kept to a minimum.
8. Suitable protective eyewear shall be worn when the laser is in use (Appendix 4).
9. The laser shall not be fired towards the door.
10. The operator shall ensure that the laser warning sign is illuminated outside the door.
11. The laser shall not be put into the ready-to-fire mode unless it is directed towards the treatment site or at a beam stop.
12. The operator shall be careful to avoid reflections of the beam from instruments (e.g. lid retractors) in close proximity to the beam.
13. The operator shall ensure that flammable substances are not introduced into the beam and that eye drops, skin preparations, etc., are non-flammable.
14. Hit the emergency off-button to switch off the laser in an emergency.
15. The laser equipment contains argon fluorine gas which is highly toxic. First indications include irritation of the eyes. If gas leakage is suspected, the operator should hit the emergency off-button, remove the patient, and evacuate the room immediately.
16. When the equipment is unattended by an authorized operator, the control panel must be switched off and the key withdrawn and placed in safe custody.
17. In the event of an incident or near-incident occurring, the laser protection adviser must be informed as soon as possible. If accidental exposure of the eye is suspected, an ophthalmic examination must be carried out within 24 hours.

out elsewhere. However, it is helpful to indicate what the hazard is. For example, it is useful for the user to know whether there is a hazard to unprotected skin as well as eyes. Also, it helps to know if there is a risk from exposure to the aiming beam.

- *Controlled and safe access.* The entry of persons into the controlled area must be considered (§19.9.2).
- *A register of authorized users.* A register should be maintained with the names of those who are permitted to fire the laser. This list should be kept with the key and be known to the keyholder.
- *Nominated keyholders.* The laser key should be kept in safe custody, for example with the key for the drugs cabinet.

Box 19.4 *(continued)*

18. The laser must only be used in accordance with these local rules.

Laser Protection Adviser: Dr LPA (telephone)

Appendix 1

Diagram of controlled area showing position and wording of warning signs.

Appendix 2

Register of authorized operators.

Appendix 3

Responsibilities and duties of the laser protection supervisor

The laser protection supervisor shall:

(1) ensure that the local rules are adhered to;

(2) inform the laser protection adviser of any concerns regarding safety or if the existing rules require amending;

(3) ensure that the correct procedure for authorization has been undertaken and that the register of authorized operators is maintained;

(4) obtain signed statements from authorized operators that they have read and understood the local rules and send copies of statements to the laser protection adviser;

(5) ensure that only authorized operators use the laser;

(6) inform the laser protection adviser as soon as possible in the event of an incident occurring;

(7) seek assistance from the laser protection adviser on the safety implications when a change in operating procedure is envisaged;

(8) provide a report, on request, on the status of laser safety to the laser protection adviser.

Appendix 4

Laser specification, MPE, NOHD, eyewear requirements

Appendix 5

Statement to be signed by all authorized operators
Hospital..
Department...
Laser details..
I have read and understood the local rules for the use of the above laser.
Name (Capitals)..
Job title..
Signature..
Date...

- *Keyholder's responsibilities.* It is extremely important that the keyholder has explicit instructions which clearly state that the key the must be given to authorized users only.
- *Need for training of all persons.* All staff involved with the laser should receive training at an appropriate level.
- *User's responsibilities.* Laser safety is ultimately in the hands of the operator. This must be understood and accepted by the laser operator, who therefore has a duty towards the safety of others who may be present when the laser is in use.
- *Methods of safe working.* The local rules should specify safe working procedures. This may include restrictions on number of visitors, use of the ready/standby button, the direction the laser beam is fired, etc.
- *Definition of simple pre-use safety checks.* With some lasers it is useful to carry out a simple check prior to admission of the patient. This may simply be a test firing against a suitable target, which may be kept as a record of the beam profile. The need for this depends on the reliability of the laser device.
- *Personal protective equipment, especially eyewear.* The need for protective eyewear should be identified in the local rules and there should be advice on the type which is required.
- *Prevention of use by unauthorized persons.* It should be clearly stated that the laser must not be used by an unauthorized person. To avoid any misunderstanding, a notice to this effect should be displayed on the laser.
- *Normal operating procedures.* Normal operating procedures should be protocolled.
- *Adverse incident procedures.* The local rules should specify the action to be taken in the event of an actual or suspected incident.
- *Contact point for the LPA.* At the very least, the name and daytime telephone number of the LPA should be given.
- *The limits of the laser controlled area.* To avoid confusion, the limits of the controlled area should be stated. Often, a sketch is helpful.

The above headings are given for guidance. The list is not exhaustive. There is no universal prescription.

19.9.4 Room layout

The first thing to determine regarding room layout is the position of the laser and the direction of the beam. Quite clearly, it is not advisable to place the laser close to a door with the beam directed towards the doorway. Wherever possible the laser should be directed away from the door and at a safe distance. This may not be possible, in which case consideration must be given to the NOHD (§19.9.2). If there is a reasonably foreseeable possibility that a hazardous beam may strike someone on entry to the controlled area, then either a barrier must be erected to protect the entrance or an interlock switch connected to the door to disable the laser if the door is opened.

There should be no shiny surfaces in close proximity to the laser beam. In most theatres, this is not a problem. A specular reflection is particularly hazardous because the beam is sent off in an unexpected direction (Figure 19.6).

Windows must also be considered. In the case of a CO_2 laser, window glass absorbs the beam. However, with visible and near-infrared laser radiation (including NdYAG laser), windows must be covered if there is a reasonable possibility that the beam may reach the window.

Flammable materials should be positioned well out of line of the laser beam. Moreover, a fire extinguisher should be readily available (§19.5.1).

19.10 Personal protection

All items of personal protective equipment are subject to legislation (Personal Protective Equipment Regulations) and must be CE-marked before they may be sold in Europe. This means that inexpensive general-purpose polycarbonate goggles, which have been widely used by hospital staff for CO_2 lasers, may not now be marketed as laser protective eyewear, unless they have been tested against an appropriate standard. In practice, this means laser protective eyewear for sale in Europe should comply with EN 207, which gives a specification for filters and equipment. Another standard provides guidance on selection, use, and maintenance of protective eyewear.

A word of warning needs to be given against the reliance which may be placed on personal protective equipment. This is always the last line of defence. First, equipment should be engineered to provide as much safety as reasonably achievable. In many hospital applications, this is limited by the nature of the application. Next comes administrative control, whereby safe systems of work are in place. This means that staff involved with the laser are adequately trained and use the laser in a way which minimizes the risk of accidental exposure. Finally, protective eyewear is worn to protect against the occurrence of an unlikely event.

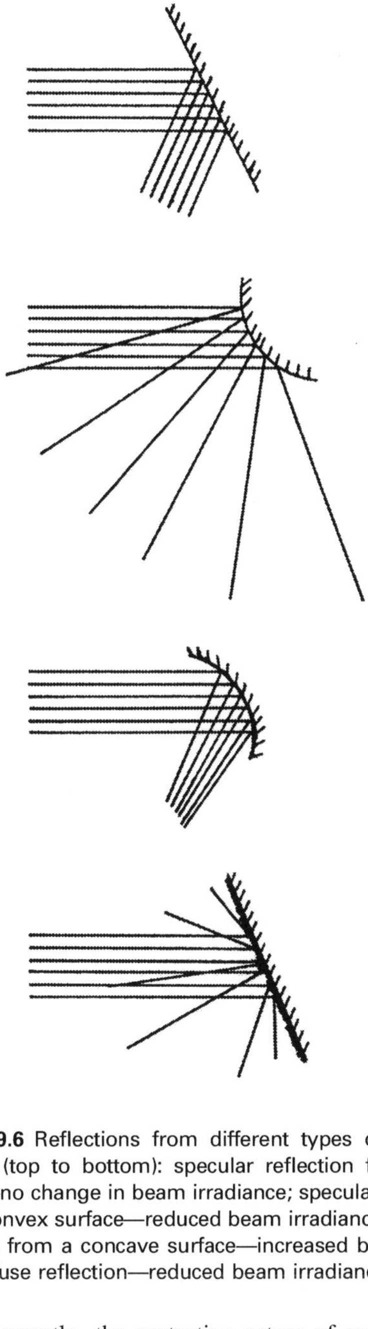

Figure 19.6 Reflections from different types of surfaces showing (top to bottom): specular reflection from a flat surface—no change in beam irradiance; specular reflection from a convex surface—reduced beam irradiance; specular reflection from a concave surface—increased beam irradiance; diffuse reflection—reduced beam irradiance.

Until recently, the protective nature of eyewear was based on the optical density of the material. Optical density (OD) required to provide protection for a particular laser is defined as

$$\mathrm{OD} = \log(H/MPE) \quad (19.3)$$

where H is the expected unprotected eye exposure level and MPE is the maximum permissible exposure level for the unprotected eye (Table 19.1) [17] (see Box 19.3). However, the OD is irrelevant if the lens material is damaged by the incident laser beam. This was demonstrated in work carried out on damage threshold of laser protective eyewear [39]. This showed the limitations of polycarbonate lenses compared to dielectric-coated or absorptive glass lenses, although polycarbonate could be suitable at lower irradiance levels. In a published study, eyewear was assessed on the basis of measured OD, labelling, peripheral protection, comfort, storage, and cleaning, and only 15 out of 48 models were rated acceptable [40].

EN 207 [32] defines a scale number (designated by the letter 'L') which is the logarithm of the inverse of the maximum spectral transmittance which shall not be exceeded at each wavelength to afford protection up to specified power or energy density levels. The L scale number is equal to the OD up to the power or energy density at which the material is damaged and laser breakthrough occurs. During testing, the spectral transmittance is measured for each laser wavelength during the course of irradiation. Exposure duration under each test condition is 10 s or 100 pulses. Marking in accordance with EN 207 requires the following:

- symbol for test condition (D = continuous; I = pulsed; R = Q switch; M = mode-coupled)
- wavelength or wavelength range (nm) in which filter provides protection
- scale number
- manufacturer's identification mark
- certification mark if applicable
- mechanical strength mark if applicable.

For example, laser goggles with a scale number 8 for CO_2 laser irradiation would carry the marking:

D 10 600 L8 X ZZ

where X is the manufacturer's identification mark and ZZ is the certification mark. The scale number L8 implies maximum spectral transmittance is 10^{-8} when the goggles are exposed to an irradiance of 10^{11} W m^{-2} for 10 s. This means that the eye would be exposed to an irradiance of 10^3 W m^{-2}, which is the MPE specified in EN 60825.

Laser eyewear should be inspected regularly and a written record kept of such inspection.

19.11 Exposure incidents

Incidents which have resulted in accidental laser exposure can often contain useful lessons. A summary of reported accidents was drawn up in a review of laser safety [41]. Incidents have been described elsewhere [42–47]. Some conclusions may be drawn from a study of laser incidents.

- High-voltage electrical power supplies have caused more deaths than the laser beam.
- Laser alignment is particularly hazardous especially when mirrors and lenses are moved through the beam.
- Pulsed lasers cause more accidents than continuous output devices.
- Every incident or near-incident should be investigated.
- Accidents usually involve relatively young and inexperienced workers.
- Failure to wear appropriate eye protection is often an important factor.
- Poor systems of work or failure to observe local rules are contributory factors.
- Failure to observe fire risks contribute to incidents.
- Unsafe equipment may result in unintentional exposure.
- Fire or explosion associated with use in close proximity to anaesthetic gases and liquids is a risk.
- Problems with beam delivery devices such as fibre optics or articulated arms lead to incidents.

A graphic description of personal injury to his own eye is given in the account of Decker [48], who was partially blinded by the reflection of a 6 mJ 10 ns pulsed NdYAG laser beam. He was not wearing goggles at the time because they were uncomfortable and interfered with normal vision. This highlights an extremely important feature in eyewear selection, namely user comfort. This is necessary to ensure compliance. When the beam struck his eye, his vision was obscured almost immediately by blood pouring into the vitreous humour. The beam struck the retina between the optic nerve and the fovea and left Decker with a blind spot. Serious as this incident was, Dr Decker was very fortunate; had the beam hit the optic nerve or the fovea, it is likely that he would have lost his sight.

In another incident which took place in a hospital, an ophthalmologist was carrying out a retinal photocoagulation procedure on a patient when he was exposed to a back-reflection of the laser beam. The equipment was operated by a foot pedal, which normally caused a filter to drop in the viewing eyepiece prior to activation of the laser. Poor maintenance resulted in failure of the protective filter. Poor equipment design meant that the laser did not fail to safety. Although the exposure at the operator's eye exceeded the MPE it was not sufficient to cause serious damage.

An engineer was making adjustments to an NdYAG laser through an opening in the top of the equipment. Because he was leaning over the equipment, his goggles slipped off his nose. The beam struck him in the eye, making a popping noise, and leaving a bright afterimage. He was left with permanent and serious loss of vision in one eye.

19.12 References

1 Ham Jr, W. T. (1983). Ocular hazards of light sources: review of current knowledge. *J. Occup. Med.*, **25**, 101–3.

2 Ham Jr, W. T., Mueller, H. A., and Sliney, D. H. (1976). Retinal sensitivity to damage from short wavelength light. *Nature*, **260**, 153–5.

3 Arden, G. B., Berninger, T., Hogg, C. R., and Perry, S (1991). A survey of color discrimination in German ophthalmologists: changes associated with the use of lasers and operating microscopes. *Ophthalmology*, **98**, 567–75.

4 American Conference of Governmental Industrial Hygienists (1993). *Threshold limit values for physical agents in the work environment.* ACGIH, Cincinnati.

5 Sliney, D. H. (1983). Standards for use of visible and nonvisible radiation on the eye. *Am. J. Optom. Physiol. Opt.*, **60**, 278–86.

6 Birngruber, R. and Gabel, V.-P. (1983). Thermal versus photochemical damage in the retina—thermal calculations for exposure limits. *Trans. Ophthalmol. Soc. UK*, **103**, 442–6.

7 Haldorsson, T. and Langerholc, J. (1978). Thermodynamic analysis of laser irradiation of biological tissue. *Appl. Opt.*, **17**, 3948–58.

8 Birngruber, R. (1991). Choroidal circulation and heat convection at the fundus of the eye. In: *Lasers: Applications in medicine and biology*, Vol. 5 (ed. M. L. Wolbarsht), pp. 277–361. Plenum Press, New York.

9 Docchio, F. (1991). Nd:YAG laser ophthalmic microsurgery: time- and space-resolved laser-induced breakdown in liquids and ocular media. In: *Lasers: Applications in medicine and biology*, Vol. 5 (ed. M. L. Wolbarsht), pp. 85–140. Plenum Press, New York.

10 Mainster, M. A., Sliney, D. H., Belcher, C. D., and Buzney, S. M. (1983). Laser photodisruptors: damage mechanisms, instrument design and safety. *Ophthalmology*, **90**, 973–91.

11 Hack, H. and Neuroth, N. (1982). Resistance of optical and colored glasses to 3-nsec laser pulses. *Appl. Opt.*, **21**, 3239–48.

12 Nuss, R. C., Puliafito, C. A., and Dehm, E. J. (1987). Unscheduled DNA synthesis following excimer laser ablation of the cornea *in vivo*. *Invest. Ophthalmol. Visual Sci.*, **28**, 287–94.

13 Trockel, S. L., Srinivasan, R., and Braren, B. (1983). Excimer laser surgery of the cornea. *Am. J. Ophthalmol.*, **96**, 710–5.

13a World Health Organisation (WHO) (1982). *Environmental Health Criteria 23, Lasers and optical radiation.* (Geneva: WHO).

14 Mainster, M. A. (1986). Wavelength selection in macular photocoagulation: tissue optics, thermal effects, and laser systems. *Ophthalmology*, **93**, 721–8.

15 Moseley, H. and Allan, D. (1987). Intensity of the flash associated with laser-induced plasma in the eye. *Phys. Med. Biol.*, **32**, 1159–66.

16 Moseley, H. and Fenner, J. A. K. (1993). Hazards associated with viewing the incandescence of lased tissue. *Lasers Med. Sci.*, **8**, 23–5.

17 BSEN 60825-1 (1994). *Radiation safety of laser products, equipment classification, requirements and user's guide.*

18 Wenig, B. L., Stevenson, K. M., Wenig, B. M., and Tracey, D. (1993). Effects of plume produced by NdYAG laser and electrocautery on the respiratory system. *Lasers Surg. Med.*, **13**, 242–5.

19 Ferenczy, A., Bergeron, C., and Richart, R. M. (1990). Human papilloma virus DNA in CO_2 laser-generated plume of smoke and its consequences to the surgeon. *Obstet. Gynaecol.*, **75**, 114–18.

20 Abramson, A. L., DiLorenzo, T. P., and Steinberg, B. M. (1990). Is papillomavirus detectable in the plume of laser-treated laryngeal papilloma? *Arch. Otolaryngol. Head Neck Surg.*, **116**, 604–7.

21 Walker, N. P. J., Matthews, J., and Newsome, S. W. B. (1986). Possible hazards from irradiation with the carbon dioxide laser. *Lasers Surg. Med.*, **6**, 84–6.

22 Byrne, P. O., Sisson, P. R., Oliver, P. D., and Ingham, H. R. (1987). Carbon dioxide laser irradiation of bacterial targets *in vitro*. *J. Hosp. Infect.*, **9**, 265–73.

23 Moseley, H., Porter, H. Q., McFarlane, H., Mellon, A., and Davis, J. A. (1992). Patient response to laser treatment. *Lasers Med. Sci.*, **7**, 127–31.

24 Vourch, G., Tannieres, M., and Frech, G. (1979). Ignition of tracheal tube during laryngeal laser surgery. *Anaesthesia*, **34**, 685.

25 Hirshman, C. A. and Smith, J. (1980). Indirect ignition of the endotracheal tube during carbon dioxide laser surgery. *Arch. Otolaryngol.*, **106**, 639–41.

26 Cozine, K. (1981). Laser-induced endotracheal tube fire. *Anaesthesiology*, **55**, 583–5.

27 Casey, K. R., Fairfax, W. R., Smith, S. J., and Dixon, J. A. (1983). Intratracheal fire ignited by the NdYAG laser during treatment of tracheal stenosis. *Chest*, **84**, 295–6.

28 The Health and Safety at Work etc. Act (1974). (England, Wales, and Scotland.)

29 The Management of Health and Safety at Work Regulations (1992). (England, Wales, and Scotland.) Amendment (1994).

30 Personal Protective Equipment at Work Regulations (1992). (England, Wales, and Scotland.)

31 BSEN 60601-2-22 (1993). *Medical electrical equipment Part 2: Particular requirements for the safety of diagnostic and therapeutic laser equipment.*

32 BSEN 207 (1999). *Personal eye protection—Filters and eye-protectors against laser radiation (laser eye-protectors).*

33 BSEN 208 (1999). *Personal eye-protection—Eye-protectors for adjustment work on lasers and laser system (laser adjustment eye-protectors).*

34 Medical Devices Agency (1995). *Guidance on the safe use of medical and dental lasers.*

35 American National Standards Institute (1996). *American national standard for safe use of lasers in health care facilities.* ANSI Z136.3. Laser Institute of America, Orlando, FL, USA.

36 American National Standards Institute (1993). *American national standard for safe use of lasers.* ANSI Z136.1. Laser Institute of America, Orlando, FL, USA.

37 McGhee, C. N. J., Craig, J., Moseley, H., and Keller, P. (1997). Laser keychains: potential for serious eye injury. *Eye News*, **4**, 17–19.

38 International Electrotechnical Commission (1999). *Safety of laser products—Part 8: Guidelines for the safe use of medical laser equipment.* IEC TR 60825-8. IEC, Geneva.

39 Fenner, J. and Moseley, H. (1989). Damage thresholds of CO_2 laser protective eyewear. *Lasers Med. Sci.*, **4**, 33–9.

40 Emergency Care Research Institute (ECRI) (1993). Laser safety eyewear. *Health Devices*, **22** (4).

41 Moseley, H. (1994). Ultraviolet and laser radiation safety. *Phys. Med. Biol.*, **39**, 1765–99.

42 Sliney, D. H. and Wolbarsht, M. (1980). *Safety with lasers and other optical sources.* Plenum, New York.

43 Wolfe, J. A. (1985). Laser retinal injury. *Military Med.*, **150**, 177–85.

44 Bandle, A. M. and Holyoak, B. (1987). Laser incidents. In: *Medical laser safety* (ed. H. Moseley and J. K. Haywood). IPSM, London.

45 Haifeng, L., Guanhuang, G., Dechang, W., Guidao, X., Liangshun, S., Jiemin, X., and Haibiao, W. (1989). Ocular injuries from accidental laser exposure. *Health Phys.*, **56**, 711–16.

46 Gabel, V.-P., Birngruber, R., Lorenz, B., and Lang, G. K. (1989). Clinical observations of six cases of laser injury to the eye. *Health Phys.*, **56**, 705–10.

47 Henderson, A. R. (1997). *A guide to laser safety.* Chapman and Hall, London.

48 Decker, C. D. (1977). An accident victim's view. *Laser Focus*, **13**, 6.

Chapter 20

Non-coherent optical radiation sources

D. K. Taylor

20.1 Introduction

Many of the hazards described in the chapter on coherent radiation are present also in non-coherent radiations and much of the advice given on coherent radiation protection remains relevant. Most non-coherent sources generate divergent radiation fields, so the power density decreases with increasing distance from the source. The normal blink, aversion, and avoidance reactions can reduce the hazards for visible and infrared radiations; however, ultraviolet, the most hazardous of the optical radiations, is not readily detected by human sense organs. In terms of the numbers of individuals at risk, and the numbers injured, the Sun is the most important source. Solar radiation at the Earth's surface is essentially non-divergent and contains a wide spectrum of hazardous wavelengths. It includes visible as well as invisible wavelengths, but is so familiar and essential to life processes that its hazards may be overlooked or ignored.

This chapter is concerned with electromagnetic radiations in the ultraviolet (UV) band (from about 100 nm wavelength) through the visible wavelengths (400 to about 780 nm) to infrared (IR) radiation (from about 780 nm to 1 mm wavelength). The subdivisions of this spectrum are summarized in Table 20.1. The arbitrary divisions in the UV waveband arise from the observed effects of the Earth's atmosphere and ozone layer on solar radiation reaching the Earth's surface, and the behaviour of normal human skin in response to the different wavelengths.

Table 20.1 UV/visible/IR optical radiation wavelength divisions

Wavelengths	Accepted or common name
100–200 nm	Vacuum UV (readily absorbed in air)
200–280 nm	UV-C (filtered from solar UV by the atmosphere and ozone layer)
280–315 nm	UV-B (erythemal or skin-reddening wavelengths)
315–400 nm	UV-A (sometimes called 'black light')
400–780 nm	Visible light: blue (shortest) to red (longest) wavelengths
780–1400 nm	IR-A (near-infrared)
1400–3000 nm	IR-B (mid-infrared)
3000 nm–1 mm	IR-C (far-infrared)

The boundary between UV-C and UV-B was chosen as the approximate wavelength below which the Earth's atmosphere and the ozone layer cut off solar UV at sea level. Shorter wavelengths can be detected at higher altitudes and in spacecraft, where atmospheric filtration is reduced or absent. They may also be emitted by artificial sources such as discharge lamps and electric arcs.

The boundary between UV-A and UV-B was chosen as the approximate wavelength at which human skin shows a marked change in response. Short UV-B wavelengths are 1000 to 10 000 times more effective at causing erythema (skin reddening, or sunburn) than similar doses of long-wavelength UV-A. The response of the skin does not alter abruptly at the boundary but changes gradually over a band of several nanometres, so that the inclusion or rejection of wavelengths near the boundary may significantly influence the estimation of a hazard.

Boundaries for the wavelength ranges have been defined by the Commission Internationale de l'Éclairage (CIE) [1], but these are not universally adopted. For example, for the crossover from UV-A to UV-B, the CIE have adopted 315 nm, but 320 nm is also widely used, especially in the USA. This is of particular importance when measuring UV doses and comparing biological effects. UV is widely used therapeutically to relieve certain skin diseases, but a therapeutic dose of UV-B, for example, may be defined differently by US and European phototherapists, who tend to use these different definitions for the bandwidth of the radiation from their UV lamps. The boundary between UV and visible is chosen to be 400 nm by nearly all workers, although at least one commercial manufacturer of dermatological UV treatment equipment has adopted 410 nm as the boundary. This is of no great importance, fortunately, since the sources commonly used for this treatment have low output around this region and contribute little to the total irradiance.

20.2 Effects of optical radiation on tissues

The hazards from UV, visible, and IR radiations are mainly to the eyes and skin, and fall into two categories–thermal damage and photochemical damage. Thermal damage arises from high-intensity radiation absorption, sufficient to raise tissue temperatures to the point where normal cell function is affected temporarily or permanently, or inhibited to the point of cell death. Photochemical damage usually results from modest energy levels, insufficient to raise tissue temperatures beyond a few degrees. The effects, however, may be much more hazardous to human tissues, often being painless at the time of the exposure and not manifesting until hours or days later, with little opportunity to reverse the changes during the intervening period.

Non-coherent electromagnetic radiations in the visible region are detectable by the eyes, and visible and IR radiations of sufficient power can be detected by thermal sense organs and pain detectors in tissues. The blink and aversion reflexes reduce the risks of thermal damage to eyes and skin, but the greater hazard arises from photochemical reactions, particularly in the shorter-wavelength, higher-energy, blue and ultraviolet regions.

20.2.1 Thermal effects

Thermal injury to eyes and skin is mostly confined to IR and is sometimes seen in foundry workers from prolonged occupational exposure to intense IR sources. Damage to skin is occasionally seen in the lower legs of older persons who habitually warmed themselves by open fires before the general availability of domestic central heating. The damage to the skin (*erythema ab igne*, literally redness from fire) arises from structural changes to the connective tissue and capillary network, and is mostly irreversible. Thermal stress and dehydration are also recognized as hazards arising from absorption of heat energy, especially in the neonate and sick or unconscious patient. Thermal damage arising from visible and UV radiations is rare, but not unknown. Photochemical effects from these wavelengths will always predominate, and cause more damage. Most incandescent sources emit large quantities of IR (whose spectrum is much wider than either UV or visible) and this overwhelms the minor contribution from the shorter wavelengths.

20.2.2 Photochemical effects

Photochemical changes can be elicited by relatively small doses of radiation, and are strongly wavelength dependent. The absorption of photons of the appropriate wavelength in biomolecules may lead to one or more chemical reactions—such as a restructuring of the molecule to make a different chemical species, a configurational change which alters its biological availability, or the release of toxic photoproducts such as singlet-state excited oxygen, one of the commonest mediators of photodamage. These effects are particularly hazardous when DNA is involved, since some of the changes may be irreversible and can interfere with normal cell division. When normal DNA repair mechanisms cannot reverse all the changes, cancer can result.

The main hazards to the eyes arise from UV radiation and blue visible light. Hazards from IR seem to be mostly confined to the near-IR wavelengths (IR-A) which are able to penetrate more deeply and cause damage to the structures of the retina beneath the focused image of IR sources. The acute effects of UV exposure, observable within hours, include photokeratitis and conjunctivitis, inflammation and soreness of the membranes covering the cornea and sclera. Welders' flash and snow-blindness are among the names applied to this condition, depending on the origin of the UV exposure. Sufferers describe the condition as sore, 'gritty' eyes, which typically lasts for 24 hours or more. Mild cases are generally reversible, although permanent damage may be observed following prolonged exposure. Longer-term changes can include discoloration or opacity of the lens (cataract). The lens absorbs most UV-A entering the eye, so in eyes without the protection provided by the lens (aphakia—perhaps following surgical removal for cataract), the retina is at greater risk and may be damaged irreversibly.

Blue light is transmitted to the retina, and is capable of causing long-term ocular damage, even blindness, due to changes in the photoreceptors. The focusing of intense blue wavelengths on the retina for as little as a few seconds can cause temporary disturbance of vision, and with longer exposure, the loss of visual function in the sensitive region. This is the main cause of damage to the eyesight arising from solar eclipse viewing without adequate protection. The total eclipse visible in the British Isles and much of Europe on 11 August 1999 was perhaps the most publicized solar event of all time, and the subject of a widespread safety publicity campaign. Solar eclipses may only be safely viewed with the naked eye during the brief period of totality. At all other times, dense solar filters must be used for direct viewing to avoid the risk of photochemical damage to the retina from the intense solar visible radiation.

The official recommendation relating to solar eclipses is to use indirect viewing by pin-hole camera or specially-adapted photographic or video equipment. Indirect viewing is also the safest means of monitoring artificial sources of intense visible radiation, and is recommended wherever possible. This is now a realistic proposition for a wide range of sources, given the ready availability of low-cost video equipment.

Filter materials exist which are adequate to filter UV and reduce visible wavelengths to acceptable levels, but these are not commonly available to the general public. The use of metallized plastic film, sunglasses, or exposed radiographic film is strongly discouraged. The optical properties of the surface coatings are easily damaged, resulting in intense localized exposure to the eye. Suppression of visible wavelengths from solar radiation may not necessarily be matched in UV. The hazard to the eye protected by certain filters could, by permitting the iris (which is unresponsive to UV) to remain dilated, be even greater than for the unprotected eye.

20.3 Short- and long-term reactions

20.3.1 Short-term effects on the skin

The main short-term hazard for human skin arises from UV radiation, and is familiar to anyone who has experienced sunburn. Acute erythema, the reddening of the skin due to vasodilation in the capillaries in the dermis, arises mostly from the UV-B wavelengths, although UV-C from artificial sources will produce the same effect in similar doses. The effect is noticeable within a few hours of the exposure.

UV-A is also able to induce erythema, but the doses required are up to 10 000 times greater than the dose of UV-B for the same result. This huge range in sensitivity is illustrated in Figure 20.1, which shows the internationally accepted erythema action spectrum for normal human skin. Note the logarithmic scale of spectral sensitivity. The function is a mathematically convenient approximation to the spectrum derived empirically [2] and is important when assessing hazards and defining UV irradiances and doses in medical phototherapy.

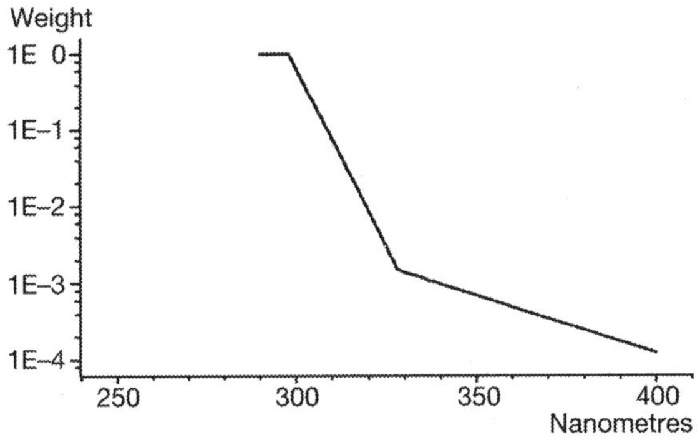

Figure 20.1 Erythema action spectrum (logarithmic plot) for UV on normal human skin.

20.3.2 Short-term effects on the eyes

The natural reaction of the eyes to high levels of visible light is eyelid blinking, head turning, and iris contraction (approximately in that order of speed). These are easily overcome by radiation of high enough intensity to deliver a large dose to the retina before the reflexes can occur. This reaction is absent for invisible UV, so that significant doses of UV can be delivered into the eye if there are no high-intensity visible components present. Sources that fall into this category include Wood's Light sources (invented by Robert Wood, an American physicist in the early twentieth century) which include a lamp emitting UV-A peaking at about 365 nm, from which visible wavelengths are almost completely removed by a dark blue nickel/chromium oxide glass filter). This is helpful in the diagnosis of parasitic infestations of the skin and certain metabolic disorders, which can be identified from the characteristic fluorescence of the skin, hair, or urine under Wood's Light. Modern semiconductor light-emitting diodes (LEDs) are also available with emission in the UV region, and may represent a hazard over long exposure periods, or if they are made up into arrays with significant irradiant power.

Cataracts have been induced in experimental animals by exposing the animals to high doses of UV-A and photosensitizers, although not conclusively demonstrated in humans, where this combination is used deliberately in psoralen and UV-A (PUVA) therapy. As a precaution, these patients are advised to use UV-suppressing eye protection after the administration of the photosensitizer, to avoid the photochemical reaction resulting from solar or artificial UV (see §20.10).

20.3.3 Long-term effects on the skin

The longer-term effects include melanogenesis, or tanning, the skin's natural protective response, which takes several days to develop, and elastosis (loss of skin elasticity or wrinkling, arising from connective tissue damage). This may not become apparent for years. Elastosis is mostly associated with longer wavelengths in the UV-A spectrum, possibly because higher doses can be tolerated, and is usually associated with regular exposure over many years, particularly from the use of cosmetic sunbeds, which emit mostly UV-A.

The long-term risk of most concern is skin cancer. Non-malignant skin cancers are now one of the highest incidence groups of cancers in humans, although fortunately rarely fatal. Squamous cell carcinoma (SCC) and basal cell carcinoma (BCC) arise in the most superficial layers of the skin and remain localized for years, so that surgical removal is usually completely successful in curing the lesion. Malignant melanoma, however, is usually invasive and metastatic, so that it is often incurable and fatal, especially if untreated for some time. It is clear that Sun exposure has an important, but not exclusive, role to play in this rising incidence, and modern dress habits, foreign holidays, and cosmetic tanning have all been offered as possible causes.

20.3.4 Long-term effects on the eyes

Since the eye is designed to admit radiation in order to function, it is difficult to separate hazardous exposure outcomes from normal ageing and deterioration. The lens stops most of the hazardous wavelengths and is therefore most at risk, with cataract as the commonest outcome—nowadays a relatively straightforward matter to correct by surgical removal and prosthetic lens insertion, but most retinal damage, caused by short exposures to hazardous wavelengths, is irreversible.

20.4 Techniques for optical radiation measurement

A typical radiometer for optical measurements in the UV and visible bands will have a detector assembly, usually

Box 20.1 Radiometric quantities

Radiant flux (ϕ) is the rate of flow of electromagnetic energy through space (W).

Irradiance (E) is the radiant flux density incident on a surface (W m^{-2}). This is the term used in phototherapy to quantify the radiant energy incident on the skin from all directions. If radiation beams of uniform intensity I are incident on a circular plane area at various angles, radiation at normal incidence will fill the area A and be entirely absorbed in the surface. A beam at angle α is absorbed not by the circular area but by the projection of the circle at angle α, an ellipse of apparent area $A/\cos\alpha$ (Figure 20.2). The energy absorbed in the area will therefore be reduced by the same cosine factor.

Radiant exposure (H) is the irradiance on a surface integrated over time (J m^{-2}). This is called the 'dose' in phototherapy.

Radiant intensity (I) is the radiant flux from a source per unit solid angle in a given direction (W sr^{-1}). It is used to quantify the spatial distribution of the radiant flux emitted by a source. For a point source emitting total radiant flux ϕ uniformly in all directions, $I = \phi/4\pi$.

Radiance (L) is the radiant intensity per unit surface area in a given direction in the plane perpendicular to that direction (W m^{-2} sr^{-1}).

The photometric analogues of these quantities are:

• Luminous flux (lumen second)	Radiant flux
• Illuminance (lumen)	Irradiance
• Luminous intensity (lm sr^{-1})	Radiant intensity
• Luminance (lm sr^{-1} m^{-2})	Radiance

It is instructive to consider briefly relationships between the various radiometric quantities (Figure B20.1). For emissions from a small area of a source A_s, emitting radiant flux ϕ into a solid angle Ω at angle θ to the perpendicular to the source surface, the radiance, L, is given by

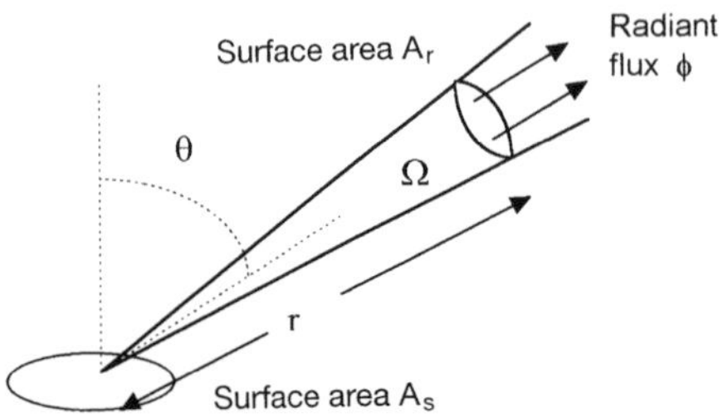

Fig. B20.1 Radiance from a source

containing a photodiode in a feedback circuit around a high-gain amplifier, filters to define the pass-band, and an optical diffuser to gather and distribute the incident radiation uniformly over the diode. The detector assembly may be separated from the rest of the electronics for reasons of convenience and flexibility, and joined by cable to the main instrument, containing an amplifier driving an analogue meter or digital display and batteries.

20.4.1 Photodiode sensors

The majority of sensors employed for optical measurements are semiconductor photodiodes. These components are cheap, robust, and readily available, with electrical characteristics that lend themselves to the construction of relatively accurate and reliable radiometers. The solid-state photodiode is basically a P–N junction, usually in doped silicon, whose electrical characteristics can be varied by incident electromagnetic radiation.

Silicon photodiodes have a reduced sensitivity at shorter UV wavelengths, so UV-B and UV-C detectors are often constructed using a more expensive and fragile device, based on an evacuated pure silica tubular envelope containing a photocathode, called a vacuum photodiode. This is larger and more expensive than a semiconductor photodiode, and results in a larger assembly, which may be less convenient to use, but has better rejection of visible and IR wavelengths than silicon.

Box 20.1 *(continued)*

$$L = I / (A_s \cos \theta) = \phi / (\Omega A_s \cos \theta).$$

If the intensity is incident perpendicularly on a surface area A_r at distance r from the source, then the radiant flux, ϕ, is given by

$$\phi = L \Omega A_s \cos \theta = (L A_r A_s \cos \theta)/r^2.$$

The irradiance, E_r, on surface A_r resulting from the emission is

$$E_r = \phi / A_r = (L A_s \cos \theta)/r^2 = L \omega$$

where ω is the solid angle subtended by the source at distance r. If A_r was an area at the eye, ω would be the solid angle subtended by the source at the eye.

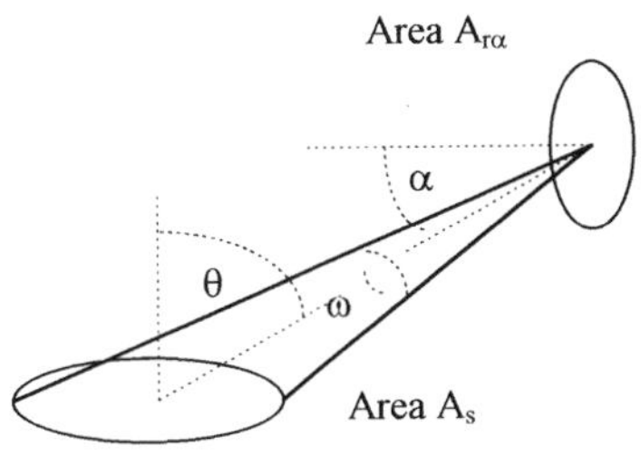

Fig B20.2 Irradiance from a source

If the perpendicular to surface $A_{r\alpha}$ was at angle α to the direction of the flux (Figure B20.2), then the irradiance would be

$$E_{r\alpha} = (L A_s \cos \theta \cos \alpha)/r^2 = L \omega \cos \alpha.$$

20.4.2 Optical filters

Silicon photodiodes have a wide range of sensitivity, from around 200 nm in the UV-C region up to the short-wavelength IR, around 1000 nm (1 μm). To ensure that only a desired waveband is permitted to illuminate the diode, filters are employed to eliminate radiation on either side of the chosen pass-band. A typical UV-A radiometer used in a phototherapy clinic, for example, will need filters to remove any UV-B present in the radiation from the source, and also to remove any visible or IR radiation present. Most UV sources have significant spectral components in the visible region as well as in the UV region, and many sources have significant IR contributions as well.

Filters do not cut off sharply at a boundary, but exhibit a change in transmission over a range of wavelengths. Out-of-band radiation, therefore, is not eliminated but is reduced with variable efficiency depending on the wavelength. This fall-off in transmission may lie entirely *outside* the desired pass-band (in which case adjacent out-of-band components may be included with the desired band) or can be selected to begin to reduce spectral components *inside* the pass-band. This ensures better rejection of unwanted out-of-band components but also compromises the performance of the meter near the limits of the intended wavelength interval.

The sharpness of the cut-off can be improved by using several filter plates with slightly different cut-off wavelengths, or interference filters, but increasing the number of plates in front of the diode usually reduces the overall transmission of the filter assembly, making the meter less sensitive to low irradiances. The design of these optical components may therefore be a compromise between pass-band performance and meter sensitivity, although most hazardous sources have intensities high enough to avoid problems of meter sensitivity.

20.4.3 Optical diffusers

The optical diffuser is designed to sum the radiation arriving at the meter from different angles, and to deliver it uniformly over the whole surface area of the photodiode, typically about 0.5 cm^2, to optimise electrical efficiency. An ideal diffuser will have low losses in the pass-band and exhibit a sensitivity to radiation arriving at any angle of incidence (α) proportional to the cosine of that angle (Box 20.1). Thus the detector of a radiometer or photometer should register as 'seeing' an irradiance E as $E \cos \alpha$ from that angle (Figure 20.2).

A major source of error, not adequately addressed in some radiometers and photometers, arises from poor angular sensitivity of the input optics, usually in the form of a diffuser or gatherer. Pye and Martin [3] examined a number of practical diffusers for deviation from true cosine weighting, and found that most transmit less than expected at non-normal incidence. A diffuser must also avoid reflections at glancing angles of incidence. Diffusers with flat polished surfaces, therefore, will tend to have a lower weighting at large angles, when specular reflection may occur. Diffusers are usually designed deliberately to increase the radiation entering the optical aperture at increasing angles of incidence to compensate. A diffuser that does not protrude into the radiation field above the plane of the sensor housing is unlikely to gather enough radiation to compensate for the losses at large angles. However, this feature may also make the meter sensitive to radiation arriving effectively from behind the sensor (i.e. at incident angles greater than 90°).

The CIE [4] defined methods of characterizing photometers to give a figure of merit (f_2) to enable comparisons to be made more easily. Pye and Martin [3] extended this idea to allow for the very wide angles of incidence commonly encountered in UV measurements. They defined a modified figure of merit which summed the deviation of the response $D(\alpha)$ from the ideal response $\cos \alpha$ (both over- and underestimated values) weighted by $\sin \alpha$ to take account of the relative contribution to a measurement:

$$f_2\% = 100\int_0^{\alpha_m} 2 \mid D(\alpha) \sin \alpha - c(\alpha) \sin \alpha \mid \mathrm{d}\alpha \quad (20.1)$$

where $c(\alpha) = \cos \alpha$ for $0 < \alpha < 90°$ and $c(\alpha) = 0$ for $\alpha > 90°$.

The figure also included contributions from incident angles greater than the CIE's limit of 85° (found to exceed 95° for some examples of protruding diffuser).

The best diffusers fitted to commercially available radiometers at the time of writing have matt surfaces, formed into thin plastic domes or tablets (usually of PTFE), which protrude into the measurement field above the plane of the sensor housing. These diffusers are less transparent than pure silica diffusers, which may be a

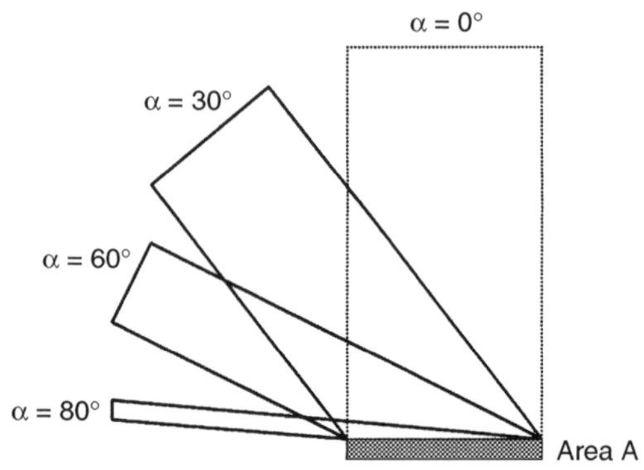

Figure 20.2 Lambert's cosine law: angular dependence of irradiance; energy falling on unit area is proportional to cosine of the angle of incidence.

problem for very low irradiances, and are more susceptible to accidental damage. The best designs had f_2 values of around 5% or less and an upper limit of 10% has been proposed for acceptable performance for typical applications [5]. Further development of the shape of the PTFE type of input diffuser may improve the cosine-weighting of low-cost radiometers (f_2 less than 5%) at minimal increase in manufacturing cost.

Precision measurements often employ an integrating sphere instead of a PTFE diffuser. This consists of a hollow sphere coated with white reflective material such as barium sulphate, pierced by an input aperture and an exit port to the detector (not in line), usually with an internal coated baffle to prevent direct transmission from input to output apertures. The aim is to gather all radiation from the input aperture and permit multiple reflections within the sphere, so that the detector at the output port 'sees' radiation from all directions equally. The effectiveness of this device is dependent on the reflection coefficient of the coating (which may be 95% or more) and the proportion of the spherical surface 'lost' to the non-reflective input and output ports, and the finite thickness of the edge of the input aperture which limits the angle of acceptance. Larger spheres reduce this proportion but make the device more bulky and therefore less convenient. Integrating spheres are available large enough for a person to enter. The use of integrating spheres is mostly confined to precision measurements in the laboratory.

20.4.4 Radiometer performance

The photocurrent from the diode is approximately proportional to the rate of energy absorption in the semiconductor, and therefore indicates irradiance (energy transfer rate per unit area, usually expressed in W m^{-2} or mW cm^{-2}; 10 W m^{-2} = 1 mW cm^{-2}). The simplest radiometers will display the signal from the photodiode directly, but more sophisticated meters may be micro-processor-controlled, with features such as auto-ranging, slope-correction, auto-zeroing, user-selectable radiation units, and user-adjustable calibration factors. This last feature is particularly useful in assessing radiation hazards from different sources, since the hazard is dependent on wavelength. Different sources may emit different spectral components and will therefore require different calibration factors. The ability to change this factor without opening the case or using tools to set a potentiometer is an advantage over other equally acceptable radiometers without this facility.

Some meters allow the interchange of the photodiode assembly, permitting several different types of measurement to be made with the same meter unit. These sensors may be designed for radiometric UV and visible measurements in radiometric units, or action/hazard spectrum-weighted units. The latter is achieved by means of filters designed to match the biological action spectrum or hazard. These sensors are useful for estimating UV and blue-light hazards, the erythemal power of UV sources, and for comparing light sources in horticulture and marine biology, using filters matching biological action spectra.

Electronic amplifiers with high gain and good linearity over several orders of magnitude are easy to design with modern semiconductors. A meter suitable for the majority of measurements to be made in the laboratory or clinic should cover the range from 1 W m^{-2} or less up to about 500 W m^{-2} or more. A meter able to resolve to 0.5 W m^{-2} or less is useful for testing radiation protection devices, such as UV-resistant visors or spectacles. A typical source will have irradiance of the order of 100 W m^{-2} so that the meter needs to resolve to at least 1 W m^{-2} to measure 1% transmission through the protective device.

20.4.5 Instruments with thermal sensors

Photodiode-based devices provide measurements of irradiance in W m^{-2} incident on a sensor for photons with wavelengths up to about 1000 nm. For longer wavelengths, where the photodiode loses efficiency, it is possible to use devices that measure the *quantity* of irradiation (its energy) falling on an absorber, by measuring the increase in temperature of the absorber. Such devices include thermopiles, pyrometers, and even the humble thermometer. The total energy absorbed usually includes all UV, visible, and IR radiation falling on the sensitive element, as the element is usually designed to be a close approximation to a perfect 'black-body'. The total over a band is an acceptable measurement (provided UV and blue-light hazards are estimated separately) as the hazards associated with long-wavelength IR are not strongly wavelength dependent.

20.4.6 Spectroradiometers

Precision radiation measurements for a wide range of radiation sources with different spectra or assessment of transmissions of protective filters for different applications requires a spectoradiometer. Such an instrument is often configurable with a range of detectors, diffraction gratings, and optical components to optimise its operation for different bands. A typical design may have an input diffuser similar to that of a simple radiometer, followed by glass filter plates (order-sorting filters) to confine the bandwidth of incoming radiation into manageable sections, and a single or double monochromator assembly. This uses diffraction gratings to separate the incoming wavelength components spatially, so that very narrow bandwidth sections of the fan of diffracted radiation may be collimated and detected.

Many spectroradiometers may be configured to measure 1 nm bandwidth or less of the incoming radiation, and reject the remainder. This requires a detector of high sensitivity, such as a photomultiplier tube, and an averaging system to improve the signal-to-noise ratio. The sequential collection of data inevitably takes a significant time to complete, which places constraints on the stability of the sources and limits the conventional spectroradiometer's ability to track rapid changes in spectrum.

A modern development of this principle employs a diffraction grating and a linear detector constructed from a charge-coupled device (CCD) detector, similar to a solid-state TV camera detector, to record the spatially dispersed radiation as stored electric charge on a photosensitive semiconductor substrate. This 'flash' conversion of radiation into stored charge may then be read sequentially like a computer memory for analysis. The advantages of high-speed conversion and instantaneous spectrum capture are offset by lower sensitivity, reduced signal-to-noise performance, limited bandwidth resolution, and limited flexibility of configuration. These limitations may be acceptable for many uses, and the technology is developing rapidly, making the pocket-sized UV and visible spectroradiometer a practical possibility. Several manufacturers now offer portable devices covering UV-B, UV-A, and blue visible, with resolution of about 1 nm.

Spectroradiometers have limitations in use, including their size and cost and the need for high-sensitivity detection systems to measure spectral irradiances of very limited bandwidth. Background noise arising from scatter of out-of-band radiation within the casing of the instrument limits the lowest intensity of wanted radiation that can be detected. Their physical size may have optical consequences when measurements are needed within three-dimensional arrays of sources (see §20.5.1).

20.5 Calibration of detectors

For a measurement of non-coherent radiation to have any meaning, it must be comparable to other similar measurements, traceable to some agreed standard, and capable of being repeated with similar results. These ideals illustrate the concepts of accuracy (getting the 'right' answer) and consistency (getting the 'same' answer), which may be quite independent properties of a measurement device.

For many practical purposes, a consistent measurement of a variable in arbitrary units is adequate. The decision to replace phototherapy lamps with fresh ones, for example, usually only depends on knowledge of the ratio of the intensity of partly used lamps to that of new ones. The device used to measure the output needs to be linear and consistent, but not necessarily calibrated to a standard, as ratios are dimensionless. A reading under standardized conditions with fresh lamps fitted can be used to establish the value (75%, for example) at which the lamps should be changed. Routine testing every few months will enable this point to be established with more accuracy than a manufacturer's quoted lamp lifetime, which may be dependent upon the pattern of use.

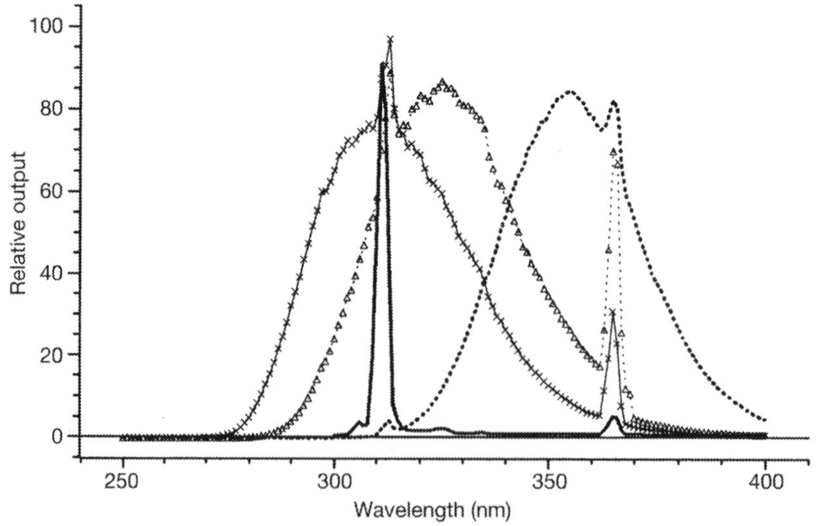

Figure 20.3 Spectral plots of four widely used UV therapy fluorescent lamps: {crosses}, Philips TL-12/Waldmann UV21 broadband UV-B; {triangles}, Waldmann UV6 broadband UV-B; {solid line}, Philips TL-01 narrowband UV-B, dots, broadband UV-A or PUVA.

20.5.1 Requirements for hazard assessment

Estimation of the hazard arising from an unknown source of radiation requires a measurement of the radiation characteristics that can be compared with published data, to determine the quantity of energy to which tissues have been exposed. For this, a measurement device which is accurate is required. It should display a value very close to that obtained by a standards laboratory, such as the National Physical Laboratory (NPL), under identical conditions.

The wavelength dependence of photochemical hazards in the UV and visible regions requires the measurement device to have accurate wavelength sensitivity and a wide dynamic range. A simple radiometer, which indicates a single value for the sum of the irradiance over a range of wavelengths, gives no indication of the presence of any peaks or troughs in the spectrum, nor where they occur. Plots of the spectral outputs of some typical UV phototherapy fluorescent lamps obtained from a spectroradiometer are shown in Figure 20.3. The total irradiance of the source is equivalent to the area beneath the spectral irradiance curve. The spectra shown could have identical areas under their spectral curves and would therefore have the same irradiance. However, there would be different proportions in the critical areas for skin erythema and risk potential, which would thus represent different hazards with different biological effects.

The wavelength dependence described above can be allowed for in simple radiometers, if the sensor has filters that shape the meter's sensitivity to match the known hazard spectrum closely. For unknown sources of radiation, a meter with 'weighted' sensitivity can indicate the magnitude of the hazard but not where the spectral components are. Where the characteristics of a hazard cannot be assumed or deduced from knowledge of the source, a spectroradiometer may be used to establish the spectral components present in the source, and thus to quantify the hazard and assist in choosing the appropriate protection methods.

20.5.2 Spectroradiometers

Spectroradiometers require calibration at individual wavelengths. A standard source with a stable power supply is required, for which constancy of radiant output and spectral emissions are well established. Measurements will be made in a standard reproducible configuration. Quartz halogen or deuterium lamp sources are normally used for UV measurement, and lamp outputs may be determined at a standards laboratory such as the NPL.

In spectroradiometers that are used in the calibration of radiometers for measurements of irradiance from large-area sources, such as phototherapy cabins, it is particularly important that the detectors have an accurate angular response ($f_2 < 10\%$) [5]. The spectroradiometer will be calibrated against a small standard source in the form of a UV-emitting lamp. A simple calibration in one configuration will only give the spectroradiometer response at essentially normal incidence. If the spectroradiometer is to be used to measure the irradiance in a phototherapy cabin giving illumination from all directions (in order to calibrate a hand-held radiometer), the percentage error in the measurement will be of the order of the value of f_2 for the diffuser/sensor assembly.

20.5.3 Radiometers for measurement of known source spectra

Most non-coherent optical sources are based on well-known physical principles. Incandescent lamps, mercury discharge lamps, and fluorescent tubes are made to stated specifications by manufacturers who exercise quality control processes. When a source has known characteristics, it is possible to calibrate a simple radiometer to read the irradiance accurately by adjusting it to display the same value as that obtained from a spectroradiometer or calibrated meter under identical measurement conditions. Provided the radiometer is only used to measure the irradiance from similar sources of the same specification, the indicated value will be accurate, within the limits of production spread and batch variability.

The meter should be adjusted to display the same value as that obtained from a calibrated meter or spectroradiometer placed in the same location in front of the radiation sources to be measured. This simple comparison is not without problems, however, and care must be taken to ensure that the measurement conditions are the same for both devices. Source lamps must be of identical type and manufacturer, or known to be direct equivalents (the manufacturer's data sheet may be helpful in verifying equivalence).

A radiometer calibrated to read the spectral output of one type of source will not measure the spectral output of another type correctly, because the peaks and troughs in the spectral curve may fall in different regions of the meter's (non-uniform) sensitivity curve. To measure more than one type of lamp correctly, a calibration factor must be determined for each and the meter adjusted for each type. This is inconvenient for a simple meter with a fixed or inaccessible calibration control, and is a good reason for choosing a meter with a readily adjustable or software-controlled factor. A radiometer constructed with limited bandwidth and calibrated in this manner will not be suitable for measuring the irradiance of unknown sources. For this purpose, a spectroradiometer is required to define the information needed to define the spectral content and spectral irradiance.

20.5.4 Calibration geometry

Ideally, the calibrating reference device (meter or spectroradiometer) should be located in the same position in a similar source configuration as will be used for measurements, or an arrangement that is as close as possible to the real configuration. This is particularly important where the radiometer sensor has an imperfect angular sensitivity to the measured wavelengths. A meter with poor sensitivity at large angles, which has been calibrated with a source of small area, will tend to underestimate the total irradiance from a large source [5].

The measurement methods used to assess hazards are also applicable to large radiation sources used for medical treatments and industrial processes (for example, UV therapy cabins for treating a patient's entire skin surface or paint-curing booths for large engineering assemblies). It is usually sufficient to place the calibrated meter sensor (or spectroradiometer input optics) in the radiation field at the location or in the plane where the irradiance is to be measured.

However, for multi-source enclosures with distributed sources and reflective backing surfaces, the presence or absence of a large opaque object within the space will change the radiation pattern by obscuring a proportion of the reflected radiation. Irradiance measurements should be made under the same conditions as those for the intentional irradiation (with a patient standing in the cabin or the production assembly in position, in the examples above). If the opaque object is removed, irradiance will increase [6]. Ideally, for phototherapy cabins, a direct measurement should be made with the person making the measurement in the cabin to simulate a patient. Where the direct measurement method is inconvenient or hazardous to an occupant in the enclosure, an indirect measurement of the unoccupied spatial field made under specified conditions is preferable for routine assessments.

A correction factor equal to the ratio of direct and indirect measured values can be applied to the unoccupied cabin measurements to obtain a true body surface irradiance. Adjustment factors have been measured in the range of about 0.7 to 0.9 depending on irradiator geometry and any deviation from the ideal angular response of the sensor(s). The same technique can be applied to other three-dimensional industrial or laboratory radiation enclosures, where occupied/unoccupied ratios depend on the geometry and characteristics of the sources and reflective surfaces inside the enclosure.

An alternative solution is to make a direct occupied cabin measurement, but use a phantom or mannequin to simulate the presence of a patient. Fulljames and Welsh [7] described a simple structure made of cardboard boxes and expanded polystyrene blocks, giving irradiance values agreeing with direct measurements on a volunteer within acceptable limits. A similar phantom could be constructed easily by any clinic wishing to make direct measurements in this manner.

20.6 Evaluation of ultraviolet optical hazards

The problems related to optical radiation measurement arising from the wavelength dependence of the erythema action spectrum for UV on normal human skin have already been alluded to in §20.2. Because this effect is strongly dependent on the wavelength of the radiation causing it, with an energy range of some 10^4 to 1 for similar erythemal effect, it is essential to know not only the amount of energy absorbed in the skin but also the radiation wavelengths. The hazard function for occupational exposure to UV shown in Figure 20.4 was proposed by the American Conference of Governmental Industrial Hygienists (ACGIH), and adopted by the National Radiation Protection Board (NRPB), as a combination of the erythema hazard to skin and the photokeratitis hazard to eyes. It is based on a daily upper limit of 30 J m^{-2} (3 mJ cm^{-2}) exposure over the UV-C and UV-B ranges in a nominal 8-hour working day. The weighting curve data are also given in tabular form, with the acceptable upper limits for daily exposure to wavelengths in the UV-B and UV-C spectrum, in Table 20.2.

Maximum permissible exposures in this band for monochromatic sources can be obtained directly from the table, and for broadband sources of unknown spectral content, the effective irradiance of the broadband radiation, E_{eff}, can be calculated by weighting the spectral irradiance components from the source, $E_s(\lambda)$,

Table 20.2 Maximum permissible occupational exposures to UV-B and UV-C wavelengths for an 8-hour working day

Wavelength (nm)	Max. permissible exposure (mJ cm^{-2})	Spectral weighting function
200	100	0.03
210	40	0.075
220	25	0.12
230	16	0.19
240	10	0.30
250	7.0	0.43
254	6.0	0.50
260	4.6	0.65
270	3.0	2.00
280	3.4	0.88
290	4.7	0.64
300	10	0.30
305	50	0.06
310	200	0.015
315	1000	0.003

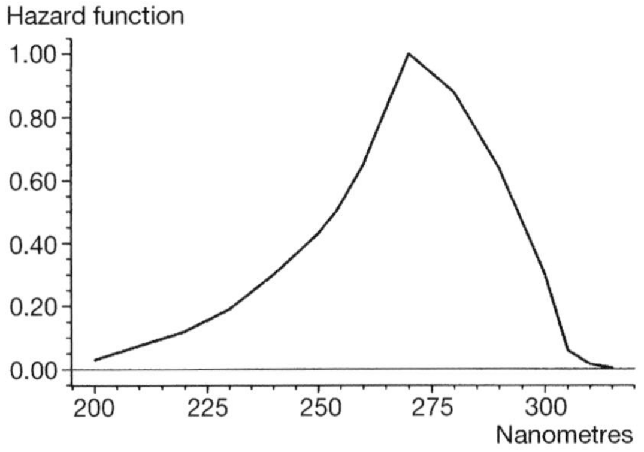

Figure 20.4 Hazard function for occupational exposure to UV-B and UV-C proposed by the ACGIH and adopted by the NRPB.

with the appropriate relative spectral effectiveness factor, $S(\lambda)$, and summing over the band:

$$E_{\text{eff}} = \sum_{200\text{ nm}}^{315\text{ nm}} E_s(\lambda)\, S(\lambda)\, \Delta\lambda \quad \text{W m}^{-2} \qquad (20.2)$$

where $\Delta\lambda$ is the bandwidth of the radiation to which each spectral value is taken to apply, and will depend on the resolution of the spectral measurements taken to calculate the effective irradiance.

The maximum permitted exposure time to this source, $t_{\max}$ – the time for delivery of 30 J m^{-2} of the effective radiation from the source – is given by:

$$t_{\max} = 30/E_{\text{eff}} \text{ seconds.} \qquad (20.3)$$

This simple summation method assumes no interactions between the various wavelengths to which the skin and eyes may be exposed, although it is not clear that this is a valid assumption.

For radiation in the UV-A band on unprotected eyes and skin, the ACGIH exposure standard proposes a limit for long exposure times (greater than 1000 s) of no more than 10 W m^{-2}. For shorter exposure times (< 1000 s) the exposure received should not exceed 10 000 J m^{-2}, equivalent to an irradiance of 10 W m^{-2} uniformly received over 1000 s.

To put UV hazards into perspective, it is useful to compare the risks from artificial sources with the natural risk from the Sun. The spectral plot in Figure 20.5 is of solar radiation on a clear cloudless July day in Gloucester, UK. The spectroradiometer detector was mounted facing vertically upwards, on a level surface outdoors, a few hundred feet above sea level. The absorption lines in the otherwise smooth spectrum are due to atmospheric water vapour and gas molecules. The absence of radiation shorter than about 300 nm is probably due to pollution and dust particles in the city environment (the hospital laboratory is within 200 m of the main railway station). The irradiance in the UV-A band is about 50 W m^{-2} and in the UV-B band about 5 W m^{-2}. Solar radiation nearer the equator rises in intensity as the Sun is higher in the sky and the thickness of atmosphere traversed decreases. Solar radiation away from polluted urban areas includes more of the shorter wavelengths.

Compare these figures with typical irradiances in UV treatment cabins of about 100 W m^{-2} UV-A and about 50 W m^{-2} UV-B. Cosmetic sunbeds, emitting mostly UV-A, have similar irradiances to therapy cabins. The difference in the hazards arises largely from the different exposure times and the cumulative doses. A therapeutic treatment course for a skin disorder may be of the order of 500 to 1000 J m^{-2}, given over 3 or 4 months. Intensive use of a cosmetic sunbed or a Mediterranean summer holiday may accumulate a similar dose in 2 weeks. Outdoor

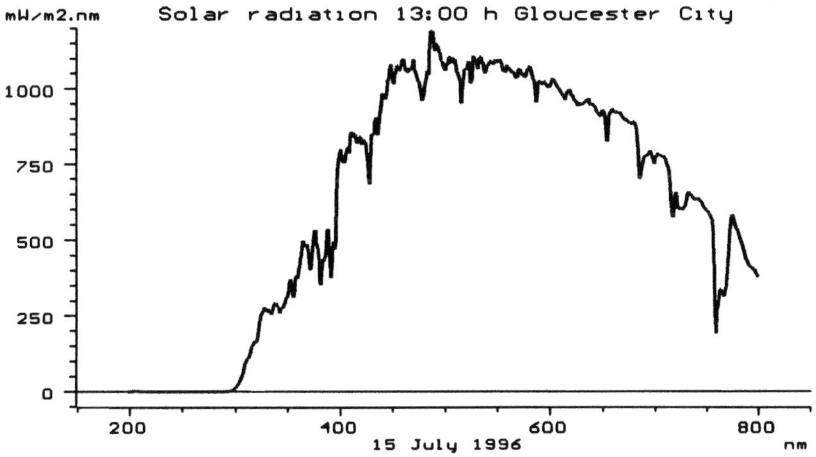

Figure 20.5 Terrestrial solar radiation spectrum.

workers may accumulate considerably more than this every year of their working lives, but indoor workers are usually well protected from solar UV.

Most adults are aware of the risks from solar and artificial UV, as a result of publicity campaigns in the press and on TV. People living in sunny climates are particularly at risk if their skin type is not similar to that of the indigenous population. For example, white ex-European Australians are at much greater risk than the Aboriginal population, whose almost black skin has adapted over millennia. There is, nevertheless, a persistent view that tanned skin is 'healthy' or 'attractive.' Government advice in the UK [8] is that cosmetic tanning is to be discouraged, that a tan is evidence of skin damage, and that there is no safe dose of UV.

20.7 Evaluation of visible radiation optical hazards

Similar methods are used for visible radiation as for UV. Simple photometer measurements are inadequate to characterize the hazard because of the strong wavelength dependency, as in the UV spectrum. The visible light hazard function curve, plotted in Figure 20.6, shows only the most hazardous part in the blue visible region. The ACGIH hazard is defined over the range 400 to 1400 nm (well into the infrared region) but the hazard is insignificant beyond 600 nm (see Table 20.3).

As for UV, there is no universally accepted standard for visible and near-infrared radiation hazard, but the ACGIH proposed and have subsequently revised occupational exposure limits based on the known effects of thermal and photochemical damage [9]. The International Commission on Non-Ionising Radiation Protection (ICNIRP) have published guidelines on exposure limits for visible and IR non-coherent radiations [10] and have also issued a statement on hazard assessment for LEDs and diode lasers [11]. LEDs have become more hazardous as technology has advanced and source sizes have diminished. Some types of LEDs emitting incoherent radiation have such small source dimensions that they share many of the hazards previously associated mostly with lasers, being able to concentrate high energy densities on the retina, and have been considered separately from other conventional light sources in safety standards [12].

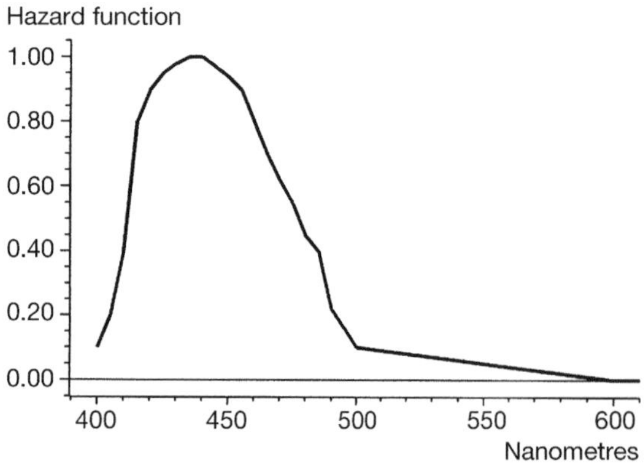

Figure 20.6 Blue-light hazard function proposed by the ACGIH.

Table 20.3 Spectral weighting functions for assessing retinal risk from broadband visible/IR radiation sources by ACGIH (1981, rev. 1999) [9]

Wavelength (nm)	Blue-light hazard function, B_λ	Thermal hazard function, R_λ
400	0.10	1.0
405	0.20	2.0
410	0.40	4.0
415	0.80	8.0
420	0.90	9.0
425	0.95	9.5
430	0.98	9.8
435	1.00	10.0
440	1.00	10.0
445	0.97	9.7
450	0.94	9.4
455	0.90	9.0
460	0.80	8.0
465	0.70	7.0
470	0.62	6.2
475	0.55	5.5
480	0.45	4.5
485	0.40	4.0
490	0.22	2.2
495	0.16	1.6
500–600	$10^{[(450-\lambda)/50]}$	1.0
600–700	0.001	1.0
700–1049	0.001	$10^{[(700-\lambda)/50]}$
1050–1400	0.001	0.2

The hazard assessment is complicated by the optical properties of the eye, which focuses incoming radiation as a small image on the retina. The hazard is thus dependent on the size of the radiation source and the diameter of the pupil of the eye, which influence the size and hence the power density of the source image on the retina. For optical hazards from extended sources, it is common to express radiation powers in units of radiance, or power density, in W m^{-2} sr^{-1}, so that the total energy entering the eye is defined by the diameter of the iris aperture.

20.7.1 Thermal effects

The calculation of risk to the retina from the thermal effects of optical radiation involves the calculation of weighted contributions to an overall radiance L_{haz} (Box 20.1) defined as:

$$L_{haz} = \sum_{400\ nm}^{1400\ nm} L_\lambda R_\lambda \Delta\lambda \quad W\ m^{-2}\ sr^{-1} \qquad (20.4)$$

where L_λ is the spectral radiance of the source, R_λ is the spectral thermal hazard function (shown in Table 20.4), and $\Delta\lambda$ is the width of the spectral measurements, depending on the resolution of the measuring device, with summation taken over the interval of 400 to 1400 nm.

For exposures within the range of 1 ms up to 10 s, the duration should not exceed a time t_{max} given by

$$t_{max} = 1/(L_{haz}\ \alpha)^2 \quad \text{seconds} \qquad (20.5)$$

where α is the angle in radians subtended at the eye by the source. This equation is empirical and not dimensionally consistent, but is an acceptable approximation for hazard assessments.

20.7.2 Photochemical effects

The photochemical hazard is calculated in a similar manner, with upper limits set for hazard-weighted radiance values. For short exposures of less than 10 000 s, the maximum radiant dose is calculated as:

$$D_{max} = \sum_{400\ nm}^{1400\ nm} L_\lambda B_\lambda t\ \Delta\lambda \quad J\ m^{-2}\ sr^{-1} \qquad (20.6)$$

where t is in seconds, placing an upper limit on this value of no more than 10^6 J m^{-2} sr^{-1}.

For exposures longer than 10 000 s, the exposure is limited through setting an upper value for the radiance as:

$$R_{max} = \sum_{400\ nm}^{1400\ nm} L_\lambda B_\lambda \Delta\lambda \quad W\ m^{-2}\ sr^{-1} \qquad (20.7)$$

In both of these expressions, the blue-light hazard function B_λ is given in Table 20.3. The calculations assume extended radiation sources, subtending solid angles of greater than 11 mrad at the eye, and a normally constricted pupil of diameter 3 mm. This may not apply to unconscious persons (undergoing surgery, for example) or the very young, whose normal eye reflexes are not fully developed. Those particularly at risk in operating theatres or receiving blue-light therapy for neonatal hyperbilirubinaemia, for example, must be given special consideration, and their eyes should be protected securely against inadvertent exposure.

20.7.3 Retinal irradiance

Retinal irradiance can be derived from a knowledge of the source brightness or radiance (Box 20.1) and the optical parameters of the human eye. The retinal irradiance E_r is given by:

$$E_r = \pi\ L_s\ \tau_{ocul}\ d_e^2/4f^2 \quad W\ m^{-2} \qquad (20.8)$$

where L_s is the source radiance, τ_{ocul} is the transmittance of the ocular media (up to 0.9 or 90% for healthy eyes), d_e is the diameter of the pupil, and f is the focal length of the cornea/lens combination. This equation is empirical and not dimensionally consistent, but is adequate for calculating irradiance values for hazard assessments. Assuming values of 17 mm for the focal length, a transmittance factor of 0.9, and a worst-case pupil diameter of 7 mm, this reduces to:

$$E_r = 0.12\ L_s \quad W\ m^{-2}. \qquad (20.9)$$

20.7.4 Hypersensitivity

All of the above assumes normal human skin and eyes, and takes no account of the possibility of hypersensitivity to radiation arising from photosensitizers ingested or applied topically to skin. Many substances have this effect, notably psoralens and photosensitizers such as δ-aminolevulinic acid (ALA) used in photodynamic therapy (PDT) to photosensitize a patient's tissues. Patients having these agents administered may be considerably more at risk from radiation hazards in the visible and UV bands, and special precautions must be taken to protect them, over and above the occupational limits described above.

Other photosensitizers can be found in cosmetics, perfumes, soaps, and several classes of drugs commonly prescribed to patients (including antibiotics, beta-blockers and non-steroidal anti-inflammatory drugs) are known to exhibit phototoxicity (the property of increasing sensitivity to visible and/or UV radiation) [13]. Patients undergoing phototherapy or PDT must be warned against using any of the known phototoxic substances, and all medications and preparations taken by the patient should be checked with the hospital pharmacy before treatment is given, to avoid possible damage to skin or eyes arising from hyper-photosensitivity.

20.8 Practical radiation protection considerations

20.8.1 Exposed groups

The hazards arising from the use of UV, visible, and IR radiations in the workplace apply to three possible groups of persons:

(1) those for whom an exposure is prescribed by a physician;

(2) laboratory, factory, or clinical personnel employed to operate radiation equipment;

(3) others in the vicinity but uninvolved with the exposure.

Hospital patients will receive a large dose of UV during their treatment series, but may evade artificial UV for months or years before requiring further treatment. These persons are explicitly excluded from the guidelines on exposure limitation, since the radiation is presumed to give benefits outweighing the risks.

Factory, laboratory, and clinical staff, however, may receive only modest doses on a daily basis, but could receive this exposure over much of their working lives, accumulating very large doses. Other persons nearby or passing through, including other workers, maintenance engineers, cleaners, visitors, and members of the public have the right to be protected from any unnecessary radiation exposure. Employers are required by law to minimize the risks from radiation hazards and to provide suitable protection for employees.

Those who elect to expose their skin to artificial and natural UV for cosmetic reasons are not included in these categories relating to the workplace, but should be informed of:

- the risks involved and of the possible consequences of their actions
- precautions they should take (protective eyewear and limitation of exposure).

Operators of establishments using UV or other sources of optical radiation, including cosmetic tanning facilities accessible to the general public, should carry out risk assessments to identify potential hazards to staff and customers from any foreseeable practice or incident, and take action to minimize the risks.

20.8.2 UV protection

For the most part, UV protection is common sense, simple to achieve and equally simple to overlook, wherein lies perhaps the greatest hazard. It is also difficult to separate occupational or clinical exposure from that received from the Sun, making it difficult to ensure that no unwanted outcomes result from the use of UV. The professional and responsible attitude is to take steps to reduce unnecessary UV exposure to the lowest possible level, and to ensure that necessary exposure (for treatment of patients' skin, for example) is always the least possible consistent with the desired clinical outcome.

There is no formal legislation on UV protection, but radiation physicists may find it useful to start with the regulations applying to ionising radiations and to relax them to some degree to suit the degree of risk and the circumstances. In clinical and industrial situations, for example, it is useful to designate a radiation controlled area, with local rules, under the control of a responsible person (such as a senior nurse, engineer, or manager). These local rules may include statements indicating

- the persons who may be present during operation of UV-emitting equipment
- the persons authorized to operate the equipment
- any protection measures that must be adopted by persons present in the controlled area.

During test or calibration procedures, others who may enter the controlled area during exposures should be warned of the presence of a hazard. Suitable eye-protection warning signs can be made or obtained from commercial sign-makers to serve as temporary or permanent warning signs outside controlled areas. Optical radiation is very easy to block, by using screens, curtains, or just by closing doors and access panels. Persons operating the equipment should employ such protective measures wherever possible. When designing or advising on the layout of a laboratory or clinic environment, it may be necessary to consider how UV-emitting equipment can be isolated from occupants of the room, by the fitting of partitions or curtains, for example. In a hospital, curtains or screens are necessary for patient privacy, and these are usually adequate for UV screening as well.

Clinic curtains are most practical when suspended from rails mounted about 2 m from floor level and hanging free of the floor by about 0.3 m. This ensures circulation of air for cooling and avoids accumulation of dirt on the curtain hem. Any partition or curtain must be compliant with the local regulations for fire prevention or evacuation of the premises, and the advice of the local fire officer or risk manager sought in any difficult cases.

Although the visible blue light emitted by UV lamps is readily reflected from decorative surfaces, UV does not reflect well from normal paint and fabric finishes, so that it is unnecessary to adopt black-out blinds or use oppressive and dark colour schemes. Operators of UV equipment are more likely to receive a higher UV dose during a working day from proximity to windows receiving sunlight.

The safest location for operators of hazardous equipment is out of the room completely, and this is to be preferred for high-powered UV-B, UV-C, and blue visible emitting equipment. This may not be practical in a clinic, for example, where contact with and supervision of patients is essential for safety. Where isolation is impractical, the staff who must remain in the same room should be protected as far as possible by screens and curtains or protective clothing. In this respect, enclosed equipment is always to be preferred over open sources. Similarly, enclosed treatment cabins for dermatology treatments are to be preferred over open lamps or columns of lamps that irradiate the whole of the space in front of them.

The UV hazard associated with the use in hospitals of canopy-type irradiation equipment is similar to that of other open irradiator devices, but the additional hazard arising from the suspension of mains-powered electrical equipment, with unprotected fragile hot glass lamps, over a patient's unclothed body should also be considered. The failure of the suspension mechanism of the canopy could result in severe injury from broken glass and electric shock to the patient from the exposed live conductors, not to mention the psychological effect on the patient unfortunate enough to be under the device at the time. The cost of litigation is likely to be far in excess of the cost of replacing obsolete devices of this type.

20.9 Protecting skin against optical radiations

After reducing the environmental radiation hazard to minimal levels, it will still be necessary to adopt protective measures for employees who operate potentially hazardous radiation equipment. Skin protection is easy to achieve with normal everyday clothing. The degree of protection depends upon the type of fibre and the weave of the cloth. Colour is not important for UV protection, but darker clothes reduce the transmission of visible wavelengths. The density and weave of the cloth are much more important, so that heavy cotton and closely woven fabrics (such as denim) are much more effective than man-made fibres in lightweight summer clothing.

Various clothing fabrics were examined by Robson and Diffey [14] for their ability to suppress solar UV irradiance on the skin. This information may be of value to persons with photosensitive diseases of the skin or to those who have been deliberately photosensitized for medical treatment purposes, such as PUVA therapy or photodynamic therapy. Any areas of skin that are not clothed but need to be protected against UV may be adequately protected with cosmetic sunblock preparations available from retail pharmacists. This is not totally reliable, however, as many sunscreens are relatively ineffective at reducing the longer wavelengths in the UV-A band, and it is always preferable to use a physical barrier whose presence is clearly visible.

Many fabrics become almost transparent to shortwave IR, and provide little protection against intense heat. Properly designed metallized suits and visors are essential if resistance to intense heat or fire is necessary.

20.10 Protecting eyes against UV

Eyes are readily protected from solar and artificial UV with approved protective spectacles and goggles (clear or tinted) designed for this purpose. Some are constructed to wrap around the face to reduce entry of UV at the edges. Others are constructed with removable side-screens, though these may be made of a different plastic with less effective UV suppression.

Dermatology patients form a large proportion of those needing UV protection for the eyes, and need to protect their eyes from UV-A as well as UV-B for up to 24 hours after ingesting psoralens. These are potent plant-derived photosensitizing chemicals used to treat various skin disorders such as psoriasis and eczema in combination with UV-A, which activates the chemical in living skin cells to form excited singlet-state oxygen. In summer, PUVA patients may choose to wear UV-protective sunglasses or one of the specially designed UV-blocking visors or goggles, but in winter, it is safer to use clear (not tinted) eye protection. Moseley *et al.* [15] examined various tinted and clear spectacles for UV-A suppression and proposed transmission criteria for adequate protection. Note that eye protection meeting EN 166 for protection against impact from flying debris is almost always made of polycarbonate plastic. This is chosen for its strength and ability to withstand shock, and is also almost perfect at suppressing UV down to 400 nm but transmits visible light, and is therefore ideal for clear lens UV-suppressing spectacle construction. Polycarbonate-lensed spectacles and visors are readily available from protective clothing suppliers, and are reasonably priced.

Many patients find standard-issue UV-protective goggles and glasses are cosmetically unacceptable, and would prefer to continue to wear their prescription lenses or corneal contact lenses. Prescription lenses made of CR39 plastic (almost all lenses of current manufacture) may be treated with chemical solutions to coat the surface and provide UV suppression down to 400 nm. Several manufacturers offer this process, which involves removal of the lenses from the frame and immersion in hot chemical solutions. It is usually effective, provided the process is carried out correctly with fresh solutions. If the lenses are not made of CR39 plastic or they have been previously coated with tints or other processes, the UV-coating process may not be effective. Patients' lenses should always be tested for negligible (less than about 2% total) UV-A transmission (with a hand-held radiometer and UV-A source) before the patient is permitted to use them outside the dermatology clinic.

In view of the rising popularity of corneal contact lenses, Anstey *et al.* [16] examined samples of nine contact lenses, whose manufacturers claimed some UV suppression, to test their suitability for protecting PUVA patients' eyes. Seven samples of lenses without such

Table 20.4 Transmission limits (%) of protective spectacles for use by PUVA patients, compared with three UV-suppressing contact lens samples; data from Moseley and Jones [17] and Anstey *et al.* [16]

Wavelength	Arbitrary limit	Lens A	Lens B	Lens C
390 nm	10	52	47	32
380 nm	5	4.4	21	10
370 nm	2	< 0.5	9.6	1.6
< 360 nm	1	< 0.5	12.6	6.4

claims were also examined as a control. The transmission factors at various UV wavelengths were determined using a stabilized broadband UV/visible lamp and a spectroradiometer, and the transmission limits [15] used as the arbitrary standard for suitability. These limits and the transmission factors for the three best-performing lenses are shown in Table 20.4. They all failed to match the performance of polycarbonate lenses and visors and the criteria set by Moseley and Jones [17], as coated prescription lenses have relatively poor suppression between 380 and 400 nm. This is not the peak region for psoralen activation, however, and it could be regarded as less critical than the shorter wavelengths, which are well suppressed. Moreover, contact lenses completely cover the cornea and, if worn throughout the normal waking day, will provide eye protection throughout daylight hours. Since spectacles can be easily taken off inadvertently or deliberately, and UV radiation can enter the eye around the edge of the frame, it could be argued that the total cover of the cornea and the continuous protection compensate for the inferior UV-suppression characteristics.

The authors concluded that adequate UV protection could probably be achieved by adjustment of the polymer and additives but that the end-product might not be economically viable. Until suitable materials have been made into lenses and shown to perform satisfactorily, it is safer to advise PUVA patients to continue to use clear polycarbonate protective glasses or polarizing sunglasses for the 24 hours following ingestion of psoralens. Others exposed to occupational UV (not photosensitized with psoralen) could, however, benefit from choosing UV-protective contact lenses to ensure optimum protection of the eyes from UV.

Where conventional spectacles or face visors are impracticable, it is possible to fabricate custom protective devices from UV-suppressing films used commercially against solar UV to protect valuable or historic items. Dawe *et al.* [18] described simple disposable face and eye shields made from such materials, requiring only scissors and moderate dexterity to make to measure.

20.11 References

1 Commission Internationale de l' Éclairage (1987). *International lighting vocabulary* (4th edn). CIE Publication No. 17.4 (E-1.1), Vienna.

2 Everett, M. A., Olson, R. L., and Sayre, R. M. (1965). Ultraviolet erythema. *Arch. Dermatol.*, **92**, 713–19.

3 Pye, S. D. and Martin, C. J. (2000). A study of the directional response of ultraviolet radiometers. I. Practical evaluation and implications for ultraviolet measurement standards. *Phys. Med. Biol.*, **45**, 2701–12.

4 Commission Internationale de l' Éclairage (1987). *Methods of characterizing illuminance meters and luminance meters: performance, characteristics and specifications.* CIE Publication No. 69, Vienna.

5 Martin, C. J. and Pye, S. D. (2000). A study of the directional response of ultraviolet radiometers. II. Implications for ultraviolet phototherapy derived from computer simulations *Phys. Med. Biol.*, **45**, 2713–29.

6 Moseley, H. (2001). *Scottish UV dosimetry guidelines. Photodermatology, Photoimmunology and Photomedicine, 17, 230–3.*

7 Fulljames, C. A. and Welsh, A. D. (2000). Measurement of patient dose in ultraviolet therapy using a phantom. *Br. J. Dermatol.*, **142**, 748–51.

8 Health and Safety Executive (1997). *Controlling health risks from the use of UV tanning equipment.* Guidance note IND(G) 209. HSE, London.

9 American Conference of Governmental Industrial Hygienists (1999). *Threshold limit values for chemical substances and physical agents and biological exposure indices.* ACGIH, Cincinnati, Ohio.

10 International Commission on Non-Ionising Radiation Protection (1997). Guidelines on limits of exposure to broad-band incoherent optical radiation (0.38 to 3 μm). *Health Phys.*, **73**, 539–54.

11 International Commission on Non-Ionising Radiation Protection (2000). Statement on light-emitting diodes and laser diodes: implication for hazard assessment. *Health Phys.*, **78**, 744–52.

12 Commission Internationale de l' Éclairage (1999). *Photobiological safety standards for lamps.* CIE 134-3-99, Report of TC 6-38.

13 Allen, J. E. (1993). Drug-induced photosensitivity. *Clin. Pharm.*, **12**, 580–7.

14 Robson, J. and Diffey, B. L. (1990). Textiles and sun protection. *Photodermatol. Photoimmunol. Photomed.*, **7**, 32–4.

15 Moseley, H., Cox, N. H., and MacKie, R. M. (1988). The suitability of sunglasses used by patients following ingestion of psoralen. *Br. J. Dermatol.*, **118**, 247–53.

16 Anstey, A. V., Taylor, D. K., Chalmers, I., and Ansari, E. (1999). Ultraviolet radiation blocking characteristics of contact lenses: relevance to eye protection for psoralen-sensitised patients. *Photodermatol. Photoimmunol. Photomed.*, **15**, 193–7.

17 Moseley, H. and Jones, S. K. (1990). Clear ultraviolet blocking lenses for use by PUVA patients. *Br. J. Dermatol.*, **123**, 775–81.

18 Dawe, R., Russell, S., and Ferguson, J. (1996). Borrowing from museums and industry: two photoprotective devices. *Br. J. Dermatol.*, **135**, 1016–17.

20.12 Further reading

Detailed accounts of the biological effects of UV and visible radiations, with particular emphasis on the uses of these radiations for various medical interventions and the consequences to human health arising from exposure to environmental and artificial sources, can be found in the following monographs:

Diffey, B. L. (1982). *Ultraviolet radiation in medicine.* Medical Physics Handbooks Series No. 11. Adam Hilger.

Diffey, B. L. and Hart, G. (1997). *Ultraviolet and blue light phototherapy –principles, sources, dosimetry and safety.* Institute of Physics and Engineering in Medicine, York.

Diffey, B. L. and Langley, F. C. (1986). *Evaluation of UV radiation hazards in hospitals.* Report 49. IPSM (now IPEM), York.

Moseley, H. (1986). *Non-ionising radiation.* Medical Physics Handbooks Series No. 18. Adam Hilger.

Parrish, J. A., Anderson, R. R., Urbach, F., and Pitts, D. (1978). *UV-A – biological effects of ultraviolet radiation with emphasis on human responses to longwave ultraviolet.* Wiley.

Chapter 21
Electromagnetic fields

J. W. Hand

21.1 Introduction

This chapter discusses aspects of radiation protection for non-ionising electromagnetic (EM) fields such as microwaves (MW), radiofrequency (RF) fields, and extremely low-frequency (ELF) electric and magnetic fields. The terms 'ELF' and 'radiofrequency' are often used in the biological effects and occupational health literature to cover the ranges from above static fields (> 0 Hz) to 3 kHz and from 3 kHz to 300 GHz, respectively.

EM fields are ubiquitous in today's environment and their sources are predominantly man-made, being inherent to communications, power, and other needs of modern society. In addition to these widespread uses, in the hospital environment EM fields are crucial to diagnosis by magnetic resonance and to various therapeutic treatments. The proliferation of RF devices has been accompanied by increased concern about ensuring the safety of their use. Throughout the world many organizations have established EM safety standards or guidelines for exposure.

When dealing with EM fields the following points should be borne in mind:

- Photon energies are insufficient to cause ionisation.
- Traditionally, the consensus of scientific opinion is that interactions with the human body are considered to be thermal, although there have been claims for other mechanisms of interaction, particularly for low-level ELF fields.
- The energy absorbed is directly related to EM fields *inside* the body and *not* those incident upon the body. These can be quite different, depending on the size and shape of the body, its electrical properties, its orientation with respect to the incident EM fields, and the frequency of the incident fields.
- Direct measurement of the incident fields is easier and more practical than measurement of the internal fields, especially in people, and so dosimetry is used to relate the internal fields to the incident fields.
- RF radiation at high power levels can be harmful because of its ability to heat biological tissue. Areas of the body that are poorly perfused (e.g. the eyes and the testes) are susceptible because of their inability to dissipate an abnormal thermal load.
- There are other effects that, although not resulting in an overall change in tissue temperature, nevertheless have a thermal basis. One example is the 'microwave auditory effect' in which, under certain specific conditions of frequency, signal modulation, and intensity, animals and humans can perceive the RF/MW signal as a buzzing or clicking sound [1]. Although a number of theories have been advanced to explain this effect, the most widely accepted explanation is that absorption of energy from the microwave field leads to a thermoelastic interaction in the auditory cortex of the brain.

The evidence for production of harmful biological effects following exposure to RF radiation at field intensities lower than those that would produce significant and measurable heating is less clear. 'Non-thermal' effects reported have included changes in the immune system, neurological effects, behavioural effects, evidence for a link between microwave exposure and the action of certain drugs and compounds, and a 'calcium efflux' effect in brain tissue [1]. There are experimental results that suggest ELF fields and microwaves might be involved in cancer promotion under certain conditions. However, contradictory experimental results have also been reported in many of these cases, and further experiments are needed to determine the generality of these effects and whether 'non-thermal' mechanisms exist that could cause harmful biological effects in animals and humans exposed to EM radiation.

Several scientific bodies have reviewed the present state of knowledge regarding untoward effects of low-level EM fields and radiation. The International Commission on Non-Ionising Radiation Protection (ICNIRP) [2], in summarizing biological effects and epidemiological studies (frequencies up to 100 kHz), concluded:

there is currently no convincing evidence for carcinogenic effects and these (experimental) data cannot be used as a basis for developing exposure guidelines.

In the absence of support from laboratory studies, the epidemiological data are insufficient to allow an exposure guideline to be established.

In the case of studies involving higher frequencies (100 kHz to 300 GHz), the ICNIRP [2] concluded:

Epidemiological studies on exposed workers and the general public have shown no major health effects associated with typical exposure environments. Although there are deficiencies in the epidemiological work, such as poor exposure assessment, the studies have yielded no convincing evidence that typical exposure levels lead to adverse reproductive outcomes or an increased cancer risk in exposed individuals.

In general, the effects of exposure of biological systems to athermal levels of amplitude-modulated electromagnetic fields are small and are very difficult to relate to potential health effects.

Recently, a working group under the auspices of the National Institute of Environmental Health Sciences (NIEHS) [3] reported that there was limited evidence (a positive association for which a causal interpretation is credible, but chance, bias, or confounding factors cannot be ruled out with reasonable confidence) that residential exposure to ELF magnetic fields is carcinogenic to children and to adults. This statement was based on results of studies on childhood leukaemia in residential environments and on studies on chronic lymphocytic leukaemia in adults in occupational settings. Overall, however, NIEHS summarized the outcome of the research it supported as follows:

Box 21.1 Basic characteristics of an electromagnetic field

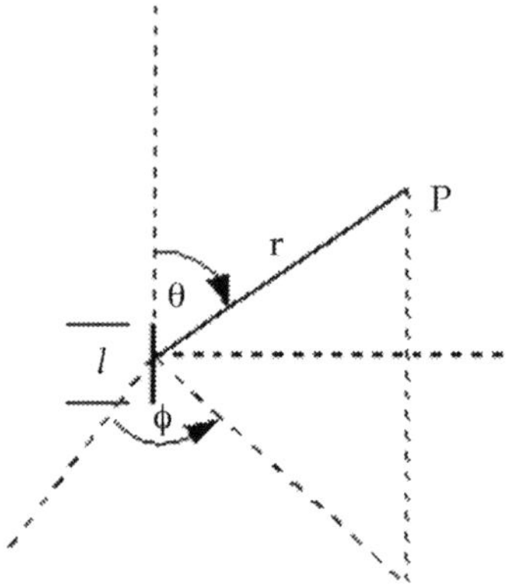

Figure 21.1 Coordinate system relating a field point P to a dipole of length *l*.

Several important points regarding the measurement and monitoring of EM fields may be identified by considering the nature of the fields from a simple source—a small dipole antenna (see Figure 21.1). In a lossless medium, the electric (E) and magnetic (M) fields associated with a dipole of length l (assumed small compared with the wavelength λ) supporting an oscillating current I at angular frequency ω are:

$$E_\theta = \frac{Il}{4\pi} sin\theta \left[\frac{j\omega\mu}{r} + \frac{1}{r^2}\sqrt{\frac{\mu}{\varepsilon}} + \frac{1}{j\omega\varepsilon r^3} \right] e^{-j\beta r} \tag{21.2}$$

$$E_r = \frac{Il}{4\pi} cos\theta \left[\frac{2}{r^2}\sqrt{\frac{\mu}{\varepsilon}} + \frac{2}{j\omega\varepsilon r^3} \right] e^{-j\beta r} \tag{21.3}$$

$$H_\phi = \frac{Il}{4\pi} sin\theta \left[\frac{j\beta}{r} + \frac{1}{r^2} \right] e^{-j\beta r} \tag{21.4}$$

where $\beta = \omega\sqrt{\mu\varepsilon}$ is the phase constant (imaginary part of the propagation constant) and μ and ε are respectively the permeability and permittivity. $\sqrt{\mu/\varepsilon} = \eta$, the intrinsic wave impedance of the medium (= $120\pi\ \Omega$ in the case of free space).

The results of the research supported by this program provide substantial evidence that there is not a robust biological effect of EM field exposure at environmentally relevant levels. These data when taken together with the National Academy of Sciences [4] report provide a basis for concluding that environmental EM field exposures at the levels to which human exposure occurs in the environment do not demonstrate an effect on critical biological processes and functions that could be expected to adversely affect human health.

Other official bodies charged with the task of reviewing the scientific evidence for potential health hazards of low-level EM fields have come to similar conclusions [5, 6]. Detailed discussions of this and related topics are to be found in several review papers [7, 8].

This chapter begins with a discussion of the characteristics of a simple EM field, leading to identification of those parameters useful for safety assessment. Having discussed which parameters should be measured, the question of how to measure them is addressed in a discussion relating to instrumentation. The concepts of dosimetry are introduced and several examples of general EM safety guidelines and standards are outlined. Topics directly relevant to clinical procedures such as magnetic resonance and thermal therapy are discussed, and the chapter closes with a consideration of interference with electromedical equipment from EM fields.

21.2 EM fields and sources

21.2.1 Characteristics of EM fields

Excellent discussions of the fundamentals of electromagnetic theory may be found in several texts [9, 10]. Only a cursory summary of the characteristics of EM fields is given here (see also Box 21.1):

Box 21.1 *(continued)*

- At large distances from the dipole ($r >> l$) the $1/r$ terms in equations (21.2)–(21.4) dominate. In this 'far-field' region
  - the field components correspond to outgoing spherical waves and these radiation fields represent propagation of energy away from the dipole
  - the approximation that wave fronts are planar is often made
  - $E_\theta / H_\phi = \eta$ and the fields are mutually orthogonal
  - the instantaneous power density is given by the Poynting vector

$$\boldsymbol{S} = \boldsymbol{E} \times \boldsymbol{H} \tag{21.5}$$

  - assuming plane waves, the average power density, given by the real part of the time-averaged Poynting vector—Re ($\frac{1}{2}$ $\boldsymbol{E}$ x $\boldsymbol{H}^*$) for sinusoidal waveforms ($\boldsymbol{H}^*$ is the complex conjugate of **H**), is given by

$$S = \frac{1}{2}\frac{E_0^2}{377} = \frac{1}{2} \cdot 377\, H_0^2$$

  where E_o, H_o are the peak values of the E and H fields.
- At points close to the dipole ($r << l$), the $1/r^3$ terms dominate and this region is known as the reactive part of the near field. In this region
  - H_ϕ is very nearly in phase with the current in the dipole and is similar to the induction field obtained from Ampère's law
  - the electric field is that associated with an electrostatic dipole.
- The region at intermediate distances from the dipole, where r is comparable with l, and the $1/r^2$ and $1/r$ terms in equations (21.2)–(21.4) become more pronounced, is often called the intermediate near field.

There is no constant relationship between E and H in the near field and the time-averaged Poynting vector is zero.

A commonly used definition for the near-field/far-field boundary is that it occurs at a distance of $2l^2/\lambda$ from the source. However, for the purpose of measurements, the region in which the power density decreases inversely as the square of the distance from the source is relevant and this may occur significantly closer to the antenna than $2l^2/\lambda$. For practical purposes the reactive near field may be assumed to be within a distance $\lambda/2$ of the source while an approximate guide regarding the far field is to assume that these conditions are present at distances greater than λ.

- Electric charge is a fundamental physical quantity and occurs in both positive and negative forms.
- A force exists between two charges which is proportional to the product of the charges, inversely proportional to the square of their separation and directed along the line joining them.
- The electric field E at some point in the vicinity of a charge or distribution of charges is defined in terms of this force, being the force per unit charge at that point.
- Magnetic fields are associated with moving charges. In addition to the electrostatic force, there is a force $\boldsymbol{F}_{\mathrm{m}}$ exerted on a moving charge which is dependent upon the velocity $\boldsymbol{v}$ of the moving charge q and a vector field quantity known as the magnetic flux density $\boldsymbol{B}$ defined by:

$$\boldsymbol{F}_{\mathrm{m}} = \mathrm{q}\ (\boldsymbol{v} \times \boldsymbol{B}). \quad (21.1)$$

- The vector product in equation (21.1) implies that $\boldsymbol{F}_{\mathrm{m}}$ is orthogonal to both $\boldsymbol{v}$ and $\boldsymbol{B}$. The magnitude of B is F_{m}/qv.
- The magnetic field intensity $\boldsymbol{H}$ is related to $\boldsymbol{B}$ through $\boldsymbol{H} = \boldsymbol{B}/\mu$, where μ is the permeability of the medium in which the fields are present. In general, the permeability of biological tissues may be assumed to be equal to that of free space, $\mu_o = 4\pi \times 10^{-7}$ H m^{-1}.

Static $\boldsymbol{E}$ and $\boldsymbol{B}$ fields can be treated independently but time-dependent $\boldsymbol{E}$ and $\boldsymbol{B}$ fields are related to each other and to their sources, charge and current density, respectively, as described in the set of equations known as Maxwell's equations. Only if the rate of change of field with time is sufficiently low may time-varying E and B fields be considered separately (so-called quasi-static approximation).

21.2.2 Characteristics of EM sources

It is important to know the characteristics of the source of the electromagnetic field when attempting to measure field parameters. These characteristics include:

- source dimensions—determine whether the measurement will be made under near-field or far-field conditions
- the range of frequencies in which power may be present
- the polarization of the field:
  - in the far field of a single source, only one polarization, which may be linear, elliptical, or circular, will be present over a broad area
  - in the near field, any one of the above polarizations may exist at any given point and the polarization may change with small changes in location.

It is important to measure both E and H fields close to an RF or microwave antenna or source because:

- the field structure may be highly inhomogeneous
- there may be considerable variation in the wave impedance $\eta(= E/H)$, the value of which may range from a few Ω to 1000s Ω
- there can be considerable spatial variations of E and H in regions out of the reactive part of the near field but still within the intermediate near field
- although the near field components do not contribute to the radiated energy, they may interact strongly with bodies located within the near-field regions, leading to energy deposition within those bodies.

21.3 Interaction between EM fields and biological materials

The interaction between $\boldsymbol{E}$ and $\boldsymbol{B}$ fields and materials in general may be considered in terms of:

- a drift of the free conduction charges in the material that results from their motion due to the superimposition of electric field forces on their random thermal motion. This conduction current is $\sigma\boldsymbol{E}$
- dielectric polarization due to
  - slight displacement of molecular positive and negative charges from their equilibrium positions due to the applied $\boldsymbol{E}$ field, resulting in a polarization charge and new fields.
  - alignment of polar molecules possessing permanent electric dipoles (e.g. water, proteins) with the applied $\boldsymbol{E}$ field which depends upon the strength of the field and is opposed by the random thermal motion of the molecules and mutual interactions between them.

Both polarization effects and conduction charge effects are accounted for by the complex permittivity ε of the material which is defined by

$$\varepsilon = \varepsilon_0\ (\varepsilon' - j\varepsilon'') \quad (21.7)$$

where ε' is known as the relative permittivity or sometimes the dielectric constant and ε'' is often known as the loss factor. The additional polarization charge is accounted for by ε', while ε'' is a measure of how much power is absorbed from the electric field, taking into account the effects of the free charges and friction associated with the changing polarization.

Magnetization, which involves the alignment of magnetic dipoles in a material in opposition to their random thermal motion, is insignificant in biological materials.

The term 'lossy' is applied to materials that absorb significant power. A related parameter is the loss tangent which is defined as $\tan\delta = \varepsilon''/\varepsilon'$.

The relationship between the ε'', σ, and Ω, the angular frequency of the field, is

$$\varepsilon'' = \sigma/\omega\,\varepsilon_o. \qquad (21.8)$$

The conductivity σ arises predominantly from mobile charges but also has a frequency-dependent part arising from dielectric polarization. Both ε' and ε'' of tissues depend upon the frequency of the applied field. Three principal regions of dispersion referred to as α (from about 1 Hz to 10 kHz), β (from about 10 kHz to 100 MHz), and γ (around 20 GHz), and a minor one (δ, which is present from around 300 MHz to 1 GHz), have been identified. Data and discussions of measurement and parametric modelling of dielectric properties of tissues are to be found in [11–13].

Predictions of forces and torques on ions and molecules and perturbation of chemical reactions through transfer of energy from ELF fields using EM theory lead to the conclusion that such effects are of extremely small magnitude at field strengths of practical relevance. However, recent studies have investigated the possibility that such small effects may be significant in modifying signal-processing structures such as receptors on cell surfaces and cellular messenger processes. Currently, all of the theories for biological effects of small-amplitude ELF fields are speculative and unproved and suffer from a lack of detailed quantitative knowledge of the process being modelled. A comprehensive survey and discussion of this topic is to be found in [3].

21.4 Monitoring for ELF fields

21.4.1 Instrumentation

It is not known with certainty which parameters are most appropriate in assessing exposure of humans to ELF fields. However, the following assumptions are usually implicit in the design of measuring instruments

- ELF electric fields couple poorly with the body.
- Biological effects that may arise from exposure to an ELF field are due to its magnetic component, or to the electric fields and currents that the magnetic field induces in the body. Thus most instruments measure the magnetic field and only a few sense the electric field.
- Frequency response is usually tailored to measure 50–60 Hz fields and harmonics up to 500–1000 Hz with the low-frequency response being limited to about 35 Hz.
- Exposure is best represented by the RMS magnitude of the field vector averaged over several cycles.
- A data logging capability is usually considered necessary to capture temporal variations in the field.

Instruments have been developed based on the use of coils, plates, and flux gates as sensors [3, 14]. In general, three approaches to field measurement are available—use of personal exposure meters, use of an instrument in a fixed location, and the taking of spot measurements at multiple locations. Assessment of exposure to ELF may also be studied in terms of the type of environment (e.g. residential, occupational, etc.) where the exposure occurs. The problem around choosing appropriate metrics for describing magnetic fields has been discussed in [15]. Although widely used, it should be remembered that time-weighted averaging fails to reflect a large number of potentially relevant exposure parameters, such as time above thresholds, intermittency, and transients.

21.4.2 Practical aspects of monitoring fields

The characteristics of the source such as fundamental frequency, potential for harmonics, temporal characteristics, anticipated field strength, and source geometry should be assessed before measurements are made. When practicable, the use of a personal monitor worn by the subject is generally the preferred method of assessing exposure since this provides a quantitative estimate of exposure to a clearly defined field. However, there may still be substantial uncertainty regarding the exposure, since factors such as changes in work tasks, intermittent use of appliances or tools, changing current loads, and variable proximity to wiring can contribute to large day-to-day variation in measurements. Personal exposure monitors can also be intrusive, causing people to alter their usual activities because they are wearing the meter. In view of the wide variation in exposure to ELF magnetic fields, a large number of measurements must be made to obtain a reasonably precise estimate of the exposure of an individual.

Some exposure meters are designed for spot measurements or stationary monitoring. These methods are relatively simple but have disadvantages in that they neglect personal activity and mobility; their most appropriate use is when mobility is restricted to a particular room or building.

If strong *E* fields are being measured, care should be taken to minimize perturbations of the field due to the presence of the probe and operator. The use of long dielectric handles or of remote fibre-optic readouts will help in this respect.

21.5 Instrumentation for RF and microwaves

21.5.1 Measurements in external media

Devices used for monitoring RF and microwave fields are known as radiation hazard meters, monitors, or survey instruments. They are designed to respond to either electric or magnetic fields and generally consist of three parts—the probe or sensor, processing and display electronics, and leads carrying the signal between them. Some discussion regarding the selection of a probe for a particular task is given in §21.5.5.

Important characteristics of probes include the following:

- The response to a particular field parameter should avoid spurious responses to other parameters. For example, an *E* field sensor should not exhibit a spurious response to *H* fields.
- The dimensions of the sensor should be small compared with the wavelength λ in the local medium in which the field parameter is to be measured at the highest operating frequency.
- Ideally, the probe's response should be constant regardless of the orientation of the probe in the field (isotropic response). This is usually achieved (approximately) in practice by using multiple dipoles or loops (Figure 21.2). Details of deviations of the probe's response from a true isotropic response should be provided by the manufacturer.

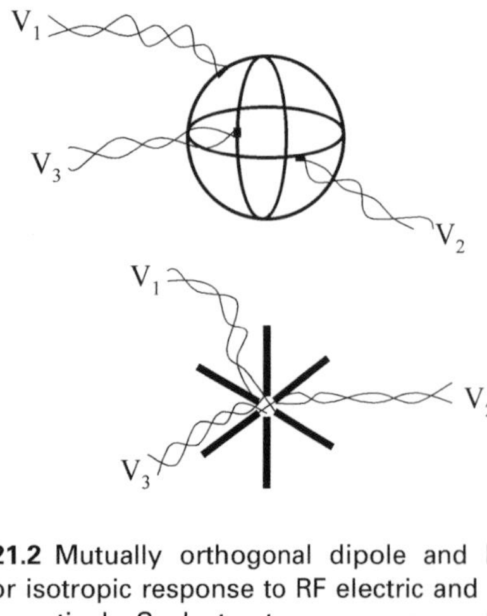

Figure 21.2 Mutually orthogonal dipole and loop elements for isotropic response to RF electric and magnetic fields, respectively. Such structures are commonly used in isotropic probes. The RF signal from each element is converted via a diode or thermocouple to provide output voltages V_1, V_2, and V_3. $\sqrt{(V_1^2 + V_2^2 + V_3^2)}$ is proportional to E_{total} or H_{total}.

- The perturbation of the field being monitored due to the leads between the sensor and other parts of the system should be minimized through the use of high resistance leads (typically 100 kΩ m^{-1}) or optical fibres.
- The readout should be in terms of one or more of the following parameters:
  - average equivalent plane-wave power density, mean-square electric field strength, mean-square magnetic field strength and energy density
  - RMS values should be indicated independent of any modulation.
- The output of the monitor should be sufficiently stable to avoid the need for re-zeroing over periods of at least 10–30 min.
- A useful dynamic range is from –10 dB with respect to the lowest value and $\pm$5 dB with respect to the maximum value stated in the RF protection guide being used (see §21.7.2).
- An acceptable level of accuracy for measurements is $\pm$1 dB (although $\pm$2 dB accuracy is acceptable for measurement of low-level fields).
- Precision should be better than 5% of the full-scale value.
- The time constant (i.e. time to respond to 90% of the final value) should be approximately 1 s.

Complete characterization of the near field is difficult to determine since three orthogonal components of the *E* field, which may have arbitrary relative phases and amplitudes, and three orthogonal components of the *H* field, again with arbitrary relative phases and amplitudes, must be measured simultaneously. Most monitoring instruments measure amplitude, but not phase information, and provide $|E|^2$ and $|H|^2$, from which average power density is inferred.

Power density is often used as a hazard indicator (far-field measurements at frequencies above about 300 MHz) but is not usually measured directly. Generally, one or more components of electric field strength, magnetic field strength, or both are measured and an equivalent plane wave power density is inferred from RMS values of *E* and *H* through equation (21.9):

$$S_{eq} = |E|^2/377 \quad \text{or} \quad S_{eq} = 377\,|H|^2. \qquad (21.9)$$

Equivalent plane wave power density is equal in magnitude to the power density of a plane wave that has the same electric or magnetic field strength.

Monitoring instrumentation of any kind requires periodic calibration. This may be carried out using either known free-space fields, guided-wave methods, or by comparison with a standard probe (transfer standard probe). Excellent discussions of these techniques are given in [16, 17].

21.5.2 Types of probe

Diode-based probes

Diode-based probes are commonly used to measure power density up to 100s of mW cm^{-2} over a frequency range of approximately 400 kHz to 12 GHz. Common characteristics include the following:

- The diode's output is:
  - proportional to power density (or to $|E|^2$ or to $|H|^2$) at low levels
  - proportional to E or H at higher levels.
- The diode is usually used at low levels (square law region) or its characteristic is electrically corrected to exhibit a square law response.
- It usually detects peak levels rather than average levels when used to measure pulsed fields. This can lead to large errors when the ratio of peak field to average field is high.
- The diode may be photosensitive. Schottky diodes exhibit some photovoltaic effect and beamlead hybrid types exhibit a larger effect. The device is encapsulated within an opaque layer to avoid potential errors arising from use in conditions of strong light.
- The variation in output from diode-based probes with varying ambient temperature is typically 0.05 dB $°C^{-1}$.

It is difficult to make broadband E and H field probes that operate at lower frequencies in the range from about 10 kHz to a few 100 MHz since the source impedance of an electrically small dipole is very high and the sensitivity of a small loop antenna is very low. Isolation of the leads from the antenna/detector is also difficult below about 100 MHz. Such problems may be overcome by using an active antenna consisting of a high-impedance RF amplifier connected directly to a monopole or loop antenna.

Thermocouple-based probes

A linear resistive dipole formed from thin-film thermocouples may be used for frequencies up to approximately 18 GHz. Such probes offer good square law characteristics. The dependence on changes in ambient temperature is typically 0.1%$°C^{-1}$. A disadvantage is that burn-out occurs at relatively low levels, typically at three times the full-scale reading.

Electro-optical sensors

Probes based on electro-optical sensors use an electro-optical modulator to amplitude-modulate an optical signal according to the instantaneous EM field. The optical signal is then detected and processed. Such devices offer the unique potential for both phase and amplitude measurements.

21.5.3 Practical aspects of monitoring fields

Information regarding the characteristics of the field should be collated and an estimate of the expected field strength made prior to making measurements (see §21.2.2). The person carrying out the survey should take appropriate safety precautions. This is particularly important when fields associated with high-power, radiating systems are being monitored. Potential hazards, in addition to those of the field itself, may include the presence of high voltages, DC magnetic fields, combustible gas, and flammable material.

It is important to select a radiation hazard meter that is best suited to the nature of the field to be measured. For example:

- An isotropic probe is to be preferred when the polarization of the field is not known, usually the case when measuring in the near field or when multi-path reflections may be present.
- An H-field probe should be selected for monitoring in an essentially inductive near-field region.
- Measurements of spatially averaged E and H fields, induced currents, and contact currents are appropriate within the frequency range 3 kHz to 100 MHz.
- Measurements of spatially averaged E and H fields are appropriate within the frequency range 100 MHz to 300 MHz.
- Measurements of the spatial average of E, H, or power density are appropriate within the frequency range 300 MHz to 300 GHz.

Further practical points that should be followed include:

- The survey should begin at a sufficient large distance from the source where the field level is expected to be low.
- The radiation hazard meter used should be set to a relatively high sensitivity range. It is important to zero the probe and to check for baseline drift during the survey. Care should be taken to avoid overexposure of the operator or burn-out of the meter as the survey proceeds to locations closer to the source.
- Care should be taken when making and interpreting measurements close to metallic objects in the field. These lead to reflections and large field gradients are also present close to edges and points of metallic objects. A distance of at least 20 cm between probe and object should be allowed in such cases.

- Care should be taken to minimize field perturbation due to the presence of the operator's body. Such effects may lead to uncertainty in measurements of equivalent plane wave power density of more than 2 dB.
- Care should be taken to minimize reflections from cables. These can lead to artefacts of approximately 1.5 dB.

Other artefacts may arise from capacitive coupling between probe and source, particularly when the frequency is below a few megahertz. Further practical details associated with surveying RF and microwave fields may be found in §5 of [17].

21.5.4 Measurements made in tissues or phantoms

In most cases, a radiation protection physicist will be faced with the task of making and interpreting field measurements made in air. However, in some cases, there may be a need to quantify the potential hazard of a near-field, or other complex field, exposure and here direct measurement of fields in tissue-like media (phantoms), or occasionally directly in tissues, may be more appropriate than an estimation based on limited sampling of the complex external field. Such examples might include the use of mobile communication systems, assessment of exposure associated with novel coils for MR procedures, exposure to fields from antennas running at reduced power during servicing procedures, etc. The quantity known as the specific absorption rate (SAR) is commonly used for dosimetric purposes for RF and MW fields.

- SAR is the time derivative of the incremental energy dW absorbed by (or dissipated in) an incremental mass dm contained in a volume element dV of density ρ, i.e.

$$\mathrm{SAR} = \mathrm{d}/\mathrm{d}t(\mathrm{d}W/\mathrm{d}m) = \mathrm{d}/\mathrm{d}t(\mathrm{d}W/\rho\, \mathrm{d}V) \qquad (21.10)$$

- SAR depends upon body shape, frequency, polarization, $\boldsymbol{E}$ and $\boldsymbol{H}$ vector fields, the presence of ground planes and reflectors, and dielectric composition.

At lower frequencies, interactions with the body are through the currents induced internally by the external fields or through internal fields. Internal currents may be determined through knowledge of the electric and magnetic flux densities. The internal electric field $\boldsymbol{E}$ and current density $\boldsymbol{J}$ are related through equation (21.11).

$$\boldsymbol{J} = \sigma \boldsymbol{E}. \qquad (21.11)$$

- RMS and peak internal electric field strength, internal current and current density are also useful dosimetric parameters.

21.5.5 Measurement of SAR

Local SAR may be measured within tissue-like phantoms or *in vivo* by determining the local change of temperature (ΔT) at one or more locations following a brief exposure ($\Delta t = 5$–30 s) to the fields using the relationship $\mathrm{SAR} = c(\Delta T/\Delta t)$ where c is the specific heat of the medium. A non-perturbing thermometer with a resolution of 0.01–0.1°C is required. The technique may be used to determine SARs greater than a few W kg^{-1} but measurements are difficult to interpret in regions of high SAR, in the presence of high SAR gradients, or in the presence of several SAR hot-spots.

SAR may also be determined using an implantable *E*-field probe. The technique, which may be used over a frequency range from about 300 MHz to 3 GHz, requires the probe to be calibrated in the tissue-like medium to better than ±1–2 dB, and knowledge of the conductivity σ and density ρ of the medium which are related to SAR through equation (21.12).

$$\mathrm{SAR} = \sigma |E_{int}|^2 / 2\rho \qquad (21.12)$$

Desirable characteristics for a miniature *E*-field probe include

- high sensitivity and linear response over a broad frequency range
- small size and a construction that is minimally perturbing to the fields
- a high degree of isotropy when used in a range of media.

In practice, response is relatively independent of the medium if

- the probe is insulated
- the relationship between the permittivity of the medium and probe insulation is $\varepsilon'_{\mathrm{medium}} \geq 5\ \varepsilon'_{\mathrm{insulation}}$.

Some guidelines and standards outline methods to be used to determine SAR. For example, two methods for the determination of SAR in relation to RF safety in MR imaging systems are outlined in [16]:

- *The pulse energy* method in which the peak power absorbed in a test object that simulates coil loading due to the patient, corrected for the power absorbed by the unloaded coil, is determined.
- *The calorimetric method* (used only to determine whole-body averaged SAR) in which a test object containing NaCl solution that simulates the coil loading observed when a 50–90 kg patient is subjected to RF pulses for a period sufficient to create a temperature increase at least 20 times the uncertainty associated with the thermometry system used.

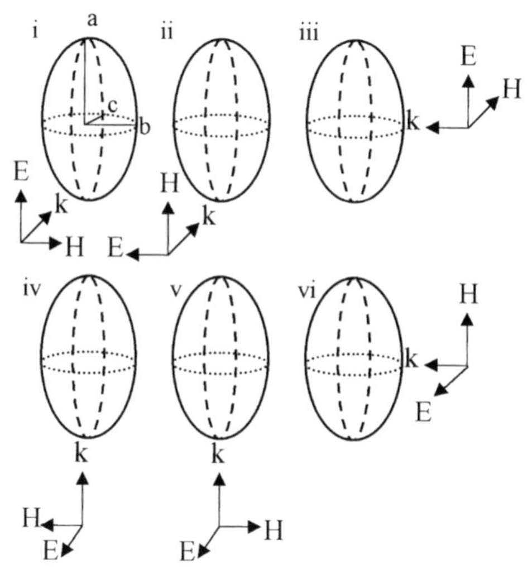

Figure 21.3 Polarization of incident fields with respect to objects that do not have circular symmetry about their long axis. The six cases are (i) EHK, (ii) HEK, (iii) EKH, (iv) KEH, (v) KHE, and (vi) HKE.

21.6 EM field dosimetry

Dosimetry of EM fields involves the determination of the energy absorbed by, and the internal fields within, an object exposed to external incident fields. Various models of humans and animals have been investigated to understand the relationships between external and internal fields. The general problem is to solve Maxwell's equations for a particular body under specific exposure conditions.

At the boundary between two media of differing dielectric properties, E fields must satisfy the boundary conditions shown in equations (21.13) and (21.14).

$$\varepsilon_1 E_{1n} = \varepsilon_2 E_{2n} \tag{21.13}$$

$$E_{1p} = E_{2p} \tag{21.14}$$

where E_{1p}, E_{2p} and E_{1n}, E_{2n} are components parallel to and normal to the boundary between the media with complex permittivities ε_1 and ε_2, respectively.

- If E_{1n} is the field in air and E_{2n} is the field in tissue, the internal field at the boundary will be much weaker than the external field at the boundary when the fields are normal to the boundary since $\varepsilon_{air} < \varepsilon_{tissue}$ (from equation 21.13)
- The external field and the internal field at the boundary are equal when the fields are parallel to the boundary (from equation 21.14)

The H fields must also satisfy boundary conditions at the interface, namely

- H_{1p}, H_{2p}, the components parallel to the boundary are continuous across it.
- $\mu_1 H_{1n} = \mu_2 H_{2n}$ where H_{1n}, H_{2n} are the normal components and μ_1, μ_2 are the complex permeabilities of the two media.

Since tissues are essentially non-magnetic, the boundary conditions for the H field are not as important for explaining relative energy absorption as those for the E field.

Considerable insight into aspects of EM dosimetry such as penetration, resonance, and coupling may be gained from solutions of canonical problems involving half-space, cylindrical, spherical, and spheroidal representation of the body or body parts. A further use of these simplified models is in the testing of the predictions of numerical models against analytical solutions. Calculations of SAR and internal fields within a large number of spheroidal models of man and animals and over a wide range of frequencies are presented in [18].

The polarization of the incident field is an important factor in determining the internal fields and SAR within an object:

- Six polarizations can be defined when the object does not possess circular symmetry (e.g. an ellipsoid with three different semi-axes (a, b, and c with $a > b > c$ in the x, y, and z directions) as shown in Figure 21.3.

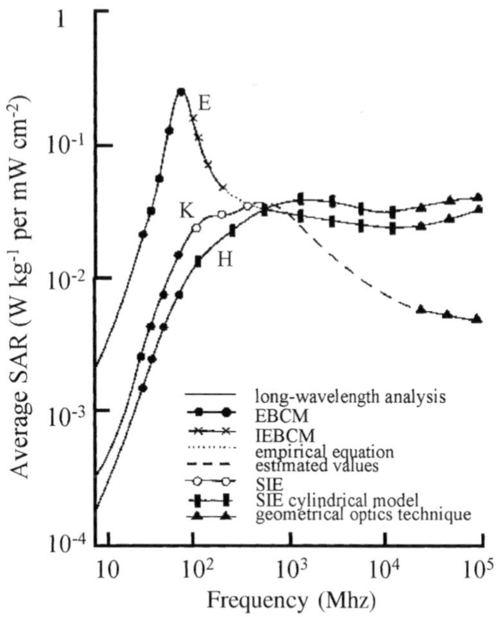

Figure 21.4 Average SAR (per mW cm^{-2}) versus frequency for models of an average man (after [18]). The various methods used for calculations are described in [18]. EBCM, extended boundary condition method; IECBM, iterative extended boundary condition method; SIE, surface integral equation method.

Box 21.2 *Bases and general structure of guidelines for exposure to time-varying electric and magnetic fields and electromagnetic radiation*

- Guidelines for limiting exposure and avoiding known adverse health effects have been drawn up by international and national bodies.
- Effects arise from both:
  - direct interaction of fields with the body
  - indirect effects—those involving interaction with an object at a different electrical potential from the body—are usually taken into account. These include stimulation of peripheral nerves and muscles, shocks and burns caused by touching conducting objects and tissue heating caused by energy absorption from the fields.
- Guidelines are often presented in terms of two levels of protection:
  - basic restrictions—based directly on established health effects
  - reference levels—derived from measurements and/or computed predictions. These provide for practical exposure assessment to determine whether the basic restrictions are likely to be exceeded.
- If a reference level is exceeded, it does not necessarily follow that the basic restriction is exceeded. However, in such cases, compliance with the basic restriction must be tested.
- Guidelines often differentiate between occupational exposure and general public exposure:
  - occupational/controlled exposures—appropriate when persons who are fully aware of the potential for exposure and can exercise control over it are exposed as a consequence of their employment. These limits also apply in situations when an individual is transient through a location where occupational/controlled limits apply provided he or she is made aware of the potential for exposure.
  - general population/uncontrolled exposures—apply when the general public may be exposed or when persons who may not be fully aware of the potential for exposure or cannot exercise control over it are exposed as a consequence of their employment.

- Polarization is defined as E, H, or K according to which incident field vector—***E***, ***H***, or ***k***–is parallel to the long axis of the body for objects that have circular symmetry about their long axis (e.g. a prolate spheroid).

The effect of polarization (E, H, and K) and frequency on average SAR within a prolate spheroidal model of an average man ($a = 0.875$ m, $b = 0.138$ m, volume = 0.07 m^3) [18] is shown in Figure 21.4. For E polarization, there is a resonance at about 70 MHz (corresponding to the height being approximately 0.4λ). In the case of children and babies this resonance occurs at a higher frequency, which may exceed

Table 21.1 ICNIRP [2] basic restrictions for electric and magnetic fields. The values given are for occupational exposures. Values relating to exposure of the general public are reduced by a factor of 5

Frequency	RMS current density for head and trunk ($mA\ m^{-2}$)	Whole-body average SAR ($W\ kg^{-1}$)	Localized SAR (head and trunk) ($W\ kg^{-1}$)	Localized SAR (limbs) ($W\ kg^{-1}$)	Power density ($W\ m^{-2}$)
Up to 1 Hz	40	–	–	–	–
1–4 Hz	40/*f*	–	–	–	–
4 Hz–1 kHz	10	–	–	–	–
1–100 kHz	*f*/100	–	–	–	–
100 kHz–10 MHz	*f*/100	0.4	10	20	–
10 MHz–10 GHz	–	0.4	10	20	–
10–300 GHz	–	–	–	–	50

f is expressed in Hz.
Current density is averaged over a cross-section of 1 cm^2 perpendicular to the current direction.
Power density is averaged over any 20 cm^2 of exposed area in any $68/f^{1.05}$-min period (*f* in GHz).
Spatial maximum power densities averaged over 1 cm^2 should not exceed 20 times the value above.

Table 21.2 ICNIRP [2] reference levels for exposure to electric and magnetic fields (unperturbed RMS values)

Frequency	*E* field ($V\ m^{-1}$)	*H* field ($A\ m^{-1}$)	*B* field (μT)	Equivalent plane wave power density S_{eq} ($W\ m^{-2}$)
Occupational exposures				
up to 1 Hz	–	163 000	200 000	–
1–8 Hz	20 000	$163\ 000/f^2$	$200\ 000/f^2$	–
8–25 Hz	20 000	$20\ 000/f$	$25\ 000/f$	–
0.025–0.82 kHz	$500/f$	$20/f$	$25/f$	–
0.82–65 kHz	610	24.4	30.7	–
0.065–1 MHz	610	$1.6/f$	$2.0/f$	–
1–10 MHz	$610/f$	$1.6/f$	$2.0/f$	–
10–400 MHz	61	0.16	0.2	10
400–2000 MHz	$3\sqrt{f}$	$0.008\sqrt{f}$	$0.01\sqrt{f}$	$f/40$
2–300 GHz	1.37	0.36	0.45	50
General public exposure				
up to 1 Hz	–	32 000	40 000	–
1–8 Hz	10 000	$32\ 000/f^2$	$40\ 000/f^2$	–
8–25 Hz	10 000	$4000/f$	$5000/f$	–
0.025–0.8 kHz	$250/f$	$4/f$	$5/f$	–
0.8–3 kHz	$250/f$	5	6.25	–
3–150 kHz	87	5	6.25	–
0.15–1 MHz	87	$0.73/f$	$0.92/f$	–
1–10 MHz	$87/\sqrt{f}$	$0.73/f$	$0.92/f$	
10–400 MHz	28	0.073	0.092	2
400–2000 MHz	$1.375\sqrt{f}$	$0.0037\sqrt{f}$	$0.0046\sqrt{f}$	$f/200$
2–300 GHz	61	0.16	0.20	10

Units of *f* as indicated in frequency column.
E^2, H^2, B^2, and S_{eq} are averaged over any 6-min period for frequencies between 100 kHz and 10 GHz and over any $68/f^{1.05}$-min period for higher frequencies.

100 MHz. When a person is standing on a perfect ground plane, the resonant frequency is reduced by about 50%. The SAR varies approximately as f^2 below resonance and as $1/f$ post-resonance. Below resonance, the SAR is highest for E polarization, intermediate for K, and lowest for H.

The rapid increase in computing power that has occurred over recent years has led to the development of anatomically and dielectrically realistic models of man and animals that provide detail regarding localized variations in fields and SAR. Examples include models of exposure to the whole body, the head, and other body parts.

21.7 EM field protection guides

21.7.1 Guidelines for exposure to static magnetic fields

Interactions between the static magnetic field and the body arise from electrical potentials and resulting currents due to movement of the body or parts of it (including movement associated with body functions) within the field and displacement of naturally generated currents within the body. Possible adverse effects include reduced aortic blood flow, increased blood pressure, cardiac arrhythmia, and impaired mental function. A comprehensive review of the effects of static magnetic fields is provided in [19].

Several guidelines have been proposed by international and national agencies based on criteria such as the need to limit currents induced by movement through the static magnetic field to levels less than those that occur naturally in the body or to limit those induced in large vessels by blood flow to below levels that result in haemodynamic or cardiovascular effects. ICNIRP [20] recommendations for limits on occupational exposure are

- short-term: whole body, 2 T; limbs, 5 T
- continuous exposure: 200 mT.

(Since these are for occupational exposure only, time-averaging is performed over the working day.)

- continuous exposure of the general public (except for those with pacemakers and other implanted devices): 40 mT
- continuous exposure of those with pacemakers and other implanted devices: 0.5 mT.

NRPB [5] recommends similar limits—2 T (whole body), 5 T (limbs), and 200 mT averaged over 24 hours–for both residential and occupational exposures.

21.7.2 Guidelines for exposure to time-varying electric fields, magnetic fields, and electromagnetic radiation

ICNIRP [2] guidelines are presented in terms of two levels of protection as summarized in Tables 21.1 and 21.2. The following conditions apply:

- All SAR values are averaged over any 6-min period and localized SAR values are averaged over a 10 g contiguous mass of tissue.
- For pulses of duration t_p, the equivalent frequency is determined by $1/(2t_p)$.
- For pulsed exposures in the frequency range 0.3–10 GHz and for localized exposure of the head, the specific absorption should not exceed 10 mJ kg^{-1}, averaged over 10 g tissue.
- For frequencies up to 100 kHz and for pulsed magnetic fields, the associated maximum current density may be determined from the rise/fall times and maximum rate of change of magnetic flux density.

ICNIRP [2] guidelines reflect current general consensus. However, other guidelines have been issued by national agencies and reflect some differences in interpretation of the data available. These include:

- NRPB [5]
  - Consists of basic restrictions and reference levels (Figures 21.5–21.8). NRPB [5, 21] does not differentiate between exposures of workers and of the general public, believing that the existing UK limits provide adequate protection. NRPB questions the scientific justification for such a blanket approach as well as the health benefits to be obtained from these further reductions in exposure.
  - Basic restrictions on exposure to static electric fields are such as to avoid annoying sensations due to surface charge effects.
  - Pulsed field conditions which invoke the microwave auditory effect in people with normal hearing should be avoided.
  - Compliance in situations where a single-frequency investigation level is not appropriate, such as magnetic fields with high harmonic content, pulsed and transient magnetic fields, and exposure to the inductive near-field of RF sources, is discussed in [22].
- Health Council of the Netherlands (HCN) [23]
  - Similar to [5] regarding basic restrictions except (i) no distinction is made between adults and children and (ii) different exposure limits for workers and the general public.
  - For $f > 10$ GHz, the use of incident power density, rather than SAR, is recommended since surface absorption dominates.
  - At 300 GHz, the recommended basic restriction level corresponds to that proposed in several laser guidelines (see Chapter 19).
  - Derived limit levels for unperturbed electric and magnetic fields (Figures 21.5–21.7):
    - envelop experimental data [5]
    - are not unnecessarily restrictive
    - are protective against indirect effects such as the sensations of perception or pain due to contact currents when touching large metallic objects in the electric field.
  - For simultaneous exposure to multiple frequencies, power densities (or $|E|^2$or $|H|^2$) should be expressed as fractions of the respective limit and summed, the total sum not exceeding unity. The same guidelines are recommended for pulsed fields as for continuous radiation.
- Federal Communications Commission [24]
  - Two levels of exposure limits based on occupational/controlled and general population/uncontrolled exposures.
  - The maximum permissible exposure (MPE) limits (Figures 21.5, 21.6, and 21.8) are generally based on recommendations of NCRP [1] and IEEE [25]). The MPE limits recommended in [25] are also shown in Figures 21.5, 21.6, and 21.8.

When the exposure involves multiple frequencies the determination of compliance with guidelines is usually complex [2, 5, 23, 25, 26].

Limits for contact currents and induced currents from several guidelines are listed in Table 21.3. These are chosen to avoid pain upon finger contact in adults [23], potential RF shock and burn [25].

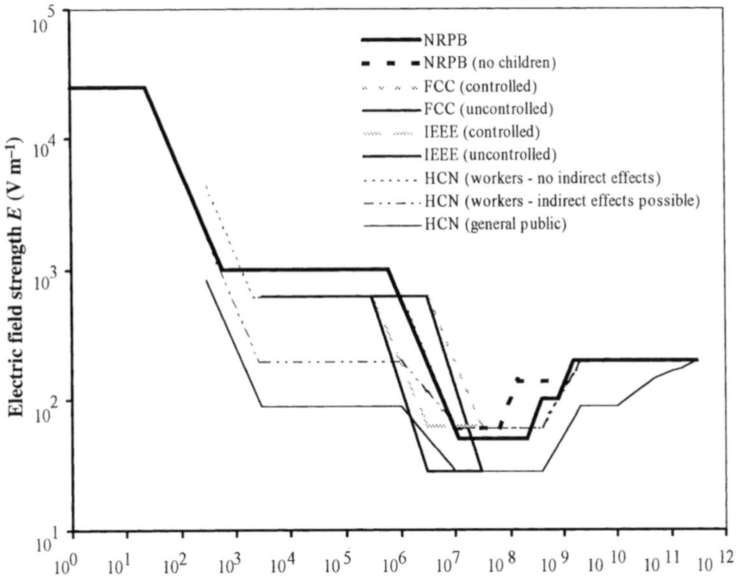

Figure 21.5 Electric field strength E (V m^{-1}) limits versus frequency as recommended by several guidelines. Data shown include NRPB [5] investigation levels (if there is no possibility of small children being exposed the higher values in the range 10 MHz–1.55 GHz may be used, FCC [24, 26] and IEEE [25] maximum permissible exposure (MPE) levels for controlled (occupational) and uncontrolled (general population) environments and HCN [23] proposed maximum field strengths for workers (both in the absence of direct effects and when direct effects are possible) and the general public. All levels are RMS values.

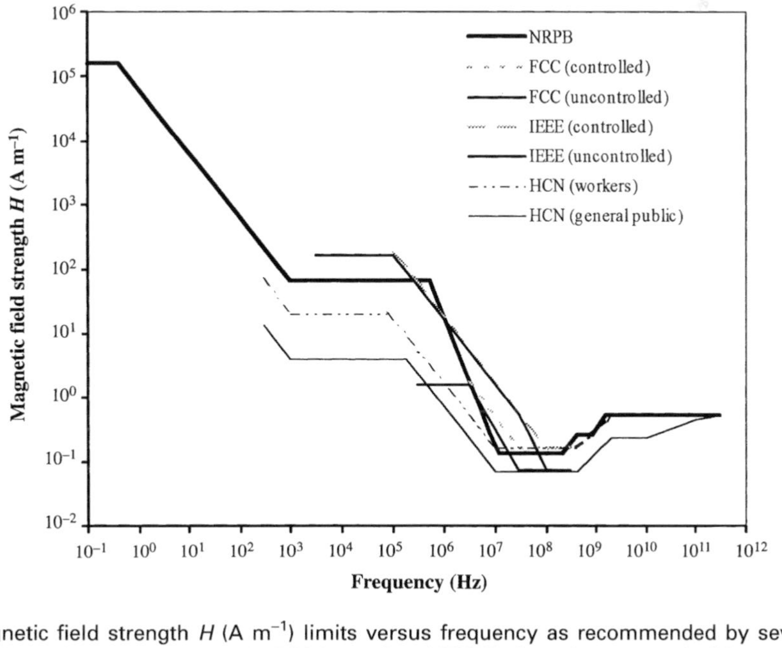

Figure 21.6 Magnetic field strength H (A m^{-1}) limits versus frequency as recommended by several guidelines. Data shown include NRPB [5] investigation levels, FCC [24, 26] and IEEE [25] maximum permissible exposure (MPE) levels for controlled and uncontrolled environments and HCN [23] proposed maximum field strengths for workers and the general public. All levels are RMS values.

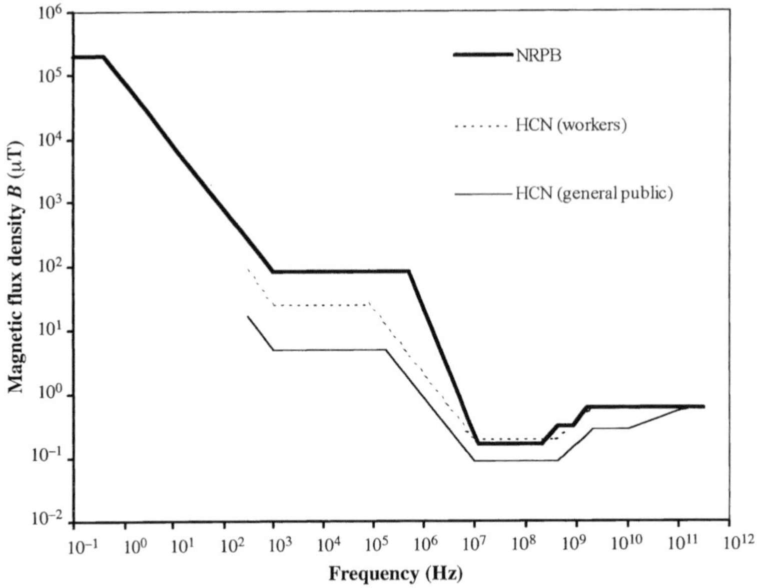

Figure 21.7 Magnetic flux density B (μT) limits versus frequency according to NRPB [5] (investigation levels) and HCN [23] (maximum levels for exposure of workers and of the general public). All levels are RMS values.

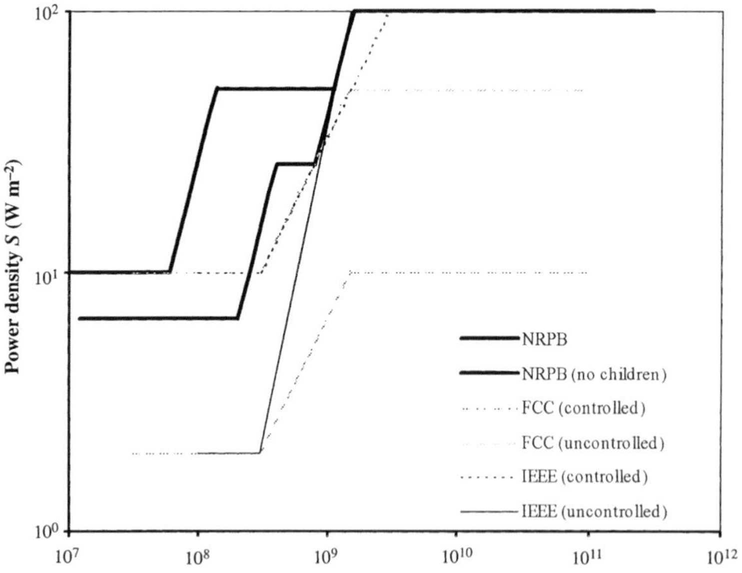

Figure 21.8 Power density S (W m^{-1}) according to NRPB [5] investigation levels (if the exposure of small children is not involved, the higher levels may be used), and FCC [24, 26] and IEEE [25] MPE levels for controlled and uncontrolled environments. In IEEE [25], in a controlled environment, $|E|^2$, $|H|^2$, and S are averaged over 6 min when $f \leq 15$ GHz and over $616\,000/f^{\,1.2}$ min (f in MHz) when 15 GHz < $f \leq$ 300 GHz. In an uncontrolled environment, the averaging times for $|E|^2$ and S are 30 min when 100 MHz $\leq f \leq$ 3 GHz, $90\,000/f$ min when 3 GHz < $f \leq$ 15 GHz, and $616\,000/f^{\,1.2}$ when 15 GHz < $f \leq$ 300 GHz. For $|H|^2$ under uncontrolled conditions, the averaging times are $0.0636f^{1.337}$ min when 30 MHz $\leq f \leq$ 100 MHz and 30 min when 100 MHz < $f \leq$ 3 GHz. In FCC [24, 26], the averaging times are 6 min and 30 min for 30 MHz $\leq f \leq$ 100 GHz in controlled and uncontrolled environments, respectively.

Table 21.3 Limits for contact currents and induced currents

Frequency	Guideline	Contact current (mA)	Maximum current in a limb (mA)
0.1 Hz–370 Hz	NRPB [5]	0.5	
370 Hz–70 kHz	NRPB [5]	$f^{0.7}$ (f in kHz)	
70 kHz–100 MHz	NRPB [5]	20	
If there is no possibility of children being exposed, the following limits may be used			
0.1 Hz–1 kHz	NRPB [5]	1.0	
1 kHz–130 kHz	NRPB [5]	$f^{0.7}$ (f in kHz)	
130 kHz–100 MHz	NRPB [5]	30	
Occupational exposure			
up to 2.5 kHz	ICNIRP [2]	1.0	
300 Hz–2.5 kHz	HCN [23]	1.0	
2.5–100 kHz	ICNIRP [2] HCN [23]	$0.4f$ (f in kHz)	
100 kHz–10 MHz	HCN [23]	40	
100 kHz–110 MHz	ICNIRP [2]	40	
10–110 MHz	ICNIRP [2]		100
General public exposure			
Except as indicated below, ICNIRP [2] and HCN [23] limits for general public exposure are half the corresponding occupational exposure limits			
10–110 MHz	ICNIRP [2]		45

21.8 Safety guidelines for magnetic resonance

Magnetic resonance (MR) is a clinical diagnostic modality that has undergone rapid development and expansion since prototype whole-body systems were introduced in the late 1970s. The basic principles of MR have been described in many publications. MR is a major activity within the hospital environment in which safety aspects of non-ionising electromagnetic fields must be considered. The potential electromagnetic hazards associated with MR arise from the static magnetic field, time-varying magnetic fields associated with gradient coils, and RF magnetic fields.

21.8.1 Static magnetic field B_0

Static magnetic fields ranging from 0.012 to 10 T are encountered in MR systems used for clinical or research purposes. Patients undergoing MR imaging or spectroscopy have the highest exposure to static magnetic fields among members of the general public (typically 0.15–2 T for periods of up to 30 min). There are safety issues both around bioeffects associated with the exposure to the static magnetic field and from the effects of the large magnetic forces that can be exerted on ferromagnetic objects in the field gradient. In this chapter only the former will be discussed; an excellent review of the latter is to be found elsewhere [27].

National and international guidelines consider the consequences of exposure to static magnetic fields as follows.

- NRPB [28]
  - Acute exposure to B_0 below about 2.5 T is unlikely to have any adverse health effects.
  - Caution is recommended when patients are exposed to $B_0 > 2.5$ T.
  - Short-term exposure to B_0 above about 4 T may produce significant detrimental health effects such as vertigo, nausea, reduced aortic blood flow, and increased blood pressure.
  - Cardiac arrhythmia and impaired mental function have been observed in primates exposed to $B_0 \approx$ 4–5 T.
  - Insufficient data are available to allow thresholds for adverse effects to be defined accurately. Therefore, a two-level approach is proposed which, with caution, provides some flexibility:
    - a lower level for which exposures, except for special cases, are considered safe and which may be exceeded under controlled circumstances
    - an upper level to exposure which the available data suggest it would be inadvisable to exceed.
  - Recommended restrictions on exposure of patients and volunteers are

Table 21.4 NRPB [28] recommended restrictions on peak rates of change of magnetic flux density for patient and volunteer exposure to gradient magnetic fields associated with MR diagnosis

Duration of field change	Peak dB/dt (T s^{-1})	
	Uncontrolled level	Upper level
$\tau > 3$ ms	20	20
120 μs $< \tau <$ 3 ms	20	$0.06/\tau$
45 μs $< \tau <$ 120 μs	$0.0024/\tau$	$0.06/\tau$
2.5 μs $< \tau <$ 45 μs	$0.0024/\tau$	1300[a,b]
$\tau <$ 2.5 μs	950[a,c]	1300[a,b]

[a]Peak dB/dt values calculated assuming tissue electrical conductivity of 0.4 S m^{-1} and an inductive loop radius of 0.15 m.
[b]Equivalent SAR is 2 W kg^{-1}.
[c]Equivalent SAR is 1 W kg^{-1}.
τ(s) is the width of a rectangular pulse or half the period of a sinusoidal dB/dt pulse.

    - trunk and head: 2.5 T (uncontrolled level) and 4.0 T (upper level)
    - limbs: 4.0 T (for both uncontrolled and upper levels).
- International Non-Ionising Radiation Committee (INIRC) of the International Radiation Protection Association (IRPA) [29]
    - No adverse effects from whole-body exposure to 2 T and of the extremities to 5 T.
    - Patients should be monitored for symptoms referable to the nervous system when using $B_0 >$ 2 T.
- The International Electrotechnical Commission (IEC) [16]
    - No scientific evidence for any adverse effect caused by chronic exposure to $B_0 <$ 2 T.
    - Short exposures to B_0 above about 4 T may produce effects such as vertigo and nausea and a degree of caution is required in these cases.
- Federal Food and Drug Administration (FDA) [30]
    - Operation of MR devices with $B_0 <$ 4 T is not associated with 'significant risk'.

The Medical Devices Directorate (MDD) of the Department of Health has issued guidelines for MR diagnostic equipment in clinical use with particular reference to safety [31]. These guidelines recommend that MR equipment is contained within an enclosed designated controlled area which encompasses the 0.5 mT contour. All unauthorized persons requiring access must be medically screened and warned of potential hazards (such as the projectile effect associated with ferromagnetic material within a strong magnetic field). Persons fitted with a heart pacemaker must not enter the controlled area. The recommended upper limits for authorized staff are 2 T (whole body) and 4 T (limbs) and maximum 8 h averages are 0.2 T. For the general public (excluding those person with pacemakers), both upper limit and the maximum 8 h average are 0.2 T. The upper limit for those with a pacemaker is 0.005 T. A similar set of requirements is described in [16].

21.8.2 Time-varying magnetic fields (gradient fields, dB/dt)

Nerve and muscle cells can be stimulated by sufficiently great current density. The implications of this for safe operation of MR systems are addressed by guidelines as follows.

- IRPA/INIRC [29]
    - Current densities of the order of 1–10 mA m^{-2} induced by continuous sinusoidal magnetic fields are of no concern while those in the range 10–100 mA m^{-2} can have effects that are strongly dependent upon frequency but are not adverse.
    - Stimulation of excitable cell membranes is observed in the range 100–1000 mA m^{-2} and health hazards are possible.
    - Threshold current densities sufficient to stimulate peripheral nerve or cardiac muscle are about 1200 mA m^{-2} at frequencies below 100 Hz.
    - If $dB/dt <$ 20 T s^{-1}, current densities are sufficiently low (a safety margin of a factor of 3 is generally achieved) to avoid stimulation. Relaxation of this restriction is possible for transverse gradient fields (those orthogonal to the static field) and for short periods of magnetic field change (< 3 ms and < 120 μs for cardiac and peripheral nerve stimulation, respectively).
    - No adverse health effects are to be expected when $dB/dt \leq 6$ T s^{-1} but electrocardiogram monitoring of the patient's cardiac function should be carried out prior to, and during, exposure to gradient fields for which $dB/dt > 6$ T s^{-1}.

- The upper limit of dB/dt should be 20 T s^{-1} to avoid peripheral nerve stimulation.
- NRPB [28, 32]
  - See Table 21.4.
- MDD [31]
  - Two-level restriction to time-varying gradient magnetic fields following NRPB except that a duration of field change less than 2.5 μs is not considered.
  - Patients or volunteers under constant clinical supervision and monitored may be exposed to the upper level limits.
- IEC [16]
  - Three operating modes with respect to dB/dt
    - *Normal operating mode*: all parameters are within recommended limits and only routine monitoring of the patient is required.

    dB/dt < 20 T s^{-1} for $\tau > 120$ μs (τ is the pulse width duration over which dB/dt occurs)
    dB/dt < 2400/τ T s^{-1} for $2.5 < \tau \leq 120$ μs
    dB/dt < 960 T s^{-1} for $\tau \leq 2.5$ μs
    - *First-level controlled operating mode*: some operating parameters reach values that may cause undue physiological stress to patients.

    dB/dt < 20 T s^{-1} for $\tau > 3000$ μs
    dB/dt < 60 000/τ T s^{-1} for $45 < \tau \leq 3000$ μs
    dB/dt < 1330 T s^{-1} for $\tau \leq 45$ μs
    - *Second-level controlled operating mode*: operating parameter values exceed the upper limit for first-level controlled mode and may produce significant risk for patients.
  - Details of how dB/dt is to be measured.

The trend in guidance to manufacturers of MR diagnostic devices provided by the FDA has been to relax restrictions on dB/dt [33–35]. FDA [35] refers to general compliance with [16] but highlights differences in limits on dB/dt. Recent data suggest that the first controlled level of [16] is too low by approximately a factor of 2 and the upper limit is well above the pain threshold. The FDA [35] also refers to specific standards for measuring performance and safety parameters for MR devices–procedures for measuring dB/dt should comply with [36].

21.8.3 RF magnetic fields

The frequency of the RF magnetic field must match the Larmor precession frequency f which is related to the static magnetic field B_o through the equation

Table 21.5 NRPB [28] recommended restrictions on whole-body temperature rise, maximum local tissue temperature, whole-body SAR, and part-body SAR for patient and volunteer exposure to RF magnetic fields associated with MR diagnosis

	Uncontrolled level	Upper level
Restrictions on whole-body temperature rise		
Whole-body temperature rise	0.5°C	1.0°C
Restrictions on whole-body SAR[a]		
Duration of exposure		
> 30 min	1 W kg^{-1}	2 W kg^{-1}
15–30 min	30 W min kg^{-1}	60 W min kg^{-1}
< 15 min	2 W kg^{-1}	4 W kg^{-1}
Restrictions on maximum local tissue temperature		
Maximum local tissue temperature	head 38°C trunk 39°C limbs 40°C	
Restrictions on part-body SAR[b]		
Duration of exposure		
> 30 min	head 2 W kg^{-1} trunk 4 W kg^{-1} limbs 6 W kg^{-1}	
15–30 min	head 60 W min kg^{-1} trunk 120 W min kg^{-1} limbs 180 W min kg^{-1}	
< 15 min	head 4 W kg^{-1} trunk 8 W kg^{-1} limbs 12 W kg^{-1}	

[a]Averaged over any 15-min period.
[b]Peak SAR in any 1 kg averaged over any 6-min period.

$$\gamma B_o = f \qquad (21.15)$$

where γ is gyromagnetic ratio. For example, for the hydrogen atom, $\gamma = 42.57$ MHz T^{-1}. Thus the RF magnetic field frequency for typical clinical systems (with B_o of 0.2–2 T) lies in the range 8.5–85.14 MHz while higher frequencies (up to about 400 MHz) are encountered in MR systems for research.

The main adverse effects that are likely to result from acute exposure to RF magnetic fields are those associated with responses to an increased thermal load and the effects of elevated body or tissue temperatures. The degree of local heating must be considered in assessing safety of MR imaging and spectroscopy examinations of body parts such as the head or abdomen. NRPB guidelines for exposure to RF fields [28] are summarized in Table 21.5.

IEC [16] defines requirements for SAR limits for three differing modes of operation and these are listed in Table 21.6. Since the ability of the body to deal with an increased thermal load is dependent upon environmental conditions, it has been recommended that the temperature and humidity of a room in which MR examinations are carried out should be no more than 24°C and 60%, respectively. If these limits are exceeded then the SAR limits should be reduced.

The FDA [35] considers the following to be 'significant risk':

- SAR > 4 W kg^{-1} whole body for 15 min
- SAR > 3 W kg^{-1} averaged over the head for 10 min
- SAR > 8 W kg^{-1} in any 1 g of tissue in the head or torso for 15 min
- SAR > 12 W kg^{-1} in any 1 g of tissue in the extremities for 15 min.

Methods for determining SAR in compliance with standards are outlined in [16, 37].

Localized peaks in RF power absorption leading to potential hot spots can arise (i) because the person undergoing a MR examination is subjected to the near field of the RF transmit coil and (ii) because of tissue inhomogeneities.

Widely used multi-echo sequences such as fast spin echo (FSE) are time-efficient but can greatly increase RF exposure when compared to conventional methods. Even in routine examinations it is not uncommon for operators to have to modify sequence parameters to remain within the limits imposed by manufacturers to ensure that scanners operate within safety guidelines. These practical limits are generally based on crude spatially averaged models. By being conservative, safety is assured but the restrictions imposed increasingly impact on routine practice. In addition, there has been a proliferation in the routine use of specialist coils with a trend towards close-coupled designs and use of local transmit systems, particularly for spectroscopy. Such trends create a pressing need to be able to model and assess localized SAR and temperature exposures in a realistic manner.

Early studies describing fields and power absorption associated with MR RF coils were often based on geometrically simple homogeneous models or inhomogeneous phantoms and these have provided valuable insight and reasonable estimates of spatially averaged power absorption during MR procedures. However, they cannot predict reliably local peak SAR levels in the dielectrically heterogeneous human body. Recently, analyses of fields and estimates of SAR produced by coils for anatomically realistic cases (e.g. the head, limbs, etc.) have been reported.

21.9 Safety of diathermy/ hyperthermia devices

There have been several reports describing surveys of electric and magnetic fields associated with diathermy equipment.

Table 21.6 IEC [16] limits on SAR

	Normal operating mode	1st level controlled operating mode	2nd level controlled operating mode
Whole body SAR	≤ 1.5 W kg^{-1} averaged over 15 minutes	≤ 4 W kg^{-1} averaged over 15 minutes	< 4 W kg^{-1} averaged over 15 minutes
Head SAR	≤ 3 W kg^{-1} averaged over 10 minutes	Not applicable	> 3 W kg^{-1} averaged over 10 minutes
Local tissue SAR		Not applicable	
head and torso	≤ 8 W kg^{-1} averaged over 5 minutes		> 8 W kg^{-1} averaged over 5 minutes
extremities	≤ 12 W kg^{-1} averaged over 5 minutes		> 12 W kg^{-1} averaged over 5 minutes

Whole body and head SARs are the values of SAR averaged over the whole body and head, respectively.
Local tissue SAR is the value of SAR averaged over any 1 g of tissue.
It is also assumed that the SAR averaged over any 10 s period does not exceed 5 times the stated time-averaged SAR limit.

Box 21.3 Basic local rules for magnetic resonance

In view of the demanding electromagnetic environment associated with MR equipment, such equipment should be located within a designated controlled area where free access is provided only to authorized staff.

- It is recommended that the 0.5 mT contour is entirely within the controlled area.
- Access to the controlled area should be through self-closing and self-locking doors.
- All unauthorized persons must be medically screened and warned of potential hazards (projectile effect, malfunctioning of some devices in the presence of a magnetic field), before entering the controlled area.
- Unauthorized persons include
  - support staff (engineering staff, nurses, portering staff, cleaning staff, emergency services staff) who should be aware of the potential hazards and should be appropriately trained
  - patients
  - volunteers for research projects who should be fully informed and have given consent
  - the general public (visitors, patients' relations or friends).
- Patients, volunteers, and the general public must be supervised by authorized staff at all times within the controlled area.
- Persons fitted with a heart pacemaker must not enter the controlled area.

It is also convenient to define an inner controlled area containing the 3 mT contour.

- All persons entering this area should remove items such as watches, credit cards, and all ferromagnetic objects from their clothing and deposit them outside the area before entering.
- No ferromagnetic object (tools, gas cylinders, trolleys, etc.) must be allowed in this inner area.
- Persons with any metallic implant should be forbidden to enter the inner controlled area until the implant has been declared safe by a suitably qualified person.
- Persons with intracranial aneurysm clips or intraorbital metallic implants should not enter the inner controlled area.
- Persons with metallic implants such as artificial joints, surgical clips, or prosthetic cardiac valves need not be excluded from MR procedures but care must be taken and the procedure terminated if discomfort or heating is experienced. A large database regarding MR compatibility and safety of implants has been compiled [27].
- It is prudent to exclude women in the first trimester of pregnancy from the inner controlled area.

Procedures for dealing with emergency situations such as cardiac arrest should be defined. Resuscitation equipment must not be taken into the inner controlled area and support staff must be fully informed of such procedures.

Care should be taken in attaching physiological monitoring equipment to the patient. High-impedance leads should be used and displays/recorders should be outside the 3 mT contour. Loops of cables should be avoided since these can lead to overheating and local burning

Adverse incidents arising from the use of MR equipment should be reported to the Medical Devices Agency. Further details regarding recommended practices in MR are given in [31].

In addition to these aspects of operational safety, working practices must ensure that exposure of patients and staff to the B_0 magnetic field, dB/dt fields, and RF fields complies with the guidelines referred to in §21.8.

- Stuchly *et al.* [38] recorded electric and magnetic fields around applicators of seven different shortwave diathermy units. Measurements were also made at the operator position and at various untreated areas of the patient during 11 treatment regimes using five types of applicators. They concluded that if the operator was behind the device console, exposure was usually within nationally recommended limits, although the intense fields within 0.5 m of the applicators and cables are a source of potential overexposure to the operator.
- Tzima and Martin [39] described fields around therapeutic and surgical diathermy equipment for many different treatments. They found that the

Box 21.4 Local rules for operation of diathermy and other thermal therapy equipment

Local rules should be drawn up to ensure compliance with national and international guidelines. They should include the following points:

- The location of shortwave and microwave diathermy or other thermal therapy equipment should be such that patients and staff not involved in the treatment are not unnecessarily close to cables, electrodes, or other applicators.
- The operator should stand at least 1 m away from electrodes and applicators when the equipment is switched on.
- The use of metallic couches or chairs and the proximity of other metallic objects within the treatment area that may be touched by the patient should be avoided. Jewellery and metallic objects on the patient's clothing should be removed before treatment.
- Cables should be positioned away from those parts of the patient's body outside the intended treatment field. Particular care should be taken to minimize exposure to the patient's eyes and testes.
- The use of other electrical equipment within 1 m of the diathermy or other thermal therapy equipment should be avoided.

highest field strengths are associated with continuous wave 27 MHz therapeutic diathermy equipment and recommended that the operator should be at least 1 m away from the applicators and cables in the case of CW capacitive treatments, 0.5–0.8 m for pulsed capacitive treatments, and 0.2 m for pulsed inductive treatments to comply with the recommendations of the NRPB. No special precautions were considered necessary for users of surgical diathermy equipment. With this type of equipment, the greatest hazard is the risk of burns to the patient due to poor contact between the dispersive electrode and the skin or due to a break in the lead to this electrode.

- The HCN [23] considers that there is evidence that its recommended exposure limits are sometimes considerably exceeded in close proximity to certain equipment used in physical therapy and therefore recommend that measurements of field strengths are made near such equipment.
- Docker *et al.* [40] and the Chartered Society of Physiotherapy [41] have produced guidelines for the safe use of shortwave and microwave therapy equipment, respectively.

Generally, fields around inductive applicators are more spatially restricted than those associated with capacitive applicators. It is important to limit the time the operator is exposed to the relatively high fields close to applicators and cables.

The addition of electromagnetically induced hyperthermia to radiotherapy or chemotherapy has been shown to improve clinical outcome in the treatment of some tumours. In addition to making analogous measurements to those made around physiotherapy equipment for devices used for superficial hyperthermia treatment, it is prudent to make measurements of stray fields around clinical devices such as those used to induce whole-body hyperthermia in view of the higher power levels employed.

- Bassen and Coakley [42] outlined a useful set of microwave safety considerations for microwave hyperthermia and diathermy devices.
- Chou [43] discusses general safety considerations for clinical hyperthermia
- Guidelines for the protection of operators have been drawn up by the Japanese Society of Hyperthermic Oncology [44].

21.10 Electromagnetic interference with medical equipment

The incidence of reports of adverse effects on medical devices from EM interference (EMI) has increased over recent years. Problems with devices such as apnea monitors, electrically powered wheelchairs, and pacemakers have been encountered and consequences have ranged from inconvenience to death.

- The IEC [45] requires a minimum immunity level of 3 V m^{-1} in the frequency range 26–1000 MHz for medical devices.
- General guidance in evaluating electromagnetic immunity of medical devices to radiofrequency fields is provided in [46, 47].

Factors that determine the level of interference include the level of coupling between device and the source and

Box 21.5 The use of emergency service radio handsets on hospital premises

- Hospitals should have a local policy regarding the use of radio handsets on their premises. The following points should be considered when formulating such policies.
- *General precautions*: awareness of the significant hazard posed by radio transmissions from emergency portable radios, disable periodic transmission of identity signal, emergency personnel to use alternative, non-transmitting communications systems such as radio-pagers during non-emergency visits to hospital premises.
- *Police/Fire Service radios*: handsets should not be used to transmit except in emergency situations. In the case of an emergency, police/fire personnel should contact the senior nurse, informing them of the use of handsets. Handsets should not be used at a distance of less than 3 m from a patient.
- *Ambulance Service radios*: handsets should not be used to establish or answer a voice call in intensive care units or cardiac care units or within 3 m of any patient connected to any form of electromedical equipment. Before transmitting from their handset, ambulance personnel should contact the senior nurse, informing them of the use of the handset.
- *Use of radios during major incidents*: areas should be identified where emergency service transmissions may be authorized subject to appropriate monitoring of patients connected to electromedical equipment that may be potentially affected. Particular attention should be given to areas adjacent to administration and accident and emergency departments.

their separation, the frequency of the carrier signal, and the nature of any modulation. Devices may be 'hardened' against the effects of interference by employing suitable shielding, grounding, and filtering. Care must be taken that any modification to the design or housing of a medical device does not result in an increased susceptibility to EM interference; similar checks should be made after servicing or repair.

There are numerous reports concerning the potential health hazard arising from EM interference with implanted pacemakers. Effects on pacemakers arising from electrocautery, radiofrequency ablation, radar, welding systems, leaking microwave ovens, and electromagnetic surveillance systems that may cause asynchronous pacing have been identified. Asynchronous pacing may be arrhythmogenic and may provoke ventricular fibrillation. Pacemakers can be affected by both electric and magnetic power-frequency (50/ 60 Hz) fields but their sensitivity and the severity of effects are very dependent on design and model.

21.10.1 Interference from mobile communication systems

The normal use of present-day mobile telephones may indirectly result in health hazards by interfering with vital medical equipment, including the normal functioning of pacemakers. It has been recommended that for patients with implanted pacemakers, hand-held telephones should be worn at least 15–20 cm from the pacemaker and preferably used with the ear contralateral to the location of the pacemaker.

Published information and guidance regarding the compatibility of mobile communication equipment with medical devices is somewhat conflicting. The MDA [48] reports the results of a large study conducted at 18 locations in which the effects of a wide range of radio handsets on 178 different medical devices were studied. Handsets were grouped as emergency radios (as used by emergency services personnel and operating between 28 and 470 MHz with power as high as 10 W), security radios (two-way radios and VHF/UHF radio handsets used by security, maintenance, and portering staff), cell phones (analogue and digital mobile phones), and cordless phones (pagers, radio computer local area networks). Overall, the medical devices suffered EMI from handsets in 23% of tests, and of these cases, 43% were considered serious since they would have had a direct impact on patient care. The likelihood of interference was strongly dependent upon the type of handset involved. At 1 m distance, 41%, 35%, and 4% of the medical devices suffered EMI from emergency radios, security radios, and cell phones, respectively. No significant effects were recorded due to the cordless phone group. Physiological monitors, defibrillators, and external pacemakers were the most severely affected.

21.10.2 Interference from emergency service vehicle radios

The two-way radios in emergency service vehicles may also interfere with electromedical devices [49]. If emergency vehicles park within 5 m of patient treatment areas where sensitive electromedical equipment is used, such as intensive care or coronary care units, a risk assessment should be performed to determine whether:

- sensitive electromedical equipment is located at points close to parked ambulances

- staff have experienced interference events
- interference events could have potentially serious consequences.

Actions taken where risks are found would include:

- display of warning notices outside the building requesting emergency service personnel not to make radio transmissions within certain areas
- display of warning notices inside the building to alert staff to the possibility of interference
- training ward staff in recognition of interference events
- where the risk is high, relocation of parking bays further from the building should be considered.

Precautions should also be taken with regard to electromedical equipment taken inside ambulances:

- to identify equipment liable to interference problems
- to identify areas with high field strengths within ambulances where equipment should not be placed
- to ensure that all staff have appropriate training
- to avoid use of handportable radios inside ambulances.

21.11 References

1 National Council on Radiation Protection and Measurements (1986). *Biological effects and exposure criteria for radiofrequency electromagnetic fields.* NCRP Report No. 86. NCRP, Bethesda, MD.

2 International Commission on Non-Ionising Protection (1998). Guidelines for limiting exposure to time-varying electric, magnetic and electromagnetic fields (up to 300 GHz). *Health Phys.*, **74**, 494–522.

3 National Institute of Environmental Health Sciences (1998). *Assessment of health effects from exposure to power-line frequency electric and magnetic fields* (ed. C. J. Portier and M. S. Wolfe). NIH Publication 98-3981. NIEHS/NIH, Research Triangle Park, NC 27709.

4 National Research Council (1997). *Possible health effects of exposure to residential electric and magnetic field.* National Academy Press, Washington, DC.

5 National Radiation Protection Board (1993). Restrictions on human exposure to static and time varying electromagnetic fields and radiation. *Doc. NRPB*, **4** (5), 1–69.

6 Health Council of the Netherlands: ELF Electromagnetic Fields Committee (1992). *Extremely low frequency electromagnetic fields and health.* Report no. 1992/07. HCN, Den Haag.

7 Moulder, J. E. (1998) Power-frequency fields and cancer. *Crit. Rev. Biomed. Eng.*, **26**, 1–116.

8 Stuchly, M. A. (1998). Biological concerns in wireless communications. *Crit. Rev. Biomed. Eng.*, **26**, 117–51.

9 National Council on Radiation Protection and Measurements (1981). *Radiofrequency electromagnetic fields: properties, quantities and units, biophysical interaction and measurements.* NCRP Report No. 67. NCRP, Bethesda, MD.

10 National Council on Radiation Protection and Measurements (1993). *A practical guide to the determination of human exposure to radiofrequency fields.* NCRP Report No. 119. NCRP, Bethesda, MD.

11 Gabriel, C., Gabriel, S., and Corthout, E. (1996). The dielectric properties of biological tissues: I. Literature survey. *Phys. Med. Biol.*, **41**, 2231–49.

12 Gabriel, S., Lau, R. W., and Gabriel, C. (1996). The dielectric properties of biological tissues: II. Measurements in the frequency range 10 Hz to 20 GHz. *Phys. Med. Biol.*, **41**, 2251–69.

13 Gabriel, S., Lau, R. W., and Gabriel, C. (1996). The dielectric properties of biological tissues: III. Parametric models for the dielectric spectrum of tissues. *Phys. Med. Biol.*, **41**, 2271–93.

14 Bowman, J., Kelsh, M., and Kaune, W. (1998). *Manual for measuring occupational electric and magnetic field exposures,* National Institute for Occupational Safety and Health, Cincinnati, OH.

15 Valberg, P., Kaune, W. T., and Wilson, B. (1995). Designing EMF experiments: what is required to characterize 'exposure'? *Bioelectromagnetics*, **16**, 396–406.

16 International Electrotechnical Committee (1995). *Medical electrical equipment–Part 2: Particular requirements for the safety of magnetic resonance equipment for medical diagnosis.* IEC 60601-2-33. IEC, Geneva.

17 Institute of Electrical and Electronics Engineers (1997). *IEEE recommended practice for the measurement of potentially hazardous electromagnetic fields–RF and microwave.* C95.3–1991. IEEE, New York.

18 Durney, C. H., Massoudi, H., and Iskander, M. F. (1986). *Radiofrequency radiation dosimetry handbook* (4th edn). USAFSAM-TR-85-73. USAF School of Aerospace Medicine, Brooks Air Force Base, TX 78235-5301.

19 Kowalzuk, C. I., Sienkiewicz, Z. J., and Saunders, R. D. (1991). *Biological effects of exposure to non-ionising electromagnetic fields and radiation: static electric and magnetic fields.* NRPB-R238. NRPB, Chilton.

20 International Commission on Non-Ionising Protection (1994). Guidelines on limits of exposure to static magnetic fields. *Health Phys.*, **66**, 100–6.

21 National Radiation Protection Board (1998). NRPB response statement: national and international exposure standards for electric and magnetic fields July 1998. *Radiological Protection Bulletin* No. 204, 26–7. NRPB, Chilton.

22 Chadwick, P. J. (1998). *Occupational exposure to electromagnetic fields: practical application of NRPB guidance.* NRPB-R301. NRPB, Chilton.

23 Health Council of the Netherlands: Radiofrequency Radiation Committee (1998). Radiofrequency electromagnetic fields (300 Hz–300 GHz): summary of an advisory report. *Health Phys.*, **75**, 51–5.

24 Federal Communications Commission (1996). *Guidelines for evaluating the environmental effects of radiofrequency radiation.* Report and Order, ET Docket 93-62, FCC 96-326, 61 Federal Register 41006.

25 Institute of Electrical and Electronics Engineers (1997). *IEEE standard for safety levels with respect to human exposure to radiofrequency electromagnetic fields, 3 kHz to 300 GHz.* C95.1-1991. IEEE, New York.

26 Federal Communications Commission (1997). *Evaluating compliance with FCC guidelines for human exposure to*

radiofrequency electromagnetic fields. FCC OET Bulletin 65 (edition 97-01).

27 Shellock, F. G. and Kanal, E. (1996). *Magnetic resonance: bioeffects, safety and patient management*. Lippincott-Raven, Philadelphia/New York.

28 National Radiological Protection Board (1991). Limits on patient and volunteer exposure during clinical magnetic resonance diagnostic procedures. *Doc. NRPB*, **2** (1), 5–29.

29 International Radiation Protection Association/International Non-Ionising Radiation Committee (1991). Protection of the patient undergoing a magnetic resonance examination. *Health Phys.*, **61**, 923–8.

30 Food and Drug Administration (1988). Magnetic resonance diagnostic device; panel recommendation and report on petitions for MR classification. *Fed. Register*, **53**, 7525–9.

31 Medical Devices Directorate (1993). *Guidelines for magnetic resonance diagnostic equipment in clinical use with particular reference to safety*. MDD, Department of Health. HMSO, London.

32 National Radiological Protection Board (1991). Principles for the protection of patients and volunteers during clinical magnetic resonance diagnostic procedures. *Doc. NRPB*, **2** (1), 1–4.

33 Food and Drug Administration (1995). *MRI guidance update for dB/dt*. Office of Device Evaluation, Center for Devices and Radiological Health, Rockville, MD.

34 Food and Drug Administration (1997). *Guidance for magnetic resonance diagnostic devices–criteria for significant risk investigations*. Center for Devices and Radiological Health, Rockville, MD.

35 Food and Drug Administration (1998).*Guidance for the submission of premarket notifications for magnetic resonance diagnostic devices*. Center for Devices and Radiological Health, Rockville. MD.

36 National Electrical Manufacturers Association (1993). *Measurement procedure for time varying gradient fields (dB/dt) for magnetic resonance imaging systems*. MS 7-1993. NEMA, Rosslyn, VA.

37 National Electrical Manufacturers Association (1993). *Characterization of the specific absorption rate for magnetic resonance imaging systems*. MS 8-1993. NEMA, Rosslyn, VA.

38 Stuchly, M. A., Repacholi, M. H., Lecuyer, D. W., and Mann, R. D. (1982). Exposure to the operator and patient during short wave diathermy treatments. *Health Phys.*, **42**, 341–66.

39 Tzima, E. and Martin, C. J. (1994). An evaluation of safe practices to restrict exposure to electric and magnetic fields from therapeutic and surgical diathermy equipment. *Physiol. Measure.*, **15**, 201–16.

40 Docker, M., Bazin, S., Dyson, M., Kirk, D. C., Kitchen S., Low, J., *et al.* (1992). Guidelines for the safe use of continuous shortwave therapy equipment. *Physiotherapy*, **78**, 755–7.

41 Chartered Society of Physiotherapy (1991). Guidelines for the safe use of microwave therapy equipment. *Physiotherapy*, **77**, 653–4.

42 Bassen, H. I. and Coakley, R. F. (1981). United States radiation safety and regulatory considerations for radiofrequency hyperthermia systems. *J. Microwave Power*, **16**, 215–26.

43 Chou, C. K. (1990). Safety considerations for clinical hyperthermia. In: *An introduction to the practical aspects of clinical hyperthermia* (ed. S. B. Field and J. W. Hand), pp. 533–64. Taylor & Francis, London.

44 Kikuchi, M., Amemiya, Y., Egawa, S., Onoyama, Y., Kato, H., Kanai, H., *et al.* (1993). Guidelines for the protection of operators occupationally-exposed personnel in hyperthermia treatment from the potential hazards to health. *Int. J. Hypertherm.*, **9**, 613–24.

45 International Electrotechnical Committee (1993). *Medical electrical equipment–Part 1: General requirements for safety*. IEC 60601-1-2. IEC, Geneva.

46 British Standards Institution (1997). BS EN 61000-4-3. *Electromagnetic compatibility (EMC). Part 4: Testing and measurement techniques. Section 3: Radiated radiofrequency, electromagnetic field immunity test*. BSI, London.

47 Institute of Electrical and Electronics Engineers (1997). *Recommended practice for an on-site ad hoc test method for estimating radiated electromagnetic immunity of medical devices to specific radio-frequency transmitters*. C63.18. IEEE, New York.

48 Medical Devices Agency (1997). *Electromagnetic compatibility of medical devices with mobile communications*. MDA Device Bulletin DB9702. MDA, Department of Health, Wetherby.

49 Medical Devices Agency (1999). *Emergency service radios and mobile data terminals: compatibility problems with medical devices*. MDA Device Bulletin DB9902. MDA, Department of Health, Wetherby.

Chapter 22
Ultrasound

S. D. Pye and B. Zeqiri

22.1 Introduction

Over the past 50 years, ultrasound has become an established technique in many areas of medicine, including diagnostic imaging, therapy, lithotripsy, and surgery. As with any technique that delivers energy to the body, risks are associated with its use and these must be assessed to ensure the overall effect on the patient is beneficial. Ultrasound can produce many bioeffects: in diagnostic applications these may be subtle, whereas in surgical techniques tissue is destroyed on a macroscopic scale. Potential biohazards of ultrasound are tissue heating, cavitation, acoustic radiation forces, and mechanical strain due to particle displacement. Risk factors are often difficult to quantify because much of our knowledge about the way ultrasound interacts with tissue is still at an early stage of development. Given this limited understanding, specific ultrasonic techniques need to be assessed individually to gauge their risks and benefits, and this chapter is organized to do that. Following a general description of ultrasound and its propagation, various bioeffects and measurement techniques are described. There are then separate sections which consider exposure, standards, and practical guidance measures for each of the four main areas of medical application.

22.2 The ultrasound field

22.2.1 Propagation of ultrasound in biological tissue

Ultrasonic radiation generated within the human body propagates through tissue as a series of time-varying local tissue compressions (pressure increases) and rarefactions (pressure decreases). Ultrasound is defined as a form of mechanical radiation in which these pressure changes occur at frequencies greater than 20 kHz. Within solid materials, two types of ultrasonic wave can be propagated and these are distinguished by the direction of motion of the individual 'elements' of the medium relative to the direction of energy transfer. If parallel to the direction of energy transfer, the ultrasound disturbance is known as a compressional or longitudinal wave; if perpendicular, it is known as a shear or transverse wave. Biological tissues are generally unable to support shear waves, so that propagation within biological materials almost exclusively involves compressional waves. Bone is an important exception because it is able to support the propagation of shear waves.

22.2.2 Ultrasound generation and the ultrasonic field

The majority of transducers for diagnostic and therapeutic applications operate in the megahertz range and use the piezoelectric principle. The transducer is coupled to the patient using water-based gel. It lies beyond the scope of this chapter to describe the complexities of the fields generated by transducers used in the full range of medical applications. This is left to more extensive texts such as Ziskin and Lewin [1]. Figure 22.1 illustrates the characteristic features of the ultrasound pulses generated by a range of different medical ultrasonic devices.

22.2.3 Finite-amplitude propagation of ultrasound

At the frequencies and acoustic pressures used for medical ultrasound, wave propagation cannot be regarded as a linear process [2]. The propagation speeds of the compressional and rarefactional half-cycles differ, resulting in the acoustic waveform undergoing progressive non-linear or finite-amplitude distortion during propagation. The resulting acoustic waveforms may be strongly 'shocked' (a very rapid change from compression to rarefaction, illustrated by the largest half-cycle of the lithotripsy pulse in Figure 22.1d). When viewed in

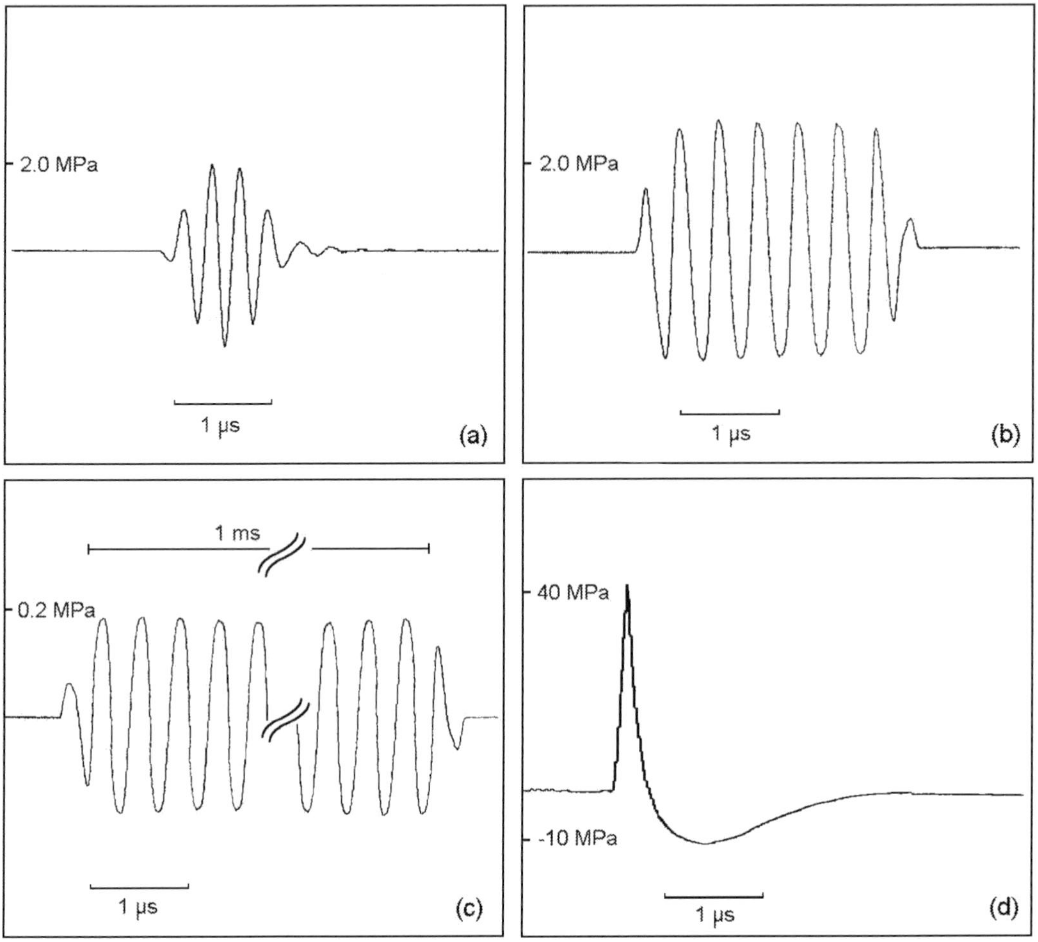

Figure 22.1 Pressure waveforms of ultrasonic devices, measured in water on the acoustic axis: (a) diagnostic scanner operating in B mode, centre frequency 3.5 MHz; (b) diagnostic scanner in pulsed Doppler mode, centre frequency 2.5 MHz; (c) physiotherapy unit in 'pulsed' mode, centre frequency 2.5 MHz; (d) extracorporeal lithotripter, centre frequency 0.5 MHz. Typical values of pressure amplitudes are shown.

the frequency domain, energy has been pumped out of the fundamental frequency into higher harmonics of the source disturbance. Even in diagnostic imaging, scanning through a full bladder or an aqueous path such as amniotic fluid may lead to shocked acoustic pulses. This is because the low absorption of the higher harmonics in the aqueous fluid leads to a progressive increase in the harmonic content of the pulse as it traverses the fluid path. One result of this may be enhanced tissue heating due to the significantly greater absorption of these higher harmonics in the tissues beyond the fluid path.

22.2.4 Concepts of exposure and dose in medical ultrasound

When considering ultrasound in relation to radiation protection, the terms *exposure* and *dose* are clearly important. Within the area of medical ultrasound, the first of these relates to the characteristics of the applied ultrasonic field which are determined under standard conditions and generally involve measurements in water. Consequent issues of applied *dose* relate to assessing the impact of this applied acoustic field on the clinical site of interest. There are several ways in which the acoustic field interacts with biological tissue and these are commonly divided into thermal and non-thermal mechanisms. Absorption of acoustic energy in tissue may generate a significant temperature increase, and these thermal mechanisms are described in §22.3.1. Alternatively, the passage of the ultrasound in a medium can lead to bubbles being generated, a process which is called cavitation and can produce cell damage. Cavitation is one of the non-thermal mechanisms described in

Table 22.1 Summary of some of the key acoustic parameters which are used to characterize the output of medical ultrasonic equipment

Parameter type	Parameter	Symbol (units)	Comments
Pressure	Peak-compressional (peak-positive)	p_+ (Pa)	Peak-positive pressure may play an important role in cavitation effects within lithotripter applications (§22.7), where pulse inversion may occur after reflection at interfaces
	Peak-rarefactional (peak-negative)	p_- (Pa)	Peak-negative pressure is related to the likelihood of cavitation occurring within a medium as it is a measure of the degree to which the medium is pulled apart (§22.3.2)
Derived intensity	Spatial-peak temporal-average intensity	I_{SPTA} (W cm^{-2})	I_{SPTA} represents an acoustic energy flow through unit area per second. Its magnitude is relevant to both thermal and non-thermal bioeffects
Power	Total acoustic power	P (W)	Total power is a key parameter influencing temperature rise and is most accurately determined using a radiation force balance (§22.4.1)
Beam properties	–6 dB beam-width	(mm)	Grid-like raster scans can be carried out to establish the spatial distribution of ultrasound, the beam area consists of all points within which the pulse-pressure-squared integral is greater than –6 dB of the peak in the scan
	–6 dB beam-area	(mm^2)	

§22.3.2. The concept of *dose* then becomes application specific because the same acoustic field (and therefore *exposure*) is applied for different clinical examinations–resulting in different *dose* levels. This arises because of the different nature of the path between the transducer generating the ultrasound field and the target site in terms of the tissues present and their acoustic and thermal properties.

22.2.5 Exposure parameters

The temporal and spatial distribution of ultrasound may be formally described through a series of parameters whose definition and measurement are embodied in international standards [3–5]. Measurement of these quantities is carried out in water, although the parameter definitions are general and are independent of the propagation medium. The interested reader is referred to these standards: here a summary of those parameters considered to be most important in assessing exposure are highlighted. Table 22.1 gives a summary of the important parameters and, wherever possible, a link is made between the observed parameter and the relevant bioeffect.

Acoustic pressures

Figure 22.1a illustrates an acoustic waveform generated by a diagnostic ultrasound system. It was determined using a calibrated hydrophone of the type described in §22.4.2. In principle, the hydrophone records the instantaneous pressure, p, at a point within the acoustic field. An important pressure-related parameter used in defining other acoustic quantities is the pulse-pressure-squared integral, p_i, which is defined as:

$$p_{\mathrm{i}} = \int p^2 \, \delta t$$

and is the time-integral of the square of the instantaneous acoustic pressure in the acoustic waveform, integrated over the whole of the waveform.

Derived acoustic intensities

It has been traditional to specify the acoustic field in terms of intensity parameters. Assuming plane-progressive acoustic waves, the instantaneous intensity may be derived directly from pressure measurements using the expression:

$$I = p^2/\rho c$$

where p is the instantaneous pressure, ρ is the density of water, and c is the propagation speed of ultrasound. The product ρc is the 'characteristic acoustic impedance' of water, and at 20°C its value is 1.48×10^6 kg m^{-2}s^{-1}.

Taking the example of the pulse waveform shown in Figure 22.1a, if we assume that all the pulses arriving at the field point at various times are identical, then the time-averaged intensity is obtained by multiplying the pulse-pressure-squared integral by the number of pulses arriving per second (the pulse repetition rate, p_{RR}) such that:

$$I_{\mathrm{TA}} = p_{\mathrm{RR}}\, p_i/\rho c$$

The maximum time-averaged intensity occurring anywhere within the acoustic field is known as the spatial-peak temporal-average intensity (I_{SPTA}).

Beam properties

In theory, the pressure distribution within an ultrasound beam can be characterized by scanning a hydrophone through the whole extent of the beam, and measuring the pressure at every point. A three-dimensional map of the pressure distribution can then be derived. In reality, a subset of parameters can usually be used to describe the pressure distribution, the most important parameter being the beam-width determined at a particular location. This is commonly defined as the –6 dB pulse beam-width, where the pulse-pressure-squared integral is determined at various positions, perpendicular to the transducer axis as shown in Figure 22.2 for a typical diagnostic ultrasound field. Figure 22.3 illustrates the relatively complex distribution of intensity generated by a physiotherapy transducer of the type which will be considered in §22.6.

Beam areas may be used to determine spatially-averaged parameters, such as the spatial-average temporal-average intensity. This is the time-averaged intensity determined over the –6 dB beam area, divided by the –6 dB beam area.

Total acoustic power

If the hydrophone is scanned in a plane perpendicular to the acoustic axis and the time-averaged intensity determined at all positions, then the total acoustic power, P, can be derived through an integration of this parameter over space such that:

$$P = \int_{\text{whole beam}} I_{\text{TA}}\ \delta A$$

22.3 Bioeffects

It is now accepted that there are two main mechanisms by which ultrasound interacts with tissue and these are commonly described as thermal and non-thermal effects. Thermal mechanisms lead to temperature rises within a medium. Non-thermal mechanisms comprise a range of mechanical effects, of which cavitation is generally considered to be the most important.

22.3.1 Thermal effects

As ultrasound propagates within tissue, its amplitude is modified by a number of processes, including diffraction, reflections at tissue boundaries, and scattering from small inhomogeneities. It will also undergo absorption, a localized process which converts ultrasonic energy to heat, leading to temperature rises whose magnitude and variation with exposure time is complex. Local temperature rise will depend on a number of parameters: the

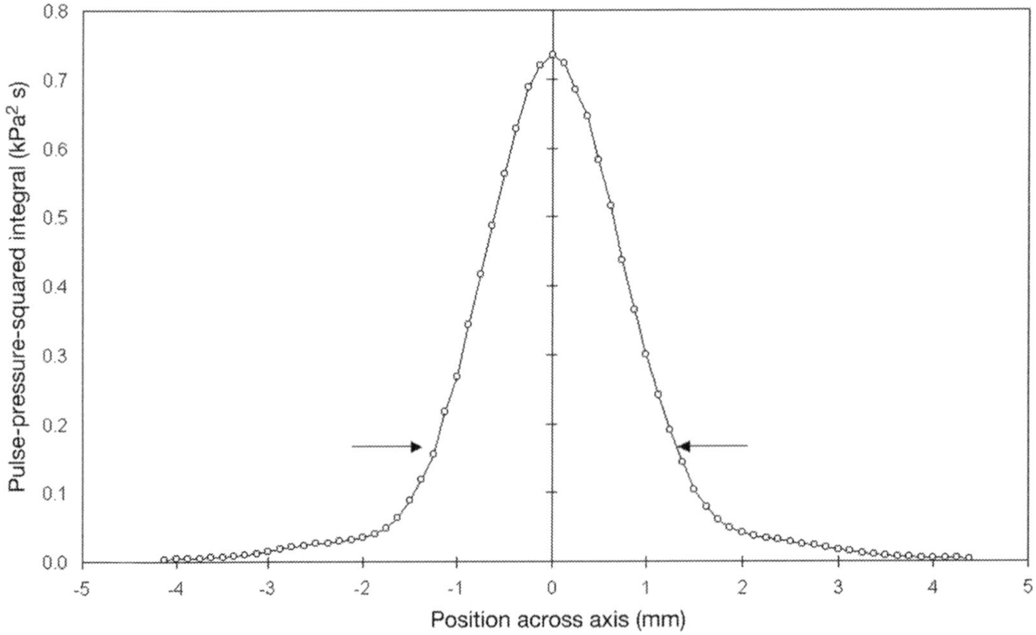

Figure 22.2 Diagram showing the distribution of acoustic energy at the focus of a typical diagnostic ultrasound scanner. The pulse-pressure-squared integral (p_i) is displayed as a function of position across the acoustic axis of the transducer. The –6 dB beam-width of the acoustic beam is indicated (as p_i is an energy-related parameter, the –6 dB point is defined when the quantity has fallen to 25% of the peak value).

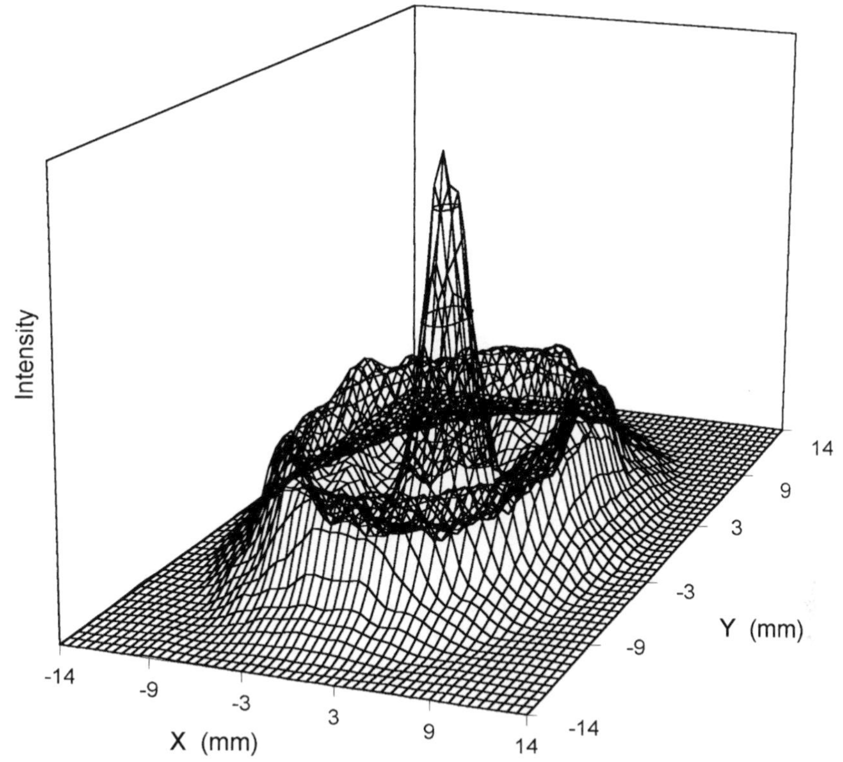

Figure 22.3 Two-dimensional raster-scan giving the distribution of intensity generated by a physiotherapy treatment head. Measurements were made using hydrophone scanning, 10 mm away from the face of the head which is vibrating at 1 MHz. Note the strong structure in the acoustic field, which arises due to interference of the ultrasound travelling from various parts of the treatment head.

characteristics of the ultrasonic field applied, such as the spatial distribution of intensity and the time-averaged power (*exposure*), the acoustic and thermal properties of the tissue, as well as perfusion processes such as blood flow which will redistribute any heat generated.

One important parameter influencing temperature rise is the ultrasonic absorption coefficient of the tissue. The magnitude of the absorption coefficient depends on macromolecular relaxation mechanisms rather than cellular level composition, and correlations have been made with the presence of collagen in tissues and high absorption coefficient values of tendon. Table 22.2 presents a listing of the absorption coefficients for several human tissues, along with a value for water presented for comparison.

The interested reader will find a number of compilations of acoustic and thermal property data for tissues, of which Bamber [6] and Duck [7] are the most recent. Care needs to be exercised when considering these values, as measurements of both the acoustic and thermal properties of tissue are difficult and large variations in values can occur. This may arise from differences in the measurement techniques but can also result from differences in specimen preparation.

In general, soft tissues have absorption coefficient values, α, which increase almost linearly with frequency, in a form commonly represented as:

$$\alpha = af^b$$

where f is the acoustic frequency and a and b are constants (b being generally in the range 1 to 1.3). While the absorption coefficients of typical soft tissues lie within the range 0.5–0.7 dB cm^{-1} MHz^{-1}, there are clearly a couple of notable exceptions in Table 22.2. Lung has an exceedingly high absorption coefficient due to the presence of air. However, for the liquid-filled lungs of the fetus, much lower absorption coefficient values can be expected, more representative of soft tissue. The second notable exception is bone, whose high absorption coefficient leads to a strong potential for heating at the bone surface. The majority of the acoustic power coupled into the bone will be absorbed in its first few millimetres, leading to heat generation at the soft-tissue–bone interface. Values given in Table 22.2 refer to adult skull bone.

Table 22.2 Tabulation of absorption coefficient values for a few human biological tissues, taken from Bamber [6]. A distinction is made within the literature between attenuation and absorption, where the former comprises contributions from both absorption and scattering. In general, the contribution of scattering to attenuation in soft tissues is small and absorption and attenuation may be taken as being approximately equal

Tissue type	Absorption coefficient (dB cm^{-1})	Frequency (MHz)
Bone (skull)	12	1
Lung	40	1
Liver	0.8	1
	5	5
Tendon	16	5
Water	0.055	5

The situation will be different for fetal bone, and this will alter as bone mineralization takes place within the uterus. By 15 weeks gestation, fetal bone is sufficiently ossified to have an absorption coefficient very similar to that of adult bone.

Although the absorption coefficient of a biological tissue plays an important role in establishing thermal risk, it is important to appreciate that an assessment of this hazard requires a clinical model representing the path from the transducer to the biological site of interest. This is because overlying tissue will attenuate the ultrasonic power reaching a target site.

22.3.2 Non-thermal effects

In addition to the effect of heating any medium through which it propagates, ultrasound has several other effects which are given the umbrella term of 'non-thermal'. These include particle displacement, cavitation, acoustic radiation forces, and fluid streaming.

Particle displacement

The simplest non-thermal effect to appreciate is particle displacement. For a typical diagnostic ultrasound pulse in the megahertz frequency range, the particle displacement amplitude is less than 100 nm. For a lithotripsy pulse with much larger amplitude and lower centre frequency, the displacement amplitude may be more than 10 µm – at least a hundred times greater than the diagnostic situation. Relative displacements cause strain within the propagation medium, and probably contribute significantly to the fragmentation of calculi and soft-tissue damage that occurs during lithotripsy.

Acoustic cavitation

In its most general sense, cavitation refers to the formation of cavities (bubbles) within a liquid medium. When an ultrasound wave passes through a liquid, bubbles may begin to form at pre-existing nucleation sites in the fluid. Expansion occurs during the rarefaction (negative pressure) phase of the wave where the tensile forces are trying to pull the medium apart. The larger the negative pressure, the longer it is sustained, and the more nucleation sites there are, the more bubbles will form. If the ultrasound wave is continuous, bubbles may grow in size over many cycles due to the process of rectified diffusion. Ultrasound pulses that only consist of a few cycles are less likely to cause bubble growth. However, even single-cycle pulses may cause bubbles to form rapidly if they have sufficiently large pressure amplitude. Bubbles that are formed very rapidly in a low-viscosity fluid expand well beyond their equilibrium size due to inertia. Their subsequent collapse can be very violent and destructive, and the gaseous contents of the bubble may be compressed enormously and reach temperatures of thousands of degrees kelvin. Free radicals may be generated. Very rapid expansion and violent collapse is termed 'inertial cavitation' because it is dominated by the inertia of the fluid set in motion when the bubble expands. Other forms of bubble formation are termed 'non-inertial' and are controlled by factors such as the surface tension and viscosity of the fluid, and the gas content of the bubbles. Bubbles that are formed over many cycles of an ultrasound wave may be driven into oscillation of large or small amplitude and set up flow in the fluid surrounding them. This is referred to as 'microstreaming'.

Both inertial and non-inertial cavitation can be induced in aerated water using therapy ultrasound devices and lithotripters. Clinically, cavitation bubbles have been detected during lithotripsy, both in the blood and within the kidney. There is currently no definitive evidence of clinically significant cavitation damage *in vivo* caused by either diagnostic or physiotherapy beams for tissues that do not contain pre-existing gas bubbles.

Radiation force, stress, and streaming

An acoustic wave exerts a net force on the medium through which it is propagating and on any surface where it is reflected or absorbed. This is known as the 'radiation force'. It arises because any finite-amplitude wave is not fully described by the simple first-order wave equation. A more rigorous analysis indicates that partial absorption or reflection results in a net transfer of momentum in the direction of wave propagation. The radiation force (or pressure) is directly proportional to the local intensity of the wave (§22.4.1).

For a diagnostic pulse or a therapy beam, the radiation pressure varies with the local intensity across the wavefront. This results in shearing forces. The stresses produced in the medium are complex and require the use of tensors to describe them adequately. For a diagnostic beam in soft tissue, the radiation pressure gradients involved are relatively small, being of the order of a few pascals per millimetre [2].

Where the propagation medium is an absorbing fluid, the radiation force exerted when ultrasonic energy is absorbed causes the fluid to move in the direction of propagation of the wave. This effect is referred to as *streaming*. Even though water has a small coefficient of absorption, it can still be caused to stream at velocities of several centimetres per second by a pulsed diagnostic ultrasound beam. Streaming and radiation stress are relatively subtle effects in diagnostic beams, but real ones nevertheless.

22.4 Measurement devices

The aim of this section is to describe those measurement devices which are used to establish the acoustic exposure parameters given in §22.2.5. Reviews of available measurement technology specifically for medical ultrasound are to be found in [1, 8]. The emphasis here will be on those methods whose use has become accepted, and upon which standardized measurement procedures are based.

22.4.1 Measurement of total acoustic power

As indicated in §22.2.5, acoustic power represents an important parameter when assessing thermal effects of ultrasound. It is generally measured by determining the radiation force generated by the beam (§22.3.2). This is defined as the time-averaged force experienced by an object, when placed within an ultrasonic field. For a plane wave which is totally absorbed by a target, the magnitude of the radiation force on the target (F) is related to the total power in the beam (P) and the propagation speed of ultrasound in the medium (c) through the simple relationship $F = P/c$. As the propagation speed in water is approximately 1480 m s^{-1} at 20°C, each watt of acoustic power will generate a radiation force of 0.67 mN, equivalent to 69 mg, which constitutes a readily measurable force. Systems which measure power on this basis are known as 'radiation force balances'.

A key component of a force balance is the nature of the object, or target, placed within the ultrasonic beam. Approximations to totally reflecting and totally absorbing force balance targets are commonly used. The former is most frequently implemented as a thin-walled stainless-steel air-backed cone of angle 90°, which represents an excellent approximation to a totally reflecting interface. A schematic of the basic set-up used for power measurements is given in Figure 22.4 for a reflecting target configuration, where the target is totally immersed in water. Ultrasound, assumed to impinge on the target at the same angle of incidence over the whole of the beam, is reflected away onto the walls of the container vessel which are coated with a sound-absorbing material. Care must be taken to ensure that the water in the force balance remains degassed. Bubbles formed in the water at high powers will cause the balance to under-read, due to scattering of the ultrasound before it reaches the target. Suitable methods for degassing water include boiling and cooling, the use of sodium sulphite solution, and bubbling helium gas through the water [9].

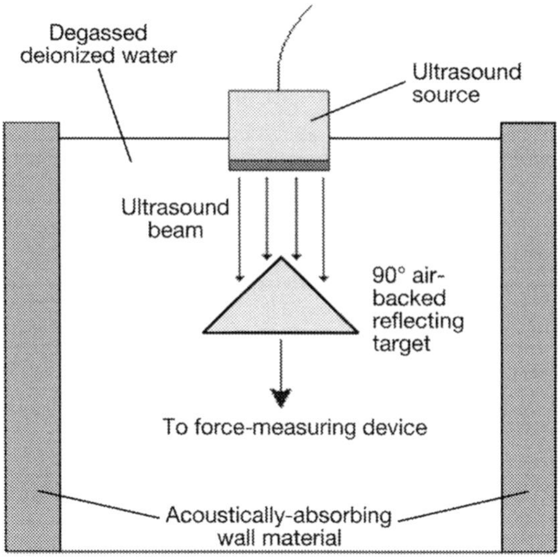

Figure 22.4 Schematic representation of a radiation force balance for determining the acoustic power of medical ultrasonic equipment. The nature of the force measurement instrument depends on the power being measured. For medical diagnostic equipment, the relatively low powers require the use of a sensitive microbalance, while for physiotherapy equipment, a top-loading chemical balance may be used.

A number of commercial force balances are now available with different sensitivities suitable for diagnostic and therapeutic power levels. They represent an important measurement tool as they are generally low-cost, portable, easy-to-use, and capable of achieving power measurements with an overall 95% uncertainty of better than ±10%. They should be traceable to national standards using an acoustic calibration technique. This may be done either through a transducer of known acoustic output, referred to as a 'checksource', or against another force balance which has itself been calibrated.

Methods of power measurement have been reviewed [1, 8] and their specification is embodied in IEC 61161 [10].

22.4.2 Measurement of acoustic pressure

While the total acoustic power delivered by a medical ultrasonic transducer is an important parameter in assessing the effect of the applied field on tissue, it provides no spatial information concerning the energy deposition. The accepted way of measuring this is to use ultrasound hydrophones to probe the temporal and spatial distribution of acoustic pressure. Their operation is based on the piezoelectric principle, where the acoustic pressure waveform incident upon a disc of piezoelectric material, such as polyvinylidene fluoride (pvdf) or the ceramic material PZT, generates a voltage waveform which in principle should be an exact replica of the incident pressure waveform. Several hydrophone types are commercially available, ranging from membrane hydrophones made from pvdf to needle-type hydrophones where the active element, made from either pvdf or PZT, is mounted on the end of a hypodermic needle [8]. The performance of the hydrophone, assessed in terms of its suitability for characterizing the acoustic field, depends sensitively on the design and how this impinges on a number of attributes of performance, including spatial resolution, directionality, stability, frequency response, linearity, and its non-perturbing nature. The suitability of a hydrophone for a specific application will also depend on the characteristics of the acoustic field being measured; for example, whether the transducer is driven in pulsed or continuous modes, as well as the magnitudes of the pressures generated.

The calibration of a hydrophone is crucial in determining absolute pressures and intensities and should be traceable to national standards. Typical sensitivities lie in the range 10 to 50 nV Pa^{-1}. The hydrophone is usually used in conjunction with a preamplifier to boost the signal level. The uncertainties achievable depend on frequency and lie within the range $\pm6\%$ to $\pm12\%$ (95% confidence) over the frequency range 1 to 20 MHz. It is worth bearing in mind that useful information can sometimes be derived from uncalibrated hydrophones; for example, beam dimensions and temporal pulse shapes for amplitude modulated waveforms (see §22.6).

The hydrophone provides one component of the measurement system. The hydrophone must be positioned at multiple locations within the acoustic field, and a sophisticated system incorporating mechanical scanning and computerized data acquisition is often required. The use of a hydrophone to characterize the acoustic output of medical ultrasonic equipment is specified in a number of standards, the main ones being IEC 61102, IEC 61220, and IEC 61157 [3–5]. These measurements are not easy, and interlaboratory comparisons have highlighted the differences that can occur.

22.5 Diagnostic ultrasound

22.5.1 Exposure

Diagnostic scanners have several different imaging modes: B mode, M mode, colour Doppler, and pulsed Doppler. Other diagnostic ultrasound devices include cardiotocographs (CTGs) and simple audio Doppler instruments for fetal heart detection. The powers, intensities, and pressures generated by CTGs and other fetal heart detectors are generally the lowest of all the diagnostic modes and are well below the levels where significant temperature rises or cavitation might occur *in vivo*. There appear to be very few structures within the body that act as natural nucleation sites for cavitation, and so the short, high-frequency pulses produced by diagnostic scanners have more potential for producing thermal effects than cavitational ones. A notable exception to this is the use of ultrasonic contrast agents. These contain millions of micron-sized bubbles and are likely to significantly reduce the threshold for cavitation *in vivo* (see also §22.3.2).

Several surveys of diagnostic instruments have been carried out over the past 30 years. They provide an indication of how machine outputs are changing as technology develops, and how exposure conditions differ between modes of operation. The overall impression is that acoustic outputs have risen steadily—perhaps by a

Table 22.3 Exposure data from 223 diagnostic transducers, measured in water, reprinted by permission of Elsevier Science from Henderson *et al.* [11]. The median value of the data is given, with the range shown in parentheses. There is a factor of approximately three in median I_{SPTA} values from B mode—to M mode—to colour Doppler—to pulsed Doppler. There is also a considerable overlap between modes, so that the highest B-mode intensity values overlap the lowest pulsed Doppler values. Median pulse amplitudes and powers are broadly similar for all modes but show a considerable range

Application	p_- (MPa)	I_{SPTA} (mW cm^{-2})	Acoustic power (mW)
Imaging and M mode	2.4 (0.45–5.5)		
B mode only		34 (0.3–991)	75 (0.3–285)
M mode only		106 (11–430)	9 (1–68)
Colour Doppler imaging	2.38 (0.46–4.25)	290 (21–2050)	90 (15–440)
Spectral pulsed Doppler	2.1 (0.67–5.3)	1180 (173–9080)	100 (10–440)

factor of three since the first surveys of the early 1970s. Some level of increase is not surprising, given the efforts of manufacturers to achieve ever better signal-to-noise ratios, especially for Doppler techniques. A factor which is likely to cause a further increase in patient exposures is a relaxation of the regulations governing the acoustic outputs of scanners sold in the United States (§22.5.2). Recent exposure data from various scanning modes are summarized in Table 22.3.

In situ exposure

In order to reliably assess the risk from ultrasound exposure, the aim must be to assess the exposure *in situ*, at particular biological sites. The estimation of *in situ* exposure from water-derived acoustic output values, such as those in Table 22.3, is not straightforward. The difficulty arises partly from the different acoustic properties of the water and tissue, which affect the propagation of ultrasound in fundamentally different ways. Furthermore, for thermal effects, there is no simple relationship between the acoustic output parameters determined in water and the resultant spatial and time variation of the temperature rise generated in tissue. There are currently two approaches to this problem:

- the use of simple theoretical models which take the water-derived acoustic parameters and provide an estimate of the temperature distribution generated in tissue (§22.5.2)
- the use of thermal test objects, fabricated from materials whose acoustic and thermal properties mimic biological tissue and within which a thermal sensor is positioned to directly record the temperature rise. Recent studies of pulsed Doppler equipment carried out by the UK National Physical Laboratory found that the temperature rises generated in soft-tissue thermal test objects were small. However, when bone mimic test objects were used, temperature rises exceeded 4°C for half of the scanning probes tested, with the highest value being in excess of 8°C.

22.5.2 Standards and guidance

One in four imaging investigations in the developed world are now carried out using diagnostic ultrasound. The organization that has exerted the most influence over acoustic outputs to date is the US Food and Drug Administration (FDA). Prior to 1993, the FDA 510(k) regulatory document required manufacturers selling ultrasound scanners in the USA to measure acoustic output parameters and control them according to arbitrary, application-specific limits. In 1993, the FDA adopted an alternative ('Track 3') method of regulation into the 510(k) document [2]. This is commonly known as the 'output display standard' or ODS. The ODS uses simple theoretical models for calculations of *in situ* exposure. In particular, ultrasonic measurements made in water are reduced ('derated') by assuming a soft-tissue attenuation coefficient of 0.3 dB $cm^{-1}MHz^{-1}$. The maximum derated I_{SPTA} must not exceed 720 mW cm^{-2}, except in ophthalmic imaging where it must not exceed 50 mW cm^{-2}.

The ODS allows manufacturers to increase acoustic intensities for almost all modes of application, so long as they provide biophysical indicators of potential hazard on the display monitor. The biophysical indicators specified in the ODS are the thermal index (TI) and the mechanical index (MI). The TI is the ratio of the total acoustic power to the acoustic power required to raise tissue temperature by 1°C, under certain defined conditions. The MI is given by the maximum derated rarefactional pressure divided by the square root of the centre frequency of the pulse. The ODS defines various conditions when TI and MI need to be displayed by the scanner.

For several years the International Electrotechnical Commission (IEC) has been grappling with the issue of developing an equipment classification scheme similar to that already in place for lasers. The idea is to define a class of equipment, Class A, which is unequivocally safe irrespective of how it is used. In contrast, Class B equipment could produce bioeffects, and the onus would be on the operator to ensure that the resultant risk was properly managed. The thresholds which would demarcate Class A and Class B equipment have been the subject of considerable and ongoing debate. Current draft standards specify Class A equipment as those systems which generate equilibrium temperature rises of less than 4°C and peak-rarefactional pressures less than 4 MPa. It is proposed that the values of these quantities for any diagnostic scanner will be determined through test method standards which are being developed in parallel. One such document will relate to the use of thermal test objects in determining equilibrium temperature rise. The 4°C temperature rise may seem high but it should be appreciated that this is not a 'whole-body' temperature rise but is applied to a highly localized volume of tissue (see Table 21.2, for comparison with temperature rises specified for EM fields).

Safety literature

Several national and international bodies have issued guidelines and safety statements concerning diagnostic ultrasound. Within Europe, the European Committee for Medical Ultrasound Safety (ECMUS) reviews the scientific literature and issues regular safety statements on behalf of the European Federation for Ultrasound in Medicine and Biology. Internationally, the World Federation for Ultrasound in Medicine and Biology has issued reviews and safety statements concerning potential thermal and non-thermal hazards of diagnostic ultrasound. These are summarized in [2].

The British Medical Ultrasound Society (BMUS) has recently published practical safety guidelines, including the action that operators should take when particular values of TI and MI are reached during scanning [12].

One of the main motivations for studies of ultrasound safety is the fact that almost 100% of fetuses in the developed world receive one or more ultrasound scans. Since the majority of fetuses scanned are entirely normal, it is extremely important to ensure that there are no significant risks associated with exposure to ultrasound. There are currently no independently confirmed epidemiological studies demonstrating adverse effects from the use of diagnostic ultrasound. The ECMUS has published a series of tutorial papers, some of which evaluate the most significant laboratory and clinical studies [13–15]. Reviews of new literature concerning safety and bioeffects are published regularly in the *European Journal of Ultrasound.*

The greatest risk to the patient is certainly that of misdiagnosis, and Wells [16] gives a graphic illustration of this. However, there is no room for complacency concerning ultrasonic bioeffects, given the trend towards higher exposures and the rapid introduction of new techniques such as endocavity imaging, contrast agents, colour Doppler, and harmonic imaging.

Current US regulations assume that users will take responsibility for interpreting the information scanners give them about potential hazards. TI and MI are intended to assist the user in reducing patient exposure. For this process to be successful, users must understand the biophysical indicators that are in use, and also know how to alter machine settings so as to reduce exposure. Both these aspects require users to receive specific training that has not generally been carried out in the past. Future IEC standards are likely to continue devolving the responsibility for exposure control from the manufacturers of ultrasound scanners to the users.

22.6 Therapy ultrasound

22.6.1 Exposure

Physiotherapists use ultrasound extensively for the treatment of acute soft-tissue injuries, and to a lesser extent for the treatment of chronic conditions. The number of therapy machines in clinical use in the UK is around 10 000 and approximately 3–4 million treatments per year are administered. Therapy is usually carried out at frequencies between 0.7 and 4 MHz, using a treatment head which contains a single disc-shaped piezoelectric transducer. Relatively low spatial-average intensities of 0.2–1.0 W cm^{-2} are favoured by physiotherapists in the UK, with the intention of minimizing tissue heating and promoting non-thermal healing effects. In other parts of the world, notably the United States and Australia, treatments at higher intensities of 1–2 W cm^{-2} are common.

A therapy head produces an unfocused beam, and is operated in either continuous or pulsed-wave mode. It should be noted that the 'pulsed' mode of therapy machines consists of bursts typically 0.5–2 ms long

Box 22.1 *Practical considerations in minimizing exposure from diagnostic ultrasound*

The operator can minimize patient exposure to ultrasound if they understand how the front panel controls of a scanner affect its acoustic output. In particular:

- The output power control should be turned down and the receiver gain increased so as to minimize acoustic output power and the potential for heating. It should be noted that acoustic power and receiver gain controls have similar effects on the appearance of the image, but are not always clearly or consistently labelled.
- The use of a narrow image sector size, 'high resolution' mode or zoom may increase scan line density and so increase exposure. This is particularly significant in colour Doppler imaging where the use of a small colour box may increase intensity values well into the range associated with pulsed Doppler.
- When using pulsed Doppler, it is important to remember that the area selected by the range gate is not necessarily the region where greatest exposure occurs: all tissues in the beam both proximal and distal to the gate will be insonated, and the user needs to be aware of any sensitive structures lying in the path of the beam.
- Check that there is no acoustic output when the image is frozen. Ultrasound probes do not convert electrical energy into acoustic energy very efficiently and so the scanning surface of the probe may become warm. This effect may also become significant during endocavity imaging, where the probe is enclosed within the body and can be almost stationary for several minutes. Transoesophageal probes may have temperature sensors fitted close to the scanning surface so as to monitor and prevent hazardous temperature rises.

Box 22.2 Checking Effective Radiating Area (ERA) of a transducer

A simplified method of measuring ERA has recently been described by Zeqiri and Hodnett [17] in which the powers transmitted through a series of special apertures are used to calculate ERA. A rapid qualitative assessment of radiating area can also be made by placing the treatment head underwater, radiating upwards, and observing the pattern of water surface levitation caused by the radiation force of the beam. The operator can protect themselves from ultrasound exposure when their hands are immersed by wearing a loose fitting rubber glove or two pairs of examination gloves. The layer of air trapped inside the gloves acts as a barrier to ultrasound transmission for frequencies in the megahertz range.

(Figure 22.1c), containing hundreds of acoustic cycles and separated by intervals of several milliseconds—unlike a diagnostic pulse. Typical pressure amplitudes for therapy machines are 100–300 kPa at 0.2–1.0 W cm^{-2}. A large treatment head may be capable of generating around 15 W of acoustic power—more than enough to cause pain and injury at superficial bone–soft-tissue interfaces. However, for treatment heads operating in pulsed mode at around 0.5 W cm^{-2}, a more typical range of acoustic powers would be 0.5–1 W for large treatment heads and 50–100 mW for small treatment heads. As can be seen from Table 22.3, this is in some instances less than the power generated by a diagnostic scanner operating in B mode.

The key acoustic parameters of ultrasound therapy beams are the total acoustic power and the effective radiating area (ERA) of the treatment head. Acoustic power can be assessed on a radiation force balance, although care must be taken to ensure that the water remains degassed (§22.4.1). In contrast to total acoustic power measurements, the ERA can be complex to determine, and may require a hydrophone and automated scanning equipment only available in a few specialized centres.

Interference effects in the near-field of a therapy treatment head result in significant non-uniformities within a few centimetres of the transducer face. The beam non-uniformity ratio (BNR) is defined as the ratio of the maximum intensity in the beam to the spatial average. Current standards set an upper limit of 8 on the BNR. The dangers associated with high BNR ('hot-spot') fields can be appreciated as follows. A field with a BNR of 8 and a spatial average intensity of 3 W cm^{-2} will have local intensity maxima of up to 24 W cm^{-2}—an intensity level more often associated with surgical applications. Physiotherapists are trained to keep the treatment head moving continuously over the surface of the skin, and so average out the effects of non-uniformities in the beam.

Safe and effective use

There is a considerable weight of evidence from animal studies that suggests that therapeutic ultrasound may produce beneficial clinical effects. However, although there are a few well-controlled trials of chronic soft-tissue conditions (for example [18]), the literature does not contain any well-controlled double-blind trials of the acute soft-tissue injuries that are commonly treated in a physiotherapy out-patient setting. Consequently, there are no generally agreed treatment regimes for such injuries. In some cases, much of the information that therapists have received during training is opinion, expressed as fact.

A further problem in achieving safe and effective treatment regimes is the notoriously poor technical performance of ultrasound therapy machines. Several studies over the last 25 years have demonstrated that a majority of machines in clinical use do not meet the appropriate performance standards, either in terms of acoustic power or ERA [19]. Of 54 new machines commissioned in the Lothian region, Scotland, between 1992 and 1995, 25% failed acceptance testing.

Good technical performance is necessary to ensure both the safety and the effectiveness of therapy. There are a number of reasons underlying the continuing poor performance of ultrasound therapy machines. First, therapists expect to purchase ultrasound machines for a relatively low cost of perhaps £500 to £1500. Most of the machines are designed with high-Q air-backed transducers for optimum efficiency and can generate maximum powers of 10–15 W. However, optimum efficiency is not compatible with optimum stability in a low-cost device. It is in fact remarkably difficult to produce a stable, high-power source of ultrasound. To further compound this problem, the majority of therapy machines contain a major design flaw, in that the front panel power/intensity display is only indirectly linked to the acoustic power of the device. This means that faults involving acoustic output are not immediately apparent to the user. In many instances the treatment head can be removed, or have the return line broken, and the machine will indicate an unchanged acoustic power, despite having no output at all. There have also been instances of therapy machines delivering excessive power, thereby causing injury to patients [19]. A further barrier to improved performance is obtaining adequately calibrated radiation force balances. There are currently few alternatives apart from direct calibration by the National Physical Laboratory, which is a relatively expensive route.

Box 22.3 Testing and calibration of therapy ultrasound equipment

Fresh guidance on the testing and calibration of therapy machines has been published by the Institute of Physics and Engineering in Medicine [9]. This document details a number of practical requirements for the safe and effective use of therapy machines, which include:

- regular user testing of equipment
- a calibration programme capable of identifying faults in both continuous and pulsed wave performance
- checks on ERA (Box 22.2)

As a result, many therapy machines have poor performance (because of inherent instability and the high cost of calibration relative to purchase price) yet remain in clinical use (because they have no direct link between the intensity display and the actual acoustic output).

22.6.2 Standards and guidance

Two international standards are directly concerned with the safety and performance of ultrasound therapy machines: IEC 60601-2-5 (2000) [20] and IEC 61689 (1996) [21]. Standard 60601-2-5 limits the effective intensity to less than 3 W cm^{-2} . This safety criterion is derived in part from the fact that the beneficial effects associated with physiotherapy ultrasound may be achieved using exposure levels less than 3 W cm^{-2}; there is therefore no justification for using higher levels. Even 3 W cm^{-2} is within the range where adverse biological effects occur. IEC 60601-2-5 also specifies that displayed intensity and power settings should be within $\pm 20\%$ of the actual output for settings between maximum and 10% of maximum. (Note that many machines in current use will have been manufactured to comply with the 1984 version of IEC 60601-2-5, which limits the tolerance to $\pm 30\%$ rather than $\pm 20\%$.)

Standard IEC 61689 defines a method for determining the ERA and BNR of therapy beams. This involves using a hydrophone to determine the area close to the face of the treatment head through which most of the acoustic power is transmitted. It also sets an upper limit of 8 on the BNR of any beam. (Note that prior to the publication of IEC 61689, most manufacturers measured ERA using a technique specified by the FDA. This involves measuring the maximum pressure in the beam close to the treatment head using a hydrophone, and then defining an area within which pressure amplitudes exceed 5% of this maximum. This has been shown to produce ERA values that are very dependent on technique and the properties of the hydrophone, but it is still used by several manufacturers [17].)

In the UK, the Chartered Society of Physiotherapy (CSP) has issued clinical guidelines for safe treatments [22]. Many of the contraindications mentioned are not based on firm evidence of hazard but are prudent measures to avoid adverse effects–particularly thermal effects–for example, avoiding exposure of the fetus, and epiphyses in children. New clinical guidelines are in preparation by the CSP.

It is difficult to justify the clinical use of ultrasound machines which have not been regularly tested. It is even harder to justify the use of such machines on physical conditions for which the benefits of ultrasound therapy have not been clearly demonstrated. Such a course of action is unlikely to result in a net benefit to patients.

22.7 Lithotripsy

22.7.1 Exposure

Lithotripsy refers to the fragmentation of calculi that form in the body. Open surgery for stone removal may cause damage to an organ such as the kidney, and is associated with high morbidity. Less traumatic non-invasive methods are preferred. Extracorporeal shock-wave lithotripsy (ESWL) involves the use of an acoustic shockwave generator sited outside the body. The focus of the shockwave generator is positioned over the stone using X-ray or ultrasound imaging and acoustic shock-waves are delivered at a pulse rate of typically 1–10 Hz. Within the kidney and ureter, stones must be fragmented to a size less than about 2 mm so that they can be washed out of the body by the natural flow of urine. Dosimetry for ESWL treatment is crude and fragmentation is often carried out at the highest shockwave setting that the patient can tolerate. Patients are often sedated in order to overcome the discomfort associated with treatment.

The relatively short pulses and long interpulse intervals mean that lithotripsy will not result in any significant thermal effects *in vivo*—except for the very localized and transient high temperatures generated by inertial cavitation. Lithotripsy pulses from ESWL machines generally have centre frequencies in the range 0.2 to 1 MHz, with peak positive pressures of 10–100 MPa and peak negative pressures of 5–10 MPa. The high amplitudes and relatively low centre frequencies of lithotripsy pulses mean that cavitation and particle displacement are the greatest potential biohazards as well as providing the most likely mechanisms for shattering the calculi.

Exposure measurements in lithotripsy fields are made particularly difficult because of the destructive nature of the acoustic field. Many hydrophones are mechanically fragile because they have been designed to cause minimal disturbance to the ultrasound field, and they may be rapidly damaged by inertial cavitation in the focal region. The large degree of non-linear distortion and the high negative pressures that may be present also make measurement artefacts increasingly prevalent.

The amplitude of a lithotripter pulse increases rapidly as it approaches the focal region, due to focusing, diffraction, and non-linear propagation. This results in a pressure waveform that looks like Figure 22.1d when measured at the focus in water. There is a large positive amplitude with a well-formed shock, followed by a smaller longer-lasting negative phase. Destructive tensile forces are exerted by the negative phase of the pulse. Phase inversion will occur if the pulse is reflected at a high-to-low acoustic impedance boundary so that the leading positive peak is inverted to become a high-amplitude negative pressure. The large amplitude of a lithotripter pulse results in relative displacements of several tens of microns over distances of a few millimetres in tissue, resulting in strains of the order of 0.5%. Because of the three-dimensional nature of the pulse, the effects of particle displacement will have components that are compressive, tensile, and shearing in nature. These are likely to contribute significantly to soft-tissue damage and stone fragmentation. Lithotripter pulses have been observed to cause inertial cavitation *in vivo* and bubble lifetimes of around 100 μs have been measured.

22.7.2 Standards and guidance

The relevant standard is IEC 61846 [23]. It specifies the acoustic parameters which should be used in the declaration of the acoustic output of ESWL equipment, and methods of measurement and characterization of the pressure field. In an attempt to cope with the destructive power of the fields, the standard defines two hydrophones classified as *field* and *focus* type. The field hydrophone should be of robust design and should be used for general field measurements, such as scanning to establish the extent of the focal region. This will reduce the exposure of the second type of hydrophone, the focus hydrophone, which will in general be more fragile and should have a wide bandwidth (0.5 to 15 MHz) to enable the full frequency content of the shockwave to be determined. The focus hydrophone is used to determine the waveform at the focus.

The ECMUS has published guidance on the safe use of ESWL [24]. This includes the following recommendations:

- Patients who have recently undergone nuclear medicine examinations should wait a time equivalent to seven half-lives of the isotope before undergoing lithotripsy. This is because radiopharmaceuticals may generate nucleation sites and increase the likelihood of inertial cavitation.
- For the same reason, patients who have had examinations involving ultrasonic microbubble contrast agents should not undergo lithotripsy until the microbubbles have been eliminated from their system.

The radiation protection physicist should be aware of a number of other safety issues in lithotripsy:

- As regards short-term patient safety, the main hazards are tissue damage due to exposing lung or gas-filled intestine to lithotripsy pulses, and vascular damage to the renal tissue itself. Pregnancy, aortic aneurysm, and hypertension are all considered contraindications for renal ESWL.
- Some lithotripters, particularly those with powerful electrohydraulic sources, are synchronized to the patient's ECG to prevent cardiac arrhythmias being induced.
- Lithotripsy is always accompanied by some degree of haematuria which usually resolves over one or two days. Patients are taken off anticoagulants prior to treatment so as to prevent excessive renal haemorrhaging, and their clotting factors are tested prior to treatment. The combination of anticoagulants and renal lithotripsy can result in haematoma and may occasionally prove fatal.
- There is a significant percentage of patients for whom lithotripsy is one of a number of clinical options. Its continued use in such patients will depend largely on whether ESWL proves to have any long-term detrimental effects, such as hypertension or impairment of renal function.
- As regards operator safety, the main concern is usually the explosive noise that accompanies the spark discharge of electrohydraulic lithotripters.

For many ESWL systems, the most difficult task that the operator has to accomplish is positioning the focal region of the lithotripter over the stone. Although the X-ray and ultrasound imaging systems of an extracorporeal lithotripter are computer linked to the therapy beam, they may not be coaxial. The focal region of a lithotripter is long and narrow, extending along the axis of the therapy beam and often projecting well outside the two-dimensional imaging plane. This often leaves the operator with a difficult problem in three-dimensional anatomy in order to avoid placing bone, bowel gas, or lung within the focal region. A written protocol should be in place to ensure that this is performed correctly.

22.8 Surgical ultrasound

22.8.1 Exposure

A review of surgical techniques may be found in [25], which describes various applications of surgical ultrasound, including the treatment of Ménière's disease. Ultrasound is applied in surgery in two main ways, the first of which uses the vibrations of a metallic tip or saw. Such tools are normally fabricated from a transducer, made of either magnetostrictive or piezoelectric material, linked to a waveguide, which is terminated in a tool shaped for a particular task. Examples of this technique include dental descalers, used for the removal of calculus and plaque, and ultrasonic scalpels. Such devices generally operate within the frequency range 20 to 60 kHz and are used to fragment, disintegrate, and aspirate unwanted tissue. The tip of the tool vibrates with displacement amplitudes of the order of 600 μm. The benefits of using such tools are that the moving tip does not stick to the tissue and the surgeon is provided with tactile feedback.

The second method of ultrasonic surgery uses focused ultrasound to generate elevated acoustic pressures and very high time-averaged intensities. These rapidly destroy tissue, principally through thermal mechanisms. Focal spot sizes of the order of 1–2 mm in width and 3–4 mm in length can be generated using frequencies in the low megahertz range, giving the ability to achieve highly localized damage to specific tissues. A number of focused ultrasound systems have undergone clinical trials, principally for use in the liver, prostate, and brain.

22.8.2 Standards and guidance

Two standards related to the operation of surgical devices exist. IEC 61205 [26] gives test methods by which the operating parameters of dental descalers are specified and measured. Principal among these parameters is the tip vibration frequency, measured using a vibrometer, and the primary tip vibration excursion which may be determined under a microscope or through the indentations made by the descaler on a glass microscope slide. Measurements are carried out under a specified load, simulating the force applied by the operator. For other ultrasonic surgical tools, the relevant standard is IEC 61847 [27]. This specifies methods for determining the operating parameters of these devices, and is also appropriate to intracorporeal lithotripters where the ultrasonic tool lies at the end of a waveguide and is placed in contact with the calculus. Key operating parameters are the primary tip excursion (again measured using either a laser vibrometer or a microscope) and the derived acoustic power (measured within a large anechoic tank using a low-frequency hydrophone operating in the kilohertz range). The standard emphasizes that this is just the low-frequency 'power' contribution, and does not include the component of power which has gone into cavitational events close to the vibrating tip. This can be estimated using a high-frequency hydrophone (operating in the megahertz range) to measure the shockwaves generated by collapsing cavitation bubbles.

The mechanisms by which surgical tools operate are in many cases poorly understood. In some applications it is likely that both particle displacement and cavitation play significant roles. In dental descaling, for instance, an irrigant fluid is normally applied to remove debris so that cleaning can be achieved even when the tip cannot make direct contact with the tooth.

As with other ultrasonic techniques, operator training is an important aspect of effective use. For example, inexperienced operators may allow a descaling tool to become hot and cause thermal injury to the teeth and gums.

22.9 Conclusion

All applications of ultrasound in medicine have an impressive safety record, be they diagnostic, therapeutic, or surgical. That the risks and benefits may vary considerably between applications can be gauged from the fact that medical ultrasonic techniques span three orders of magnitude in frequency, from surgical techniques operating at tens of kHz to high-resolution imaging operating at tens of MHz. A number of key issues have been discussed in the text. The interaction of ultrasound with biological tissues is complex. Even the most classical interaction–tissue heating–is difficult to predict because of the computationally demanding nature of the numerical modelling and our lack of knowledge about the thermal and acoustic parameters of individual human tissues, especially those of the developing fetus. Given the requirement to establish that the net effect on the patient is a beneficial one, there is considerable motivation to elucidate the bioeffects of ultrasound on tissue–both beneficial and detrimental. Despite the emotive nature of diagnostic fetal scanning, and the significant levels of soft-tissue damage caused by lithotripsy, it is perhaps surprising that the 3 W cm^{-2} limit for therapeutic ultrasound is the only safety criterion that has been formally adopted into current international standards.

22.10 References

1 Ziskin, M. C. and Lewin, P. A. (ed.) (1993). *Ultrasonic exposimetry*. CRC Press, Boca Raton.

2 ter Haar, G. and Duck, F. A. (ed.) (2000). *The safe use of ultrasound in medical diagnosis*. BMUS/BIR, London, UK.

3 International Electrotechnical Commission (1993). IEC 61220. *Ultrasonics–Fields–Guidance for the measurement and characterisation of ultrasonic fields generated by medical ultrasonic equipment using hydrophones in the frequency range 0.5 MHz to 15 MHz*. IEC, Geneva, Switzerland.

4 International Electrotechnical Commission (1991). IEC 61102. *Measurement and characterisation of ultrasonic fields in the frequency range 0.5 MHz to 15 MHz*. IEC, Geneva, Switzerland.

5 International Electrotechnical Commission (1992). IEC 61157. *Requirements for the declaration of the acoustic output of medical diagnostic ultrasonic equipment*. IEC, Geneva, Switzerland.

6 Bamber, J. C. (1986). Attenuation and absorption. In: *Physical principles of medical ultrasonics* (ed. C. R. Hill), pp. 118–99. Ellis Horwood, Chichester, UK.

7 Duck, F. A. (1990). *Physical properties of tissue*. Academic Press, London.

8 Preston, R. C. (ed.) (1991). *Output measurements for medical ultrasound*. Springer Verlag, London.

9 Pye, S. D. and Zeqiri, B. (2001). Guidelines for the testing and calibration of physiotherapy ultrasound machines. Report 84, Institute of Physics and Engineering in Medicine, York, UK.

10 International Electrotechnical Commission (1992). IEC 61161. *Ultrasonic power measurement in liquids in the frequency range 0.5 MHz to 25 MHz*. IEC, Geneva, Switzerland.

11 Henderson, J., Willson, K., Jago, J. R., and Whittingham, T. A. (1995). A survey of the acoustic outputs of diagnostic ultrasound equipment in current clinical use in the Northern Region. *Ultrasound Med. Biol.*, **21**, 699–705.

12 British Medical Ultrasound Society (2000). BMUS safety guidelines and safety statement. *BMUS Bulletin.*, **8** (3), 29–33.

13 European Committee for Medical Ultrasound Safety (1994). Diagnostic ultrasound: genetic aspects. *Eur. J. Ultrasound*, **1**, 91–2.

14 European Committee for Medical Ultrasound Safety (1996). Epidemiological studies of diagnostic ultrasound exposure during human pregnancies. *Eur. J. Ultrasound*, **4**, 69–73.

15 European Committee for Medical Ultrasound Safety (1999). Tutorial papers. In: *EFSUMB Newsletter*, **13** (1).

16 Wells, P. N. T. (1999). Safety issues in diagnostic ultrasound. In: *Clinical diagnostic ultrasound* (2nd edn) (ed. G. Baxter, P. Allan, and P. Morley), pp. 73–81. Blackwell Science, Oxford, UK.

17 Zeqiri, B. and Hodnett, M. (1998). A new method for measuring the radiating area of physiotherapy treatment heads. *Ultrasound Med. Biol.*, **24**, 761–70.

18 Ebenbichler, G. R., Resch, K. L., Nicolakis, P., Wiesinger, G. F., Uhl, F., Ghanem, A., *et al.* (1998). Ultrasound treatment for treating the carpel tunnel syndrome: randomised 'sham' controlled trial. *Br. Med. J.*, **316**, 731–5.

19 Pye, S. D. (1996). Ultrasound therapy equipment: does it perform? *Physiotherapy*, **82**, 39–44.

20 International Electrotechnical Commission (2000). IEC 60601-2-5. *Medical electrical equipment: particular requirements for the safety of ultrasonic therapy equipment*. IEC, Geneva, Switzerland.

21 International Electrotechnical Commission (1996). IEC 61689. *Ultrasonics – Physiotherapy systems – Performance requirements and methods of measurement in the frequency range 0.5 MHz to 5 MHz*. IEC, Geneva, Switzerland.

22 The Chartered Society of Physiotherapy, Safety of Electrotherapy Equipment Working Group (1990). Guidelines for the safe use of ultrasound therapy equipment. *Physiotherapy*, **76**, 683–4.

23 International Electrotechnical Commission (1998). IEC 61846. *Ultrasonics–Pressure pulse lithotripters–Characteristics of fields*. IEC, Geneva, Switzerland.

24 European Committee for Medical Ultrasound Safety (1994). Guidelines for the safe use of extracorporeal shockwave lithotripsy devices. *Eur. J. Ultrasound*, **3**, 315–16.

25 ter Haar, G. R. (1986). Therapeutic and surgical applications. In: *Physical principles of medical ultrasonics* (ed. C. R. Hill), pp. 436–61. Ellis Horwood, Chichester, UK.

26 International Electrotechnical Commission (1993). IEC 61205. *Ultrasonics–Dental descaler systems–Measurement and declaration of the output characteristics*. IEC, Geneva, Switzerland.

27 International Electrotechnical Commission (1998). IEC 61847. *Ultrasonics–Surgical systems–Measurement and declaration of the basic output characteristics*. IEC, Geneva, Switzerland.

22.11 Further reading

Barnett, S. B. and Kossoff, G. (ed.) (1998). *Safety of diagnostic ultrasound*. Parthenon Publishing, UK.

Baxter, G., Allan, P., and Morley, P. (ed.) (1999). *Clinical diagnostic ultrasound*. Blackwell, London.

ter Haar, G. and Duck, F. A. (ed.) (2000). *The safe use of ultrasound in medical diagnosis*. BMUS/BIR, London.

22.12 Organizations

British Medical Ultrasound Society, 36, Portland Place, London W1N 3DG, UK.

European Federation of Societies for Ultrasound in Medicine and Biology (EFSUMB). Secretariat: Carpenters Court, 4a Lewes Rd, Bromley, Kent BR1 2RN, UK.

Index